PENN
Clinical Manual of Urology

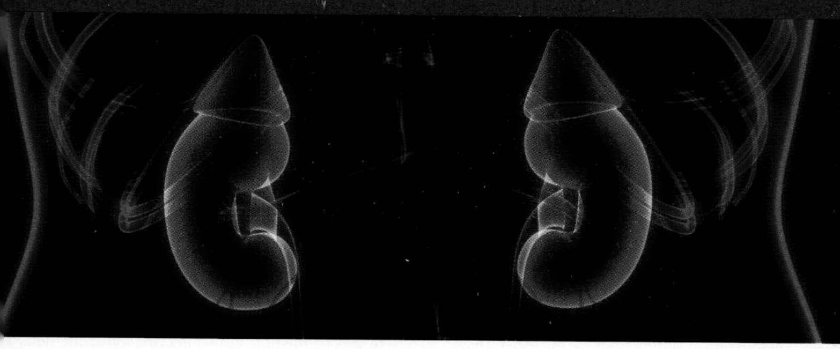

PENN Clinical Manual of Urology

THIRD EDITION

Thomas J. Guzzo, MD, MPH
Associate Professor of Urology in Surgery
Chief, Urology
Associate Program Director, Urology
University of Pennsylvania Health System
Philadelphia, Pennsylvania

Alan J. Wein, MD, PhD (Hon), FACS
Professor and Chair, Co-Director, Urologic Oncology Program
Co-Director, Voiding Function and Dysfunction Program
Founders Professor in Urology
University of Pennsylvania Health System
Philadelphia, Pennsylvania

Robert C. Kovell, MD
Department of Urology
Penn Medicine
Philadelphia, Pennsylvania

Dana A. Weiss, MD
Assistant Professor, Department of Urology
University of Pennsylvania
Attending Physician
Department of Urology
Children's Hospital of Philadelphia
Philadelphia, Pennsylvania

Justin B. Ziemba, MD, MSEd
Assistant Professor
Division of Urology, Department of Surgery
Perelman School of Medicine
University of Pennsylvania
Philadelphia, Pennsylvania

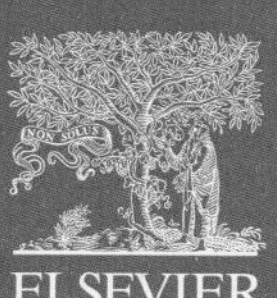

ELSEVIER

Elsevier
1600 John F. Kennedy Blvd.
Ste 1800
Philadelphia, PA 19103-2899

PENN CLINICAL MANUAL OF UROLOGY, THIRD EDITION ISBN: 978-0-323-77575-5

Senior Content Strategist: Belinda Kuhn
Senior Content Development Specialist: Priyadarshini Pandey
Publishing Services Manager: Deepthi Unni
Project Manager: Nayagi Anandan
Design Direction: Brian Salisbury

Printed in India

Last digit is the print number: 9 8 7 6 5 4 3 2 1

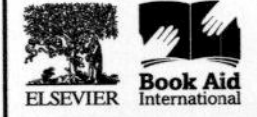

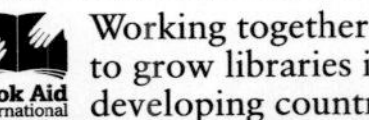

On May 30, 2022, Penn Urology lost one of our brightest lights and most exemplary individuals. Douglas A. Canning (Doug) became our Chief of Pediatric Urology in 1997. Doug was a charismatic, exhaustively active, and exceptionally productive chief who demanded excellence in every area of clinical practice, research, administration, and development, significantly enlarging Penn Pediatric Urology in all of these areas. As we sat around later that week at a meeting called to talk about our emotions and thoughts regarding this tragedy, numerous anecdotes were recounted, which reminded us of the many positive influences he had on each of us in so many areas of life and practice. In his professional life, next to his devotion to his patients came his dedication to the residents and fellows, specifically their education and quality of life. With the greatest respect for his many talents and the way he led his life, we humbly dedicate this edition of the *Penn Clinical Manual of Urology* to him.

The Editors

Christina W. Augdelo, MD
Department of Urology
Penn Medicine, University of Pennsylvania Health System
Philadelphia, Pennsylvania

Raju Chelluri, MD
Department of Urology
Penn Medicine, University of Pennsylvania Health System
Philadelphia, Pennsylvania

George W. Drach, MD
Professor Emeritus of Urology in Surgery
Department of Surgery
University of Pennsylvania
Philadelphia, Pennsylvania

Katherine M. Fischer, MD
Assistant Professor
Division of Urology
Department of Surgery
The Children's Hospital of Philadelphia
Philadelphia, Pennsylvania

Zoe S. Gan, MD
Resident Physician Division of Urology
Department of Surgery
University of Pennsylvania
Philadelphia, Pennsylvania

Harcharan Gill, MD, FRCS
Professor
Department of Urology
Stanford University
Stanford, California

Karl Godlewski, MD
Resident Physician
Division of Urology
University of Pennsylvania
Philadelphia, Pennsylvania

Akshya Gupta, MD
Assistant Professor
Department of Imaging Sciences (Radiology)
University of Rochester
Rochester, New York

Thomas J. Guzzo, MD, MPH
Associate Professor of Urology in Surgery
Chief
Division of Urology
Associate Program Director
Penn Urology Residency
University of Pennsylvania Health System
Philadelphia, Pennsylvania

Philip M. Hanno, MD, MPH
Clinical Professor
Department of Urology
Stanford University
Stanford, California
Professor Emeritus
Division of Urology
Hospital of the University of Pennsylvania
Philadelphia, Pennsylvania

Joseph F. Harryhill, MD, MSEd
Clinical Associate Professor of Urology
Department of Surgery
Perelman School of Medicine
University of Pennsylvania
Staff Urologist
Department of Surgery
Penn Presbyterian Medical Center
Philadelphia, Pennsylvania

Hanna Jia, BA
Medical Student
Perelman School of Medicine
University of Pennsylvania
Philadelphia, Pennsylvania

Thomas F. Kolon, MD, MS
Professor of Urology in Surgery
Perelman School of Medicine at University of Pennsylvania
Howard M. Snyder III MD Chair in Pediatric Urology
Children's Hospital of Philadelphia
Philadelphia, Pennsylvania

Robert C. Kovell, MD
Division of Urology
Penn Medicine
Philadelphia, Pennsylvania

Alexander Kutikov, MD
Professor and Chief
Division of Urology and Urologic Oncology
Roberta R. Scheller Chair in Urologic Oncology
Fox Chase Cancer Center
Philadelphia, Pennsylvania

Hyezo Kwun, MD, MPH, BA
Division of Urology
Penn Medicine
Philadelphia, Pennsylvania

Michael J. LaRiviere, MD
Assistant Professor
Department of Radiation Oncology
University of Pennsylvania and Children's Hospital of Philadelphia
Philadelphia, Pennsylvania

Daniel J. Lee, MD
Assistant Professor of Urologic Oncology
Department of Urology
Penn Medicine
University of Pennsylvania Health System
Philadelphia, Pennsylvania

Caitlin Lim, DO, MS
Clinical Instructor
Department of Urology
Medical University of South Carolina
Charleston, South Carolina

Christopher J. Long, MD
Assistant Professor of Urology
Division of Urology
Department of Surgery
Children's Hospital of Philadelphia
Philadelphia, Pennsylvania

Aseem Malhotra, MD
Department of Urology
Penn Medicine
University of Pennsylvania Health System
Philadelphia, Pennsylvania

Puneet Masson, MD
Director of Male Reproductive Medicine and Surgery
Division of Reproductive Endocrinology and Infertility
Department of Obstetrics and Gynecology
Penn Medicine
Philadelphia, Pennsylvania

Sameer Mittal, MD, MS, FAAP
Assistant Professor
Division of Urology
Department of Surgery
Children's Hospital of Philadelphia
Philadelphia, Pennsylvania

Thomas F. Monaghan, MD, PhD
Resident
Department of Urology
University of Texas
Southwestern Medical Center
Dallas, Texas

Phillip Mucksavage, MD
Associate Professor
Division of Urology
University of Pennsylvania
Philadelphia, Pennsylvania

Diane K. Newman, DNP, ANP-BC, FAAN
Research Investigator Senior
Adjunct Professor of Urology in Surgery
Division of Urology
Perelman School of Medicine
Co-Director
Penn Center for Continence and Pelvic Health
Division of Urology
Penn Medicine
Philadelphia, Pennsylvania

Esther Nivasch Turner MD, MBE
Department of Urology
Penn Medicine
University of Pennsylvania Health System
Philadelphia, Pennsylvania

Daisy Obiora, MD
Fellow in Urologic Oncology
University of Pittsburgh Medical Center
Pittsburgh, PA
Former Resident in Urology
Cooper Medical School of Rowan University
Camden, New Jersey

Parvati Ramchandani, MD
Professor of Radiology and Surgery
Department of Radiology
Perelman School of Medicine
University of Pennsylvania
Philadelphia, Pennsylvania

Ingride Richardson, MD
Assistant Professor of Clinical Urology
Department of Surgery
University of Pennsylvania
Philadelphia, Pennsylvania

Daniel Roberson, MD
Resident Physician
Division of Urology
Department of Surgery
University of Pennsylvania
Philadelphia, Pennsylvania

Eric S. Rovner, MD
Professor
Department of Urology
Medical University of South Carolina
Charleston, South Carolina

Allen D. Seftel, MD
Chief, Division of Urology
Cooper University Hospital
Camden, NJ
Professor of Urology
Cooper Medical School of Rowan University Camden, NJ
Adjunct Professor of Surgery (Urology)
MD Anderson Cancer Center, Houston, Texas

Ankur A. Shah, MD, MBA
Resident Physician
Division of Urology
Penn Medicine
Philadelphia, Pennsylvania

Alexander J. Skokan, MD
Assistant Professor
Department of Urology
University of Washington
Seattle, Washington

Ariana L. Smith, MD
Professor of Urology
Division of Urology
University of Pennsylvania
Philadelphia, Pennsylvania

Zachary L. Smith, MD
Assistant Professor of Surgery
Division of Urologic Surgery
Washington University in St. Louis
St. Louis, Missouri

Arun K. Srinivasan, MD
Pediatric Urologist
Division of Urology
Department of Surgery
Children's Hospital of Philadelphia
Associate Professor of Urology in Surgery
Perelman School of Medicine
University of Pennsylvania
Philadelphia, Pennsylvania

Marshall Strother, MD
Assistant Professor
Department of Urology
Oregon Health and Science University
Portland, Oregon

Kiran Sury, MD
Resident Physician
Division of Urology
University of Pennsylvania
Philadelphia, Pennsylvania

Ruchika Talwar, MD
Resident Physician
Division of Urology
Associate Fellow
Leonard Davis Institute for Health Economics
University of Pennsylvania
Philadelphia, Pennsylvania

Gregory E. Tasian, MD, MSc, MSCE
Associate Professor of Surgery
Division of Urology
Department of Surgery
Department of Biostatistics and Epidemiology
Perelman School of Medicine
University of Pennsylvania
Attending Physician
Division of Urology
Children's Hospital of Philadelphia
Philadelphia, Pennsylvania

Keith N. Van Arsdalen, MD
Professor
Division of Urology
Department of Surgery
University of Pennsylvania
Chief
Department of Urology
Philadelphia VAMC
Philadelphia, Pennsylvania

Jason P. Van Batavia, MD
Assistant Professor
Division of Urology
Children's Hospital of Philadelphia
Philadelphia, Pennsylvania

Neha Vapiwala, MD
Professor
Department of Radiation Oncology
University of Pennsylvania
Philadelphia, Pennsylvania

David J. Vaughn, MD
GU Medical Oncology Professor
Vice Chief for Clinical Affairs
Division of Hematology/Oncology
Hospital of the University of Pennsylvania
Department of Urology
Penn Medicine
University of Pennsylvania Health System
Philadelphia, Pennsylvania

John K. Weaver, MD
Fellow
Division of Urology
Children's Hospital of Philadelphia
Philadelphia, Pennsylvania

Alan J. Wein, MD, PhD (Hon), FACS
Founders Professor and Emeritus Chief of Urology
Division of Urology
Department of Surgery
Penn Medicine
Perelman School of Medicine
University of Pennsylvania Health System
Associate Director
Residency Program in Urology
Division of Urology
University of Pennsylvania School of Medicine
Philadelphia, Pennsylvania

Dana A. Weiss, MD
Assistant Professor of Urology in Surgery
Division of Urology
Perelman School of Medicine
University of Pennsylvania
Attending Physician
The Children's Hospital of Philadelphia
Philadelphia, Pennsylvania

Jeffrey P. Weiss, MD, PhD, FACS
Professor and Chair
Department of Urology
SUNY Downstate Health Sciences University
Brooklyn, New York

Hunter Wessells, MD, FACS
Professor and Nelson Chair, Department of Urology
Adjunct Professor, Department of Surgery
Affiliate Member, Harborview Injury Prevention and Research Center
Member, Diabetes Research Center
University of Washington
Seattle, Washington

Stephen Zderic, MD
The John W. Duckett Jr. Endowed Chair in Pediatric Urology
Division of Urology
Children's Hospital of Philadelphia
Professor of Urology in Surgery
Division of Urology
Perelman School of Medicine
University of Pennsylvania
Philadelphia, Pennsylvania

Justin B. Ziemba, MD, MSEd
Assistant Professor of Urology in Surgery
Division of Urology
Department of Surgery
Perelman School of Medicine
University of Pennsylvania
Philadelphia, Pennsylvania

Stephen Mock, MD
Fellow in Female Pelvic Medicine and Reconstructive Surgery
Vanderbilt University Medical Center
Nashville, Tennessee

Roger R. Dmochowski, MD, MMHC
Professor of Urology and Surgery
Department of Urology
Vanderbilt University Medical Center
Nashville Tennessee

Zachary Winnegrad, MD
Resident in Urology
Cooper Medical School of Rowan University
Camden, New Jersey

Anisleidy Fombona, MD
Department of Urology
Penn Medicine
University of Pennsylvania Health System
Philadelphia, Pennsylvania

Hailiu Yang, MD
Division of Urology
Gould Medical Group
Modesto, California
Former Resident in Urology
Cooper Medical School of
Rowan University
Camden, New Jersey

In 1987, the faculty of Penn Urology first put together a basic Urology text designed for the busy student and house officer. This current edition of the *Penn Clinical Manual of Urology* (the seventh in total; third with the current publisher) represents our latest effort to present a useful introductory text. Rather than provide a heavily referenced compendium, we have tried to present a framework that program directors and faculty can use as an educational foundation to allow them to reflect individual practices at their own institution and allow their own philosophies to be placed in the perspective of the field of Urology in general. We hope the book will appeal also to nonurologic providers who routinely see patients with urologic problems: the primary care physician, gynecologist, nurse practitioner, and the urologic nurse specialist. For those studying for certification and recertification in Urology, it will hopefully be a useful and compact source of information that spans the discipline. Although the practices and philosophies of Penn Urology will no doubt be evident, more so in some sections then in others, we have tried to keep dogma to a minimum and thus allow the addition of other opinions without the intellectual disruption to the reader of major disagreements. Algorithms, Suggested Core Readings, Clinical Pearls, and Self-Assessment Questions are part of each chapter. From physical examination to magnetic resonance (MR) imaging, and from the identification and treatment of simple issues to more complex topics, we have tried to encapsulate the major issues in virtually all subspecialty areas. It is our hope that this text will find a place not only on the office desk but also on the clinic book shelf and in the house staff coat pocket, as a trusted resource and ready reference.

Our thanks to the contributors and to the publisher, Belinda Kuhn in particular, for making this edition possible.

Thomas J. Guzzo, MD, MPH
Alan J. Wein, MD, PhD (Hon), FACS
Robert C. Kovell, MD
Dana A. Weiss, MD
Justin B. Ziemba, MD, MSEd

Signs and Symptoms: The Initial Examination

Keith N. Van Arsdalen, MD

Background

DEFINITION

Urology is a surgical specialty devoted to the study and treatment of disorders of the genitourinary tract of the male and the urinary tract of the female. The urologist surgically corrects acquired and congenital abnormalities and diagnoses and treats many medical disorders of the genitourinary tract.

IMPORTANCE TO OTHER BRANCHES OF MEDICINE

1. Approximately 15% of patients initially presenting to a physician will have a urologic complaint or abnormality.
2. There is a wide overlap with other specialties, and urologists have frequent interaction with other physicians, including family practitioners, internists, pediatricians, geriatricians, endocrinologists, nephrologists, neurologists, obstetricians and gynecologists, and general, vascular, and trauma surgeons.
3. It is important that all physicians be aware of the specific diagnostic and therapeutic measures that are available within this specialty.

Urologic Manifestations of Disease

DIRECT

The most obvious manifestations of urologic disease are those signs and symptoms that are directly related to the urinary tract of the male and female or to the genitalia of the male. Hematuria and scrotal swelling are examples in this category.

REFERRED MANIFESTATIONS

1. Symptoms from the genitourinary tract may be referred to other areas within the genitourinary tract or to contiguous organ systems.
   a. A stone in the kidney or upper ureter may produce ipsilateral testicular pain.
   b. This same stone may be associated with symptoms of nausea and vomiting.
   c. The gastrointestinal (GI) tract is probably the most common site to manifest symptoms from primary urologic problems. This is most probably due to the common innervation of these systems and the close direct relationship between the various component organs.
2. Primary urologic disorders may also be manifest in different organ systems and by seemingly unrelated signs and symptoms. Bone pain and pathologic fractures secondary to metastatic carcinoma arising in the genitourinary tract are examples.
3. Similarly, primary disease in other organ systems may result in secondary urologic signs and symptoms that initially lead the patient to the urologist. Diabetes may be detected by finding glucosuria in a patient presenting with frequency and nocturia. Other signs and symptoms mimicking urologic disease are related to inflammatory or neoplastic processes arising in the:
   a. Lower lobes of the lungs
   b. GI tract
   c. Female internal genitalia

SYSTEMIC

Fever, weight loss, and malaise can be nonspecific systemic manifestations of acute and chronic inflammatory disorders, renal failure, and genitourinary carcinoma with or without metastases.

ASYMPTOMATIC

Localized or extensive disease may exist within the genitourinary tract without any signs or symptoms being manifest.

1. Renal calculi or neoplasms may be found during other examinations. **Up to 60% of renal masses are detected incidentally.**
2. Sixty percent of prostate cancers are detected secondary to prostate-specific antigen (PSA) elevations only without palpable abnormalities of the prostate.
3. Far-advanced renal deterioration may occur prior to the detection of silent reflux or obstruction.

History

SYMPTOMS

1. A symptom is any departure from normal appearance, function, or sensation as experienced by the patient. Symptoms are reported to the physician or uncovered by careful history taking, with varying degrees of importance and/or significance attached to each symptom by both parties.
   a. The chief complaint, history of the present illness, and past medical history are delineated in a standard fashion.
   b. The character, onset, duration, and progression of the symptom are carefully defined. It is important to note what factors exacerbate or ameliorate the problem.
2. Urologic symptoms are generally related to:
   a. Pain and discomfort
   b. Alterations of micturition
   c. Changes in the gross appearance of the urine
   d. Abnormal appearance and/or function of the external genitalia

PAIN

1. Pain within the genitourinary tract generally arises from distention or inflammation of a part or parts of the genitourinary system. Pain can be experienced directly in the involved organ or referred as noted previously. Referred pain is a relatively common symptom of genitourinary disease.
2. Renal pain
   a. The kidney and its capsule are innervated by sensory fibers traveling to the T10-L1 aspect of the spinal cord.
   b. The etiology of renal pain may be due either to capsular distention or inflammation or to distention of the renal collecting system.

c. Renal pain can be a dull, aching sensation felt primarily in the area of the costovertebral angle or pain of a sharp, colicky nature felt in the area of the flank, with radiation around the abdomen into the groin and ipsilateral testicle or labium. The latter is due to the common innervation.
d. The nature of the primary disease process within the kidney often determines the type of sensation that is experienced and depends on the degree and rapidity of capsular and/or collecting system distention.

3. Ureteral pain
   a. The upper ureter is innervated in a similar fashion to that for the kidney. Therefore upper ureteral pain has a similar distribution to that of renal pain.
   b. The lower ureter, however, sends sensory fibers to the cord through ganglia subserving the major pelvic organs. Therefore pain derived from the lower ureter is generally felt in the suprapubic area, bladder, penis, or urethra.
   c. The most common etiologic mechanism for ureteral pain is sudden obstruction and ureteral distention.
   d. Acute renal and ureteral colic are among the most severe types of pain known to humankind.
4. Bladder pain
   a. Pain within the bladder may be derived from retention of urine with overdistention or from inflammatory processes.
   b. The pain of overdistention is generally felt within the suprapubic area, resulting in severe local discomfort.
   c. The pain due to bladder inflammation is generally felt as a sharp, burning pain that is often referred to the tip of the penile urethra in males and the entire urethra in females.
5. Prostate pain
   a. Sensory fibers from the prostate mostly enter the sacral aspect of the spinal cord.
   b. Prostate pain is most commonly due to acute inflammation and is generally perceived as discomfort in the lower back, rectum, and perineum.
   c. Irritative symptoms arising from the bladder may overshadow the purely prostate symptoms.
6. Penile pain
   a. Penile and urethral pain are generally directly related to a site of inflammation.

7. Scrotal pain
   a. Pain within the scrotum generally arises from disorders of the testis and/or epididymis.
   b. The most common etiologic factors include trauma, torsion of the spermatic cord, torsion of the appendix testis or appendix epididymis, and acute inflammation, particularly epididymitis. The pain in these cases is generally of rapid onset, if not sudden, and severe in nature.
   c. Hydroceles, varicoceles, and testicular tumors can also be associated with scrotal discomfort but are generally of a more insidious nature and less severe in most cases.

ALTERATIONS OF MICTURITION

1. Definitions and problems
   a. Specific terms have been developed to describe alterations related to the act of micturition. This section defines a variety of these terms.
   b. It must be emphasized that a variety of disease processes can result in similar symptoms at the level of the lower urinary tract, and although these terms are used to describe specific symptoms in this area, they do not necessarily pertain to specific etiologies.
2. Changes in urine volume
   a. ***Anuria* and *oliguria* are terms that refer to the varying degrees of decreased urinary output that may be secondary to prerenal, renal, or postrenal factors.** In all cases, it is essential to rule out urethral and/or ureteral obstruction as postrenal causes for these problems.
   b. ***Polyuria* refers to an increase in the volume of urine excreted on a daily basis.** The etiologic mechanisms include increased fluid intake, exogenous or endogenous diuretics, and abnormal states of central or peripheral osmoregulation.
3. Irritative symptoms
   a. *Dysuria* is a term that refers simply to painful or difficult urination. The burning sensation that occurs during micturition associated with either bladder, urethral, or prostatic inflammation is generally used synonymously. This discomfort is generally felt in the entire urethra in females and in the distal urethra in males.

b. *Strangury* is a subtype of dysuria in which intense discomfort accompanies frequent voiding of small amounts of urine.
c. *Frequency* refers to the increased number of times one feels the need to urinate. This can be secondary to a true decrease in bladder capacity from a loss of elasticity or edema due to inflammation, or it can be secondary to a decrease in the effective bladder capacity due to a failure of the bladder to empty completely with persistence of a large amount of residual urine.
d. *Nocturia* is essentially the nighttime equivalent of urinary frequency, that is, a decreased real or effective bladder capacity forces the patient to arise at night to urinate.
e. ***Nycturia* refers to the excretion of larger volumes of urine at night than during the day and is secondary to mobilization of dependent fluid that accumulated when the patient was in the upright position.** Nycturia can result in nocturia even in the presence of a normal bladder capacity if large quantities of fluid are mobilized.
f. *Urgency* refers to the sudden, severe urge to void that may or may not be controllable.
g. The irritative symptoms noted previously are most commonly associated with inflammation of the lower urinary tract, that is, bladder and prostate. Acute bacterial infections probably represent the most common etiologic mechanism. It should be noted, however, that the irritative symptoms may be secondary to the presence of a foreign body, nonspecific inflammation, radiation therapy or chemotherapy, neoplasms, and neurogenic bladder dysfunction.
h. The term *overactive bladder* refers to the symptoms of frequency and urgency, with or without urge or reflex incontinence, in the absence of local pathologic or metabolic factors that would account for these symptoms. The urodynamic-based definition of overactive bladder requires the demonstration of involuntary bladder contractions.

4. Bladder outlet obstructive symptoms
   a. *Hesitancy* refers to the prolonged interval necessary to voluntarily initiate the urinary stream.

b. *Straining* refers to the need to increase intraabdominal pressure to initiate voiding.
c. *Decreased force* and *caliber* of the urinary stream refer to the physical changes of the urinary stream that may be noted due to increased urethral resistance.
d. *Terminal dribbling* refers to the prolonged dribbling of urine from the meatus after the completion of micturition.
e. *Sense of residual urine* is the complaint of a sensation of incomplete emptying of the bladder that the patient recognizes after micturition.
f. *Prostatism.* All of the previous symptoms may be noted with any type of bladder outlet obstruction, that is, secondary to benign prostatic hypertrophy (BPH), prostate carcinoma, or urethral stricture disease. The most common cause of these symptoms, however, is benign prostatic enlargement, and hence this complex of symptoms has often been referred to as *prostatism.*
g. *Urinary retention.* Acute urinary retention may be associated with severe suprapubic discomfort. Alternatively, the chronic retention of urine within the bladder may occur on a gradual basis due to progressive obstruction and bladder decompensation, and large amounts of urine may be retained with minor changes in symptomatology.
h. *Interruption* of the urinary stream. Sudden painful interruption of the urinary stream can be secondary to the presence of a bladder calculus that ball valves into the bladder neck, causing abrupt blockage of the urinary flow.
i. *Bifurcation* of the urinary stream. The symptom of a double stream or spraying of the urinary stream can be secondary to urethral stricture disease or can occur intermittently without any obvious pathology.

5. Incontinence
   a. *True* or *total incontinence* occurs when constant dribbling of urine comes from the bladder. It may be due to the configuration of the bladder, such as with extrophy or epispadias, to ectopia of the ureteral orifices distal to the bladder neck in females, or to a fistula, usually between the bladder and the vagina. The most common cause, however, is secondary to injury to the sphincter mechanisms of the bladder neck and urethra

due to trauma, surgery, or childbirth. Neurogenic disorders affecting the bladder outlet can also have similar effects.

b. *False* or *overflow incontinence* is seen with total bladder decompensation in which the bladder acts as a fixed reservoir and the only outflow of urine is an overflow phenomenon with constant dribbling through the bladder outlet.

c. *Urgency incontinence* results when the sensation of urgency becomes so severe that involuntary bladder emptying occurs. This is commonly secondary to severe inflammation of the urinary bladder. This type of incontinence can also be due to involuntary bladder contractions without inflammation (see definition of overactive bladder on Page X).

d. *Stress incontinence* is secondary to distortion of the normal anatomic relationship between the bladder and the urethra such that sudden increases in intraabdominal pressure (laughing, straining) are transmitted unequally to the bladder and the urethra, resulting in elevated bladder pressure without a concomitant rise in urethral pressure. Most commonly, this is related to laxity of the pelvic floor, particularly following childbirth, but it may also be noted in women who have not had children. It is also a frequent sequel of radical prostatectomy surgery for prostate cancer.

e. **It is important to differentiate the various types of incontinence because each is treated differently. Historical factors are very important in separating these different entities.**

6. *Enuresis* refers to involuntary urination and bed-wetting that occurs during sleep.
7. Quantification of voiding symptoms

a. **The American Urological Association (AUA) Symptom Index and the International Prostate Symptom Score (IPSS) are self-administered questionnaires consisting of seven questions relating to symptoms of lower urinary tract voiding dysfunction** (Table 1.1). The IPSS includes a quality-of-life question to assess the degree of bother experienced by the patient.

b. Symptoms are classified as mild (0–7), moderate (8–19), or severe (20–35).

c. The symptom score is an integral part of the clinical practice guidelines for treatment planning and follow-up for BPH management.

TABLE 1.1 The AUA Symptom Index

Question	Not at All	Less Than 1 Time in 5	Less Than Half the Time	About Half the Time	More Than Half the Time	Almost Always
1. During the last month or so, how often have you had a sensation of not emptying your bladder completely after you finished urinating?	0	1	2	3	4	5
2. During the last month or so, how often have you had to urinate again less than 2 hours after you finished urinating?	0	1	2	3	4	5
3. During the last month or so, how often have you found you stopped and started again several times when you urinated?	0	1	2	3	4	5
4. During the last month or so, how often have you found it difficult to postpone urination?	0	1	2	3	4	5
5. During the last month or so, how often have you had a weak urinary stream?	0	1	2	3	4	5
6. During the last month or so, how often have you had to push or strain to begin urination?	0	1	2	3	4	5
7. During the last month, how many times did you most typically get up to urinate from the time you went to bed at night until the time you got up in the morning?	None 0	1 time 1	2 times 2	3 times 3	4 times 4	5 or more times 5
AUA symptoms score = sum of questions 1 to 7.						

d. The symptom score is not specific for or diagnostic of BPH. It can be used in men and women for general assessment of voiding symptoms.

CHANGES IN THE GROSS APPEARANCE OF THE URINE

1. Cloudy urine
   a. Cloudy urine is most commonly due to the benign process of precipitation of phosphates in an alkaline urine (phosphaturia). This may be noted after meals or after consumption of large quantities of milk and is generally intermittent in nature. Patients are otherwise asymptomatic. Acidification of the urine with acetic acid at the time of urinalysis causes prompt clearing of the specimen.
   b. *Pyuria* refers to the finding of large quantities of white blood cells that cause urine to have a cloudy appearance. Microscopic examination of the urine sample will demonstrate the inflammatory nature that is usually secondary to an infection.
   c. *Chyluria* refers to the presence of lymph fluid mixed with the urine. It is an unusual cause of cloudy urine.
2. *Pneumaturia* refers to the passage of gas along with urine while voiding. There may be associated pyuria or frank fecal contamination of the urine, as this phenomenon is almost exclusively due to the presence of a fistula between the GI and urinary tracts. On occasion, the presence of a gas-forming infection within the urinary tract can produce similar symptoms, although this is very unusual.
3. Hematuria
   a. The passage of bloody urine is always alarming, and generally the patient makes a prompt visit to the physician. Investigation is always warranted, including a properly performed urinalysis to be certain that the red discoloration of the urine is indeed secondary to the presence of blood. For a differential diagnosis of the causes of red urine, see Page X.
   b. Although hematuria is always a danger signal, a clue to its significance may lie in whether there is associated pain or whether the bleeding is essentially painless. Pain that occurs in association with cystitis or passage of a urinary

tract calculus may indicate that the bleeding is in fact benign in nature. **Painless hematuria, however, is always believed to be secondary to a urinary tract neoplasm until proven otherwise.** This differentiation is not infallible, and therefore all urinary tract bleeding warrants investigation to be certain that there is not an associated neoplasm in addition to the more obvious cause for painful bleeding.

c. The probable site of bleeding within the urinary tract may be ascertained by determining whether the bleeding is initial (at the beginning of the stream only), terminal (at the end of the stream only), or total (throughout the entire stream). Initial hematuria generally indicates some type of anterior urethral bleeding that is flushed out by the initial passage of the bladder urine through the urethra. Terminal hematuria is often secondary to posterior urethral, bladder neck, or trigone bleeding and is noted when the bladder finally compresses these areas at the end of micturition. Total hematuria indicates that the bleeding occurs at the level of the bladder or above, such that all of the urine is mixed with blood and is therefore bloody throughout the entire stream.

4. *Colored urine* may result from a variety of foods, medications, and medical disorders. The colors may range from almost clear to black, with all other colors of the spectrum noted in between. (See Table 1.2 for common causes of colorful urine.)

ABNORMAL APPEARANCE AND FUNCTION OF THE MALE EXTERNAL GENITALIA

1. Sexual dysfunction
2. Infertility
3. Penile problems
   a. *Cutaneous lesions.* A variety of exophytic and ulcerative lesions may be noted by the patient. The relationship of the onset of these lesions to recent sexual activity should be explored. The physical characteristics of these lesions should be noted at the time of physical examination. The combination of historical and physical factors and associated physical findings such as adenopathy will

TABLE 1.2 Common Causes of Colorful Urine

Colorless	Very dilute urine
	Overhydration
Cloudy/milky	Phosphaturia
	Pyuria
	Chyluria
Red	Hematuria
	Hemoglobin/myoglobinuria
	Anthocyanin in beets and blackberries
	Chronic lead and mercury poisoning
	Phenolphthalein (in bowel evacuants)
	Phenothiazines (Compazine, etc.)
	Rifampin
Orange	Dehydration
	Phenazopyridine (Pyridium)
	Sulfasalazine (Azulfidine)
Yellow	Normal
	Phenacetin
	Riboflavin
Green-blue	Biliverdin
	Indicanuria (tryptophan indole metabolites)
	Amitriptyline (Elavil)
	Indigo carmine
	Methylene blue
	Phenols (IV cimetidine [Tagamet], IV promethazine [Phenergan], etc.)
	Resorcinol
	Triamterene (Dyrenium)
Brown	Urobilinogen
	Porphyria
	Aloe, fava beans, and rhubarb
	Chloroquine and primaquine
	Furazolidone (Furoxone)
	Metronidazole (Flagyl)
	Nitrofurantoin (Furadantin)
Brown-black	Alcaptonuria (homogentisic acid)
	Hemorrhage
	Melanin
	Tyrosinosis (hydroxyphenylpyruvic acid)
	Cascara, senna (laxatives)
	Methocarbamol (Robaxin)
	Methyldopa (Aldomet)
	Sorbitol

provide a working diagnosis for the treatment of these lesions.

b. *Penile curvature*. Bending of the penis, particularly during erection, is noted in association with scarring and fibrosis of the tunica albuginea. These plaque-like structures may be noted on physical examination. The process is essentially idiopathic and has been referred to as *Peyronie disease*. Congenital curvature is usually in a ventral direction and is not associated with fibrosis or formation of a plaque.
c. *Urethral discharge*. The character of the urethral discharge and its onset in relation to sexual activity should be described. The presence of the discharge should be confirmed on physical examination, a microscopic examination performed, and a culture obtained.
d. *Bloody ejaculate*. Like hematuria, this is also a frightening experience that usually causes the patient to seek prompt attention. This problem, however, is generally secondary to benign congestion and/or inflammation of the seminal vesicles. The process is usually self-limited or treatable with antibiotics and does not initially require an extensive evaluation.

4. Scrotal problems
   a. *Cutaneous lesions*. The hair-bearing skin of the scrotum is susceptible to skin diseases that can occur anywhere else on the body. Fungal infections and venereal warts may also be noted commonly.
   b. *Scrotal swelling* and *masses*. The presence of scrotal swelling and/or a scrotal mass may be noted incidentally by the patient while bathing or performing a self-examination or due to the presence of associated discomfort. A variety of lesions can produce unilateral or bilateral scrotal enlargement. These range from normal structures that are misinterpreted by the patient to testicular neoplasms. The differential diagnosis is as noted in the following box. A combination of historical information, particularly with regard to onset of the mass, progression, and associated pain, and the physical examination is helpful in differentiating some of the more confusing lesions.

DIFFERENTIAL DIAGNOSIS

Scrotal Swelling

Structure Involved	Pathology
Scrotal wall	Hematoma
	Urinary extravasation
	Edema from cardiac, hepatic, or renal failure
Testis	Carcinoma
	Torsion of testes or appendix testis
Epididymis	Epididymitis
	Tumor
	Torsion of appendix epididymis
Spermatic cord	Hydrocele surrounding testis of involving cord only
	Hematocele
	Hernia
	Varicocele
	Lipoma

The Physical Examination

GENERAL INFORMATION

1. The problems delineated in the history will determine how extensive the physical examination should be. A complete physical examination is obviously necessary for someone who will undergo some type of urologic surgery; in most instances, however, a limited examination of the genitourinary tract is usually sufficient at the time of the initial examination.
2. The commonly taught techniques of physical examination, including inspection, palpation, percussion, and auscultation, are also used during the urologic examination. Each has varying degrees of usefulness, depending on the organ being evaluated. Particular aspects of the physical examination will be noted later.

KIDNEYS AND FLANKS

1. *Inspection.* Inspection of the flanks is best carried out with the patient in the sitting or standing position facing straight ahead and the examiner located behind the patient facing the area in question. Scoliosis may be evident in the patient with an inflammatory process directly or indirectly involving the psoas

muscle with resultant spasm. Bulging of the flank may be noted if an underlying mass exists, although this is evident in most cases only if the mass is extremely large or the patient is very thin. Edema of the flank may be noted if there is an underlying inflammatory process.

2. *Palpation* and *percussion*. A method of bimanual renal palpation has been described with the patient in the supine position (Fig. 1.1). The examiner lifts the flank by placing one hand beneath this area and subsequently palpates deeply beneath the ipsilateral costal margin anteriorly. This technique is successful in children and thin adults but generally yields little information under most other circumstances. A large mass may be palpable. Percussion is a useful technique, particularly in the area of the costovertebral angle, to elicit tenderness due to underlying capsular inflammation or distention (Fig. 1.2).

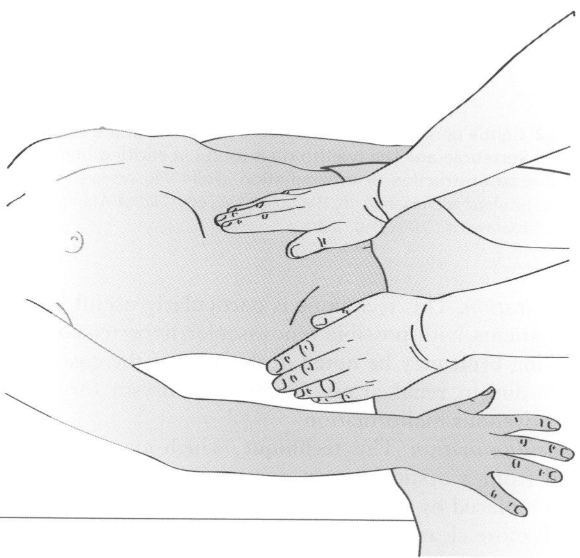

FIGURE 1.1 With the patient in the supine position, one hand is used to raise the flank while the abdominal hand palpates deeply beneath the costal margin. (From Van Arsdalen K. Signs and symptoms: the initial examination. In: Hanno P, et al., eds. *Clinical Manual of Urology*. New York: McGraw-Hill; 2001, Fig. 2-1.)

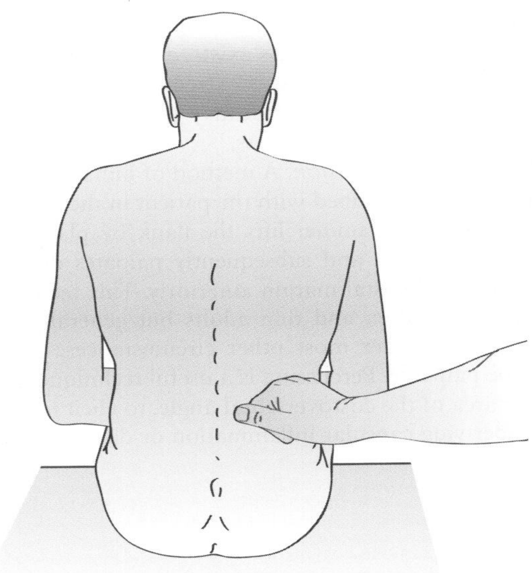

FIGURE 1.2 Gentle percussion with the heel of the hand in the angle between the lumbar vertebrae and the twelfth rib is useful in eliciting underlying tenderness due to obstruction or inflammation. (From Van Arsdalen K. Signs and symptoms: the initial examination. In: Hanno P, et al., eds. *Clinical Manual of Urology.* New York: McGraw-Hill; 2001, Fig. 2-2.)

3. *Auscultation.* This technique is particularly useful in evaluating patients with possible renovascular hypertension. An underlying bruit may be noted in the area of the costovertebral angle due to renal artery stenosis, aneurysm formation, or arteriovenous malformation.
4. *Transillumination.* This technique, which may differentiate a solid from a cystic mass in neonates or infants, has largely been replaced by ultrasonography, which defines these lesions much more clearly.

ABDOMEN AND BLADDER

1. *Inspection.* The abdominal and bladder examinations are best carried out with the patient in the supine position. The full or

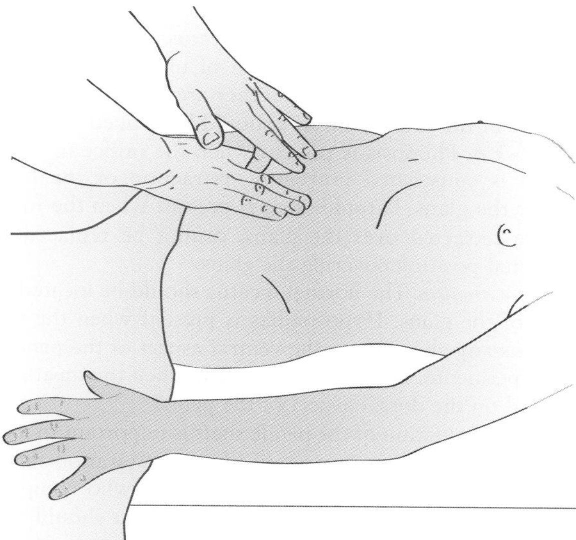

FIGURE 1.3 Percussion over the bladder may be particularly useful when palpation is difficult due either to obesity or failure of the patient to relax during the examination. The bladder may be percussed if it contains greater than 150 mL of urine in the adult. (From Van Arsdalen K. Signs and symptoms: the initial examination. In: Hanno P, et al., eds. *Clinical Manual of Urology.* New York: McGraw-Hill; 2001, Fig. 2-3.)

overdistended bladder may be visible on general inspection of the abdomen with the patient in this position.

2. *Palpation* and *percussion.* It is generally possible to palpate or percuss the bladder above the level of the symphysis pubis if it contains 150 mL or more of urine (Fig. 1.3). It should be remembered that in the child, the bladder *may* be percussible or palpable with much smaller volumes of urine due to the fact that it is more of an intraabdominal organ in the child than the true pelvic organ it is in the adult.

PENIS

1. *Inspection.* Inspection of the penis will reveal obvious lesions of the skin and will define whether the patient has been circumcised. If the patient has been circumcised, the glans penis

and meatus can be inspected directly. In the uncircumcised patient, the foreskin, glans, and meatus should then be inspected. The number and position of ulcerative and/or exophytic lesions should be noted if they are present. The position and size of the urinary meatus should be defined.

a. *Foreskin.* Phimosis is present when the orifice of the foreskin is constricted preventing retraction of the foreskin over the glans. Paraphimosis is present when the foreskin, once retracted over the glans, cannot be replaced to its normal position covering the glans.
b. *Penile meatus.* The normal meatus should be located at the tip of the glans. Hypospadias is present when the meatus opens anywhere along the ventral aspect of the penis or in the perineum. Epispadias is present when the meatus is located on the dorsal aspect of the penis.

2. *Palpation.* Palpation of the penile shaft is important to identify and define the limits of areas of fibrous induration that may be found in patients with Peyronie disease who complain of penile curvature during erection. The urethra should also be palpated for areas of induration that may be associated with periurethritis and urethral stricture disease. The urethra can also be "stripped" from the penile-scrotal junction toward the meatus to look for a urethral discharge that can then be collected for microscopic examination and culture.

SCROTUM AND SCROTAL CONTENTS

1. *Inspection.* The inspection of the scrotum and the remainder of this portion of the physical examination are best carried out with the patient initially in the standing position. Lesions of the scrotal skin are readily evident in this position. The examiner also generally notes that if two testicles are present, one usually hangs lower than the other. In most cases, the left testicle is lower than the right. In cases of congenital absence or failure of descent of one or both testicles, the involved side may demonstrate hypoplastic scrotal development. It is always important to note the presence or absence of the testes. Scrotal masses and the "bag of worms" appearance of an underlying large varicocele may be identified on initial inspection.
2. *Palpation.* The contents of each hemiscrotum should be palpated in an orderly fashion. First, the testes should be

examined, then the epididymides, then the cord structures, and finally the area of the external inguinal ring to check for the presence of an inguinal hernia (Fig. 1.4).

a. Each testis should be in the dependent portion of the scrotum when the patient is relaxed and in a warm environment. The long axis of the testicle should be in a vertical direction, and the size of the testis should normally be greater than or equal to 4 cm in adult males.
b. Each epididymis is adherent to the posterolateral aspect of the testicle. The head of the epididymis is noted to be near

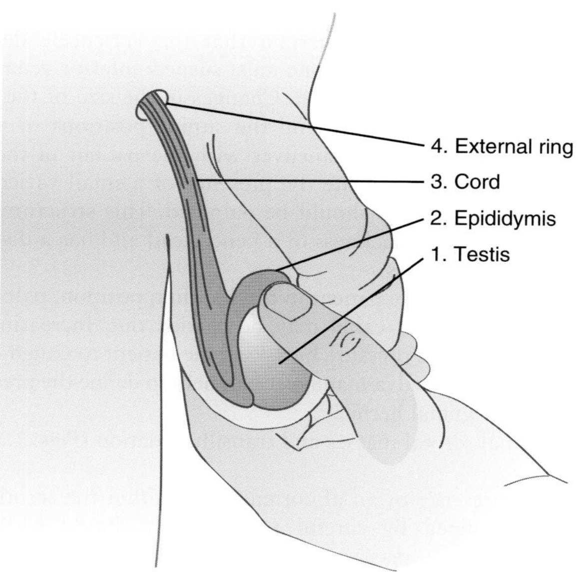

FIGURE 1.4 Palpation of the scrotal contents should be carried out in an orderly, routine fashion. One should begin palpating the testes, followed by the epididymides, the cord structures, and finally the external rings. Palpating each structure from side to side is useful for detecting differences in testicular size and identifying varicoceles. All of the scrotal structures may be examined between the thumb and the index and middle fingers. (From Van Arsdalen K. Signs and symptoms: the initial examination. In: Hanno P, et al., eds. *Clinical Manual of Urology.* New York: McGraw-Hill; 2001, Fig. 2-4.)

the superior pole of the testicle, the body of the epididymis is near the middle portion of the testicle, and the tail of the epididymis represents the most inferior aspect of this structure. The examiner should palpate each portion of the epididymis, looking primarily for areas of tenderness or induration.

c. The spermatic cord varies somewhat in thickness, and often this depends on the presence or absence of what has been termed a *lipoma of the cord*. The examiner should be particularly attentive to the presence or absence of enlarged venous structures (i.e., a varicocele). If a varicocele is detected, the patient should also be examined in the supine position to be certain that the varicocele decompresses. If it does not, one must suspect inferior vena cava or renal vein obstruction. Changes in the size of the cord between the standing and the supine positions or when using the Valsalva maneuver with the patient in the upright position indicate the presence of a small varicocele. The vas deferens should be palpated. This structure normally has the thickness of a pencil lead and has a distinct, smooth firmness.

d. Finally, with the patient in the standing position, palpation of the inguinal canal may be carried out. Increasing intraabdominal pressure by asking the patient to cough or by using the Valsalva maneuver will help to define the presence of an inguinal hernia.

3. Abnormal scrotal masses and transillumination (Figs. 1.5 and 1.6).

   a. The presence of an abnormal mass within the scrotum is best defined by careful palpation. It should be noted whether the mass arises from the testicle, is contained within the testicle, arises from the epididymis, is located in the cord, or tends to surround most of the scrotal structures. It is important to note the character of the mass, that is, whether it is hard, firm, or cystic in nature.

   b. **All scrotal masses should be transilluminated, and this can be accomplished with a small penlight.** Any mass that radiates a reddish glow of light through the lesion represents a cystic, fluid-filled structure. Caution is advised in defining

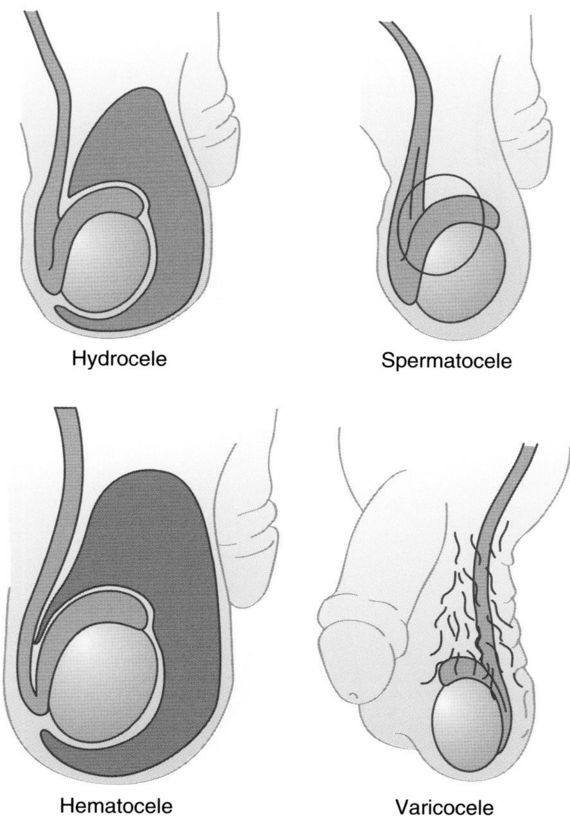

FIGURE 1.5 A variety of fluid-filled masses develops within the scrotum. Hydroceles and spermatoceles (and occasionally bowel in the hernia sac) will transilluminate. Hydrocele fluid is contained within the tunica vaginalis and essentially surrounds the testicle. A spermatocele generally occurs above or adjacent to the upper pole of the testis and represents a cyst of the rete testis or epididymis. A hematocele is a collection of blood within the tunica vaginalis due usually to trauma or surgery. Occasionally bleeding will occur spontaneously that is associated with bleeding disorders. A varicocele represents dilated veins of the pampiniform plexus. Hematoceles and varicoceles will not transilluminate. (From Van Arsdalen K. Signs and symptoms: the initial examination. In: Hanno P, et al., eds. *Clinical Manual of Urology*. New York: McGraw-Hill; 2001, Fig. 2-5.)

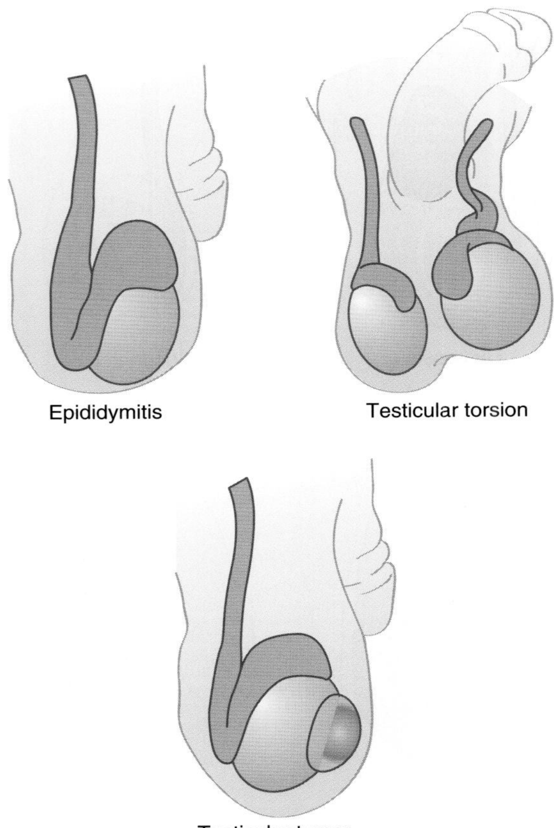

FIGURE 1.6 Solid scrotal masses may be painful or painless and may involve the testis, epididymis, or both. (From Van Arsdalen K. Signs and symptoms: the initial examination. In: Hanno P, et al., eds. *Clinical Manual of Urology.* New York: McGraw-Hill; 2001, Fig. 2-6.)

the benignity of these lesions, however, in that benign and malignant lesions can coexist. A hydrocele surrounding a testicular tumor is an example.

c. See the following box for a differential diagnosis of scrotal masses.

DIFFERENTIAL DIAGNOSIS

Scrotal Discomfort and Solid Mass Lesions

	Torsion	Epididymitis	Tumor
AGE	Birth to 20 years	Puberty to old age	15 to 35 years
PAIN			
Onset	Sudden	Rapid	Gradual
Degree	Severe	Increasing severity	Mild or absent
Nausea/ vomiting	Yes	No	No
EXAMINATION			
Testis	Swollen	Normal early	Mass
Epididymis	together and both tender	Swollen, tender	Normal
Spermatic cord	Shortened	Thickened, often tender as high as inguinal canal	
URINALYSIS	Normal	Often infection	Normal

THE RECTUM AND PROSTATE

1. *Position.* Various positions have been described for performing a digital rectal examination (DRE). Having the patient lie on the examining table in the lateral decubitus position with the legs flexed at the hips and knees and the uppermost leg pulled higher toward the chest than the lowermost leg creates a comfortable position for the patient and the examiner (Fig. 1.7). Alternatively, the patient can bend over the examining table while in the standing position so that the weight of his upper body rests on his elbows. The lateral decubitus position typically allows for deeper penetration of the rectum to feel the prostate in obese patients or to feel the top of large glands. Probably more important than the position, however, is that the gloved examining finger be adequately lubricated and slow, gentle pressure be applied as the finger traverses the anal sphincter. A rectal examination can be an extremely painful or a painless experience, depending on the skill and patience of the examiner. It is important at the time of the examination, not only to palpate the prostate gland, but to palpate the entire inside of the rectum in search of other abnormalities.

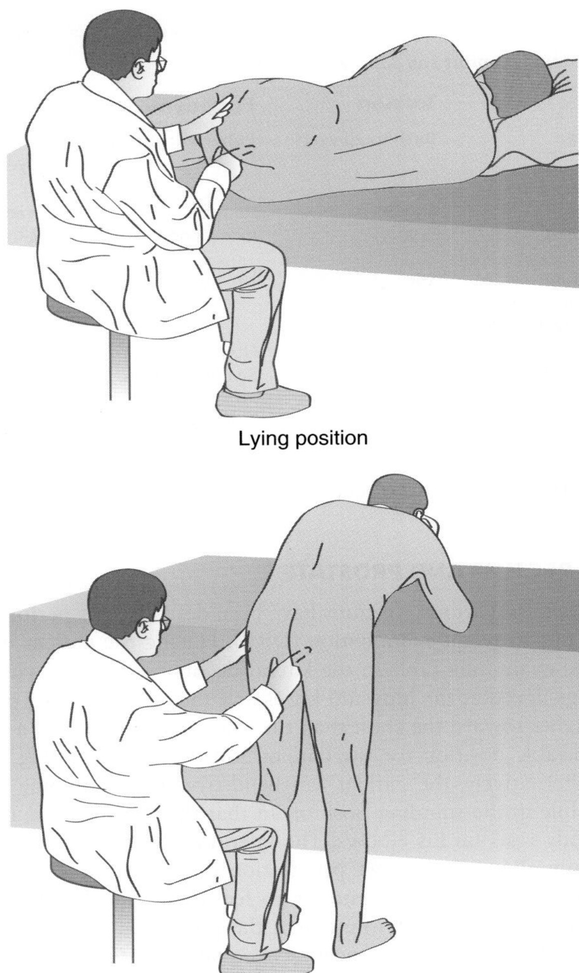

FIGURE 1.7 **Two positions are illustrated for performing the digital rectal examination.** (From Van Arsdalen K. Signs and symptoms: the initial examination. In: Hanno P, et al., eds. *Clinical Manual of Urology.* New York: McGraw-Hill; 2001, Fig. 2-7.)

2. *Prostate*. During the rectal examination, the posterior aspect of the prostate is palpated (Fig. 1.8). The significance of this part of the general physical examination cannot be overemphasized. Most types of prostate carcinoma begin in the posterior lobe of the prostate, which is very accessible to the examining finger.

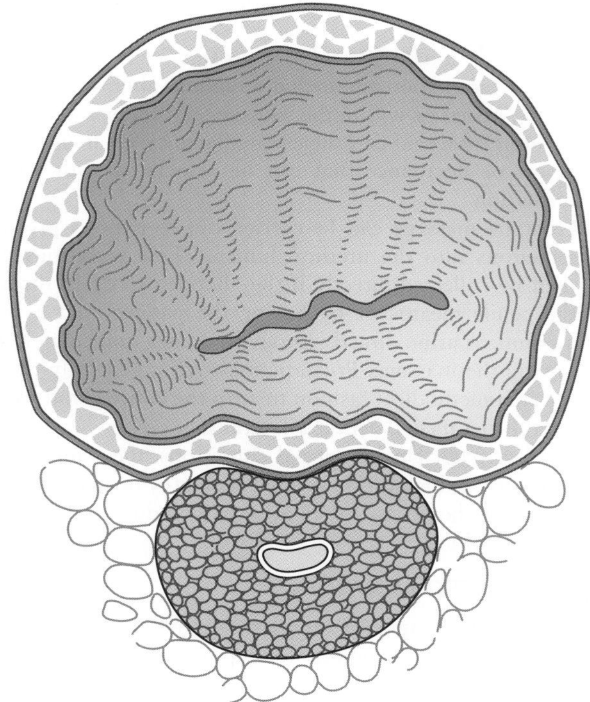

FIGURE 1.8 The posterior aspect of the prostate is palpable on rectal examination. The surface is normally smooth, rubbery, and approximately 4 × 4 cm in size. The median furrow may be lost with diffuse enlargement of the gland, and the lateral sulci may be either accentuated or obscured. Deviations from normal contour, consistency, or size should be carefully described. Stating that an area is "hard" implies the presence of carcinoma. The seminal vesicles are not normally palpable. *Remember:* Check the entire rectum. Do not miss an occult rectal carcinoma. (From Smith DR. *General Urology*. 11th ed., New York: McGraw-Hill; 1984.)

a. **The prostate gland is normally a small, walnut-sized structure with a flattened, heart-shaped configuration.** A median furrow runs down the longitudinal axis of the prostate. There are two lateral sulci, where the rectal mucosa folds back on itself after reflecting off the prostate. The consistency of the normal prostate is generally described as "rubbery" in nature and has been likened to the consistency of the thenar eminence when one opposes the thumb and fifth finger.
b. Abnormal consistency of the prostate may be noted on rectal examination and includes nodular abnormalities that can be raised or within the substance of the prostate, areas of induration that can suggest malignancy, or areas of bogginess or fluctuance that can be associated with abscess formation.
c. Prostatic massage can be carried out to express prostatic secretions into the urethral lumen. These secretions may then be collected directly if they happen to drain through the penile meatus or by having the patient void a small amount of urine directly into a container immediately following the massage. Prostatic massage is generally carried out in a methodical fashion to strip the entire gland from a lateral to a medial aspect bilaterally.

3. *Seminal vesicles.* Under normal conditions, the seminal vesicles are not palpable. They can become evident on a rectal examination, however, if they are enlarged due to obstruction or inflammation.

THE VAGINAL EXAMINATION

1. *Inspection.* The vaginal examination is best performed with the patient in the relaxed lithotomy position. Inspection of the vulva may reveal a variety of venereal and nonvenereal lesions. The urinary meatus should be identified and its position and size noted. An erythematous tender lesion arising from the meatus may represent a benign urethral caruncle or possibly a urethral carcinoma. The character of the vaginal mucosa at the introitus should be noted. The examiner *may* also note the presence of a cystocele or a rectocele while examining the patient in this position. These structures may be accentuated with increases in intraabdominal pressure such as those that

occur with coughing or straining. In fact, this maneuver may elicit some leakage of urine in patients with stress urinary incontinence.

2. *Palpation.* Palpation of the urethra to the level of the bladder neck and trigone may be accomplished during examination of the anterior vaginal wall. Bimanual palpation is useful to define the internal genitalia and to define further the size and consistency of the urinary bladder.

The Urinalysis and Culture

COLLECTION

Proper collection and prompt examination of the urine are essential to gain the most information from the routinely collected specimen.

1. Males
   a. A midstream urine collection is most commonly obtained in men for routine examination. With this technique, the male patient is instructed to retract the foreskin if he is uncircumcised and to gently cleanse the glans. He begins to urinate into the toilet, subsequently inserting a sterile glass container into the urinary stream to collect a urine sample. The container is then removed and the act of voiding is completed.
   b. A variety of other collection techniques affords more information with regard to localization of infection within the urinary tract. Four such specimens may be obtained and analyzed separately by routine microscopic evaluation and culture techniques. These have been designated the VB-1, VB-2, EPS, and VB-3 specimens, according to Stamey. The VB-1 is the initial 5 to 10 mL of the stream, which contains bladder urine mixed with urethral contents that are initially washed from the urethra. The VB-2 specimen is essentially the midstream portion of the collection. The EPS specimen represents the expressed prostatic secretions following prostatic massage. Finally, the VB-3 specimen represents a small voided specimen that mixes bladder urine with the contents contained in the urethra immediately following the expression of prostatic secretions. This collection is particularly useful if inadequate amounts of secretion from

the prostate are expressed during the prostatic massage. The value of these cultures for localization of urinary tract infection is that the VB-1 represents urethral flora, the VB-2 represents bladder flora, and the EPS and VB-3 represent prostatic flora.

2. Females
   a. The midstream urine collection in females is somewhat more difficult to accomplish and is often considered to be inadequate for even the most routine examination. With this technique, the vulva is cleansed and the stream is initiated into the toilet with subsequent insertion of a collecting container as described previously for the male. If this specimen is grossly contaminated or appears infected, then one of the collection methods noted later may be necessary to differentiate these two possibilities. However, if the collection has been done with reasonable care and the specimen is essentially negative on microscopic examination, then this technique is generally considered adequate.
   b. A more proper method of midstream urine collection has been described in which the patient is placed in the lithotomy position and then asked to void. The nurse holds the labia apart to prevent contamination and collects a midstream specimen. This is often awkward, if not difficult, for both the patient and the nurse, and this method of collection is not recommended.
   c. If there is any question with regard to the problem of contamination versus infection of the midstream specimen as noted previously, then catheterization to obtain a true bladder specimen is the preferred technique. An examiner should not hesitate to use this method to properly categorize a patient's problem.
3. Children
   a. Percutaneous suprapubic aspiration of urine from neonates and infants is a particularly useful method of obtaining a truly uncontaminated specimen of urine from the bladder. With this technique, the suprapubic area is cleansed with an antiseptic solution and percutaneous aspiration is performed with a fine-gauge needle. The specimen can then be examined for urinalysis and sent for culture.

b. A variety of sterile plastic bags is available with adhesive collars that surround the male and female infant's genitalia. They are particularly useful for routine screening urinalysis, but as with the collection of midstream specimens from women, it may be difficult at times to differentiate a truly infected urine specimen from a contaminated one due to this collection technique.
c. Older boys and girls may have urine collected in a fashion similar to that described previously for their adult counterparts. One is generally quite hesitant, however, to catheterize young boys due to the possibility of urethral trauma. It is easier and safer to perform this in girls and may be used if necessary.

PHYSICAL ASPECTS OF URINE

1. *Color.* The color of urine is generally a clear, light yellow, but a wide range of colors has been described. The changes in color can be secondary to foods and medications and to intrinsic disease processes. Table 1.2 describes the etiologic factors in relationship to abnormal urine color.
2. *pH.* The normal pH of urine ranges from 4.5 to 8.0. Urine is described as having an acid pH if it ranges between 4.5 and 5.5. It has an alkaline pH if it ranges between 6.5 and 8.0.
3. *Specific gravity.* The specific gravity can be determined in the office by relatively simple techniques and gives some idea of the concentrating ability of the kidneys and their ability to excrete waste products. A variety of substances within the urine, such as intravenous contrast material, can detract from the value of this test. The osmolality of the urine is a better indicator of renal function but requires standard laboratory methods.

DIPSTICK TESTS

1. A variety of dipsticks is available to evaluate the urine sample. These consist of short plastic strips with small pads that are impregnated with a variety of reagents that react with abnormal substances within the urine.
2. In addition to determination of urinary pH, the most sophisticated dipsticks now contain reagents for the determination of the following:
   a. Protein
   b. Glucose

c. Ketones
d. Urobilinogen
e. Bilirubin
f. Blood
g. Hemoglobin
h. Leukocytes
i. Nitrites

MICROSCOPIC EXAMINATION

1. A small portion of the collected urine sample is placed in a test tube and centrifuged at approximately 5000 rpm for 5 minutes. The supernate is then poured from the tube, and the remaining sediment is resuspended in the small quantity of urine that drains back down the side of the tube to the sediment. A drop of the resuspended sediment is placed on a glass slide followed by a cover slip.
2. The wet specimen is then examined under low and high power for the presence and number of epithelial cells, red blood cells, white blood cells, bacteria, and casts.

URINE CULTURE

1. **If a urine culture is desired, it should be promptly plated in the office or sent immediately to the laboratory to prevent overgrowth of bacteria and falsely elevated bacterial counts.**
2. The value of localization cultures has been noted previously.

Initial Point-of-Care Imaging

ULTRASOUND

1. Diagnostic ultrasound has been refined over the past half century and is widely used and available not only in Radiology Departments but also in Emergency Departments, on surgical and medical floors, and in many specialty clinics.
2. The use and type of ultrasound used by Urologists varies dramatically based upon training, level of experience and type of disease state needing evaluation.

BLADDER SCANNING

1. Bladder scanning is a safe, painless, noninvasive method to determine bladder urine volume without the use of a urinary catheter.

A Bladder Scanner is a device made by several manufacturers that makes the volume determination using different ultrasound frequencies with real-time or non–real-time displays. It generally requires minimal training to be used effectively and is used commonly by medical practitioners, nurses, techs and trainees.

2. The use of a Bladder Scanner to measure urine volume in the bladder related to the evaluation and management of lower urinary tract voiding dysfunction is probably the most common and the most ubiquitous form of ultrasound used outside of Radiology Departments. Bladder scanning is used primarily after Foley catheter removal to confirm the adequacy of bladder emptying, or conversely, to measure residual urine volume in states of incomplete bladder emptying.

Blood Tests

PANEL 7 (OR SIMILAR DESIGNATION)

1. Serum electrolytes (Na, K, Cl, CO_2) are useful indicators of maintenance of homeostasis for which the kidney plays a significant role.
2. Glucose levels in the serum may be variable relative to the presence of glucosuria.
   a. Diabetes is a significant risk factor for voiding and sexual dysfunction.
3. Blood urea nitrogen (BUN) and creatinine are indicators of renal function.

PSA LEVEL

1. PSA is a protein kinase produced by the prostatic epithelium.
   a. It is a normal component of the ejaculate responsible for liquification of the semen.
   b. Normally found in very low levels in serum (0–4.0 ng/mL).
2. Causes of PSA elevation
   a. Prostate cancer
   b. BPH
   c. Prostatitis (acute and chronic)
   d. Instrumentation (catheterization, cystoscopy, biopsy)
   e. Urinary retention
   f. Vigorous prostatic massage, probably little elevation for routine DRE

3. PSA as a tumor marker
   a. Limitations due to prostate organ specific but not cancer specific.
   b. Substantial overlap of values for men with prostate cancer and benign conditions.
   c. Absolute value greater than 10 ng/mL has more than 60% predictive risk of prostate cancer.
   d. Sixty percent of current prostate cancer diagnoses are made due to an elevated PSA level.
   e. Useful marker for following efficacy of treatment for prostate cancer.
4. Recommendations
   a. One must be familiar with the guidelines and controversies for prostate cancer screening using PSA levels.

Summary

The surgical subspecialty of urology deals with a well-defined organ system within the body. The urologist diagnoses and treats a wide variety of medical and surgical disorders that may have local or systemic ramifications for the patient. The history, physical examination, and urinalysis serve as the cornerstones of the initial evaluation of these patients. In addition, a variety of unique diagnostic and therapeutic instruments are available for use in the office or outpatient setting to aid in caring for those with urologic diseases. The frequency with which these problems are seen by generalists and other specialists necessitates that all practitioners have some familiarity with this field.

CLINICAL PEARLS

1. A stone in the kidney or upper ureter may produce ipsilateral testicular pain.
2. Pain derived from the lower ureter is generally felt in the suprapubic area, bladder, penis, or urethra.
3. Although hematuria is always a danger signal, a clue to its significance may lie in whether there is associated pain or whether the bleeding is essentially painless.
4. Congenital curvature is usually in a ventral direction and, unlike Peyronie disease, is not associated with fibrosis or formation of a plaque.

Additional content, including Self-Assessment Questions and Suggested Readings, may be accessed at www.ExpertConsult.com.

Diagnostic and Interventional Uroradiology

Akshya Gupta, MD, and Parvati Ramchandani, MD

DIAGNOSTIC URORADIOLOGY

The imaging techniques used to evaluate the urinary tract are dictated by the indication for which the diagnostic evaluation is being performed. Modalities currently in use include conventional abdominal plain film radiography, ultrasonography, computed tomography (CT), magnetic resonance imaging (MRI), radionuclide studies, and positron emission tomography (PET). In this chapter, the role of these different imaging modalities in the management of patients will be addressed, starting with the most commonly used techniques.

Plain Films (Kidney, Ureters, and Bladder Plain Radiography)

X-ray films are rarely used currently, having been entirely replaced by digital imaging; a digital image is technically not a *radiograph* or a film, although the term continues to be used in common clinical parlance. *Computed radiograph* of the abdomen is one term used for an x-ray examination of the abdomen and the term KUB simply denotes an examination of the kidney, ureters, and bladder performed without intravenous contrast. Radiation exposure for an abdominal radiograph is low and is approximately 0.53 millisieverts (mSv). For comparison purposes, radiation exposure from natural background radiation is about 3 mSv per year.

INDICATIONS

A radiograph of the abdomen is an essential tool in the evaluation of patients with gastrointestinal (GI) or genitourinary (GU) symptoms and in postoperative patients, after virtually any surgery, who present with symptoms suspected to be due to bowel ileus or obstruction. Abdominal radiography may be necessary to specifically evaluate the urinary tract in the following circumstances:

- To assess for the presence of radiopaque calculi
- To assess the results of therapy for calculi (shockwave lithotripsy [SWL] or percutaneous techniques)
- To evaluate urinary stents for their position and for complications such as encrustation (Fig. 2.1)

As bowel content overlies the renal fossae, small or faintly opaque stones may be challenging to identify. Calculi that project over the bony pelvis may also be difficult to identify and potentially be obscured by the bony trabeculae. Oblique images are often helpful in such cases, because the obliquity allows the kidney or ureter to be rotated off the overlying bowel or bone, thus facilitating the visualization of small and faintly opaque calculi.

Ultrasonography

Ultrasound (US) can be used to image most parts of the GU system, making it the preferred first-line imaging modality, not only to evaluate renal pathology, the presence or absence of urinary obstruction, but also to glean functional and morphologic information about the bladder. Portable techniques allow for use in patients who are too unstable to undergo other cross-sectional studies such as CT or MRI; it is not uncommon to examine patients in the intensive care unit, for example.

Ultrasound as an imaging modality has the significant advantages of being a noninvasive examination with no radiation exposure. It is important to recognize that the quality of an ultrasound examination is highly dependent on the expertise of the sonographer performing the examination, as well the body habitus of the patient; imaging may be suboptimal or limited in large and obese patients. The increasing availability of US contrast agents can enhance the diagnostic yield of the examination, and US contrast is proving to be a safe and effective way to characterize renal masses, both for diagnosis and to guide tissue sampling.

Characteristics of blood flow can also be determined by US, discussed later in further detail.

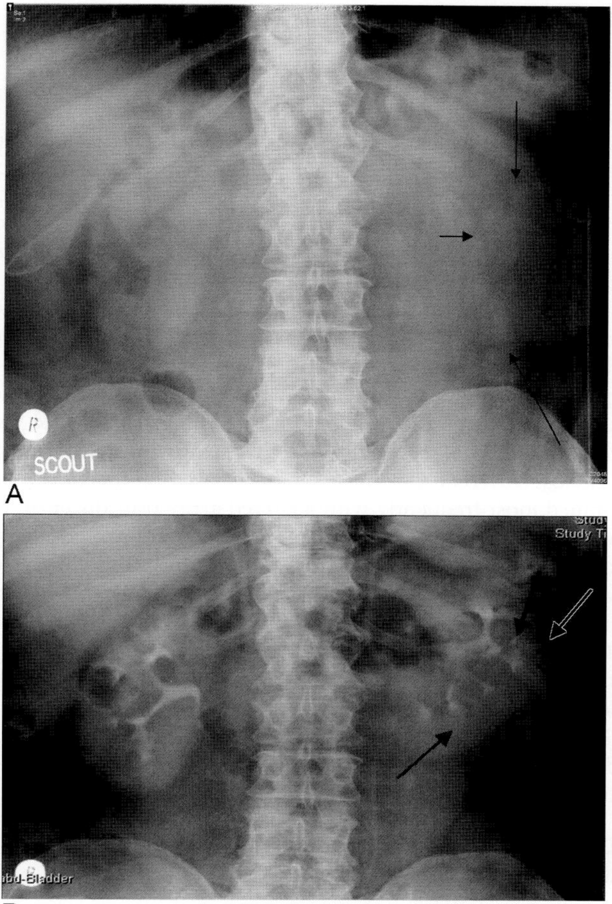

A

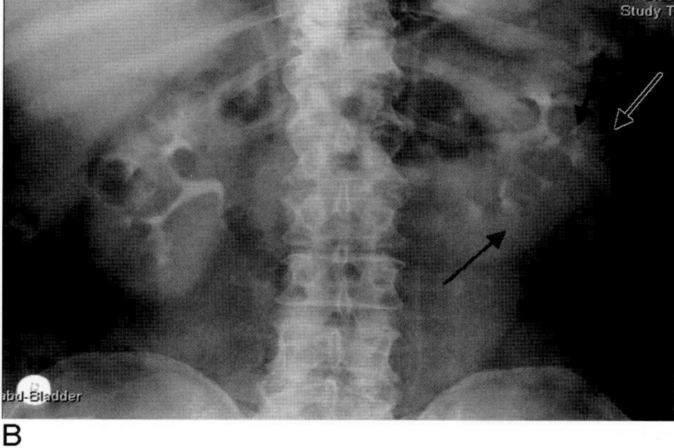

B

FIGURE 2.1 Large bilateral staghorn calculi in a 25-year-old female. (A) Abdominal radiograph centered over the kidneys and (B) radiograph of the entire abdomen demonstrates a large right staghorn calculus, a percutaneous nephrostomy catheter, and a ureteral stent on the right side. On the left side, there is a large calculus primarily in the renal pelvis and a nephroureteral stent in place. Note additional smaller calculi in the lower poles of both kidneys as well as encrusted on the right ureteral stent.

TECHNIQUE

Gray-scale and color Doppler imaging are commonly used in combination to identify the anatomy and morphology of the organ of interest, and subsequently any normal or abnormal vascularity. Imaging is dynamic and obtaining high-quality diagnostic images typically requires changes in patient position, respiration, and attention to technical components such as the transducer being used, or the transducer pressure being applied. Cine loops are often obtained to help mimic real-time visualization, and to highlight areas of interest. If ultrasound contrast is utilized, intravenous access is required. The kidneys are examined most commonly in longitudinal and transverse scan planes, with the transducer positioned in the flanks. Patients may need to be placed in different positions and asked to change respiration (such as deep inspiration or expiration) to allow complete visualization of the kidneys and avoid the shadowing related to the lower ribs. Different transducers may be used, but the kidneys are examined most frequently with a curved array transducer of 3 to 6 MHz frequency; higher frequency transducers provide higher resolution images and are used in patients with normal habitus. Lower frequency transducers are usually needed in larger patients to image the kidneys.

Color Doppler or flow imaging is used to assess the vascularity of the organ and any masses and is usually combined with real-time gray-scale imaging.

Newer advances in US such as three-dimensional (3D) imaging and extended field of view imaging may facilitate the depiction of spatial relationships.

INDICATIONS FOR US EXAMINATION IN THE URINARY TRACT

Kidneys

1. Renal insufficiency: US is the first-line imaging modality to identify obstruction as a possible cause of acute renal failure. The absence of frank hydronephrosis helps narrow the etiology of renal dysfunction to prerenal causes or renal pathology. Alteration in the normal echogenicity of the kidneys is seen in patients with medical renal disease—the kidneys may be smaller and more echogenic than normal. The presence of

renal atrophy, cortical thinning, or increased parenchymal echogenicity indicates chronic renal insufficiency.

2. Renal mass evaluation: US is often the first study used to evaluate for the presence of a renal mass in patients with hematuria. It is also very useful to characterize a renal mass, particularly where expensive techniques such as CT or MRI may be difficult to access. The ability to identify, characterize, and stage a renal mass is dependent on the depth of the lesion beneath the skin and the body habitus of the patient.

   Renal cysts are fluid filled masses with no internal echogenicity, and demonstrate excellent through transmission of the ultrasound beam. US can detect cysts of all sizes with more than 98% accuracy. Solid renal masses that are larger than 1 cm in diameter are also routinely identified, especially if they are located in the renal cortex. US is a useful tool in characterizing renal lesions as the appearance of cysts and solid masses is quite distinct; cysts can be readily distinguished from angiomyolipomas, and other benign or malignant enhancing solid renal neoplasms, particularly when over 1 cm in size. Solid masses are typically heterogeneous, and the ultrasound beam is poorly transmitted through the mass. Color Doppler imaging, as well as contrast-enhanced ultrasound, can help to definitively characterize lesions as solid or cystic and solid. The diagnosis of a renal neoplasm requires the demonstration of flow within the mass by color-flow or power Doppler.

3. Renal colic: Ultrasound can identify renal calculi that are large enough to cause acoustic shadowing or demonstrate twinkling artifact (Fig. 2.2); typically stones larger than 7 mm in size can be identified on US. Ureteral calculi may sometimes be identified as an echogenic focus in a dilated fluid filled proximal ureter. Calculi at the ureterovesicular junction may sometimes be seen as echogenic foci. The absence of a ureteral jet may indicate high-grade obstruction from a ureteral stone while the presence of a jet indicates that the obstruction is incomplete.

4. Pyelonephritis: Although most patients who have pyelonephritis have a normal sonogram, complications such as a renal abscess may be identified with ultrasound.

5. Renal intervention: Ultrasound is used routinely to visualize the kidneys and help guide needle placement for percutaneous biopsy or for percutaneous nephrostomy (PCN) tube placement.

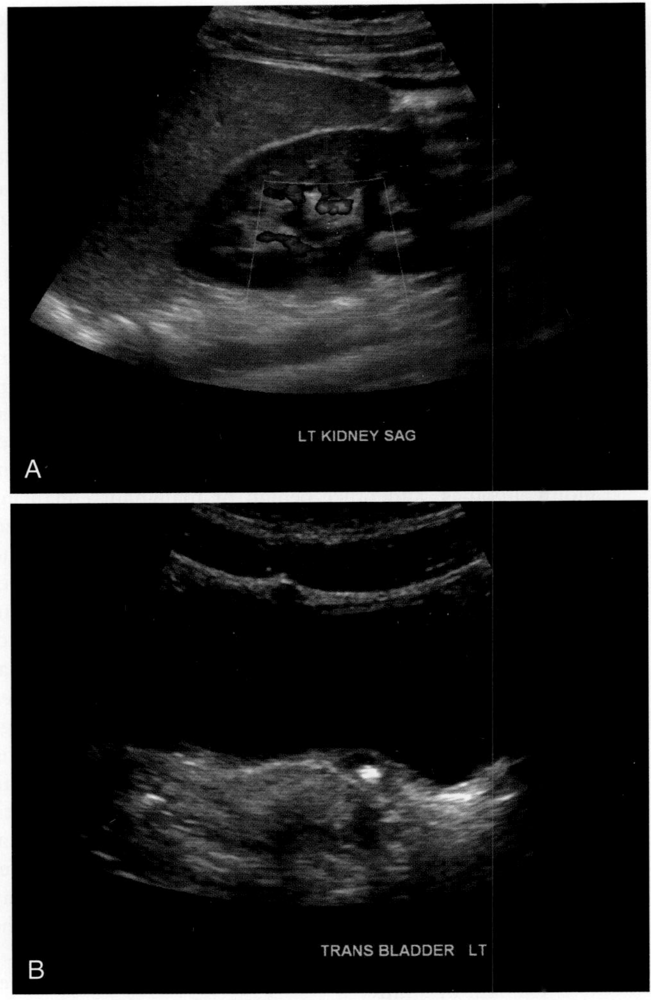

FIGURE 2.2 Hydronephrosis due to a distal ureteral stone. (A) Renal ultrasound shows mild left hydronephrosis. (B) A shadowing echogenic focus is identified in the distal left ureter, compatible with obstructing calculus.

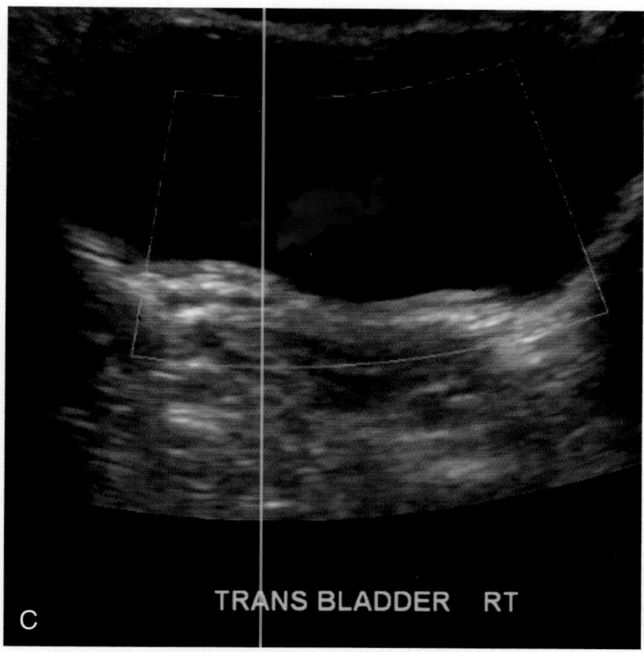

FIGURE 2.2, cont'd (C) A right ureteral jet is visualized; however, left ureteral jet is absent due to ureteral obstruction.

6. Renal artery stenosis: Color and spectral Doppler is often used to screen for renal artery stenosis (RAS), particularly in a patient with unexplained hypertension. Elevated velocities, gradients across the artery, and downstream abnormal vascular waveforms can all help identify hemodynamically significant stenosis. Other vascular malformations such as pseudoaneurysms and arteriovenous fistulas can also be identified using these techniques.
7. Renal transplant evaluation: The transplanted kidney, because of its superficial position in the pelvis, is particularly well suited for US evaluation. The combination of Doppler and gray-scale sonography (duplex Doppler) makes it possible to evaluate renal allografts for such complications as renal arterial stenosis, and arterial or venous thrombi. Surgical complications

such as hydronephrosis and lymphocele formation are also easily assessed by US. US is routinely used to guide biopsy of the allograft on patients with suspected acute or chronic rejection, as well as to guide percutaneous interventions in patients with suspected obstruction of the transplant ureter.

8. Fetal renal US: The detection of fetal hydronephrosis alerts physicians to the need for additional urologic evaluation in the early neonatal period. The availability of fetal therapy is an exciting development and still in early stages.

Ureter

US has limited usefulness in ureteral evaluation, as the ureter is obscured by overlying bowel in most of its lumbar, sacral, and pelvic course. Dilated ureters may be visualized in the proximal lumbar region in the vicinity of the ureteropelvic region, and in the juxta vesicular segments; small calculi may be visualized within the dilated fluid filled ureter in these segments. A congenital abnormality—ureterocele—may be demonstrated within the bladder. Color-flow demonstration of asymmetric jets of urine from the ureteral orifices in the bladder may be an indication of ureteral obstruction.

Urinary Bladder

1. Bladder morphology: Ultrasound can identify anatomic abnormalities in the bladder, for example, a thick walled and trabeculated bladder indicates changes due to bladder outlet obstruction (often due to an enlarged prostate in older men). Dynamic pre- and postvoid imaging provides useful clinical information regarding postvoid residual and thus, the adequacy of bladder emptying.
2. Bladder filling defects: Most commonly, filling defects in the bladder represent clots due to hemorrhage from different causes such as anticoagulation or traumatic catheterization. Asymmetric wall thickening or polypoid solid lesions can indicate underlying neoplasm. Changes in positioning can differentiate mobile pathology such as a clot from nonmobile pathology such as a tumor.

Prostate and Seminal Vesicles

1. Benign prostatic hypertrophy: Transrectal ultrasound (TRUS) can be used to evaluate prostate size and is generally more accurate than transabdominal ultrasound.

2. Prostate carcinoma: TRUS, with or without fusion of MRI, is widely used to localize a suspicious prostate lesion for transrectal biopsy in the evaluation for prostate cancer.
3. TRUS and pelvic US are also useful in the evaluation of a pelvic mass and to guide aspiration of cystic lesions such as seminal vesicle cysts.

Scrotum and External Genitalia

1. Acute pain: US is the primary imaging modality used to evaluate men presenting with acute scrotal pain. Acute pathology such as testicular torsion, epididymitis, and traumatic injury to the testicle or scrotum are all readily identified by US. Color-flow Doppler is very helpful in the scrotum and external genitalia. Perfusion patterns may help to differentiate inflammation from neoplasms and to substantiate a diagnosis of torsion or infarction.
2. Palpable lump: US can usually differentiate intratesticular from extratesticular masses, which is an important clinical issue as most intratesticular masses represent primary testicular neoplasms. US can also distinguish cystic from solid lesions. Some benign pathologies such as an epidermoid cyst have a characteristic appearance on US, which may allow a definitive diagnosis. Vascular abnormalities such as scrotal varicoceles can also be evaluated by US.
3. Undescended testicles can often be identified in the inguinal canal. To localize cryptorchid intraabdominal testes, MRI or CT scan is usually required.
4. In male sexual dysfunction, inadequacies of flow in the cavernosal arteries are readily identified, and this technique has become a standard part of the evaluation of erectile dysfunction. Fibrous or calcified plaques in the tunica albuginea in Peyronie disease can be easily identified. In women, translabial or endoluminal (endourethral) US has been used to identify urethral diverticula but is not favored by most urologists and radiologists over voiding cystourethrography and MRI.
5. Intraoperative ultrasound: This technique is often used to assist in partial nephrectomy in patients with one or more small renal tumors. It is particularly helpful in localizing small tumors that are intrarenal with little or no exophytic component.

Pitfalls of Ultrasound

Many pitfalls can occur while using ultrasound. Normal or benign findings can be mischaracterized; for example, renal sinus cysts can be mistaken for hydronephrosis and prominent lobulation of the renal contour can be mistaken for a renal cortical mass. Technical pitfalls such as suboptimal angle correction or inaccurate spectral gate placement can lead to erroneous vascular interpretations.

Computed Tomography

BASIC PRINCIPLES

CT is the diagnostic imaging workhorse that is used in the evaluation of most GU pathology. From acute flank pain to cancer staging, CT provides valuable information with a broad field of view that cannot be matched by ultrasound, and with speed and relative ease of acquisition that cannot be matched by MRI.

TECHNIQUE

A collimated x-ray beam is used to generate images as the patient moves through the CT scanner. Oral and intravenous contrast are often used to enhance visualization of enteric and vascular structures, respectively. Images are commonly acquired prior to and at different intervals following intravenous contrast administration to better characterize arterial or venous pathology, lesional enhancement, or to assess the collecting system.

INDICATIONS

Renal

CT is very useful in the assessment of many renal pathologies including renal mass evaluation, evaluation of suspected urinary obstruction, renal or ureteral calculi, and in suspected pyelonephritis.

Renal Mass Evaluation

1. Diagnosis of a renal mass: CT is very accurate in both detecting and characterizing renal masses (Fig. 2.3), distinguishing renal masses from renal pseudotumors (an appearance usually caused by compensatory renal hypertrophy after severe renal

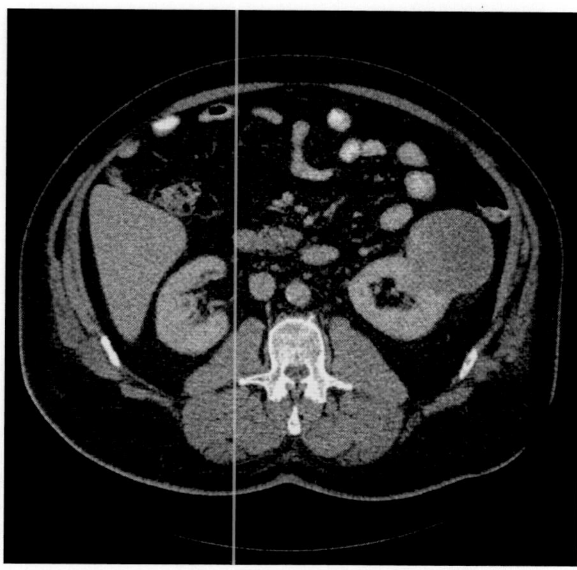

FIGURE 2.3 CT of renal cell carcinoma. A large mass is seen arising from the anterolateral aspect of the left kidney. Note that the density within the mass is similar to the enhanced renal parenchyma, suggesting enhancement and therefore a malignant neoplasm. *CT,* Computed tomography.

scarring) and in differentiating simple and complicated cystic masses from solid lesions of the kidney. CT can differentiate a non-enhancing mass (indicating a benign etiology) from enhancing renal lesions; the diagnosis of renal neoplasm is suggested when a lesion enhances after contrast administration and thus increases in density. Some benign renal masses such as a fat-containing angiomyolipoma, demonstrate fat within the lesion, allowing a specific diagnosis. Other lesions such as lipid-poor angiomyolipomas and oncocytomas may be difficult to differentiate from renal cell carcinoma by their CT appearance alone; with the increasing application of CT for all manner of abdominal symptoms, there is increasing serendipitous diagnosis of small renal masses ranging in size from <1 to 3 cm (Fig. 2.4). As smaller renal masses are diagnosed and resected, it is becoming apparent that these small benign tumors,

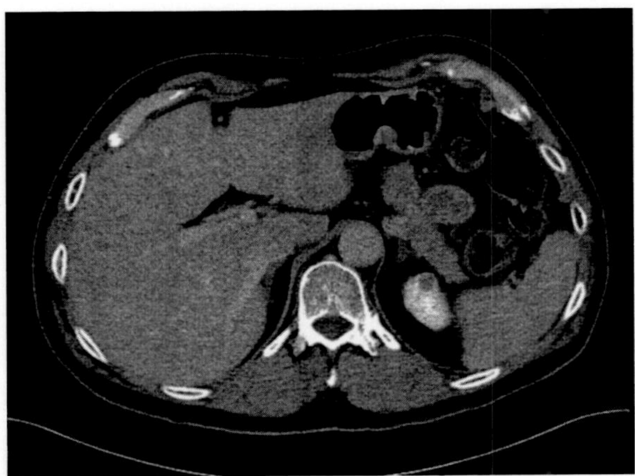

FIGURE 2.4 CT scan done for non-specific abdominal pain shows a small, left, upper-pole renal mass, which was an incidental finding. This small lesion proved to be a small renal cell cancer. Accurate characterization of small lesions can be challenging and short interval follow-up imaging may be recommended in such patients. *CT*, Computed tomography.

particularly small lipid-poor angiomyolipomas, may be indistinguishable from renal cell cancers (RCCs) on imaging. These benign lesions demonstrate enhancement, and may require percutaneous biopsy or serial follow-up to demonstrate stability in appearance, before a certain diagnosis can be made.

2. Staging of renal neoplasms: CT is the most common imaging modality utilized to stage renal or urothelial malignancy. CT is superb at demonstrating perinephric extension; evidence of renal vein or inferior vena cava (IVC) tumor thrombus; regional and abdominal lymphadenopathy; and the presence of lung, liver, or adrenal metastases. CT is also used in the surveillance of patients undergoing locoregional, surgical, or systemic therapies.
3. Postoperative evaluation: CT can detect local or distant intraabdominal recurrence of neoplasm after partial or total nephrectomy for malignant disease, or after thermal ablative therapy such as radiofrequency ablation (RFA) or cryotherapy.
4. Characterizing renal cysts: A cyst with homogeneous low attenuation (< 20 HU) and thin, imperceptible walls represents

a simple renal cyst (see Fig. 2.5), whereas nodular enhancement of walls, thick irregular septations, and central enhancement are indicative of a malignancy. Benign cysts complicated by hemorrhage may be difficult to distinguish from malignant cystic neoplasms on CT and US. MRI is often helpful in evaluation of such indeterminate lesions because subtle enhancement of the lesion may be detectable on MRI but not on CT.

Hematuria

CT urography (CTU) allows for complete evaluation of the GU tract to identify benign or malignant etiologies of hematuria. Scans are obtained prior to and following the administration of intravenous contrast, and during the excretory phase. CTU is helpful in the diagnosis of urolithiasis, renal masses, and the collecting system for urothelial malignancy.

Urolithiasis

CT is the study of choice in the evaluation of a patient presenting with suspected acute renal colic, with extremely high sensitivity and specificity for detecting renal and ureteral stones (Fig. 2.6). No oral or intravenous contrast is required and the diagnosis is available in a few minutes from the start of the scan. Low-dose scans are also now widely used, sacrificing a small degree of image quality in exchange for obtaining diagnostic information at lower radiation levels. Definitive diagnosis requires identification of a stone in the ureter with proximal hydronephrosis. Perinephric fluid or stranding may also be seen.

Nearly all stones are dense on CT, with the notable exception being a drug calculus, as in patients on protease-inhibitor therapy for HIV infection.

As CT becomes more widely used to evaluate a patient presenting with abdominal or flank pain, unsuspected renal and nonrenal diagnoses that may masquerade clinically as renal colic are often diagnosed. These include aortic aneurysms, spinal problems, renal vein thrombosis, diverticulitis, appendicitis, and acute pyelonephritis. The diagnosis of pyelonephritis and renal vein thrombosis may be difficult on noncontrast scans and may require the administration of intravenous contrast.

The increasing use of CT in the emergency room setting is raising concerns about the radiation exposure to patients with

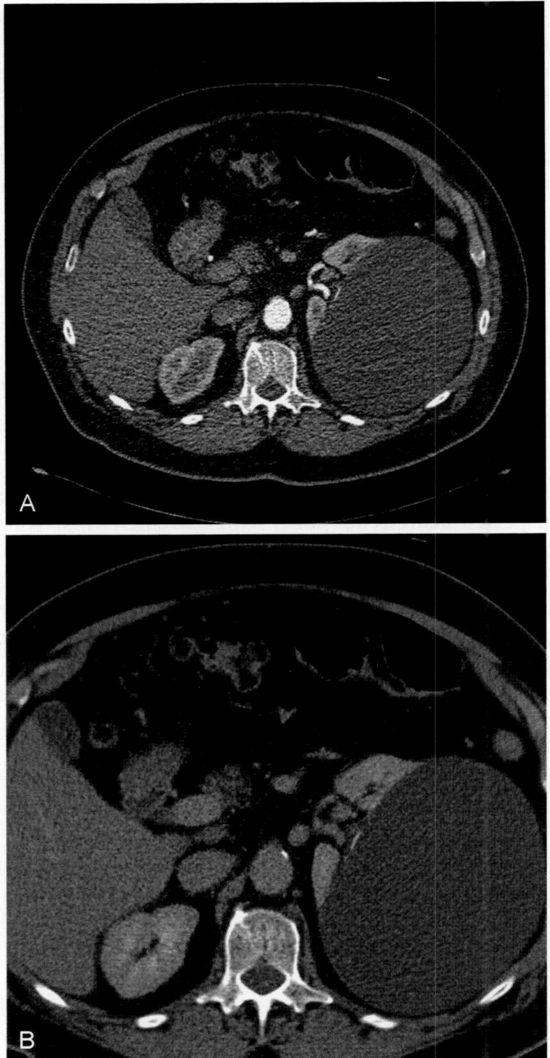

FIGURE 2.5 Left renal cyst. (A) Arterial phase. (B) Homogeneous nephrographic phase. The large left renal cyst does not enhance, indicating it is benign. There is a small linear calcification on the medial aspect of the cyst.

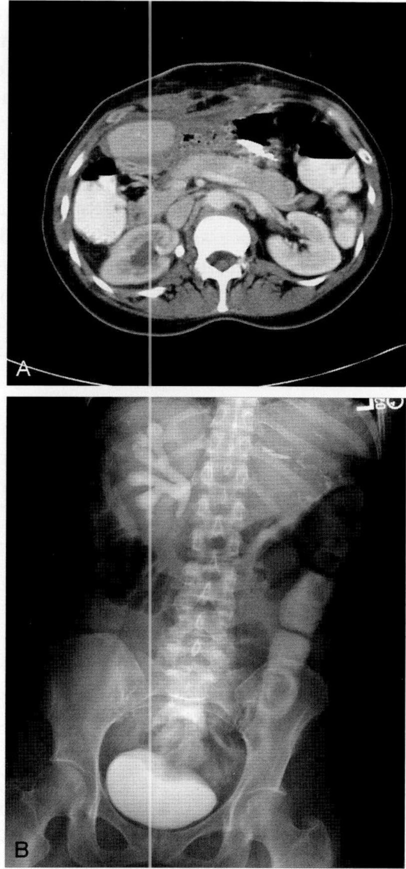

FIGURE 2.6 Patient with acute abdominal pain due to a right proximal ureteral calculus. The patient was given contrast because the emergency room physician did not think the patient's symptoms suggested renal colic. (A) CT scan demonstrates a large calculus in the proximal right ureter. The right nephrogram is delayed indicating that the obstruction is urodynamically significant. (B) Abdominal film obtained immediately after the CT scan shows contrast within the dilated right collecting system indicating impaired drainage due to the stone. Although well seen on CT, the stone was nonopaque on plain abdominal radiographs (not shown). It is important to keep in mind that even radiopaque stones will not be visible in a collecting system that is filled with contrast. *CT*, Computed tomography.

urolithiasis who have a chronic and recurrent disease and may present repeatedly with symptoms of colic which then leads to imaging. Vigilance on the part of the physicians and personnel taking care of such patients is recommended, so that patients receive no more radiation than absolutely necessary. As mentioned earlier, low-dose techniques should be used whenever feasible, to minimize radiation dose.

In pregnant patients with suspected stone disease in whom imaging confirmation is necessary, an ultrasound is typically the first-line imaging modality used to identify hydronephrosis. However, a low-dose noncontrast CT may be needed to establish the diagnosis. MRI is also used in the evaluation of a pregnant patient with acute abdominal or flank pain, but is still less widely available compared to CT.

Trauma

CT is the imaging modality of choice in the assessment of renal trauma. Parenchymal, vascular, and collecting system injuries are readily identified. Excretory phase imaging may be necessary for the assessment of urine leak.

Urinary Bladder

Bladder Carcinoma

CT is useful in staging tumors confined to the urinary bladder when the perivesical fat planes are preserved. However, perivesical stranding could be attributable to previous bladder biopsy or tumor extension, thereby limiting the staging value of CT. Enlarged lymph nodes are easily detected on CT. MRI surpasses CT as the dominant imaging study in staging bladder cancer. Both techniques are limited, however, by their inability to detect small or microscopic metastases in normal-sized lymph nodes and minimal or microscopic tumor invasion of peripelvic fat and contiguous surfaces.

Trauma

CT and CT cystogram are valuable diagnostic tools in evaluation of the bladder in a patient who has sustained blunt or penetrating trauma to the abdomen and pelvis. Extraperitoneal versus intraperitoneal injury to the bladder is readily distinguished in most cases, permitting the appropriate management.

CT cystography is also useful to assess for leak from the bladder or a urinary pouch following surgery on the bladder or after cystectomy and urinary pouch creation.

Prostate and Seminal Vesicles

CT can identify congenital prostatic anomalies and prostatic abscess. However, MRI has largely replaced CT in the evaluation of the prostate gland, particularly for prostate carcinoma.

Adrenal Gland

Adrenal masses are a common finding on abdominal CT scans, and the vast majority represent benign adenomas, even in patients with a known underlying primary malignancy. An adrenal mass that measures less than 10 HU in density on unenhanced scans is most likely to represent an adrenal adenoma, and no further workup is necessary. Masses that are greater than 10 HU on noncontrast CT are indeterminate in nature and can represent either lipid-poor adenomas or malignant lesions. The addition of delayed imaging at 15 minutes after contrast administration is helpful to evaluate washout. If there is greater than 66% calculated washout of contrast from a lesion, it most likely represents an adenoma.

Adrenal myelolipoma is a benign lesion that may contain macroscopic fat (areas with density measurements less than 10 HU) (Fig. 2.7).

Adrenal carcinomas are usually large lesions at diagnosis.

PITFALLS OF COMPUTED TOMOGRAPHY EVALUATION

Low-grade enhancement of renal lesions may be equivocal by CT and require either MRI or tissue sampling for diagnosis. Complex cystic lesions may be difficult to characterize adequately as benign or malignant.

Lack of bladder distention frequently limits assessment of the urinary bladder for leaks.

MAGNETIC RESONANCE IMAGING

Basic Principles

MRI is a valuable adjunct and problem solver in imaging urinary tract pathology. The high-contrast resolution of MRI permits tissue characterization. Some advantages of MRI over CT are the

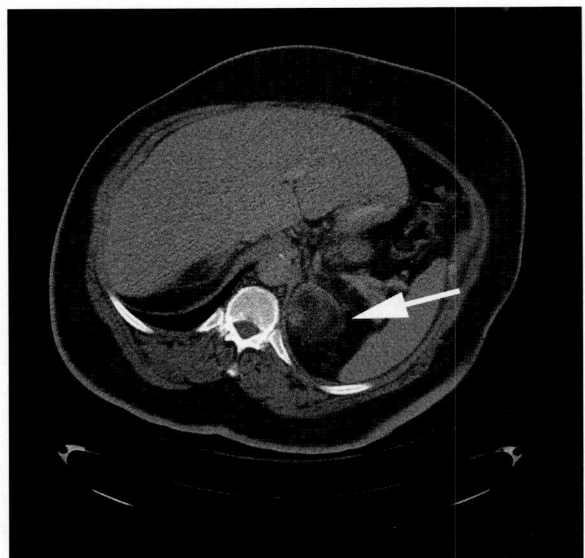

FIGURE 2.7 CT of left adrenal myelolipoma. Left adrenal lesion *(arrow)* has low attenuation within it which represents fat, indicating that it is a myelolipoma. *CT*, Computed tomography.

lack of ionizing radiation in MR examinations and the ability to perform contrast-enhanced imaging in patients with chronic kidney disease or history of adverse reaction to contrast agents used for CT; MRI contrast can be used in such patients.

The technical details of MRI are beyond the scope of this review.

MRI exams can be challenging for a patient, requiring longer scan times and breath holds than CT.

Complications

Nephrogenic systemic fibrosis (NSF) has been documented with gadolinium-based contrast agents. However, there are no confirmed cases of NSF with newer agents, at standard weight-based doses.

Gadolinium-based contrast agents are classified as Category C by the Food and Drug Administration (FDA) for use in pregnant patients.

The high magnetic field strength precludes examination of patients with certain types of metal and certain medical devices. Patients must be carefully screened to ensure that any hardware or implanted medical devices are MRI compatible.

Indications for Magnetic Resonance Imaging

Renal

1. Renal mass: Renal lesions are well evaluated by MRI. Nodular septations, small enhancing components, and low-grade enhancement are all well visualized by MRI.
2. Renal colic: US and CT are the mainstays in evaluating for urolithiasis; however, MRI can play a role in evaluating select patient populations, such as pediatric or pregnant patients, for whom radiation is a concern.
3. Hematuria: Magnetic resonance urography (MRU) can be performed in the assessment of hematuria. Typically, multiple sequences are obtained in the coronal plane as contrast is excreted into the urinary tract. Urothelial evaluation for small masses is usually limited on MR; CTU remains the modality of choice for urothelial evaluation.

Bladder

MRI is not often used in bladder cancer staging as cystoscopy and CT typically provide all of the necessary information. However, MRI has superior tissue contrast and can be used as a problem-solving imaging modality in patients with indeterminate bladder lesions, concerns for bladder fistulae, or in the evaluation of local bladder invasion by non-GU tumors such as rectal or cervical cancer.

Prostate

MRI has evolved to become integral in the diagnosis and management of patients with prostate cancer. MRI can provide valuable staging information including seminal vesicle involvement or extracapsular extension, involvement of the neurovascular bundle, and locoregional osseous or nodal metastases. MRI may also be obtained to evaluate for potential sites of biopsy in patients with elevated prostate-specific antigen (PSA), to screen patients who are under active surveillance, and to evaluate the prostate bed in patients with biochemically recurrent prostate carcinoma. The use of an endorectal coil to improve image resolution is institution or practice dependent.

Adrenal Glands

When lipid-poor adrenal lesions cannot be adequately characterized on an adrenal protocol CT examination, MR may be helpful in characterizing the lesion.

Pitfalls

There are a number of artifacts which may limit the diagnostic yield. In the abdomen, respiratory motion and bowel peristalsis, as well as signal degradation from surgical hardware, can frequently impact image quality.

Intravenous Urography

The intravenous urogram (IVU), also referred to as *excretory urogram (EU)* or *intravenous pyelogram (IVP)*, was the basic diagnostic radiologic study to evaluate the upper urinary tract for many decades. Its role in the assessment of many urologic conditions is now very limited due to the advantages offered by cross-sectional imaging modalities. IVU requires intravenous injection of radiographic contrast medium, followed by a sequence of films. Radiation exposure for an IVU (6 images) is approximately 2.5 mSv.

INDICATIONS

1. Hematuria (macroscopic and microscopic): IVU provides evaluation of both the renal parenchyma and the collecting system in patents with gross or microscopic hematuria. However, CT is indisputably more sensitive for detecting renal masses compared to an IVU. Although large masses are identifiable on an IVU, it is well recognized that renal masses smaller than 2 cm are often missed. CTU is sensitive in detecting urothelial abnormalities and is the study most commonly used for a complete assessment of the urinary tract in patients with a history of hematuria. CT is also more sensitive than IVU in detecting urolithiasis; both small stones and those that are faintly opaque are often not detectable on an IVU.

2. Upper urinary tract surveillance in patients with a history of a urothelial malignancy, such as bladder cancer, or positive urine cytology: As mentioned earlier, CTU has nearly completely superseded conventional IVU for this indication (Fig. 2.8).
3. Preoperative evaluation for select endourological procedures such as endopyelotomy: However, CT is increasingly being used even for this indication as 3D reconstructions can be performed with high spatial resolution, allowing display of the vascular structures and their relationship to the collecting system. Additionally, the collecting system can also be displayed in a manner similar to that seen on an IVU.
4. Postoperative evaluation following urologic procedures: An IVU may be performed 6 to 8 weeks after a urologic procedure to assess the urinary tract for complications, such as clinically unsuspected obstruction, and to have a baseline postoperative examination. This is likely the most common indication for an IVU in the current era.

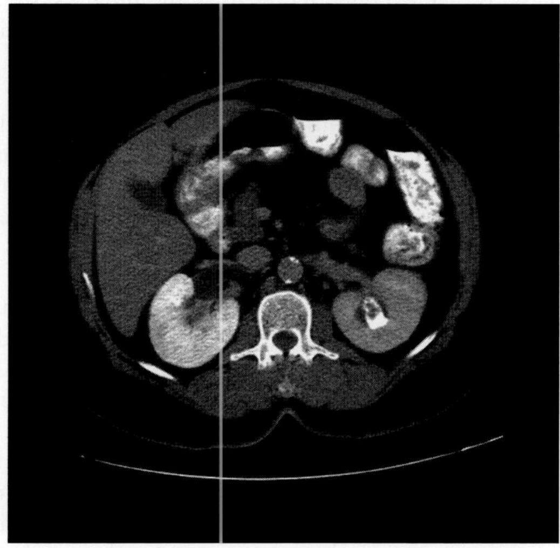

FIGURE 2.8 Urothelial cancer on CTU. Note the filling defect in the opacific left renal pelvis which proved to be a urothelial cancer in this patient with a prior history of bladder cancer. *CTU*, Computed tomography urography.

5. Stone disease: Patients who present with acute renal colic are best evaluated with noncontrast CT (no oral or intravenous contrast is necessary), which is acknowledged to be the most sensitive and specific study to exclude an obstructing ureteral calculus as the cause of the abdominal pain.

RADIOGRAPHIC IODINATED CONTRAST AGENTS

Radiographic contrast media (CM) consist of three atoms of iodine attached to a benzene ring. Low-osmolarity or iso-osmolar nonionic contrast medium are used for intravascular administration. Contrast agents used in the past were of high osmolarity (HOCM) and are referred to as *ionic contrast agents,* but these are no longer used in most clinical practices. Multiple studies have shown that the frequency of reactions is lower with the low osmolar contrast media (LOCM) as compared to the HOCM when given intravenously in both the general population and in patients at higher risk for contrast reaction.

The majority of injected contrast is excreted almost entirely by glomerular filtration. A small amount may be bound to serum albumin and is then excreted by the liver and biliary system and is known as *vicarious excretion*. Patients with renal insufficiency or obstruction frequently have vicarious excretion (Fig. 2.9).

In patients with a history of adverse reaction to the administration of contrast medium in whom a contrast-enhanced examination is deemed essential, premedication with corticosteroids and antihistamines is mandatory. One example of a premedication regimen in clinical use for an elective examination is prednisone 50 mg orally, given 12, 6, and 1 hour before the examination, and diphenhydramine 50 mg 1 hour before the examination, orally or by intramuscular injection. Institutional and practice variations in the exact premedication regimen exist. For emergent contrast administration, 200 mg hydrocortisone is given intravenously five hours and one hour prior to exam.

Patients at increased risk for adverse reactions include those with a history of prior contrast reactions (four times increased risk), or a history of allergies or asthma (two to three times increased risk), as compared to patients who do not have such histories. Premedicating such patients prior to contrast administration is prudent.

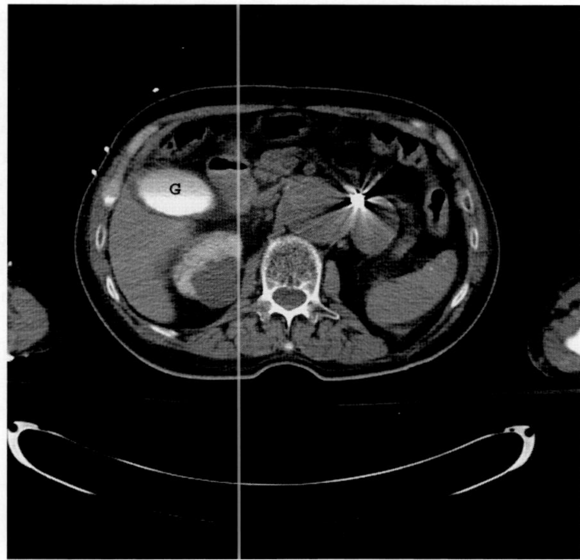

FIGURE 2.9 Noncontrast CT examination shows vicarious excretion into the gall bladder. Patient with a solitary right kidney had received multiple contrast loads in a short time period for cardiac catheterization, and developed contrast-induced nephrotoxicity. The left kidney was removed for benign disease many years ago. Noncontrast CT scan demonstrates that the right kidney has a dense, persistent nephrogram from contrast given 48 hours previously for cardiac catheterization. There is opacification of the gallbladder *(G)*, indicating vicarious excretion of contrast into the gallbladder. The abdominal aorta is aneurysmal. *CT*, Computed tomography.

Symptoms of nausea, vomiting, or sensation of heat after contrast administration are considered to be side effects of the contrast and not allergic reactions. Shellfish allergy has no particular significance for contrast administration and is managed the same way as other noncontrast allergies (e.g., allergy to bee sting, penicillin, or peanuts).

Multiple myeloma was long considered a risk factor for contrast induced nephropathy (CIN) with the cause believed to be precipitation of protein-contrast aggregates in the renal tubules. However, it is now acknowledged that myeloma does not increase the risk of CIN if the patient is well hydrated.

In patients with cardiac disease, CM administration can cause worsening of congestive heart failure due to the osmotic load.

Patients who are on metformin, an oral hypoglycemic agent (trade names Glucophage, Glucovance, Avandamet, and Metaglip), and who also have acute kidney injury or severe chronic kidney disease, should discontinue the drug when they receive contrast and not resume taking their medication until 48 hours after contrast administration. Although metformin itself does not have an adverse effect on renal function, patients who develop worsening renal function due to contrast administration can have impaired drug clearance and can rarely develop lactic acidosis that can be fatal.

Delayed reactions, defined as those occurring more than 1 hour after contrast administration, can be seen with all contrast agents; they occur in 0.5% to 23% of patients and tend to be skin reactions.

Retrograde Pyeloureterography

INDICATIONS

1. To further evaluate lesions of the renal collecting system and ureter that cannot be adequately defined by CTU.
2. To visualize the collecting systems and ureters when intravenous contrast administration is contraindicated (renal insufficiency or severe prior contrast reaction).
3. To demonstrate the collecting systems and ureters in their entirety when CTU fails to do so in a patient with a prior history of urothelial cancer or persistent hematuria (Fig. 2.10).
4. To visualize the ureteral stump remaining after nephrectomy in a patient with hematuria, positive urinary cytology or history of urothelial cancer.

CONTRAINDICATIONS

1. Untreated UTI.
2. Patients who cannot or should not be cystoscoped (e.g., patients recovering from recent bladder or urethral surgery).

TECHNIQUES

1. Preliminary cystoscopy is required.

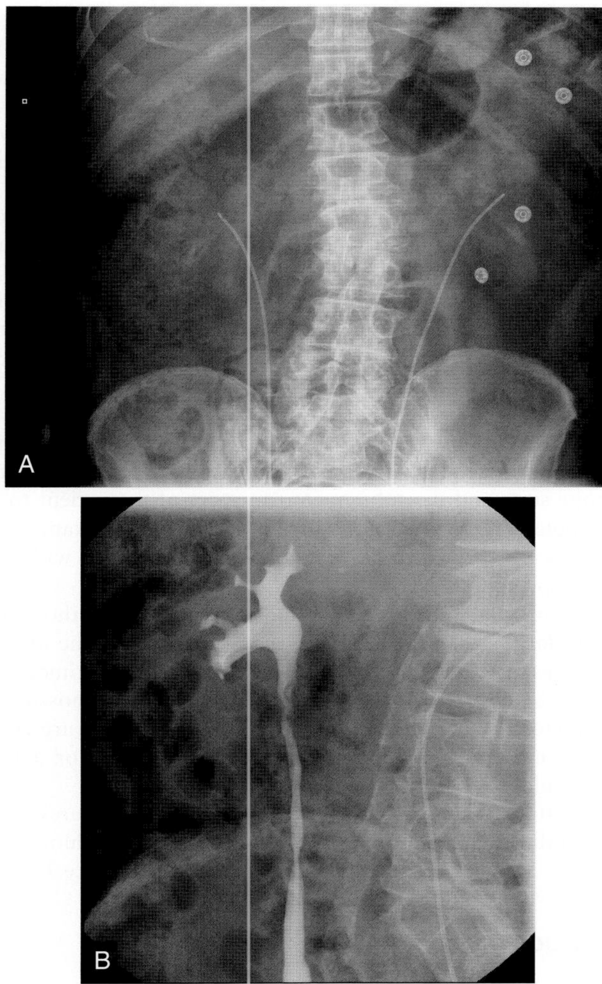

FIGURE 2.10 Retrograde pyelogram in a patient with previous history of bladder cancer. CTU failed to demonstrate the collecting systems adequately, necessitating a retrograde pyelogram. (A) Preliminary image demonstrates bilateral retrograde catheters ascending from the bladder. (B) Contrast injection demonstrates small filling defects in the proximal ureter which proved to be urothelial cancer. *CTU*, Computed tomography urography.

2. A ureteral orifice is identified and catheterized with a catheter, usually 5 French in size. The catheter is advanced to the renal pelvis, and contrast is instilled. The same contrast agent employed for CT is used for retrograde pyelography. To opacify the ureter alone, the ureteral orifice is occluded with a bulb occlusion catheter and contrast injected while a film is obtained.
3. Images: A preliminary image is essential to document the position of the retrograde catheters. After contrast injection, fluoroscopic images are obtained to delineate the unopacified or poorly seen portions of the collecting system or ureter in question (Fig. 2.10). If obstruction is suspected, an image is also obtained several minutes after removal of the ureteral catheter to evaluate the drainage of the collecting system.
4. The use of fluoroscopy is an important adjunct to retrograde pyeloureterography (RPG). In most hospital settings, however, this requires the placement of a ureteral catheter in the cystoscopy suite and the subsequent transport of the patient to the radiology department for catheter injection. The examination can be performed in an operating room equipped with fluoroscopy equipment.
5. RPG may be impossible in some patients, such as those with very large prostates, in whom the gland overlies the ureteral orifices, preventing proper catheter placement. At times, even though the orifice is identifiable, it may not be possible to catheterize it, such as may occur with tortuous ureters or after ureteral reimplantation in a native system or a renal transplant.
6. Radiation exposure with all fluoroscopic procedures varies with the equipment, size, body habitus of patient, fluoroscopy times, and factors such as collimation and distance between x-ray source and the patient.

COMPLICATIONS

1. Perforation of the ureter is uncommon. When it does occur, there is usually no serious sequela. Contrast extravasation outside the collecting system does not usually result in any harm. In some cases of perforation associated with a large amount of urine leakage, diversion of urine with a ureteral stent may be required for a few weeks.

2. A too-vigorous injection of contrast material in an infected urinary tract may disseminate bacteria into the bloodstream and kidney, causing bacteremia and rarely pyelonephritis. This risk increases in the presence of a urinary tract obstruction. Fortunately, the normal antegrade flow of urine is usually enough to wash out any bacteria that may have been introduced during the procedure. Patients usually receive prophylactic periprocedural antibiotics as well.
3. Absorption of contrast agent can occur if there is perforation of the collecting system or pyelosinus extravasation due to overdistention. In patients truly allergic to CM, the retrograde approach does not obviate a systemic contrast reaction, although reactions are much less common than after IV injection. Patients with a history of contrast allergy should receive premedication with corticosteroids and antihistamines.

Antegrade Pyelography

INDICATIONS

1. In patients with a history of urothelial malignancy and high-grade obstruction of a collecting system, an antegrade pyelogram may be the only way to evaluate the urothelium of the collecting system and ureter. Contrast excretion is impaired in an obstructed system, and thus intravenous contrast administration for CTU will not depict the collecting system well enough to exclude upper urinary tract urothelial lesions. It is important to note that larger urothelial lesions may be visualized as enhancing regions of mucosal irregularity on a routine contrast-enhanced CT, even if there is no contrast excretion.
2. In patients with renal transplants who have azotemia in association with a dilated collecting system, antegrade pyelogram can help determine whether the transplant collecting system is obstructed or not. The ureteroneocystostomy created to drain a renal transplant is often difficult to cannulate cystoscopically.

CONTRAINDICATIONS

Coagulation abnormalities and bleeding diathesis.

TECHNIQUE

The renal pelvis is percutaneously punctured with a 20- or 21-gauge thin-walled needle from a posterior or posterolateral approach. Localization of the dilated collecting system is usually provided by ultrasound. A sample of urine is sent for culture and sensitivity determination, after which contrast is injected, and images obtained under fluoroscopic control. For a renal transplant, the anterior approach is used.

COMPLICATIONS

These are similar to a PCN.

1. Inadvertent puncture of neighboring structures may occur. Although puncture of the renal vein, kidney, parenchyma, or liver and spleen is possible, few if any complications result because of the small size of the needle.
2. Some extravasation of contrast or urine outside the collecting system usually occurs with many antegrade pyelograms. However, the puncture site is very small and seals rapidly after the needle is removed.
3. Entry into a nondilated collecting system may be difficult and time consuming and, on rare occasions, may fail completely.

Cystography

INDICATIONS

1. Suspected bladder trauma.
2. Bladder opacification by contrast excreted during CT is unreliable in assessment for bladder ruptures. To reliably exclude a bladder rupture, the bladder should be opacified through a catheter placed in the bladder, and sufficient contrast injected until a detrusor contraction is elicited. The study should not be terminated at a predetermined volume of contrast, as a detrusor contraction may occur at variable intravesical volumes in different individuals. It is important that the bladder should be filled until a detrusor contraction occurs.
3. Evaluation of fistulae involving the urinary bladder (Fig. 2.11).
4. Evaluation of healing following bladder or distal ureteral surgery.

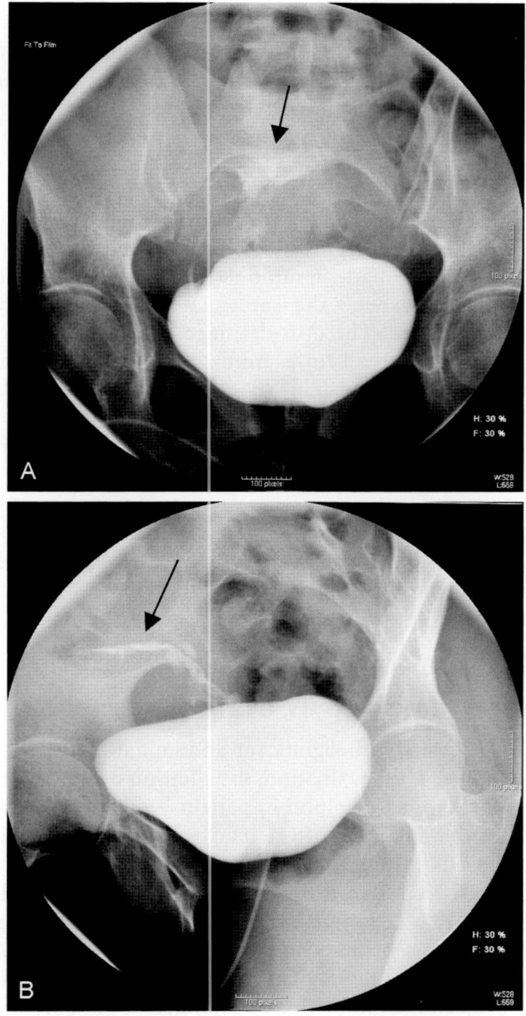

FIGURE 2.11 (A and B) Frontal and oblique views of cystogram in a woman with vaginal leakage a few weeks after cesarean section delivery. Opacification of the uterus *(arrow)* from the urinary bladder is seen.

CONTRAINDICATIONS

There are no contraindications to cystography itself. When a patient has sustained significant pelvic trauma, the integrity of the urethra must first be established before passing a urethral catheter. This may often require that retrograde urethrography precede cystography.

TECHNIQUE

1. After a preliminary image, a urethral catheter is passed into the bladder, and CM is instilled into the bladder. Images of the filled bladder are made in multiple projections. The bladder is then emptied through the catheter, after which a drainage image is obtained. The post-drainage image is extremely important because small leaks from the posterior wall may be obscured by a contrast-filled bladder and be visible only after the bladder has been drained of contrast.
2. Cystography may also be performed through an existing cystostomy tube or via suprapubic puncture.

COMPLICATIONS

Complications of cystography are rare. Excessively forceful injection may result in disruption of a fresh suture line.

Modifications of Cystography

COMPUTED TOMOGRAPHY CYSTOGRAM

Since most patients with significant abdominal or pelvic trauma undergo a CT scan for evaluation, the addition of a CT cystogram to assess the bladder is helpful in patients with significant pelvic injury. After the initial set of CT images have been obtained, diluted contrast is injected through an indwelling Foley catheter, and scanning is repeated through the pelvis. Most published reports indicate that CT cystograms and conventional cystograms have comparable sensitivity in detecting bladder injury. An advantage of CT is that the patient does not have to be turned into different projections (an obvious advantage in patients with pelvic fractures) for optimal evaluation, and a post-drainage image is unnecessary because the entire anterior and posterior wall of the bladder is well seen on a CT.

When evaluating a patient for a suspected fistula involving the bladder, a CT cystogram helps in demonstrating the fistula well. CT is the most sensitive imaging technique in patients with suspected colovesical fistulae due to complications of diverticulitis.

Voiding Cystourethrogram

Voiding cystourethrogram (VCUG) demonstrates the anatomy of the lower urinary tract during micturition and allows assessment for vesicoureteral reflux, which may occur only during voiding.

INDICATIONS

1. Recurrent urinary tract infections, especially in children, in whom reflux is not uncommon.
2. Evaluation of the posterior urethra in the male and the entire urethra in the female.
3. VCUG is used to evaluate urethral stricture disease, posterior urethral valves in the infant male, and the postoperative urethra (Fig. 2.12). In the female, it is a primary method of evaluating for suspected urethral diverticula.
4. Evaluation of certain voiding dysfunctions (e.g., detrusor-external sphincter dyssynergia, neurogenic bladder).
5. VCUG can be combined with simultaneous pressure-flow recordings for a study known as *videourodynamics*.
6. For the evaluation of an ectopic ureter thought to insert into the urethra; reflux into such ectopic ureters is fairly common.

CONTRAINDICATIONS

Acute urinary tract infection.

TECHNIQUES

1. This procedure is best performed under fluoroscopic control.
2. The bladder is catheterized and filled with water-soluble CM. HOCM is usually used for this study because a large amount of contrast is required (300–600 mL), and adverse reactions with contrast injection into the bladder are uncommon. When

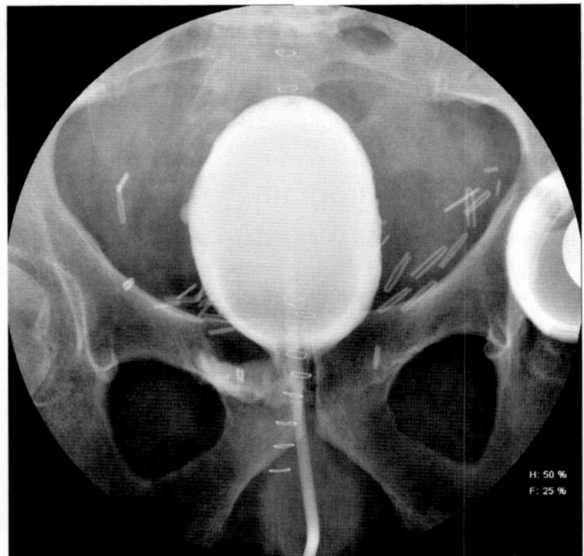

FIGURE 2.12 VCUG 10 days after radical retropubic prostatectomy demonstrates leak from the right posterior aspect of the anastomosis. Follow-up examination a week later (not shown) showed healing of the leak. *VCUG*, Voiding cystourethrogram.

the patient has a strong desire to void, the catheter is withdrawn and the patient voids. Fluoroscopic images are obtained during voiding, and an estimate of the completeness of bladder emptying is made. In patients who have undergone recent bladder-neck or urethral surgery, voiding around an indwelling urethral catheter is initially performed to look for contrast extravasation. If none is seen fluoroscopically, the urethral catheter may be removed and another void documented fluoroscopically.

3. Although the bladder is filled with the patient recumbent, voiding is usually performed with the patient standing.

COMPLICATIONS

These are the same as those listed under cystography.

Retrograde Urethrogram

PURPOSE

Retrograde urethrogram (RUG) provides detailed visualization of the anterior urethra in the male. The procedure has little or no application in the female. On a RUG, the posterior urethra is incompletely visualized, because the closed external urethral sphincter resists the retrograde flow of contrast into the posterior urethra. Complete evaluation of the anterior and posterior urethra in a male requires both a VCUG and a RUG (Fig. 2.13). Although the anterior urethra is seen on a VCUG, a diseased anterior urethra is optimally evaluated on a RUG.

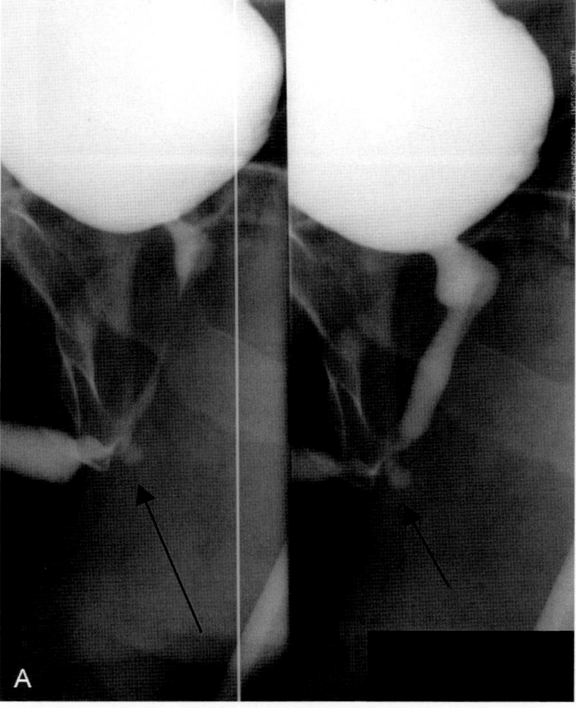

FIGURE 2.13 Straddle injury. (A) VCUG through a suprapubic catheter demonstrates irregularity of the bulbar urethra at injury site *(arrows)*.

Continued

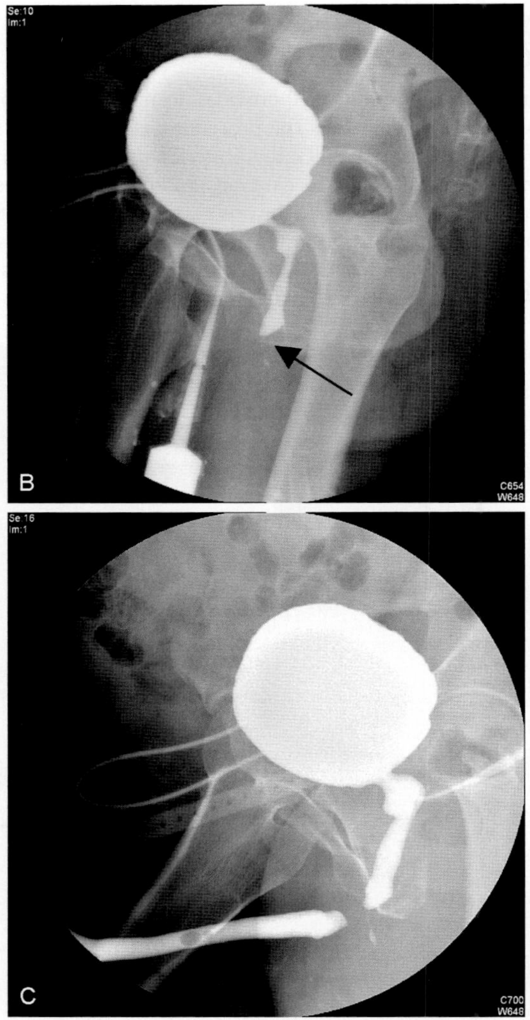

FIGURE 2.13, cont'd (B) VCUG demonstrates urethral occlusion at injury site *(arrow)* 5 weeks later. (C) Combined VCUG and RUG help in assessing the length of occlusion more optimally. *VCUG*, Voiding cystourethrogram.

INDICATIONS

1. Detailed delineation of suspected or known urethral stricture (most common indication).
2. The study is also useful postoperatively, to assess the results of surgery for urethral stricture repair.
3. Suspected urethral trauma.
4. RUG should be routinely performed before attempting passage of a urethral catheter in a male patient with a pelvic fracture.
5. Demonstration of urethral diverticula, fistulae, and neoplasms.

CONTRAINDICATIONS

1. Acute urethritis, as discussed later.
2. Patients who are allergic to contrast should be pretreated. LOCM should be employed in this situation.

TECHNIQUE

1. A Foley catheter is placed with sterile technique, and the Foley balloon is inflated in the fossa navicularis. Approximately 1 to 2 mL of contrast is sufficient to seat the balloon in a stable fashion in the urethra. It is preferable to use contrast to fill the balloon because air is more compressible than fluid, and an air-filled balloon can inadvertently extrude during the study.
2. LOCM is then injected, and fluoroscopic images of the fully distended urethra are taken.

COMPLICATIONS

Reflux or intravasation of contrast from the urethra into the surrounding corpus spongiosum can occur during RUG. Such reflux is usually minimal and without clinical consequence except in the presence of urethritis when bacteria may be forced into the bloodstream. In patients with venereal warts, the procedure should not be performed until the active infection has been controlled, in order to avoid spreading the infection to the urethra. Intravasation into the corpus spongiosum is more apt to occur in patients with high-grade urethral strictures.

Loopogram and Pouchogram

Following cystectomy for urothelial tumor, anastomosis of the ureters to an isolated intact segment of ileum or transverse colon (loop) or to a detubularized large or small bowel segment (pouch) is the most common method of establishing permanent urinary diversion (Fig. 2.14). The isolated bowel loop serves as a conduit to propel urine outward toward the stoma, and a urine collection bag is applied to the stoma to collect the urine. A detubularized pouch functions as a continent reservoir rather than a conduit. Pouches can be connected to a cutaneous stoma or be anastomosed to the urethra (orthotopic diversion). Cutaneous continent pouches require intermittent catheterization for emptying, whereas patients with orthotopic pouches void by increasing abdominal pressure to empty the pouch. Radiologic examination of urinary diversions is referred to as *loopography* or *pouchography*.

INDICATIONS

1. To evaluate the bowel conduit or reservoir for suspected intrinsic disease (e.g., filling defect, anastomotic or other leaks, loop stenosis), capacity, or peristaltic activity.
2. To visualize the upper urinary tract by reflux.
3. Reflux is normal with ileal conduits but unpredictable in continent diversions. If a patient with a continent diversion requires urothelial evaluation beyond that provided by CTU, antegrade pyelogram is usually the next step.
4. To evaluate patients with loop diversion whose upper urinary tracts show deterioration on serial CT or ultrasonogram (i.e., worsening hydronephrosis, renal calculi, or renal scarring) or whose renal function is diminishing. In such patients, the absence of reflux from the ileal loop into the ureters may indicate ureteroileal anastomotic obstruction.

CONTRAINDICATIONS

There are no contraindications to the retrograde study of a urinary conduit or reservoir other than active urinary tract infection. Because the urinary tract of patients with urinary diversions is usually colonized with bacteria, prophylactic antibiotics are administered prior to the procedure to prevent bacteremia after the procedure.

TECHNIQUE

1. A preliminary image is obtained. Using aseptic technique, the stoma of an ileal conduit is catheterized with a 14 or 16 French Foley catheter. The balloon is inflated just below the

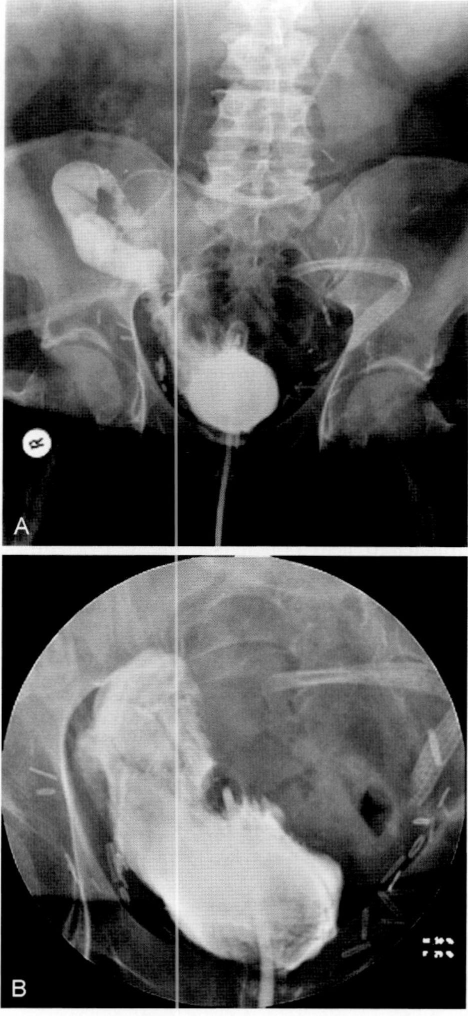

FIGURE 2.14 Normal examination of a Studer pouch 3 weeks after surgery. (A) An image taken early in the filling process. (B) An image after the pouch is filled. Note that early filling image better demonstrates the afferent limb than the image taken when the pouch is fully distended.

anterior abdominal wall, and the conduit is filled with LOCM until the ileum is well distended. Fluoroscopic images are obtained with particular attention given to the presence or absence of reflux. Images of the collecting systems and ureters are obtained to evaluate for urothelial abnormalities. The catheter is then removed and the conduit and upper urinary tracts evaluated for emptying.

2. A continent urinary pouch or reservoir is also evaluated fluoroscopically. The stoma (for a cutaneous diversion) or urethra (for an orthotopic diversion) is catheterized and a Foley catheter placed into the reservoir. The reservoir is opacified with CM to capacity, which varies with time. At maturity, it should accommodate several hundred milliliters of fluid. Filling defects and leaks are documented if present. Nonopaque mucus in the reservoir is an expected finding and will be seen as irregular filing defects.

Although many pouches do not normally allow for ureteral reflux, reflux may be observed with a Studer pouch in which the ureters are anastomosed to an isoperistaltic afferent loop of ileum, which drains into a detubularized ileal pouch (see Fig. 2.14). Although reflux does not occur in a normally functioning Studer pouch, the elevated intraluminal pressures generated during retrograde pouch opacification may fill the isoperistaltic afferent limb and diverted ureters.

COMPLICATIONS

Pyelonephritis may accompany forceful reflux of infected urine.

Angiography

Angiography refers to the radiologic study of both the arterial and venous systems. Studies pertinent to the study of the urinary tract include:

1. Arterial: aortography, renal arteriography, and adrenal arteriography
2. Venous: inferior venacavography, renal phlebography, adrenal phlebography, and gonadal phlebography

INDICATIONS FOR RENAL ARTERIOGRAPHY

1. To evaluate for suspected RAS, which is a cause of potentially reversible hypertension and renal insufficiency, particularly in

elderly patients. Many screening tests have been used in an effort to noninvasively diagnose RAS. CT angiography and MR angiography are the most frequently used imaging techniques; the latter is preferred in patients with renal insufficiency to reduce the risks of contrast-induced nephrotoxicity, which is more frequent with iodinated contrast materials than with gadolinium-based contrast agents used for MR. Patients with significant truncal stenosis of the renal artery and fibromuscular dysplasia are treated with angioplasty. Lesions at the renal artery ostia are resistant to angioplasty and require primary stenting. Randomized trials that compared renal artery angioplasty with best medical therapy do not indicate that angioplasty is a convincingly superior treatment.

2. Neoplasms: Since the development of CT and MRI, angiography has almost never been used in the diagnosis of renal masses. It is still used occasionally for the preoperative embolization of large, hypervascular renal cell carcinomas and for prophylactic embolization of angiomyolipomas that are larger than 4 cm in size, to prevent spontaneous hemorrhage.
3. Renal trauma: Most traumatic parenchymal and vascular lesions can be satisfactorily imaged by CT. Angiography is usually reserved to demonstrate an arterial bleeder or arteriovenous communication prior to embolization.
4. For the evaluation (and potential ablation) of vascular abnormalities such as aneurysms and arteriovenous malformations suspected on other imaging studies.
5. CT angiography or MR angiography are preferable over catheter angiography to provide a preoperative arterial "road map" for surgery when there is a high risk of anomalous vascular supply, such as in a horseshoe kidney or an ectopic kidney.
6. Preoperative evaluation of potential renal donors; CT angiography, and MR angiography have supplanted catheter angiography in most institutions.

INDICATIONS FOR ADRENAL GLAND ANGIOGRAPHY

1. Ablation of adrenal function by embolization
2. For adrenal vein sampling to diagnose functioning adrenal tumors

INDICATIONS FOR GONADAL PHLEBOGRAPHY

1. Gonadal phlebography is valuable in evaluating varicoceles and in treating them by means of venous occlusion with balloons, coils, or sclerosing agents.
2. High-resolution CT and MRI are preferred to gonadal phlebography to search for a nonpalpable undescended testis.

Radionuclide Imaging

INDICATIONS

1. Assessment of renal function: Following a bolus injection of radionuclide, computer analysis of radioactivity plotted against time allows analysis of blood clearance rates to determine the glomerular filtration rate and effective renal function. Ascertaining the relative function of the kidneys is especially important when decisions regarding nephrectomy versus salvage operation must be made in patients with renal malignancies. In cases of severe hydronephrosis, split renal functions before and after a period of nephrostomy drainage allow assessment of residual renal functional in the previously obstructed kidney.
2. Hypertension: Differential renal blood flow studies (performed before and after the administration of an angiotensin-converting enzyme inhibitor [ACEI] such as captopril) detect approximately 85% of cases of renal vascular disease. Difficulties with isotope screening in hypertension include problems in distinguishing unilateral renovascular lesions from unilateral renal parenchymal disease and problems recognizing bilateral vascular stenoses. The accuracy of the examination is decreased in patients with renal insufficiency, bilateral renal artery stenoses, and with chronic use of ACEIs.
3. Evaluation of renal transplant failure: Isotopic methods of imaging the kidney are very helpful in evaluating renal transplant complications, including obstruction, extravasation, and stenosis of the arterial anastomosis. Differentiation between acute tubular necrosis and transplant rejection is a more difficult task and may sometimes require biopsy of the renal transplant.
4. Questionable or intermittent obstruction: The presence of intermittent obstruction, especially at the ureteropelvic junction

(UPJ), is often difficult to evaluate and confirm. Using radionuclide methods, the rate of emptying of the collecting system after a diuretic challenge (also known as washout or Lasix renogram) can be evaluated and compared to standard emptying profiles. A normal kidney puts out over 76% of the activity that enters it within 20 minutes.

5. Evaluate for urine leak: Small urinary leaks in patients who cannot receive iodinated contrast can be detected readily with radionuclide studies. Renal transplant patients with impaired renal function and suspected urinary leak are the classic case where radionuclide studies are very helpful in evaluating for urinary leak.
6. Evaluate for vesicoureteral reflux: VCUG is used for initial evaluation of suspected reflux in children, so that the anatomy of the lower urinary tract can also be assessed, a task not possible with radionuclide imaging. However, radionuclide cystogram is the follow-up procedure of choice for proven reflux because it is more sensitive than VCUG and imposes less of a radiation burden on the patient. Using agents such as ^{99m}Tc-DMSA, renal scarring, which is often the consequence of reflux, can also be demonstrated.
7. Adrenal gland: ^{131}Iodine metaiodobenzylguanidine (MIBG), an adrenal medullary imaging agent, can readily and easily localize pheochromocytomas. Cholesterol analogues (Iodine-131 NP-59) have also been synthesized and have proven helpful in localizing hyperfunctioning and hypofunctioning adrenal lesions.
8. PET scanning: In urogenital imaging, the most widely used tracer is ^{18}F-fluorodeoxyglucose (FDG), which is taken into cells through glucose transporters. Many tumors have increased glucose uptake, and therefore concentrate FDG. FDG is normally excreted by the kidneys through urine, which limits its utility in evaluating the kidneys. Modern machines have a CT scanner incorporated into the PET machine, allowing accurate localization of sites of increased uptake. To date, FDG-PET has not shown much value in the initial staging of prostate, renal, urothelial, or bladder cancer when compared to conventional imaging modalities. However newer radionuclides have shown promise in the evaluation of patients with biochemically recurrent prostate carcinoma. For example,

^{18}F-sodium fluoride is a marker for osteoblastic activity and C11-Choline PET scans have shown increased sensitivity in the identification of nodal metastases when compared to CT or MRI. Prostate-specific membrane antigen (PSMA) PET scans have shown superiority to conventional imaging, with clinical trials currently underway to evaluate potential therapeutic radiopharmaceuticals in patients with metastatic prostate carcinoma.

9. Radionuclide bone scans are useful for detecting bone metastases, particularly in prostate cancer staging and follow-up.

CONTRAINDICATIONS

Radionuclides should not be administered during pregnancy. There are no other contraindications to the use of radionuclide studies for diagnostic purposes.

TECHNIQUE

Techniques vary depending on the information desired. In general, a tracer dose of radioactive isotope bound to a specific pharmaceutical agent is administered and the patient is placed beneath a gamma camera where images (scans, scintigrams) are generated at intervals depending on the information sought. For flow studies, images are taken as frequently as every few seconds. For anatomic information, images are obtained by accumulating counts for several minutes. These images may be taken sequentially for as long as several hours, and under certain circumstances may even be delayed up to 24 or 48 hours. Recently, techniques for obtaining tomographic scintigraphy (single-photon emission computed tomography [SPECT]) have considerably improved the anatomic information provided by radionuclide images. When evaluating renal function, small radiation detectors or gamma cameras placed directly over the kidneys can be used to generate time-radioactivity curves. This is known as a *renogram*.

COMPLICATIONS

There are no complications of nuclear medicine diagnostic procedures. The radiation doses involved are modest and often less than those for comparable conventional radiographic studies or CT.

INTERVENTIONAL URORADIOLOGY

This section will discuss commonly performed nonvascular interventional procedures in the urinary tract.

Percutaneous Nephrostomy

PCN refers to the percutaneous placement of a drainage catheter or access sheath into the kidney, using radiologic guidance.

INDICATIONS FOR PCN

PCN is performed to relieve urinary obstruction, to gain access to the collecting system for therapeutic and diagnostic procedures, to divert urine to allow closure of a ureteral fistula or a dehiscent urinary tract anastomosis, and to allow assessment of residual recoverable function in a chronically obstructed kidney. These indications are further elaborated as follows.

1. To relieve urinary obstruction. PCN is most often requested in patients in whom imaging studies demonstrate hydroureteronephrosis; these studies may indicate the etiology and the anatomic level of the obstruction. Calculus disease is responsible for obstruction in approximately one-third of patients with urinary obstruction who undergo PCN, and malignancy in the rest, with carcinoma of the bladder, cervix, and colon being the most common primary tumors to cause urinary obstruction. When ureteral obstruction results in renal impairment, noncontrast computed tomography (NCCT) appears to be the best imaging modality to identify calculus causes of obstruction, whereas MRU is superior for identifying noncalculus causes of obstruction. In patients with normal renal function, contrast-enhanced CT can identify the presence and cause of hydronephrosis in nearly all cases. MRU is particularly helpful in delineating the anatomy in patients with urinary diversion to bowel conduits.
2. It is important to attempt, or at least consider, the periurethral retrograde approach for renal drainage (ureteral intubation with cystoscopic guidance) in a patient with urinary obstruction before resorting to a PCN. Percutaneous drainage should ideally be reserved for patients in whom retrograde attempts are either unsuccessful or not feasible in ureteral stent placement.

3. In patients with obstruction, accompanied by signs or symptoms of urosepsis, PCN drainage provides rapid decompression of the obstructed collecting system and defervescence of urosepsis. However, when obstruction and infection are due to renal or ureteral calculi, retrograde ureteral drainage is as effective in draining the collecting system as is PCN. In these cases, the decision to perform PCN or retrograde ureteral catheter drainage should be made by assessing what the best therapy for the stone would be. For instance, patients who have large renal calculi that would be best managed by percutaneous methods should have a PCN performed; patients with smaller ureteral calculi that would be amenable to SWL should be drained by a ureteral catheter placed by a retrograde periurethral approach with cystoscopic guidance (Box 2.1).
4. PCN drainage can help to preserve or improve renal function until the cause of obstruction can be relieved in patients in whom the obstruction is expected to respond to treatment, such as chemotherapy, radiation therapy, or surgery. For patients with terminal malignancies and bilateral obstruction in whom ureteral stents cannot be placed, unilateral PCN drainage is usually preferred to bilateral drainage to avoid the inconvenience of two externally draining nephrostomy bags.

BOX 2.1 Indications for Percutaneous Therapy for Stone Disease[a]

1. Size
   a. Large stones (>2–2.5 cm)
   b. Most staghorn calculi
2. Composition: cystine calculi
3. Anatomical considerations
   a. Compromised urine drainage (includes ureteropelvic junction obstruction, ureteral strictures, stones in dependent calices, and stones in caliceal diverticula)
   b. Abnormal body habitus (scoliosis, myelomeningocele)
   c. Congenital abnormalities such as horseshoe kidneys, fusion anomalies
   d. Postoperative states—urinary diversion, renal transplant
4. Miscellaneous indications
   a. Certain removal of all calculous material important (airline pilots)
   b. Stones for which other treatment modalities have failed

[a]These clinical scenarios could also be considered to be contraindications for shockwave lithotripsy.

Unilateral drainage suffices in most patients to maintain renal function at an acceptable level, and the less affected kidney (as judged by less hydronephrotic changes or parenchymal atrophy on imaging studies) is chosen for drainage (Figs 2.15 and 2.16).

5. To gain access to the collecting system. PCN is often just the first step in performing a variety of other interventional procedures in the kidney and ureter. Some examples of procedures that can be performed through a PCN track include the treatment of renal or ureteral calculi (stone fragmentation, removal, or chemolysis), ureteral interventions such as stricture dilation or stent placement, retrieval of foreign bodies such as fractured stent fragments, nephroscopic surgery such as endopyelotomy for ureteropelvic junction obstruction (UPJO), and brush biopsy or percutaneous therapy of urothelial tumors.

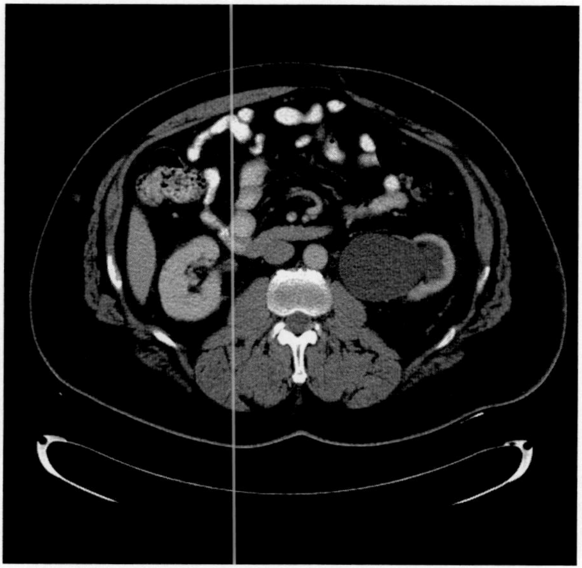

FIGURE 2.15 CT shows chronic hydronephrotic atrophy of left kidney due to colon cancer. Patient developed right hydronephrosis a few months later, necessitating a right nephrostomy. *CT*, Computed tomography.

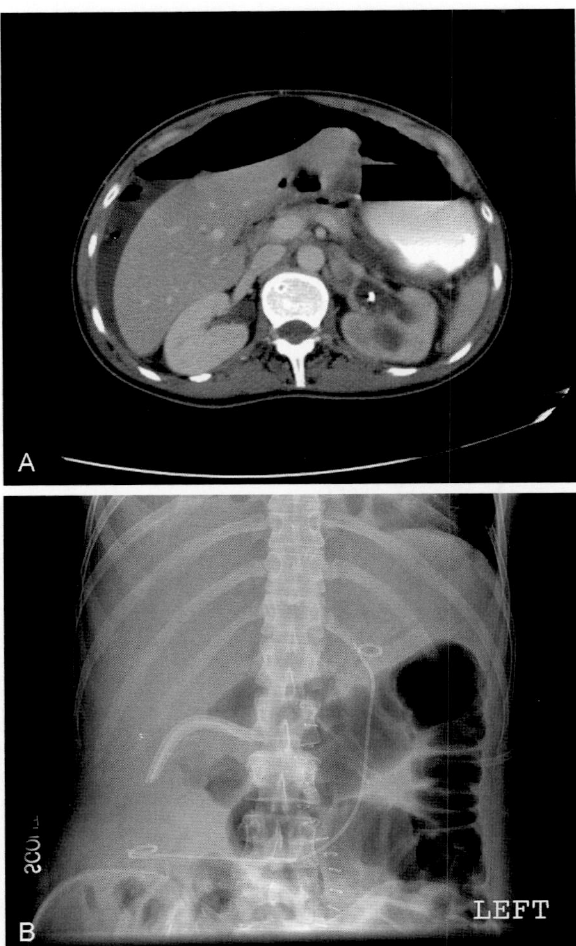

FIGURE 2.16 Percutaneous nephrostomy in patient with continent urinary diversion and occluded internalized stent. (A) CT shows left-sided obstruction with delayed nephrogram. (B) Abdominal film demonstrates an internalized stent in the continent pouch. Patient was febrile with urinary tract infection. The distal end of the stent could not be found even with pouch-endoscopy in the operating room.

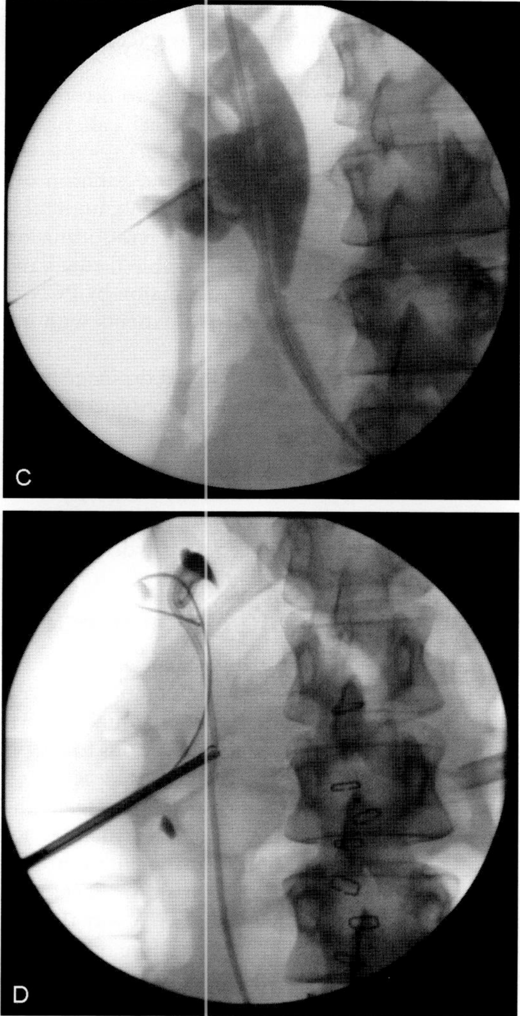

FIGURE 2.16, cont'd (C) Percutaneous nephrostomy of the hydronephrotic left kidney. Patient was allowed to defervesce for a few days. Grossly purulent urine was aspirated. (D) When patient was afebrile, the left ureteral stent was removed through the nephrostomy track. *CT*, Computed tomography.

Interventions can often be done at the same sitting as the PCN if the procedure is not complicated by excessive bleeding and if there is no infection.

6. To divert urine. PCN is often performed to divert the urine to allow closure of a ureteral fistula, ureteral leak, or a dehiscent urinary tract anastomosis. PCN drainage alone is rarely successful in totally diverting the urine; the addition of ureteral stenting is usually required to bridge leaking ureteral segments or dehiscent anastomoses, whereas ureteral occlusion is usually necessary in patients with intractable fistulae, most commonly vesicovaginal fistula. Urine diversion by PCN alone has been used with some success to treat patients with intractable hemorrhagic cystitis.
7. To assess residual renal function. Renal drainage by PCN may allow assessment of residual recoverable function in a chronically obstructed kidney that appears to be either nonfunctioning or poorly functioning. The presence of renal parenchymal atrophy on CT or renal US does not necessarily predict a poor potential for functional recovery after drainage with a PCN, although a kidney that is reduced to a hydronephrotic shell is unlikely to recover function significantly.

PREPROCEDURAL EVALUATION PRIOR TO PCN

Preprocedural evaluation in patients being considered for PCN includes a clinical history to identify a potential bleeder and routine laboratory tests of coagulation and renal function. This is discussed further in the section on contraindications to the procedure.

Prophylactic antibiotics are beneficial in decreasing the development of sepsis in both high-risk patients (e.g., those with struvite stones, diabetes, urinary tract obstruction, indwelling catheters, previous manipulation, instrumentation of the urinary tract) and in patients with a low risk for developing sepsis. Antibiotics should be administered in such a way that maximum blood levels are attained during the procedure, immediately prior to or less than 2 hours before the procedure, and should be continued after the procedure for 24 to 48 hours in low-risk groups and for 48 to 72 hours in high-risk groups. In patients with urinary obstruction, antibiotic therapy should be continued until satisfactory renal drainage is assured to avoid postprocedural bacteremia.

The risk of periprocedural sepsis is increased in the elderly, diabetics, and in patients with indwelling catheters, stones, ureterointestinal anastomosis, or the clinical presence of infection; septic shock can occur in as many as 7% of patients with pyonephrosis. The organisms that commonly infect the GU tract are gram-negative rods and include *Escherichia coli*, *Proteus*, *Klebsiella*, and *Enterococcus*. Antibiotic prophylaxis ideally should be based on culture results. For patients with obstruction and overt clinical infection in whom a specific organism has not yet been identified, broad-spectrum antibiotic therapy active against the common urinary pathogens is prudent.

CONTRAINDICATIONS TO PCN

The only absolute contraindication to PCN is the presence of an uncorrectable bleeding disorder; however, if the bleeding diathesis is due to a coagulopathy caused by urosepsis, urinary drainage will be necessary before the bleeding abnormality can be corrected. Correction of abnormal coagulation is needed if the international normalized ratio (INR) and the activated partial thromboplastin time (PTT) are greater than 1.5 times above the normal range; standard protocols are used for this. Platelet transfusion will correct drug-induced prolongation of the bleeding time if needed. Platelet counts greater than 50,000/dL are a safe value for most patients.

PCNs are often performed as an inpatient procedure but may be performed on an outpatient basis. Patients who may not be suitable candidates for outpatient PCN include those with hypertension, untreated urinary tract infection, coagulopathy, and staghorn calculi because these patients may be more likely to have complications such as procedure-related sepsis or bleeding.

TECHNIQUE

1. Monitoring of patients. Continuous electrocardiogram monitoring during the procedure is advisable. Large-bore and secure intravenous access should be routinely established before the procedure so that intravenous sedation and analgesia can be administered during the procedure and intravenous access is readily available if other medications need to be administered. Intravenous sedation combined with local anesthesia is sufficient to keep most patients comfortable; such patients require transcutaneous oximetry.

2. Localization of collecting system. The renal collecting system is localized by US if it is hydronephrotic. In a moderately or severely dilated collecting system, US guidance is successful in aiding entry into the collecting system in 85% to 95% of patients; conversely, in mildly dilated collecting systems, the success rate may be as low as 50%.
   Fluoroscopic guidance is used for the procedure if a radiopaque stone can serve as a target for puncture, or if the collecting system can be opacified with contrast. If renal function is normal (as in a patient with a urinary fistula), the collecting system can be opacified with contrast excreted after intravenous administration. Opacification of the collecting system by injecting through a retrograde catheter is helpful in patients with nonopaque calculi, for planned percutaneous endopyelotomy, and in patients with nondilated collecting systems and urinary stones. Blind punctures of the kidney using anatomic landmarks are apt to require multiple punctures for optimal entry and should be measures of last resort; ultrasound guidance can facilitate appropriate and safe puncture of the collecting system with the fewest number of sticks.
3. The patients are positioned in either a prone or a prone oblique position with the ipsilateral side elevated 20 to 30 degrees; however, if the patient cannot lie prone, the procedure can be performed in a supine oblique position. CT guidance is particularly helpful in this case. Initial puncture can be performed with CT guidance, and the subsequent manipulations for catheter placement are performed with fluoroscopic guidance. Preprocedural CT or MR scanning is necessary and highly recommended in patients with aberrant anatomy (e.g., severe scoliosis, congenital abnormalities) so that the relationship of the kidney to the liver, spleen, colon, gallbladder, and pleural space can be determined.
4. The flank is cleansed, and a subcostal skin entry site in the posterior axillary line is anesthetized. A needle is advanced into the collecting system from the flank, urine aspirated, contrast material injected, and a guidewire inserted through the needle into the kidney. The procedure is monitored fluoroscopically.
5. The needle is removed and the nephrocutaneous track enlarged by passing fascial dilators over the guidewire.

6. A drainage catheter, usually an 8 French "pigtail" catheter with a self-retaining mechanism, is passed over the guidewire and positioned in the renal pelvis. The guidewire is removed and the catheter secured to the skin and attached to a closed gravity drainage bag.

RESULTS

1. A PCN catheter can be successfully placed in 98% to 99% of patients with obstructed kidneys and dilated collecting systems.
2. Nondilated collecting systems or complex stone cases are technically challenging, with reported success rates of catheter placement in 85% to 90%.
3. When obstruction is complicated by urosepsis or azotemia, the response to renal decompression is marked and often immediate, with fever and flank pain improving in 24 to 48 hours after PCN drainage. As mentioned earlier, when obstruction and infection are due to ureteral calculi, retrograde ureteral catheterization and PCN are equally effective in relieving the obstruction and infection; neither technique is superior to the other in promoting rapid drainage or clinical defervescence.
4. In patients with azotemia secondary to obstruction, PCN returns renal function to normal or near normal levels in 7 to 14 days and can improve renal function enough to obviate dialysis in 28% to 30%. In patients with malignancies, the ureters can be obstructed by contiguous involvement or extrinsic compression. The need for external nephrostomy drainage is often permanent in such patients because ureteral stents often fail in adequately draining patients with extrinsic obstruction. Long-term survival after palliative diversion for malignant ureteral obstruction is poor, with only 25% of patients alive at 1 year. Our approach in patients with bilateral obstruction due to malignancies is to initially drain the symptomatic side, if there is one, or drain the kidney which appears to have more preserved renal parenchyma as gauged by cross-sectional imaging. The contralateral kidney is drained only if there is suspected infection, or if unilateral drainage does not improve renal function enough to administer the necessary chemotherapy.

COMPLICATIONS

1. The overall serious complication rate of PCN is low, with a mortality of 0.2% compared to a surgical mortality of 6%. Major complications include hemorrhage and sepsis.
2. Hemorrhage requiring transfusion or other therapy is a complication in less than 1% to 2.4% of patients and is related to renal arterial pseudoaneurysms or arteriovenous fistulas due to laceration of lobar arteries. Most hemorrhage associated with nephrostomy placement is transient and self-limited; it is not uncommon to have pink or slightly bloody urine drainage for several days after a nephrostomy, and this is not considered a complication. Serious vascular trauma is suspected if the urine continues to be grossly bloody after 3 to 5 days, if new intrapelvic clots are observed on nephrostograms, or if there is a significant drop in the hematocrit. If the drop in the hematocrit is out of proportion to the urine blood loss, a retroperitoneal hematoma should be suspected and a CT scan obtained. Angiography and possible arterial embolization should be considered in patients who have significant continuous or recurrent bleeding for longer than 4 to 5 days after PCN placement.
3. Sepsis can occur after nephrostomy tube placement, particularly in patients with stone disease. Patients with pyonephrosis are more prone to this complication and may develop postprocedure fever or even septic shock, despite the use of aminoglycoside prophylaxis. Forceful opacification of the collecting system to visualize the site and cause of obstruction should be deferred in all patients with urinary obstruction until the collecting system has been adequately decompressed for 24 to 48 hours and the patient is afebrile.
4. Inadvertent injury of adjacent organs is uncommon. The colon may lie posterior or posterolateral to the kidney and can be entered during a PCN. Retrorenal position of the colon is more common in patients who are thin and have little retrorenal fat, who have colonic dilation, or have abnormal anatomy such as marked kyphosis or scoliosis. When doubt about safe access exists, preprocedure CT to delineate the anatomy is prudent. The complication can often be managed conservatively, with drainage of both the kidney and the colon by separate catheters until the nephrocolic fistula heals.

5. An intercostal approach (often required for access to the upper poles of the kidneys) causes more thoracic complications than a subcostal puncture. In expiration, a posterior intercostal approach between the 11th and 12th ribs poses little risk of injury to the spleen and liver, but the lungs remain vulnerable to puncture in many patients. Other thoracic complications include pleural effusion, pneumonia, atelectasis, hydrothorax, and pneumothorax.
6. Minor complications that may occur are catheter dislodgment and urine extravasation. Dislodgement is more common in obese patients and in disoriented patients and can be minimized by using self-retaining drainage catheters, routinely exchanged every few months. Dislodgement in the first week after placement often necessitates a fresh track. Renal pelvic perforation is unusual in a routine PCN performed for drainage of an obstructed collecting system and is more likely to occur in patients with large staghorn stones. It is usually a self-limiting complication.

PERCUTANEOUS NEPHROSTOMY FOR NONOBSTRUCTIVE INDICATIONS

Management of Upper Urinary Tract Calculi

Percutaneous management of urinary tract calculi is indicated in patients who are not candidates for SWL or ureteroscopy. Percutaneous techniques are also used to salvage SWL or ureteroscopic failures. SWL is the treatment of choice for most renal and ureteral calculi. Stone-free success is greatly influenced by the stone size, with stones that are 1 cm or less in size representing the ideal for SWL. Stone-free rates of 85% to 87% have been reported for stones that are 1 to 2 cm in size. Distal ureteral calculi are managed by retrograde ureteroscopy or, in select cases, extracorporeal SWL.

Stone size: In patients with large calculi, over 2 to 3 cm in size, SWL has a poor chance of complete success, a high probability of requiring adjunctive therapy, and a significant incidence of complications. With stones larger than 2.5 to 3 cm, only 30% to 35% of patients may be stone-free with SWL, compared to 70% to 90% of those treated with percutaneous nephrostolithotomy (PCNL).

Staghorn stones: The primary approach to these stones should be by PCNL. Branched staghorn stones that fill the majority of the collecting system pose special problems because stones may be located deep in infundibula and calices that may be difficult to reach from the initial percutaneous tract. PCNL is initially used to rapidly remove large volumes of easily accessible stone with ultrasonic or electrohydraulic lithotripsy ("debulking"). If infundibulocaliceal fragments are inaccessible from the nephrostomy tract using the usual endourological techniques, SWL is used to break up the small volumes of remaining stones, followed by PCNL to remove the residual fragments.

Urinary obstruction, compromised urinary drainage: Urinary stasis can predispose to calculus formation. The most common examples of stones in association with obstruction are in UPJ obstruction, caliceal diverticula, malrotated kidneys, ectopic kidneys, horseshoe kidneys, and obstruction due to renal cysts or other renal masses. Although SWL can successfully break up the symptomatic calculi in these situations, the fragments are unlikely to be able to successfully pass even if the stone debris is adequately fragmented. In these cases, percutaneous stone therapy is combined with endourologic treatment for the underlying obstructive process, such as endopyelotomy for UPJ stenosis or balloon dilation for infundibular or ureteral strictures.

Stone composition: The composition of a calculus is critical to decide on the best method of management. Certain calculi (e.g., cystine calculi) are readily fragmented by ultrasonic lithotripsy but are refractory to SWL, making PCNL the treatment of choice. On the other hand, uric acid calculi respond well to SWL but not to ultrasonic lithotripsy. For stones larger than 2 cm, proceeding directly to PCNL is the best option. All stone material must be removed at the time of the percutaneous procedure to ensure that the patient will remain stone-free.

Stones composed of calcium oxalate dihydrate and struvite break up well with SWL or any other form of power lithotripsy, whereas stones composed either partially or completely of calcium oxalate monohydrate do not respond well to SWL. With these stones, the volume of the stone is the main determinant of the most desirable mode of therapy.

Stones that do not adequately fragment with SWL or that are inaccessible by ureteroscopy require a PCN for percutaneous ultrasonic lithotripsy. PCNL is also indicated in patients in whom certain removal of a stone is important (such as airline pilots) because residual stone fragments persist in a significant percentage of patients following SWL.

TECHNIQUE FOR PERCUTANEOUS NEPHROSTOLITHOTOMY

Two primary components in the percutaneous therapy of upper urinary tract calculi are the establishment of an access tract and the actual stone removal itself. Accurate access is the essential underpinning of a successful PCNL because a poorly placed track may make it impossible to remove even the most accessible of calculi. Fluoroscopic control is usually preferred for the procedure, especially if the calculi are radiopaque. CT is useful in preprocedural planning in patients with aberrant anatomy, so that the liver, spleen, colon, and pleural space can be avoided by the proposed track. If the calculi are faintly opaque or the collecting system is not dilated, placement of a retrograde catheter prior to the puncture is invaluable and allows both opacification and distension of the collecting system. Local anesthesia and intravenous sedation are generally sufficient for establishing the track.

Subsequently, track dilation and stone extraction are performed in the operating room. Experience has proven that tracts can be dilated acutely to 24 to 30 French with no adverse effects. After the procedure, the collecting system is inspected to ensure a stone-free state. It is standard practice to leave in a nephrostomy tube after the procedure to provide reliable drainage of urine, but many endourologists place small-bore catheters or a ureteral stent only following the stone removal. The nephrostomy catheter is removed 48 hours to 1 week later, after a nephrostogram demonstrates no leaks from the collecting system and no residual stones.

When the calculus is located in a calix or diverticulum, access should be obtained through that particular calix or diverticulum.

CONTRAINDICATIONS

An uncorrected bleeding abnormality is the only absolute contraindication. The procedure should not be performed if a stone-bearing kidney is uninfected and nonfunctioning. A relative contraindication is the inability to establish a safe access track.

COMPLICATIONS

1. Bleeding. Significant arterial bleeding occurs in 0.5% to 1.5% of patients. Vascular injury during the placement of the access track or track dilation can lead to pseudoaneurysms, arteriovenous fistulas, perinephric hematomas, and loss of functional parenchyma. Initial puncture into a calix, rather than an infundibulum or the renal pelvis, is the least likely to cause major vascular injury and is the preferable site of puncture. If excessive bleeding occurs during or after PCNL, the nephrostomy tube can be clamped to tamponade the track and the collecting system. If that fails, a larger nephrostomy catheter can be placed, which will tamponade the track better and also allow blood clots and residual calculus fragments to pass. Selective angiography and embolization should be considered if the aforementioned measures fail.
2. Injury to adjacent organs. The colon can be nicked if it is positioned posterior to the kidney. The colonic injury may not be obvious until the postprocedure nephrostogram demonstrates colonic filling with contrast. If the nick is small, the injuries can be managed conservatively by draining the kidneys with a double pigtail ureteral stent placed from below, pulling the nephrostomy tube into the colon, and leaving it to act as a colostomy tube. The track usually seals in a few days. If a more serious injury occurs, open repair may be required.

   Injury to the duodenum, liver, and spleen is uncommon. Pleural and lung injuries may occur with supracostal punctures.
3. Sepsis. PCNL is considered to be a clean-contaminated procedure in patients with sterile urine preoperatively, but a rise in temperature is common after stone removal. Postoperative bacteremia can occur, and some of the factors affecting the development of postoperative fever are the duration of surgery and the amount of irrigant fluid.
4. Perforation. During the process of stone removal, the renal pelvis can be perforated by a sharp fragment of stone or by one of the instruments (such as the ultrasound probe) in as many as 10% of cases. Most such perforations heal within 12 to 24 hours as long as good urine drainage is maintained. Serial

nephrostograms will show that even sizable renal pelvic and ureteral lacerations heal in a few days without stricture formation.

5. A calculus can extrude through a urothelial tear. Renal pelvic extrusions should be treated with nephrostomy drainage, whereas ureteral tears should be treated with stenting for a few weeks. In the absence of infection, extrusion of calculus material into the perinephric and periureteral tissues appears to be of no clinical consequence.

TREATMENT OF URETERAL CALCULI

SWL is the treatment of choice for upper ureteral calculi and has higher success rates if the stone can be pushed back into the kidney. These calculi can also be approached in a percutaneous, antegrade fashion. In the midureter, most authorities favor ureteroscopic extraction of calculi or retrograde displacement of the calculus into the kidney followed by SWL. For distal ureteral stones, ureteroscopic extraction is probably the technique of choice because of its high initial success rate, the rare need for secondary treatments and postureteroscopic interventions, and the low complication rate of ureteroscopy in the distal ureter.

Ureterolithotomy for stone removal is unusual and performed on the rare occasion for stones that are impacted or embedded in the ureter and require open surgical removal.

OTHER PROCEDURES PERFORMED THROUGH A PCN ACCESS TRACK

In patients with **UPJ obstruction**, PCNL can be often combined with an endopyelotomy. The percutaneous route is also well suited to the **removal of foreign bodies** (e.g., broken stents, guidewire fragments, internal ureteral stents, fungus balls) from the renal pelvis and/or ureter. Stents that have not been changed in the recommended period may encrust, become brittle, and fracture; fractures are best approached with a combined percutaneous-endoscopic technique.

Ureteral Stenting

PRINCIPLES

1. Percutaneous ureteral stenting provides urinary diversion without the need for an external collection device when retrograde insertion of a ureteral stent is not possible or practical.

2. Most patients find a ureteral stent catheter more acceptable and convenient than a nephrostomy catheter.

INDICATIONS

1. Long-term stenting (months to years) is most frequently performed to bypass a ureteral obstruction.
2. Short-term stenting (weeks to months)
   a. Facilitates healing of postoperative or traumatic pyeloureteral leaks or ureteral fistulae by diverting the urinary stream
   b. Prevents stricture formation as ureteral injuries or implantations (native or allograft ureters) heal by providing a mold around which ureteral epithelialization is facilitated
   c. Maintains ureteral caliber following balloon dilation or incision of benign ureteral strictures
3. Catheters percutaneously placed into the ureters facilitate intraoperative ureteral identification during difficult surgical dissections (e.g., revision of an obstructed ureteroileal diversion).

CONTRAINDICATIONS

1. The presence of active renal infection
2. Markedly diseased bladder that would be intolerant of a stent (e.g., radiation cystitis, bladder invasion by adjacent neoplasm)
3. Bladder fistulae

TECHNIQUE

1. Following PCN, a guidewire and catheter are manipulated through the abnormal (often stenotic) ureteral segment into the urinary bladder, or bowel conduit, or urinary reservoir.
2. The catheter is replaced with a ureteral stent in which multiple side holes have been created where the stent will eventually be positioned in the renal pelvis. Kidney urine enters the stent through these side holes, travels through the catheter, and exits from its distal pigtail segment. Depending on ureteral caliber, urine may also flow around the stent. The proximal end of the stent protrudes from the skin and is obturated externally. This is an external ureteral stent catheter.
3. An external ureteral stent can be periodically changed from the flank over a guide wire.
4. Urinary drainage can be totally internalized by placing an internal ureteral stent with a pigtail configuration at both ends.

The proximal pigtail is positioned in the renal pelvis and the distal pigtail in the bladder. Double pigtail stents must be periodically changed (at least every 6 months) cystoscopically.

5. Patients who require ureteral stenting following ureteral diversion to a bowel conduit should have an external ureteral stent inserted in combined antegrade/retrograde fashion. A guide wire and catheter are first manipulated beyond the abnormal ureteral segment, through the bowel conduit, and out the stoma rather than into the bladder. The catheter is removed, and a single pigtail drainage catheter is passed retrograde into the renal pelvis. The distal end of this catheter protrudes through the stoma to drain into the urostomy collection bag. Internal ureteral stents should not be used in patients with ureteroenterostomies or continent urinary diversion reservoirs.
6. If retrograde endoscopic attempts to pass catheters beyond ureteral obstructions and fistulae are unsuccessful, fluoroscopically guided retrograde periurethral catheter manipulations are often successful in the radiology department. This approach employs standard interventional equipment (e.g., catheters, guide wires, sheaths) passed through or over partially inserted ureteral catheters.

RESULTS

1. Both internal and external ureteral stents allow patients to lead as active a life as their underlying condition will permit.
2. Ureteral obstructions can often be negotiated in antegrade (percutaneous) fashion even if retrograde cystoscopic catheterization is not possible (e.g., neoplastic obstruction of a ureteral orifice, distal ureteral angulation secondary to prostatic enlargement, spread of prostatic malignancy, ureteral reimplantation, tight ureteral stenoses, urethral stricture).
3. Approximately 85% to 90% of ureteral obstructions and fistulae can be stented percutaneously. Very tightly obstructed ureters and ureters that are both tortuous and encased by tumor or fibrosis are the most frequent causes of failure of antegrade stent placement.
4. Internal ureteral stents may not drain kidneys as well as a PCN, especially when ureteral obstruction is caused by extrinsic compression or if intravesical pressure is elevated at rest or during micturition.

COMPLICATIONS

1. Improperly positioned stents will not provide optimal urinary drainage. This problem can be rectified with percutaneous, cystoscopic, or ureteroscopic techniques. Proximal stent migration can lead to perforation of the renal pelvis or calyces, which can result in a urinoma or even catastrophic exsanguination due to erosion of the stent tip into a renal vessel. Stents that have migrated up into the kidney above a lower ureteral stricture or anastomosis can be extracted through a nephrostomy track under fluoroscopic guidance. A second approach is to use ureteroscopy to reposition the caudal end of the stent within the bladder. A stent that is positioned too far cephalad (so that the distal end is no longer within the urinary bladder) is usually related to placement of too short a stent rather than to cephalad migration.
2. Symptoms attributable to the intravesical coil of the stent (even when properly positioned) occur commonly, including microscopic hematuria, pyuria, lower abdominal pain, dysuria, urinary frequency, nocturia, and flank pain on voiding (due to renal reflux of bladder urine).
3. Fatigue fractures and encrustation of ureteral stents may occur if stents are not periodically replaced. This should be carried out at least every 6 months and more often in patients who form stones.

Dilation of Ureteral and Urethral Stenoses

PRINCIPLES

1. Chronic ureteral stenting is not the optimal therapy for benign postoperative ureteral strictures, although it may be appropriate for malignant ureteral obstructions.
2. Many benign ureteral strictures are amenable to balloon catheter dilation or endourologic incision.
3. These procedures, if successful, can spare patients the nuisance of chronic indwelling stents or the risks of additional surgery.

INDICATIONS

1. An attempt at balloon catheter dilation of all benign ureteral strictures should be made before relegating patients to additional surgery or to chronic PCN or indwelling ureteral stent drainage.

2. Endoscopic incision, employed alone or in combination with balloon dilation and ureteral stenting, can relieve certain UPJ obstructions (both congenital and acquired) and postoperative ureteroenteral anastomotic strictures.
3. Balloon dilation of ureters encircled by sutures sometimes results in disruption of the offending ligature, thus saving the patient an operation.
4. Balloon dilation of vesicourethral anastomotic strictures that develop after radical prostatectomy is a nonoperative alternative to endoscopic incision and appears to be less likely to cause urinary incontinence.

CONTRAINDICATIONS

1. Ureteral strictures caused by malignant disease, either primary or recurrent.
2. Inflammatory or traumatic urethral strictures appear to be more amenable to optical internal urethrotomy than to balloon dilation.

TECHNIQUE

1. The strictured ureter is cannulated as described earlier.
2. Biopsies and/or other imaging studies are obtained to confirm that the stricture is of benign etiology.
3. A catheter with an inflatable balloon capable of withstanding high pressure (15–17 atmospheres of pressure) and inflated diameter of 6 to 10 mm (18–14 French) is used. Ureteral stenoses are generally inflated to 6 to 8 mm, whereas urethral stenoses are dilated with 8- to 10-mm balloons (24–30 French). The catheter is advanced across the stricture and the balloon inflated with diluted contrast material. A waist or narrowing is seen initially in the inflated balloon at the stricture site which should disappear with continued or repeated inflations if the balloon dilation is technically correct.
4. Following dilation, a ureteral stent is placed, which remains in situ for 6 to 8 weeks to maintain luminal patency while the ureteral musculature heals. Stenting is accomplished with the largest catheter that can be comfortably accommodated. This is generally 10 French if the stent traverses the intramural

ureter, but it may be larger if a ureteroenterostomy stricture is dilated and stented.

5. After 6 to 8 weeks, the stent is exchanged for a PCN, and the efficacy of the dilation is assessed by a nephrostogram and urodynamic studies prior to catheter removal.
6. If the ureteral stricture has been dilated and stented in a retrograde fashion per urethra with an internalized double pigtail catheter (usually 7–8 French in size), assessment of efficacy of balloon dilation is performed with an IVU obtained at 1, 6, and 12 months after stent removal.
7. Similar techniques have been adapted to treat congenital UPJ obstructions by balloon dilation, endoscopic incision, and stenting.

RESULTS

1. Approximately 58% of all benign ureteral strictures can be successfully dilated with balloon catheters, usually with one attempt.
2. If there is poor response to the first attempt at balloon dilation, a second attempt at balloon dilation is worthwhile because some strictures will respond favorably to a second similar procedure.
3. The etiology and age of the stricture seem to influence the outcome of dilation therapy. Strictures not associated with ischemia or dense fibrosis may be successfully dilated (including those that occur in renal allograft recipients). Those associated with radiotherapy or surgical devascularization have a much lower rate of success. Strictures that have been present for less than 3 months respond much better to dilation therapy than those that are more chronic in nature.
4. Endoscopic incision followed by balloon dilation and ureteral stenting is more effective than balloon catheter dilation alone for ureteroenteral anastomotic strictures and UPJ strictures.
5. Unsuccessful balloon dilation does not adversely affect other therapeutic options, including chronic indwelling ureteral stenting, surgical revision, or insertion of a metallic expandable ureteral stent (Wallstent or similar device). Although favorable short-term results have been reported with metallic ureteral stents, the long-term efficacy of metallic stents has not been stellar.

COMPLICATIONS

No known permanent sequelae have resulted from unsuccessful dilation therapy. Laceration of ureteral mucosa or wall may occur with balloon dilation. These perforations heal uneventfully if the ureter is adequately stented and probably do not affect the outcome of dilation therapy.

Percutaneous Drainage of Renal and Related Retroperitoneal Fluid Collections

PRINCIPLES

Percutaneous drainage of renal and related retroperitoneal abscesses almost always obviates the need for surgical drainage. Cross-sectional imaging is used for guidance for the drainage. Most patients who present with acute pyelonephritis do not require imaging, but contrast-enhanced cross-sectional imaging is indicated when patients do not respond to appropriate antibiotics with a few days—in such cases, CT or MR allows evaluation for complications such as abscess formation.

INDICATIONS

Renal abscess or infected renal cyst that fails to improve with broad-spectrum antibiotics or a large infected renal or retroperitoneal fluid collection that requires drainage.

CONTRAINDICATIONS

1. Absence of a safe percutaneous drainage route.
2. Small renal abscesses (less than 3 cm in diameter) can often be effectively treated with a course of intravenous antibiotics and may not require drainage.
3. Abnormal coagulation parameters.

TECHNIQUE

1. The anatomic relationship of the fluid collection to its surrounding structures is assessed by cross-sectional imaging (CT or, less commonly, US). A safe, extraperitoneal route that avoids puncture of viscera, pleura, and major vessels is planned for diagnostic needle aspiration and catheter placement.

2. Diagnostic aspiration is performed with a 20- or 21-gauge needle to confirm the diagnosis.
3. If diagnostic aspiration yields infected material, a catheter is introduced into the collection under fluoroscopic control, the abscess drained completely, and the catheter securely sutured in place to provide continuous drainage. Injection of contrast medium (to evaluate the size and appearance of the abscess and assess whether it communicates with the collecting system) is minimized at the time of the drainage to reduce the chances of inciting bacteremia or septic shock.
4. Septa within an abscess can usually be perforated with catheters and guide wires so that locules intercommunicate. Even so, multiloculated abscesses may require more than one catheter for complete drainage.
5. Multiple drainage catheters may be needed for renal abscesses that have spread retroperitoneally (one catheter for each component). Abscesses associated with ureteral obstruction require a PCN catheter in addition to the abscess drainage catheter.
6. Abscesses related to the urinary tract have less viscous contents than those that originate from the pancreas or GI tract. Gravity drainage with 10 to 14 French pigtail or Malecot catheters is effective in draining most urinary tract abscesses. If the abscess contents are very viscous, large sump catheters placed to suction and periodic irrigation with saline may be required.
7. When there is clinical defervescence to the percutaneous drainage, patients can be switched to oral antibiotics from parenteral therapy, discharged from the hospital with their drainage catheters in place, and followed as outpatients. Periodic follow-up catheter studies and CT scans are usually obtained at 1- to 2-week intervals to ensure that the catheter remains patent. Follow-up CT scans also demonstrate if undrained locules exist.
8. If a patient fails to improve on antibiotics and catheter drainage, a CT scan is obtained to detect undrained locules, enteric communications, or misplaced catheters.
9. Indications for catheter removal include the following:
   a. A satisfactory clinical response with defervescence of clinical signs of infection
   b. Return of white blood cell count to normal
   c. Cessation of drainage
   d. Obliteration of the abscess cavity

10. Drainage catheters usually need to remain in place for an average of 2 to 4 weeks for most urinary abscesses. Renal abscesses usually resolve in less time than those that have spread extrarenally. The track will close following catheter removal if all infected material has been evacuated.
11. Perinephric abscesses are almost always associated with an underlying anatomic abnormality such as stones or strictures which have to be treated after the abscess has resolved.

RESULTS

Percutaneous abscess drainage can be expected to cure approximately 72% of renal and related retroperitoneal abscesses. This is a significant improvement compared to the results of surgical drainage and is due to the use of cross-sectional imaging techniques for evaluation, which allows the diagnosis of abscesses earlier in their development, needle aspiration to confirm the nature of a fluid collection, and also the efficacy of percutaneous drainage techniques.

COMPLICATIONS

1. Many patients develop transient bacteremia, febrile episodes, and even septic shock after percutaneous abscess drainage. These complications can be minimized by limiting catheter manipulation, lavage of the cavity, and/or contrast opacification of the abscess at the time of drainage. Definitive study of the abscess cavity should be deferred until the abscess has been effectively drained for several days.
2. Unsatisfactory clinical response may be due to partial drainage of septated collections or premature catheter removal.
3. An infected, obstructed calyceal diverticulum may be mistaken for a renal parenchymal abscess and continue to drain urine after the infection has cleared. Specific measures must then be directed toward dilating or occluding the neck of the diverticulum to prevent recurrence.

PERCUTANEOUS DRAINAGE OF LYMPHOCELES

1. Lymphoceles that occur after renal transplantation or pelvic surgery can be drained percutaneously but usually recur if only simple drainage is performed.

2. Sclerotherapy of the lymphocele cavity appears to be more effective in preventing fluid reaccumulation than simple catheter drainage alone. Agents used for sclerotherapy include tetracycline, with povidone-iodine (Betadine), or absolute alcohol in combination with Betadine. However, the therapy requires several weeks of treatment and is making laparoscopic surgery (to create a peritoneal window) the procedure of choice.

PERCUTANEOUS DRAINAGE OF URINOMAS

1. Urinomas are urine collections that result from extravasation of urine due to obstruction of the renal collecting system, surgery, or trauma and are often contained within a fibrous pseudocapsule.
2. Urinomas may cause secondary ureteral obstruction.
3. Large urinomas can be aspirated or drained in conjunction with management of the cause of the urine leak with PCN and ureteral stenting. However, not all urinomas require drainage because small (and occasionally large) urinomas will usually resorb spontaneously if the urinary obstruction is relieved.

Renal Cyst Aspiration and Ablation

INDICATIONS

Primary indication for this procedure is to decompress and/or obliterate a symptomatic benign simple renal cyst. Percutaneous ablation of a renal cyst is indicated if the lesion is producing pain, obstructive hydronephrosis, or segmental compression of portions of the collecting system with stasis of urine resulting in stone formation. Pain is the most common indication to perform renal cyst ablation.

CONTRAINDICATIONS

1. An uncorrected bleeding diathesis.
2. Aspiration and ablation of cysts in autosomal dominant polycystic kidney disease is rarely performed because of the difficulty in localizing a specific cyst or locule that may be causing the symptoms. Here again, the most common indication is flank pain.

TECHNIQUE

1. Renal cysts are aspirated with a 20-gauge needle, using CT, or, most often, US guidance.
2. If the cyst is being punctured to ascertain whether it is responsible for the patient's flank or back pain, as much fluid as possible is aspirated from the lesion for a therapeutic trial. Ablation is deferred for a few weeks to see if the patient's flank pain responds to the cyst decompression, and if it recurs when fluid reaccumulates within the cyst.
3. For cyst ablation, a small catheter or sheath is placed in the lesion, the majority of the cyst fluid is aspirated, and a sclerosing agent is then instilled into the cyst. The agent is left in for approximately a half hour and then aspirated before the catheter is removed.
4. Many sclerosing agents can obliterate renal cysts. Absolute alcohol is most often used because it appears to be the most consistent in its action.

RESULTS

1. Most renal cysts reaccumulate after diagnostic aspiration, even if the cyst is drained completely.
2. The majority of renal cysts can be permanently obliterated, thereby relieving the symptoms that prompted the intervention.

COMPLICATIONS

1. Improper needle placement may cause perinephric hemorrhage, inadvertent puncture of adjacent organs (e.g., lung, GI tract), infection, arteriovenous fistula, and urinoma formation.
2. Extravasation of sclerosing agents into the perinephric tissues can cause fat necrosis, soft tissue fibrosis, or a febrile reaction.

Urinary Tract Biopsy Techniques

1. Soft tissue and visceral lesions related to the urinary tract and suspicious nodal lesions can readily be sampled for cytologic or histologic analysis when necessary for patient management. Prostate needle biopsy is considered elsewhere in this book.
2. Biopsies can be obtained with needles percutaneously placed into lesions (to biopsy renal masses, retroperitoneal masses, or

nodes). Biopsy of urothelial lesions can be performed through percutaneously placed catheters or through retrograde catheters placed with cystoscopic guidance.

INDICATIONS

1. Evaluation of renal and adrenal masses in patients with a history of malignancy.
2. A significant number, approximately 20%, of small renal masses may be benign but indistinguishable from RCC by imaging criteria. Interest is increasing in biopsy of these masses for management decisions because the availability of immunohistochemistry often makes a definitive diagnosis possible on very small specimens.
3. Evaluation of urothelial irregularity or filling defects in patients with a past history of bladder or upper tract urothelial cancer, or with hematuria.

CONTRAINDICATIONS

1. Contraindications to needle aspiration biopsy include the following:
   a. Hemorrhagic diathesis
   b. Suspicion of an arteriovenous malformation in the area to be biopsied
2. There are no contraindications to transcatheter brush biopsy.

TECHNIQUE

1. Needle biopsy
   a. Most percutaneous biopsies are guided by CT or US, some by MRI, with operator preference, lesion size and location, and machine availability determining the modality used for guidance.
   b. Biopsies performed with small (21- to 22-gauge), thin-walled needles yield samples for cytologic evaluation. Larger needles (14- to 20-gauge), often used in conjunction with automated, spring-loaded biopsy devices, yield specimens for histologic evaluation.
   c. Aspiration biopsies are obtained and evaluated immediately by a cytopathologist to ascertain the adequacy of tissue sampling. Additional biopsies are performed until diagnostic material is obtained.

d. Large needles provide tissue cores of sufficient size for conventional histopathologic examination.

2. Transcatheter biopsy
   a. This approach is most frequently used to obtain a brush biopsy of a pyelocalyceal or ureteral lesion suspicious for transitional cell carcinoma on noninvasive imaging studies.
   b. An open-ended catheter is passed cytoscopically into the ureter or kidney. A guide wire on which a nylon brush is mounted is then passed through the catheter and the suspicious abnormality "brushed" under fluoroscopy. Exfoliated cells retrieved by the brush are subjected to cytologic analysis. A variety of brush configurations are available for approaching lesions through the collecting system and ureter. Other biopsy instruments, including forceps and snares, can be passed through larger catheters or sheaths inserted into the upper urinary tract.

RESULTS

1. Transcatheter and percutaneous brush biopsies yield true positive results in over 90% of cases. False positive results are very infrequent.
2. Cytologic demonstration of malignant cells generally alters patient management by obviating the need for more invasive diagnostic techniques (including ureteroscopy), surgical biopsy, or staging procedures.
3. Negative findings do not exclude the presence of malignancy because they may represent sampling error. Therefore thin-needle aspiration or transcatheter brush biopsy is of value only when positive results are obtained.
4. Tissue-core biopsies analyzed histologically may have fewer false negative results.

COMPLICATIONS

1. Complications include the following:
   a. Blood vessel injury with bleeding, pseudoaneurysm, or arteriovenous fistula formation.
   b. Peritonitis due to bowel leak.
   c. Pneumothorax.
   d. Seeding of the needle track with malignant cells.
   This may be more a theoretical than an actual risk. Only a handful of cases of spread of renal malignancy following

aspiration biopsy has been reported. Nonetheless, because of the propensity for urothelial (but not parenchymal) tumors to spread along epithelial surfaces, suspected urothelial malignancies should not be biopsied percutaneously.

2. Brush biopsy is rarely associated with complications.
   a. Patient discomfort and hematuria related to catheter manipulation and vigorous "brushing" of friable lesions.
   b. It is best to perform these biopsies with conscious sedation to keep the patient comfortable.
   c. Collecting system or ureteral perforation with catheters or guide wires can occur but are innocuous if adequate urinary drainage, usually with a retrograde ureteral catheter, is maintained for a day or two after the procedure.

IMAGE-GUIDED ABLATION OF RENAL TUMORS

Percutaneous tumor ablation is a viable option for patients with RCC in whom nephron-sparing surgery is contraindicated because of significant comorbidities. The role of percutaneous ablation therapy in patients without surgical contraindications is still unclear. The techniques in current use include RFA, microwave ablation, and cryotherapy. Although RFA was initially the most widely used technique, cryotherapy has the advantage that the zone of necrosis can be visualized as the procedure is performed. Cryoablation also can be used to treat larger tumors than with RFA, and it is associated with fewer complications when treating central tumors near the collecting system.

RADIOFREQUENCY ABLATION

Electrodes are placed percutaneously in the tumor with CT guidance, and a high-frequency alternating current is applied to heat the tumor to 50°C, which coagulates the tissues. Tumors that can be successfully ablated are usually less than 5 cm in diameter and located in the periphery of the kidney. Centrally located tumors are more resistant to RFA than peripheral tumors because the large vessels in the renal hilus disperse the heat, resulting in incomplete ablation. Ablation of centrally located tumors is also associated with a higher risk of injury to the collecting system. Anteriorly located tumors are often in proximity to the colon, and special maneuvers are necessary to prevent thermal injury to the colon. Tumor ablation is assessed by lack of enhancement of the lesion on follow-up contrast-enhanced studies, whereas foci of enhancing tissue indicate the presence of a viable tumor.

CRYOABLATION

Cryoablation has been used with open surgery and percutaneously. Cell death is produced by producing extracellular and intracellular ice crystal formation, and this "ice ball" can be visualized with imaging as the procedure is performed.

Other techniques that are being investigated for renal tumor ablation include high-intensity focused ultrasound, microwave therapy, and renal ablation.

Additional content, including Self-Assessment Questions and Suggested Readings, may be accessed at www.ExpertConsult.com.

Lower Urinary Tract Infections in Women and Pyelonephritis

Zoe S. Gan, MD, and Ariana L. Smith, MD

Lower Urinary Tract Infection

DEFINITION

The lower urinary tract, even in healthy, asymptomatic individuals, hosts a local microbial community that likely plays a role in maintaining normal bladder function. While all individuals likely have some degree of *bacteriuria*, or presence of bacteria in the urine, this usually is nonpathologic and goes undetected with the sensitivity of commonly used urine culture tests. When bacteria are detected in the urine, the clinical picture should be used to determine whether its presence is pathogenic and warrants treatment.

Bacteriuria can be symptomatic or asymptomatic. *Cystitis* refers to the symptoms of dysuria, urgency, frequency, and/or suprapubic pain. Lower urinary tract infection (UTI) (*bacterial cystitis*) is only one of many causes of this symptomatology, but one which is generally easy to prove or disprove with urine testing. *Pyuria* is the presence of white blood cells in the urine and, when seen in conjunction with bacteriuria, is indicative of an inflammatory response that may signify true infection. Urine culture determines if a specific bacterial pathogen is present at a threshold to indicate true infection. *Asymptomatic bacteriuria* (ASB) is the isolation of bacteria from the urine in significant quantities consistent with infection, but without the local or systemic genitourinary signs or symptoms. The presence of ASB in the absence of symptoms or pyuria is often referred to as *colonization*. Colonization is often mistaken for infection and treated with antibiotics, potentially contributing to antibiotic resistance, changes in normal intestinal and urogenital flora, and emergence of pathologic organisms in the host.

DIFFERENTIAL DIAGNOSIS

Includes, but is not limited to:
Vaginitis
Urethritis
Interstitial cystitis/bladder pain syndrome
Radiation cystitis
Bladder calculi
Overactive bladder
Bladder cancer

Other important definitions include:

1. Recurrent urinary tract infection (rUTI): At least two UTIs (i.e., distinct, symptomatic episodes) in 6 months or at least three UTIs in 1 year.
2. Pyelonephritis: Infection of the upper urinary tract including the renal pelvis and kidney parenchyma.
3. Prophylactic antimicrobial therapy: Prevention of infection in a urinary tract with a negative urine culture by administration of antimicrobial medications.
4. Suppressive antimicrobial therapy: Prevention of a clinically symptomatic infection in an asymptomatic patient whose urinary tract is colonized with bacteria identified on urine culture.
5. Nosocomial UTI: Those that occur in hospitalized or institutionalized patients.

CLASSIFICATION SCHEMA

UTIs can be classified according to their *site of origin*. Cystitis refers to the nonspecific clinical syndrome of dysuria, urinary frequency, urgency, and suprapubic pressure. Fever, chills, and flank pain can indicate the presence of pyelonephritis, an interstitial inflammation caused by bacterial infection of the renal parenchyma. **Surprisingly, based on symptoms, it can be remarkably difficult to differentiate infection involving the upper tracts from bacteriuria confined to the bladder.** Many patients with pure lower tract symptoms will have positive cultures of renal pelvic and ureteral urine if catheterization of the upper tracts is performed. Conversely, some patients with flank pain will be found to have only cystitis on differential urine cultures. Fortunately, from a practical standpoint, it is not generally an important distinction, and localizing the site of infection in clinically uncomplicated infections is unnecessary.

UTIs can also be classified in terms of the *anatomic or functional status of the urinary tract* and the overall health of the patient. An uncomplicated infection indicates it is occurring in an otherwise normal urinary tract in a healthy individual. A complicated infection is one occurring in a functionally or structurally abnormal urinary tract, in a host with a compromised immune system, or an infection with bacteria of increased virulence or antimicrobial resistance (i.e., nosocomial UTI).

While the definition of rUTI varies in the current literature, the Food and Drug Administration (FDA) criteria currently defines it as two or more symptomatic episodes in 6 months or three episodes in 1 year. This definition is endorsed by the American Urological Association (AUA) and Society for Urodynamics, Female Pelvic Medicine and Urogenital Reconstruction (SUFU) joint guidelines. Symptomatic episodes are considered distinct with resolution of symptoms in between episodes.

EPIDEMIOLOGY

UTIs are considered to be the most common bacterial infection. They are generally associated with minimal morbidity except among specific subpopulations. Eleven percent of women report having had a UTI during any given year, and more than half of all women have had at least one UTI in their lifetime. One in three women have had a UTI before the age of 24 years. This contrasts with men, in whom infection is uncommon until after the age of 50 when the problem of an enlarged prostate and outlet obstruction may occur. Between 3.5 and 7 million office visits a year are the result of UTI, and direct costs exceed $1.6 billion. It is difficult to assess the true incidence of UTI because urine cultures are not often done in the outpatient setting, and symptoms are variable.

In women with a first UTI, 24% will have a second episode within 6 months, and up to half of women will have a second infection within a year. The risk of recurrent uncomplicated bacterial cystitis remains unchanged whether the initial episode is left untreated to clear spontaneously, or treated with short-term, long-term, or prophylactic antimicrobial therapy. Symptomatic episodes in the healthy population are more of a nuisance than a threat to health. **No association between recurrent infections and renal scarring, hypertension, or renal failure has been established in patients with uncomplicated, simple recurrent UTI.** Symptomatic UTI is especially common among sexually active women. Modifiable behavioral risk factors include the use of a diaphragm and spermicides for contraception and frequency of sexual intercourse among premenopausal women. Estrogen deficiency is another risk factor, as is antimicrobial use itself.

While UTI in the nonobstructed, nonpregnant female adult acts as a benign illness with no long-term sequelae, this is not true in other populations, as noted in Box 3.1.

Catheter-associated urinary tract infection (CAUTI) is the most common nosocomial infection. The risk of bacterial colonization increases with the duration of catheterization, approaching 100% at 30 days. UTI accounts for 25% of infections in the noninstitutionalized elderly. Diabetes increases the risk of UTI and bacteriuria among female but not male patients. UTIs in ambulatory patients with diabetes are considered complicated, with a heightened risk for pyelonephritis and severe complications if left untreated. UTI is more common in the multiple sclerosis population and can herald acute exacerbations and progression of the disease. Additional risk factors for UTI include immunosuppression and instrumentation of the genitourinary system.

ASB is present in 3% of women in their early 20s, rising from 1% with the onset of intercourse in the late teenage years. It increases 1% per decade. Approximately 11% to 25% of elderly,

BOX 3.1 Subpopulations at Increased Risk From Urinary Tract Infection

1. Infants
2. Pregnant women
3. Elderly
4. Spinal cord injury
5. Indwelling catheters
6. Diabetes
7. Multiple sclerosis
8. Acquired immunodeficiency disease
9. Underlying urologic abnormalities

noncatheterized patients can develop transient ASB, and persistent colonization in the elderly may affect up to 50% of geriatric women and be extremely difficult to eradicate. The incidence of ASB in the pregnant population is similar to the nonpregnant population, but the implications are more concerning. The risk during pregnancy for pyelonephritis is increased substantially in those harboring bacteria in the urinary tract, especially during the end of the second and beginning of the third trimester. Studies suggest a 20% to 40% incidence of pyelonephritis if ASB is untreated in this population.

PATHOPHYSIOLOGY

The paradigm of uncomplicated UTIs is that bacterial virulence appears to be crucial for overcoming normal host defenses. With complicated UTI, the paradigm is reversed, in that bacterial virulence is much less important, and host factors tend to be critical.

The bacteria responsible for UTIs are normally present in the bowel. *Escherichia coli* is the most common, accounting for 85% of community-acquired infections and up to 50% of nosocomial infections. *E. coli* commonly seeds the urine in the presence of introital or vaginal colonization. The female urethra is short, and bacteria generally enter the bladder in an ascending fashion. Less commonly, *E. coli* may directly invade the bladder superficial cells in the absence of local colonization.

The intracellular bacteria mature into biofilms that provide an internal reservoir of bacteria capable of causing clinical bacterial cystitis. Other common organisms include *Proteus* sp., *Klebsiella* sp., *Enterococcus faecalis*, and *Staphylococcus saprophyticus*. *S. saprophyticus* and enterobacterial species adhere to uroepithelial cells through different adhesive mechanisms than *E. coli*. After attachment, *Proteus* spp., *K. pneumoniae*, and *S. saprophyticus* each produce urease, which catalyzes the hydrolysis of urea in urine and causes the release of ammonia and CO_2. This elevates the urinary pH and can lead to the formation of bladder or kidney stones.

Vaginal mucosal introital colonization that generally precedes infection is determined by bacterial adherence, the receptive characteristics of the epithelial surface, and the fluid that bathes both surfaces. Estrogens and pH affect attachment and colonization of the vaginal mucosa. Host defense mechanisms include the antiadherence properties of the vaginal and bladder mucosa, the hydrokinetic clearance of bacteria through voiding, and changes in urine pH and composition that may inhibit bacterial growth. The female urethra is lined by cells identical to those of the vagina that respond readily to estrogens. The normally functioning urethra may help to protect the bladder from cystitis through the shedding of uropathogens bound to exfoliating urethral cells; trapping of bacteria by mucus secreted by the paraurethral glands; intermittent washout by urine, local production of immunoglobulins, cytokines and defensins; and mobilization of leukocytes.

It is generally believed that some failure with the host defense mechanism allows for colonization of the introitus and vaginal mucosa in women subject to recurrent bacterial infection from reinfection outside the urinary tract. While colonized, these women can experience repeated infections for 6 to 12 months or more, each readily treated with antibiotics, but recurring within weeks or months. This introital colonization is of limited duration, and may resolve after 1 or 2 years and leave the patient asymptomatic until the next episode of colonization when subsequent bouts of infection begin. In addition, women with recurrent UTIs demonstrate increased adherence of bacteria in vitro to uroepithelial cells when compared to findings in women who have never had an infection. Studies suggest that this may be genetically determined.

Several factors predispose to vaginal colonization and UTI through alteration of the normal vaginal flora. The vaginal microbiome is largely lactobacillus-dominant and has been found to be altered both before and after episodes of acute UTI. Microbiome health may influence not only susceptibility to UTI, but also severity of symptoms and recovery. Disrupting agents include spermicide, harsh cleansers, and antibiotics. The ABO-blood group nonsecretor phenotype is at increased risk for vaginal colonization with uropathogenic bacteria. Low estrogen levels allow vaginal pH to rise, resulting in a higher likelihood of vaginal colonization with *E. coli*. Such factors may be implicated in cases of recurrent UTI in the peri- and postmenopausal women and during lactation. Conversely, the use of oral contraceptive agents is unrelated. Personal hygiene habits are not generally related to recurrent UTI, and it is wise to assure patients that this represents a biologic phenomenon rather than a result of poor cleanliness.

DIFFERENTIAL DIAGNOSIS: SIGNS AND SYMPTOMS, DIAGNOSTIC STUDIES

The history is a critical component in the diagnosis of UTI. The diagnosis is often made on history alone. The probability of bacterial cystitis in a woman with dysuria, urinary frequency, or gross hematuria is about 50% in the primary care setting. Urethritis and vaginitis can also cause acute dysuria in women. Cystitis is usually caused by enteric gram-negative bacilli or *S. saprophyticus*. Urethritis is caused by *Chlamydia trachomatis*, *Neisseria gonorrhoeae*, or herpes simplex virus. Vaginitis is caused by *Candida* species or *Trichomonas vaginalis*. Pyuria is rare in vaginitis but common in urethritis and cystitis. A positive urine culture is usually present in bacterial cystitis. Symptoms of cystitis are usually severe and more acute than those in urethritis, which can be mild, gradual in onset, and include vaginal discharge.

Symptoms suggesting vaginitis such as vaginal irritation or discharge reduce the likelihood of a diagnosis of cystitis by 20%. Dysuria and frequency in the absence of vaginal discharge raise the probability of acute UTI to 90%. If the woman has a history of culture-documented bacterial cystitis and experiences similar symptoms, the chance of a true infection approaches 90%.

Urologic investigation is not routinely indicated in women with isolated episodes of acute urinary frequency, dysuria, and urgency suggestive of lower UTI. Diagnosis is often empiric; however, a urinalysis and/or culture can provide helpful documentation of the true diagnosis and responsible organism (Table 3.1). Examination of urine sediment after centrifugation will show microscopic bacteriuria in more than 90% of infections. Pyuria will be seen in 80% to 95% of infections, and microhematuria in about 50%. False positive urinalyses are commonly caused by normal vaginal flora appearing to be gram-negative bacteria on urinalysis, and pyuria that can be the result of a variety of other inflammatory conditions of the urinary tract. Alternatively, a false negative urinalysis is commonly the result of urinary dilution from a high fluid intake in the symptomatic patient and frequent voiding, which prevents the bacteria in the bladder from multiplying to the high counts commonly associated with UTI. A meta-analysis suggests that urine dipstick findings of nitrituria increase the odds of a positive culture by a factor of 11, whereas

TABLE 3.1 Diagnosis of UTI

Test	Sensitivity	Specificity
Pyuria	95%	71%
Bacteriuria	40%–70%	85%–95%
Dipstick nitrite + or leukocyte esterase + midstream clean-catch pure culture	75%	82%
Greater than 100,000 bacteria/mL	50%	80%
Greater than 1,000 bacteria/mL	70%–90%	High if dysuria

UTI, Urinary tract infection.

A positive dipstick (nitrite or leukocyte esterase positive) indicates that the likelihood of infection is 25% higher than the pretest probability. A negative test indicates that it is 25% lower. A positive dipstick in the setting of consistent symptoms suggests treatment can be instituted without urine culture, provided there is an absence of factors associated with upper tract or complicated infection. A negative dipstick does not rule out infection when the pretest likelihood is high, and a urine culture in necessary in this situation. Culture is also critical in patients who do not respond to standard or initial therapy for UTI.

(Adapted from Fihn SD. Acute uncomplicated urinary tract infection in women. *NEJM*. 2003;349:259-266.)

a dipstick finding of leukocyte esterase increases the likelihood of a culture documented infection by a factor of over 3.

If a urine culture is performed, it should be a carefully collected, midstream specimen to decrease the likelihood of any vaginal contamination. While the cutoff for clinically significant bacteriuria has traditionally been 10^5 colony forming units (CFU)/mL, this standard was published over 60 years ago based on a study comparing bacteriuria between clean and catheterized specimens in asymptomatic individuals. Approximately one-third of women with acute symptomatic cystitis caused by *E. coli*, *S. saprophyticus*, or *Proteus* sp. have colony counts of midstream urine specimens ranging from 10^2 to 10^4 CFU/mL. Thus, a positive culture in the presence of symptoms must be considered significant, regardless of colony count.

Clues in the history that may suggest an increased risk of complicated UTI include childhood bladder or kidney infections, previous urologic surgery or instrumentation, an unusual causative organism, urolithiasis, or the presence of diabetes. If hematuria is noted, the physician is obligated to be sure that it is no longer present after treatment of infection. If it persists, a urologic imaging study and cystoscopy are necessary to rule out other urologic pathology. If a complicated UTI is suspected by history, a similar evaluation may be required.

Additional studies and/or imaging should be considered in the following situations:

1. Women with febrile infections
2. Men
3. If urinary tract obstruction and/or urinary stasis is suspected due to a history of:
   a. Urinary tract calculi
   b. Urinary tract malignancy
   c. Ureteral stricture
   d. Congenital ureteropelvic junction obstruction or anomalies of the urinary tract (e.g., horseshoe kidney, atrophic kidneys, ureterocele)
   e. Previous urologic surgery or instrumentation
   f. Diabetes or neurologic disease
4. Persistent symptoms despite several days of appropriate antibiotic therapy
5. Persistence or rapid recurrence of infection after apparently successful treatment.

Ultrasonography is an excellent initial screening test when imaging is indicated. It is noninvasive, does not cause radiation exposure, does not risk contrast reaction, and is generally readily available. It can identify stones of moderate size, obstruction of the urinary tract, abscess, bladder dilation, and many congenital abnormalities. Bladder scanners provide a noninvasive method of assessing emptying function of the bladder. Computed tomography (CT) and magnetic resonance imaging (MRI) provide the best anatomic data on the site, cause, and extent of infection. **The key point to remember is that in the vast majority of symptomatic lower UTIs, imaging does not have a role to play in diagnosis or treatment.**

THERAPY: GENERAL CONSIDERATIONS

The management of UTIs is complicated by the increasing prevalence of antibiotic-resistant strains of *E. coli* and other common uropathogens. In the past, antibiotic resistance had been a problem only in the management of complicated nosocomial urinary infections. This resistance has now spread to uncomplicated community-acquired UTIs. In many countries, the resistance of

E. coli for trimethoprim has already exceeded the threshold for empiric therapy of 20%, and resistance for fluoroquinolones is also rising, approaching 30% in urologic populations. Ampicillin resistance rates are among the highest, and ampicillin is not recommended for empiric therapy. Of course, once cultures are obtained, and/or if therapy is initiated after sensitivity data are available, the least expensive and most limited-spectrum antibiotic with appropriate sensitivities would be preferred. Resistance development tends to be very local and follow usage patterns. Therefore, it is helpful to know the patterns of microbial resistance in your city and even in your hospital and surrounding outpatient clinics in order to make an informed decision on empiric therapy.

Persistent symptoms following treatment for UTI necessitate urine culture and sensitivity testing prior to prescribing additional antibiotics. Additional treatment should be guided based on initial and repeat culture results. In the absence of persistent symptoms, test of cure culturing is generally not recommended. Furthermore, urine levels of antibiotic are much more important than serum levels in determining efficacy for treating UTI, and many antibiotics that appear to be poor choices based on sensitivity data relating to serum levels may eradicate UTI when administered because of high urinary excretion rates. Table 3.2 offers a guide to choosing an antimicrobial for specific UTI circumstances.

UNCOMPLICATED ISOLATED CYSTITIS

Multiple randomized controlled trials have demonstrated that treating acute cystitis with antibiotics offers mildly faster improvement in symptoms compared to placebo. However, antibiotic treatment remains common practice due in part to a small risk of progression to pyelonephritis without treatment. Treatment of isolated cystitis is often empirical and not based on culture data. A drug should be chosen based on the following criteria:

1. The relative likelihood that it will be active against enteric bacteria that commonly produce UTIs.
2. Ability to achieve high concentrations in the urine.
3. Tendency not to alter the bowel or vaginal flora or to select for resistant bacteria.
4. Limited toxicity.
5. Availability at reasonable cost to the patient.

TABLE 3.2 Guide to antimicrobial choice for UTI in women

First line (uncomplicated lower UTI)	Nitrofurantoin 100 mg BID × 5 days[a] TMP-SMX 160/800 mg BID × 3 days[b] Fosfomycin 3 gm × 1[a,c]
If allergies to above	Fluoroquinolone × 3 days[d] Beta lactams × 3–7 days[c,e]
One-time postcoital prophylaxis	TMP-SMX 40/200 mg or 80/400 mg Nitrofurantoin 50–100 mg Cephalexin 250 mg
Continuous prophylaxis	TMP 100 mg daily TMP-SMX 40/200 mg daily or 3 times a week Nitrofurantoin 50–100 mg daily Cephalexin 125–250 mg daily Fosfomycin 3 gm every 10 days
Suspected pyelonephritis (outpatient) IV/IM agents	CTX 1 gm × 1 Aminoglycoside consolidated 24h dose Ciprofloxacin 500 mg BID × 7 days[f], ± initial 400 mg IV dose
PO agents	Ciprofloxacin 1000 mg ER daily × 7 days Levofloxacin 750 mg daily × 5 days TMP-SMX 160/800 mg BID × 14 days[g] Beta lactams × 10–14 days[c] + initial IV agent
Suspected pyelonephritis (inpatient)	Fluoroquinolone Aminoglycoside ± ampicillin ES cephalosporin ± aminoglycoside ES penicillin ± aminoglycoside Carbapenem

BID, Twice daily; *CTX*, ceftriaxone; *ER*, extended release; *ES*, extended spectrum; *gm*, gram; *IM*, intramuscular; *IV*, intravenous; *mg*, milligram; *PO*, by mouth; *TMP-SMX*, trimethoprim-sulfamethoxazole; *UTI*, urinary tract infection.

[a]Avoid if pyelo suspected.

[b]Avoid if local resistance > 20% or if used for UTI in past 3 months.

[c]Lower efficacy than some other recommended agents.

[d]Resistance high in some areas.

[e]Avoid ampicillin or amoxicillin alone.

[f]Avoid if local resistance > 10%.

[g]If susceptibility unknown, give initial IV agent.

(Adapted from Figure 1 from Gupta, K., et al. International clinical practice guidelines for the treatment of acute uncomplicated cystitis and pyelonephritis in women: A 2010 update by the Infectious Diseases Society of America and the European Society for Microbiology and Infectious Diseases. *Clin Infect Dis*. 2011;52(5):e103-20. Additional information incorporated from Anger, J., et al. Recurrent Uncomplicated Urinary Tract Infections in Women: AUA/CUA/SUFU Guideline. *J Urol*. 2019;202(2):282-289.)

Because organisms causing isolated UTI in the community are generally pansensitive to antibiotics, cost and convenience are major factors in drug selection. First-line agents for the treatment of uncomplicated lower UTI have been established using the above considerations by the Infectious Diseases Society of America (IDSA). These include trimethoprim-sulfamethoxazole (TMP-SMX) (3 days), nitrofurantoin (5 days), and fosfomycin (single dose). In the vast majority of cases, these options will prove to be adequate to treat the infection, will be much less expensive for the patient, and will result in less chance of community bacteria acquiring resistance to powerful alternative antibiotics that can be lifesaving when used in appropriate situations.

Nonsteroidal antiinflammatory drugs (NSAIDs) have shown some promise compared to antibiotics for the treatment of uncomplicated UTIs in a few randomized controlled trials. While their efficacy in symptom management compared to antibiotics is debatable, they appear to decrease short-term UTI recurrence and antibiotic use in a few studies (see Suggested Readings). However, Kronenberg et al. showed a significantly higher risk of pyelonephritis (5% vs. 0%). Given risks and benefits of both agents, further research is warranted to clarify the role of NSAIDs as a stand-alone agent or in conjunction with antibiotics for treating uncomplicated UTIs.

RECURRENT URINARY TRACT INFECTION

After confirming a diagnosis of rUTI—at least two culture-positive, distinct UTIs in 6 months or at least three in one year—a thorough history and physical exam is critical in order to identify any complicating factors that may warrant additional testing. These are listed in the accompanying management algorithm (Fig. 3.1). Culture history, including cultures obtained in the setting of persistent symptoms after treatment, can help differentiate reinfection from a site outside the urinary tract from reinfection from a site of bacterial persistence within the urinary tract. The former accounts for over 95% of cases of rUTI. In the latter case, sterilization of the urine based on culture is short-lived, and within weeks, a relapse with the identical organism occurs. Infections in the setting of bacterial persistence may indicate a site of persistent infection within the urinary tract that could be a manifestation of an infected staghorn calculus,

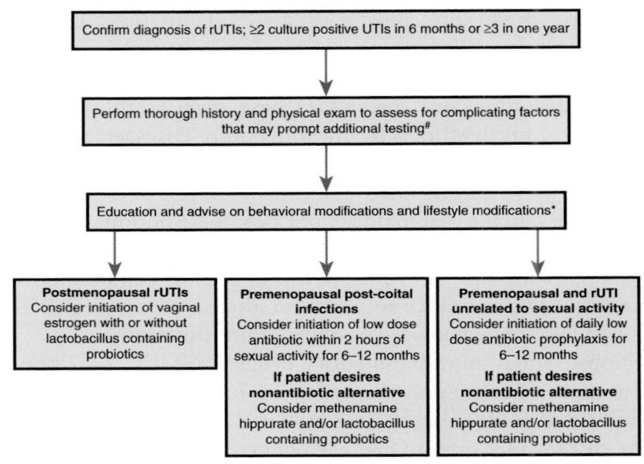

Antibiotic choice should take into account patient's prior organism identification and susceptibility profile, drug allergies, and antibiotic stewardship. Nitrofurantoin 50 mg, trimethoprim-sulfamethoxazole 40/200 mg, trimethoprim 100 mg are preferred over fluoroquinolones and/or cephalosporins. Rotating antibiotics at 3-month intervals can be considered to avoid selection of antimicrobial resistance.

Complicating factors include: Congenital abnormalities of urinary tract, spinal cord injury, transplant recipients, neurogenic bladder, immunosuppression, chemotherapy, nephrolithiasis or recent surgery

* Behavioral/lifestyle modifications include: Controlling blood glucose in diabetics, avoiding disruption of normal vaginal flora with spermicides and/ or harsh cleansers, avoiding prolonged antibiotic courses (>5 days), broad spectrum or unnecessary antibiotics, maintaining adequate hydration, voiding after intercourse, avoiding prolonged holding of urine, and avoiding sequential anal and vaginal intercourse.

FIGURE 3.1 A clinical algorithm for prevention of recurrent urinary tract infections *(rUTIs)* in women. (Reprinted with permission from Smith AL et al. Treatment and prevention of recurrent lower urinary tract infections in women: A rapid review with practice recommendations. *J Urol.* 2018 Dec;200(6):1174-1191.)

enterovesical fistula, or infected anatomic anomaly such as a diverticulum in the urinary tract.

A pelvic examination is needed to evaluate for purulent discharge or abscess in the vagina, periurethral fullness suggestive of urethral diverticulum or cyst, foreign body in the vagina from prior surgery or birth control method, and vaginal atrophy. Workup may include a bedside bladder scan to assess for low postvoid residual urine. If the patient's history elicits risk factors for anatomic abnormalities of the urinary tract or review of culture data demonstrates persistence of the same pathologic organism, a renal and bladder ultrasound can be obtained to confirm normal anatomy, exclude moderate-to-large-sized stones, and assess for hydronephrosis. Cystoscopy should be reserved for those patients where there is suspicion of a fistula, foreign body from prior surgery (e.g., infected suture, mesh), or voiding dysfunction that may be related to functional or anatomic obstruction.

Once it is clear that the patient's problem represents recurrent cystitis from reinfection from a site outside the urinary tract, usually gram-negative introital colonization, one can discuss treatment strategies with the patient. The patient should be reassured that the problem is largely one of controlling the symptoms, and is not a threat to their urologic health. It is a treatable nuisance that most patients can manage on their own without numerous visits to physicians' offices.

Treatment for acute cystitis episodes in patients with a history of rUTI should be based on available culture data. Culture-directed rather than empiric therapy for rUTI is associated with both fewer UTI-related hospitalizations and lower rates of intravenous antibiotic use, thus emphasizing the importance of obtaining urine cultures prior to initiation of therapy in these individuals. Antibiotics can be offered after cultures are obtained and can be based on results of the prior culture until the new data are available. Importantly, ASB should not be treated in patients with rUTI, as this practice predisposes to additional episodes of symptomatic cystitis, antibiotic resistance, pyelonephritis, and poorer quality of life. The exception to this rule is when the patient is undergoing a procedure or surgery on the urinary tract, in which case the urine should be sterilized prior.

Behavioral strategies for rUTI prevention with supporting indirect data include avoiding disturbance of normal vaginal flora with harsh cleansers; avoiding antibiotics that are unnecessary, broad-spectrum, or prescribed for a prolonged course, as such practices may be associated with the disruption of vaginal and periurethral microbiota and subsequent increases in rUTI; and controlling blood glucose in diabetic patients. Despite limited evidence to support their recommendation, local hygiene practices are generally advised since they make intuitive sense and cause no harm to the patient. Such practices include maintaining adequate hydration, avoiding prolonged holding of urine, voiding after intercourse, and refraining from sequential anal and vaginal intercourse.

Cranberry has been used as a folk remedy to prevent rUTI for many years. In the 1920s it was thought the mechanism was urinary acidification. Sixty years later, cranberry was found to interfere with the attachment of bacteria to uroepithelial cells. Despite its historical use and theoretical benefits, there is insufficient clinical evidence that cranberry prevents rUTI. A recent Cochrane review recommended against using cranberry juice for this purpose and advised standardizing the active ingredient in different cranberry products for future research. The AUA-SUFU guidelines, however, make a conditional recommendation that clinicians may offer cranberry prophylaxis to women with rUTIs, concluding that it carries little risk apart from high sugar content limiting use in diabetic patients.

Methenamine hippurate has also been used to prevent rUTI because of its bacteriostatic properties. It is absorbed from the gut and passes into the urine where it releases the chemical formaldehyde if the urine is acidic. It is administered (1 gm twice daily) with vitamin C to acidify the urine. Formaldehyde causes the breakdown of proteins essential to the bacteria, which ultimately results in their death. A Cochrane Review found weak evidence supporting the use of methenamine hippurate in preventing rUTIs and concluded that the adverse event rate was low. The authors support the usage of methanamine hippurate in select patients with rUTI, including those who harbor residual urine which allows the medication to release formaldehyde and keeps bladder urine colony counts low, thus decreasing incidence of symptomatic infection. It is an ideal drug for patients on intermittent catheterization who present with recurrent symptomatic UTI. It may also be helpful in other women by reducing antibiotic use through placebo effect, reduction of bacterial load, and therefore reducing intensity or duration of symptoms allowing avoidance of antibiotic, or by truly decreasing infection rates. While further studies are needed to justify cost, side effects are low. It is best to sterilize the urine with an appropriate antibiotic before initiating prevention therapy.

Meta-analyses support 6 to 12 months of antimicrobial prophylaxis for rUTI, although the quality of existing studies is fair to poor. Furthermore, antimicrobial prophylaxis in general does not appear to show long-term improvement in the rates of rUTI and is associated with multiple adverse events in high-powered studies, including nausea, vomiting, diarrhea, vaginal candidiasis, and skin rashes. Intermittent antibiotic use has therefore been employed to decrease such adverse events as well as antimicrobial resistance. "Self-start" therapy involves patients starting antibiotics at the onset of urinary symptoms, presuming that symptom episodes in the past have been confirmed to be infectious by culture. Self-start therapy has been shown to be less effective than daily prophylaxis but can be considered in patients who can reliably obtain urine samples for culture prior to initiating therapy. Alternatively, in sexually active women, low dose antimicrobial therapy immediately after intercourse appears to be equally effective as daily prophylaxis. Thus, prophylaxis upon experiencing conditions that predispose to UTI may be preferred over starting therapy after the onset of symptoms. In addition, per AUA-SUFU guidelines, rUTI patients experiencing an episode of acute cystitis should be treated with as short of a course of antibiotics as appropriate, generally no more than 7 days. No evidence exists to support increasing dosing, broadening coverage, or extending the course of coverage in rUTI patients presenting with acute cystitis.

In peri- and postmenopausal women, topical estrogen therapy decreases rUTIs by reducing vaginal pH, restoring the lactobacillus-dominant environment, and reducing gram-negative colonization. Topical estrogen does not appear to increase the serum estrogen and subsequent risks of breast cancer recurrence, endometrial hyperplasia, or endometrial carcinoma. It is, however, associated with vaginal irritation and poor patient adherence possibly due to the aforementioned concerns. Interestingly, systemic estrogen has not been shown to reduce rUTI.

Prevention modalities for rUTI for which there is insufficient supporting evidence include D-mannose, which inhibits bacterial adhesion to urothelial cells; hyaluronic acid, a glycosaminoglycan that restores and protects the urothelium; probiotics, although existing studies are limited by poor quality and variable dosing; acupuncture; and herbal medicine. Based on small trials, a vaginal vaccine (Product B; not commercially available) consisting of 10 uropathogenic bacteria, including six heat-killed strains of *E. coli*, may reduce UTIs in sexually active women younger than 52 years old when given as a booster but not a primary dose. Larger trials are warranted to confirm these findings. An oral vaccine, OM-89 (Uro-Vaxom; available in Europe but not the United States), consists of freeze-dried lysate of 18 strains of *E. coli* and effectively reduces rUTIs for 6 to 12 months compared with placebo based on meta-analyses.

CHOICE OF ANTIBIOTIC

A variety of excellent, inexpensive, first-line antimicrobials can be considered for the treatment of uncomplicated lower UTIs in women. **Nitrofurantoin, while not effective against *Pseudomonas* and *Proteus* species, does cover the vast majority of pathogens encountered, and development of resistance over the last 30 years has not been a problem.** It has high urine levels, a short half-life in the blood, and minimal effect on resident fecal and vaginal flora. It seems ideal for short-term use. It should not be administered to patients with known G6PD deficiency or creatinine clearance below 30 mL/min. A rare pulmonary toxicity limits its use for long-term, low-dose continuous prophylaxis.

Trimethoprim with or without sulfamethoxazole is another widely used and very effective treatment for UTI. While resistance to TMP-SMX has increased in the last decade, this antibiotic is still an appropriate choice if local resistance rates do not exceed 20%, and treatment can be changed if symptoms prove unresponsive or cultures show bacterial resistance. Alone or in combination, these drugs will not eradicate *Enterococcus* and *Pseudomonas* species. They are inexpensive and can clear the vaginal flora of gram-negative uropathogens, although the clinical significance of this is questionable. Skin rashes and gastrointestinal side effects prove the main drawbacks.

Fosfomycin, a naturally occurring antibiotic originally described under the name *phosphomycin* in 1969, is commonly used for UTI in many parts of the world. A single 3-gram dose of fosfomycin trometamol has been recommended for the empiric therapy of uncomplicated cystitis in women. The low level of *E. coli* resistance does not seem to be jeopardized by its high consumption in some areas. In countries where it has been used for many years, about 3% of bacterial pathogens are resistant to fosfomycin, and this percentage has been stable for several years. It gives very high and sustained urinary concentrations that rapidly kill bacteria reducing the opportunity for mutant selection. Availability of the agent and cost can sometimes limit use.

Cephalosporins, as a group, have poor activity against *Enterococcus*. First-generation drugs are reasonable to treat uncomplicated UTI, but the second- and third-generation members of this group should be reserved for culture-documented infections requiring their broader coverage. **Ampicillin and amoxicillin, traditionally regarded as inexpensive first-line therapy, have generally fallen out of favor due to their interference with the fecal flora and the resultant emergence of resistant strains such that these drugs are now ineffective against as many as 30% of common urinary isolates.**

Although the fluoroquinolones have a very broad spectrum of activity against most urinary pathogens, including *Pseudomonas aeruginosa*, their routine use for treatment of uncomplicated UTI is to be avoided. Gram-positive activity is limited, and efficacy against *Enterococcus* is poor. As of 2006, quinolones had surpassed sulfas as the most common class of antibiotics prescribed for isolated outpatient UTI in women. The increasing use of a potentially lifesaving, broad-spectrum antibiotic for what is, in most patients, a "symptomatic nuisance," raised concerns about increases in resistance to this important class of antimicrobials in the future. The question arose as to whether it was better to potentially undertreat 5% to 20% of patients with recurrent UTI with empiric first-line agents, and subsequently change antibiotics after 2 days if needed when culture data became available, than to overtreat the with a quinolone. That question was answered in 2016 when fluoroquinolones lost their indication as first-line agents for lower UTIs. Despite this and their rising rate of resistance, they are still in common use for this indication today. Alarming reports of community-acquired UTIs caused by fluoroquinolones-resistant *E. coli* strains in some parts of the world suggest that we will continue to see an evolution of resistance to these agents just as we have with sulfonamides, ampicillin, oral cephalosporins, and TMP-SMX unless a much more aggressive approach to the control of antimicrobial resistance in taken. The fluoroquinolones remain a valuable class of antibiotic, best restricted to complicated UTIs, pseudomonal infections, or treatment of resistant organisms.

CATHETER-ASSOCIATED URINARY TRACT INFECTION

Patients with an indwelling urethral or suprapubic catheter, on intermittent catheterization, or with a catheter removed in the previous 48 hours may qualify as having a CAUTI if they have signs and/or symptoms compatible with UTI, bacteriuria, and no other identifiable source of infection. Apart from typical cystitis symptoms (i.e., dysuria, frequency, urgency) in patients with recently removed catheters, the 2009 IDSA guidelines for CAUTI also include the following as signs or symptoms of UTI in catheterized patients: fevers, rigors, altered mental status, lethargy, flank pain or costovertebral angle tenderness, pelvic discomfort, and acute hematuria. Patients with spinal cord injury may have autonomic dysreflexia or increased spasticity. Notably, the presence of cloudy or odorous urine alone does not indicate infection.

CAUTI follows formation of a biofilm on both the internal and external catheter surface. The biofilm is protective against antibacterials and also against the host immune response. **Antimicrobial treatment of asymptomatic catheter-acquired infection (colonization) should be discouraged because treatment in the presence of an indwelling catheter is unlikely to sterilize the urinary tract and acts to promote emergence of more resistant organisms, complicating management when subsequent symptomatic infection occurs.** Treatment should be reserved for symptomatic infections only.

The IDSA guidelines recommend 7 days of antimicrobial treatment for patients with CAUTI whose symptoms promptly resolve and 10 to 14 days for those who have a delayed response. Alternatively, patients who are not severely ill may receive 5 days of levofloxacin, and women aged 65 or younger who develop lower UTI symptoms after removal of an indwelling catheter may receive 3 days of antibiotics. If a patient develops a CAUTI and still requires a catheter, and the catheter has been in place for over 2 weeks, then it is appropriate to replace the catheter.

The most effective method for preventing CAUTI is reducing the use of unnecessary urinary catheterization and removing the catheter as soon as clinically appropriate. Intermittent catheterization provides an alternative to both short- and long-term catheterization for reducing CAUTI. Systemic antimicrobial prophylaxis should not be routinely employed given the risk of developing antimicrobial resistance. In addition, there is insufficient evidence to suggest a benefit from routine antimicrobial prophylaxis at the time of catheter placement, removal, or replacement.

ASYMPTOMATIC BACTERIURIA

The 2019 IDSA guidelines for ASB recommend against screening for or treating ASB in healthy, nonpregnant women; patients with diabetes; patients with either short-term or long-term indwelling catheters; patients with spinal cord injury; patients with renal transplants more than 1 month prior; and patients with nonrenal solid organ transplants. For patients with renal transplants within 1 month, and for patients with high-risk neutropenia (absolute neutrophil count <100 cells/mm^3) on prophylactic antimicrobial therapy per current standards of care, there exists insufficient evidence to recommend for or against screening for or treating ASB.

In cognitively and/or functionally impaired elderly patients with bacteriuria, delirium, and no local genitourinary symptoms or systemic signs of infection (fever, hemodynamic instability), the IDSA makes a strong recommendation based on very low-quality evidence to avoid antibiotic treatment and instead assess for other causes of infection and employ careful observation. It is not uncommon for courses of antibiotics to be unsuccessful in long-term management of bacteriuria in this group of patients. Studies suggest that noncatheterized male and female residents with bacteriuria living in nursing homes have no higher frequency of courses of antimicrobial treatment, infections, or hospitalizations than those without persistent bacteriuria. Furthermore, treatment of ASB in the setting of delirium does not appear to improve behavioral scores in older residents in long-term care facilities or mortality in hospitalized patients. Pyuria accompanying ASB is not an indication for antimicrobial treatment. Clearly, symptomatic UTIs in the elderly patient should be appropriately treated. **Otherwise, the routine treatment of ASB in the elderly appears unjustified and is often ineffective.**

Pregnancy merits particular attention with regard to screening for bacteriuria. The prevalence of bacteriuria identified by screening is no higher in pregnant females than nonpregnant females of the same age. However, pregnancy results in physiologic changes that have important implications with regard to ASB and progression of infection. With pregnancy comes an increase in renal size, augmented renal function, hydroureteronephrosis, and anterosuperior displacement of the bladder. The frequency of acute pyelonephritis in pregnant women is significantly higher than in their nonpregnant counterparts. Studies suggest a 20% to 40% incidence of pyelonephritis if ASB is untreated in this population. In addition, bacterial pyelonephritis in pregnancy has been associated with infant prematurity and perinatal mortality. These factors make it prudent to screen for ASB in pregnancy, treat it aggressively, and obtain follow-up cultures. The IDSA guidelines make a weak recommendation for a 4- to 7-day course of antibiotics based on low-quality evidence and conclude that the shortest effective course should be used. If an initial negative screening urine culture is negative, or if a positive culture is treated, there is insufficient evidence for or against repeating screening at a later point during the pregnancy.

Additional considerations must be made for patients undergoing urologic procedures. One should screen for and treat ASB in patients planning to undergo endoscopic procedures given associated mucosal trauma. A short course (1–2 doses) initiated 30 to 60 minutes before the procedure is appropriate. Patients undergoing placement of a penile prosthesis or artificial urinary sphincter should receive standard perioperative prophylaxis, although the IDSA makes a weak recommendation against screening or treatment for ASB in this population based on very low-quality evidence. Although antibiotic prophylaxis at the time of removing indwelling catheters may prevent symptomatic UTI in some patients, it is unclear whether patients with ASB have greater benefit.

Pyelonephritis

Infection of the upper urinary tract including the renal pelvis and kidney parenchyma is referred to as pyelonephritis. Acute pyelonephritis is characterized by acute suppuration accompanied by fever, flank pain, bacteriuria, and pyuria. Repeated attacks of acute pyelonephritis may result in chronic pyelonephritis, characterized by progressive renal scarring that can be asymmetric and involve both the cortex and pelvicalyceal system.

Several potential routes of upper tract infection are:

1. Ascending: Bacteria that reach the renal pelvis gain entry through the collecting ducts at the papillary tips and make their ascent through the collecting tubules. The presence of reflux of urine from the bladder or increased intrapelvic pressures from lower tract obstruction can facilitate upper tract infection, especially in the presence of intrarenal reflux.
2. Hematogenous: This is uncommon but can be a result of *staphylococcus aureus* septicemia or *Candida* in the blood stream.

3. Lymphatic: This is a very unusual form of extension to the renal parenchyma from an intraperitoneal infectious process (i.e., abscess).

CLINICAL PRESENTATION

The classic clinical scenario is the acute onset of fever, chills, and flank pain in a patient with obviously infected urine on urinalysis, subsequently proven on urine culture. One must keep in mind that some patients with flank pain and UTI do not have upper tract infection and that patients can have pyelonephritis in the absence of local or systemic symptoms. A high index of suspicion is required in a patient with one of the known risk factors for pyelonephritis (Box 3.2).

Additional symptoms of acute pyelonephritis may include systemic malaise, nausea, and vomiting. Lower tract symptoms including dysuria and urinary frequency are commonly present. Pyelonephritis can result in sepsis, hypotension, and death, especially in the scenario of infection behind an unrecognized upper tract obstruction.

On physical examination, flank tenderness may be a prominent finding. An infected urine with the presence of large amounts of granular or leukocyte casts in the sediment is also suggestive of the diagnosis. *E. coli* possesses special virulence factors and accounts for 80% of cases of acute pyelonephritis. *Pseudomonas*, *Serratia*, *Enterobacter*, and *Citrobacter* are sometimes identified as causative microorganisms in complex cases with a history of urinary tract instrumentation, nosocomial infection, indwelling catheters, and/or ureteral stents.

Suspect *Proteus* or *Klebsiella* in patients with stone disease. *Proteus mirabilis* and some strains of *Klebsiella* contain the

BOX 3.2 Potential Risk Factors for Pyelonephritis

1. Vesicoureteral reflux
2. Obstruction of the urinary tract (congenital ureteropelvic junction obstruction, stone disease, pregnancy)
3. Genitourinary tract instrumentation
4. Diabetes mellitus
5. Voiding dysfunction6.Age (renal scarring rarely begins in adulthood but is generally related to intrarenal reflux in children)
7. Female gender

enzyme urease, which is capable of splitting urea with the production of ammonia and an alkaline environment. The latter is favorable for precipitation of the salt struvite (magnesium ammonium phosphate). Struvite may form branched calculi that harbor bacteria in the interstices of the stone. These so-called *staghorn calculi* can cause chronic renal infection, abscess, or chronic lower tract infection. The infection is difficult to cure unless the stone itself is removed.

The intravenous urogram may be normal or can show renal enlargement secondary to edema. Focal enlargement must be distinguished from a renal mass or abscess. Inflammation may cause a diminished nephrogram or delayed appearance of the pyelogram on the affected side. One of the most important aspects of any imaging study is to rule out the presence of urolithiasis and/or obstruction, which can lead to a life-threatening situation if not appreciated and relieved. Ultrasound can demonstrate many of the above findings and help to rule out an obstructive process. CT is also useful in some cases, and may show patchy decreased enhancement suggesting focal renal involvement (Figs. 3.2 and 3.3).

COMPLICATIONS

1. **Xanthogranulomatous pyelonephritis** (XGP) is an unusual, often severe, chronic renal infection that destroys the

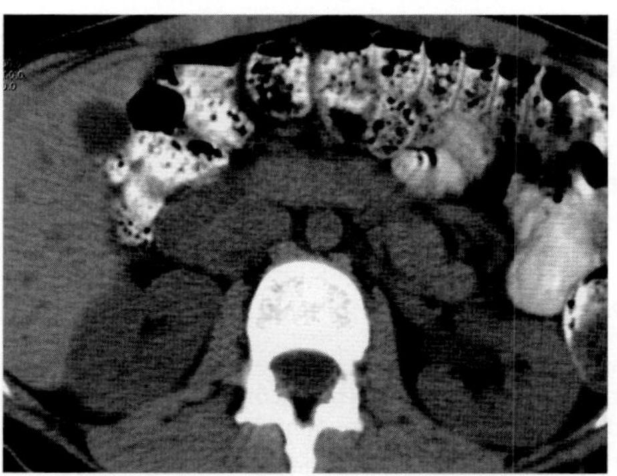

FIGURE 3.2 Acute pyelonephritis in 26-year-old female. Precontrast CT does not help in making diagnosis. *CT,* Computed tomography. (Courtesy Parvi Ramchandani, MD.)

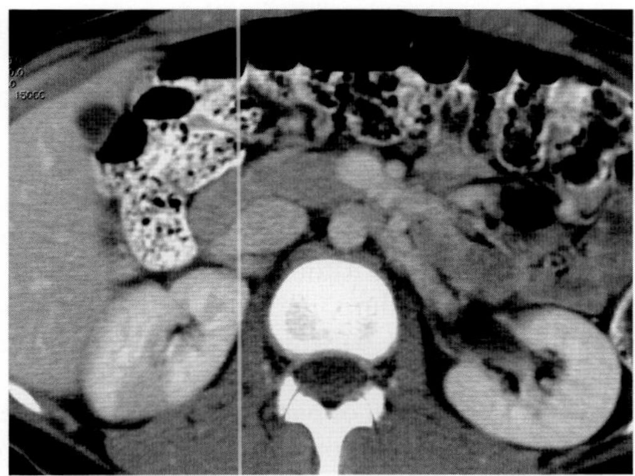

FIGURE 3.3 Postcontrast CT shows patchy decreased enhancement in right kidney. *CT*, Computed tomography. (Courtesy Parvi Ramchandani, MD.)

kidney. It is generally unilateral, associated with obstructing calculi, and results in an enlarged, nonfunctioning kidney that must be differentiated from malignancy. Perirenal fat may be involved with adjacent subcapsular inflammatory response. *Proteus* and *E. coli* are the primary microbes responsible for initiating the inflammatory process. Pathologically, the kidneys consist of yellow-white nodules, pyonephrosis, and hemorrhage. Granulomatous inflammation with lipid-laden macrophages known as *xanthoma cells* is seen histologically. Suspect XGP in the patient with persistent bacteriuria accompanied by flank pain, fever, and chills in the presence of an enlarged, nonfunctioning kidney with a stone or solid mass lesion. CT and ultrasound aid in diagnosis. Treatment is generally nephrectomy, removing the entire inflammatory mass.

2. **Chronic pyelonephritis** is rare in the absence of underlying functional or structural abnormalities of the urinary tract. The symptoms are those of the chronic renal failure it produces, and a history of recurrent acute pyelonephritis may be elicited. Urine cultures may be negative. A localized scar over a deformed calyx is a classic presentation on imaging studies. Pathologically, the kidneys are often diffusely contracted,

scarred, and pitted. Histologically, periglomerular fibrosis is common in conjunction with atrophied tubules.

3. **Renal insufficiency** is a rare complication of acute pyelonephritis.
4. **Hypertension** is noted in over 50% of patients with chronic pyelonephritis. This may be due to fibrosis of the renal parenchyma with resulting ischemia and secondary activation of the renin-angiotensin system. Although hypertension can accelerate progressive renal failure, the fact that nephrectomy cures hypertension in selected patients suggests that the reverse is also true.
5. **Renal abscess,** a collection of purulent material confined to the renal parenchyma, may follow insufficient treatment of focal bacterial nephritis (lobar nephronia). Diagnosis is with CT and ultrasound. Needle aspiration and drainage of the abscess and prolonged antibiotic treatment often preclude the need for surgical drainage.
6. **Infected hydronephrosis** denotes the bacterial infection of a hydronephrotic kidney. When associated with suppurative destruction of renal parenchyma, the term *pyonephrosis* is used. Ultrasound and CT can usually make the diagnosis, and emergent drainage is required, usually by ureteral catheter or percutaneous catheter placement, until definitive relief of the obstruction is attempted.
7. **Perinephric abscess** can result from rupture of a cortical abscess or hematogenous seeding from another infected site. The primary treatment is drainage.
8. **Emphysematous pyelonephritis** is an acute necrotizing parenchymal and perirenal infection caused by gas-forming uropathogens. Diabetic patients are at increased risk. Complicating factors can include urinary tract obstruction secondary to calculi or sloughed necrotic papillae. Women are affected more commonly than men. Fever, vomiting, and flank pain constitute the classic triad of symptoms. The diagnosis is established by the finding on plain x-ray, CT, or ultrasound of intrarenal parenchymal gas. The disease can be fatal, and aggressive percutaneous renal and perirenal drainage or immediate nephrectomy, in combination with appropriate antibiotics, is critical. Most cases are associated with *E. coli*, though *Proteus*, *Klebsiella*, and *Candida albicans* can be responsible pathogens.

MANAGEMENT (FIG. 3.4)

Acute pyelonephritis can be managed on an outpatient basis with oral antibiotics in the patient who is not septic and does not suffer from nausea and vomiting. Fluoroquinolone is a good choice pending culture results. Many physicians administer a single parenteral dose of ceftriaxone, gentamicin, or a fluoroquinolone before initiating oral therapy.

Dehydration, vomiting, or sepsis may require hospitalization and parenteral administration of antibiotics (Box 3.3). A parenteral fluoroquinolone, a combination of ampicillin and gentamicin, or an extended-spectrum cephalosporin with or without an

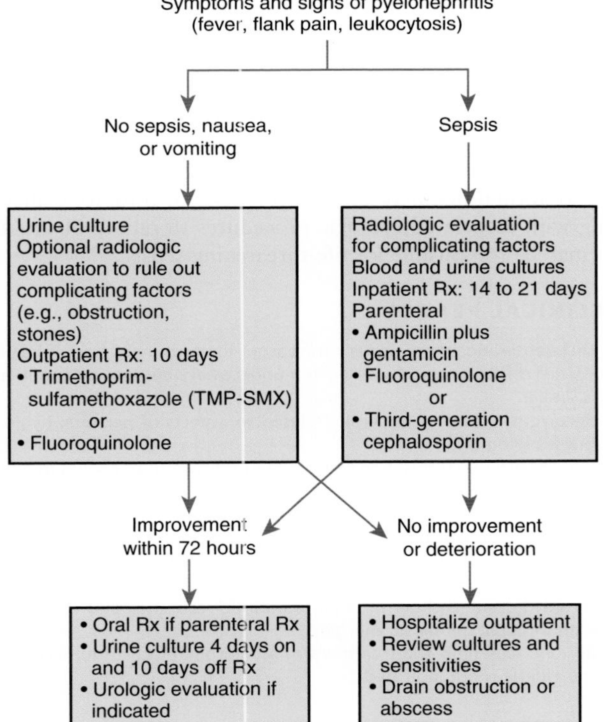

FIGURE 3.4 Management of acute pyelonephritis. (From Schaeffer AJ, Schaeffer EM. Infections of the urinary tract. In: Wein AJ, Kavoussi LR, Novick AC, et al., eds. *Campbell-Walsh Urology*. 10th ed. Philadelphia: Saunders; 2012.)

BOX 3.3 Guidelines for Parenteral Treatment of Pyelonephritis

1. Clinical severity of infection, suspected urosepsis
2. Presence of underlying anatomical urinary tract abnormality
3. Inadequate access to follow-up care
4. Renal failure
5. Presence of urinary tract obstruction (infection behind an obstruction can be a lethal combination)
6. Immunocompromised and/or elderly host
7. Failed outpatient management on oral antimicrobials

aminoglycoside is recommended. Antibiotics should be administered parenterally until the patient is afebrile. They can then be switched to oral therapy. In the pregnant patient, ceftriaxone, aztreonam, or a combination of ampicillin and gentamicin can be administered with conversion to an oral cephalosporin when the patient is afebrile.

Therapy for uncomplicated pyelonephritis is generally recommended for 10 days, and a full 2-week course is recommended for those who present with sepsis. Complicated infection associated with hospitalization, catheterization, urologic surgery, or urinary tract abnormalities may require 3 weeks of antibiotic therapy along with associated urologic procedures to relieve obstruction that may be responsible for life-threatening sepsis.

CLINICAL PEARLS

1. Differentiating upper urinary tract from lower urinary tract infection (UTI) is difficult clinically and often unnecessary because management is similar.
2. Recurrent UTI is not generally related to aspects of personal hygiene but is biological in origin.
3. Retroperitoneal ultrasonography is the best overall screening imaging study when investigating UTI.
4. Nitrofurantoin remains an excellent antibiotic for the short-term treatment of recurrent urinary infection but should not be used for long-term prophylaxis because of the slight risk of pulmonary fibrosis.
5. Do not forget fosfomycin as an excellent antibiotic, especially when sensitivity panels show multiple antibiotic resistance and in patients with multiple antibiotic allergies.
6. Routine screening and treatment of asymptomatic bacteriuria (ASB) in the elderly is not indicated.

Additional content, including Self-Assessment Questions and Suggested Readings, may be accessed at www.ExpertConsult.com.

Lower Urinary Tract Infection in Males

Joseph F. Harryhill, MD, MSEd,
Aseem Malhotra, MD, and Hanna Jia, BA

Introduction

INCIDENCE AND EPIDEMIOLOGY

Lower urinary tract infections (UTIs) and nonbacterial inflammatory processes in men can involve the bladder and all parts of the genital tract, primarily the urethra, prostate, epididymis, and testes. Lower UTIs are common, with a lifetime risk of 12%. In the United States alone, UTIs account for over 10 million office visits and 2 to 3 million emergency department visits per year. Rates of UTI are rising, as increasing fluoroquinolone resistance is contributing to decreased antibiotic efficacy and increased rates of "recurrent" UTI. Lower UTIs must be treated appropriately to prevent complications such as upper tract damage, sepsis, and even possible mortality.

Notably, the lower urinary tract and genital systems are openly connected, and infection can spread from one component to another, for example, from prostate to epididymis. This chapter will focus on bacterial cystitis, prostatitis, prostatic abscess, epididymitis, and orchitis.

ETIOLOGY, PATHOPHYSIOLOGY, BACTERIAL ORGANISMS

UTIs are less common in men due to the length of the male urethra, which provides relative protection from ascending pathogens. However, the incidence of UTI after age 50 is similar in men and women. Older men are at higher risk of UTI due to predisposing risk factors such as incomplete emptying from bladder outlet obstruction, voiding dysfunction, bladder diverticula, indwelling urinary catheters, and instrumentation.

The most common pathogens causing UTI are uropathogenic *Escherichia coli*, *Klebsiella pneumoniae*, *Enterococcus* spp., Group B Streptococcus, *Proteus mirabilis*, *Pseudomonas aeruginosa*, *Staphylococcus aureus*, and *Candida* spp. Knowledge of the most common pathogens to cause UTI is critical for appropriate antibiotic choice to improve treatment outcomes.

Bacterial Cystitis

DIAGNOSIS

Cystitis presents as a constellation of symptoms including dysuria, frequency, urgency, suprapubic pain, and/or hematuria. Notably, elderly men may present only with vague symptoms, such as failure to thrive or change in mental status.

Diagnosis begins with a detailed history and physical exam, and is confirmed with urinalysis and urine culture with antimicrobial sensitivities. A false negative urinalysis is possible in early phases of bacterial cystitis. On the other hand, false positives are possible due to contamination when collecting the urine specimen. A clean-catch midstream specimen is the most common collection method for culture, but has a higher contamination rate than urethral catheterization or suprapubic aspiration.

Urinalysis findings in bacterial cystitis include positive dipstick for nitrites (sensitivity of 50%, specificity of >95%), positive leukocyte esterase (sensitivity of approximately 80%, specificity of approximately 75%), and pyuria on microscopy (more than 6–10 WBC per high-powered field). If urine dipstick tests positive for both nitrite and leukocyte esterase, the specificity reaches 98%–100%, but sensitivity declines to under 50%.

Active bacterial infection will usually yield a colony count of greater than 100 colony forming units/mL. If a culture is positive for multiple organisms, contamination should be suspected. Finally, antibiotic sensitivities are reported to help select appropriate antibiotic therapy. Urinary tract instrumentation, hospitalization, and recent treatment with broad-spectrum antibiotics all increase the risk for resistant organisms.

MANAGEMENT

An important role of the urologist is to recognize when a patient with UTI should be admitted to the hospital. The presence of fever, tachycardia, or toxic appearance are indications for admission, and upper tract imaging should be performed to rule out obstruction. Patients may also require admission for management of UTI if they are unable to tolerate liquids, are immunocompromised, or have significant comorbidity, especially diabetes mellitus.

In general, antibiotic treatment for bacterial cystitis should be prescribed for 7 to 10 days. In the outpatient setting, the most commonly prescribed antibiotics are trimethoprim-sulfamethoxazole (TMP-SMX) double strength tablet twice daily, ciprofloxacin 500 mg twice daily, and levofloxacin 250 to 500 mg once daily. For patients with fungal cystitis with *Candida albicans* (more common in diabetics, immunocompromised patients, or those with indwelling urinary catheters), oral fluconazole 50 to 100 mg daily is prescribed for 5 to 7 days.

In men under age 50 who are not sexually active, further workup may be indicated to search for an underlying urinary tract abnormality causing urinary obstruction or stasis. This may include cystoscopy as well as imaging studies to assess the upper tracts and postvoid views of the bladder.

Prostatitis

INCIDENCE

Prostatitis is one of the most common urologic problems for men, occurring in 5% of men between the age of 20 and 50. It is the single most common urologic diagnosis for men less than 50 years of age, and the third most common for men greater than 50 years old.

ETIOLOGY AND RISK FACTORS

The etiology of prostatitis is multifactorial. Risk factors include:

1. Bacteria: same as those causing bacterial cystitis (65%–80% *E. coli*; 10%–15% combination of *Pseudomonas*, *Serratia*, *Klebsiella*, *Enterobacter*)
2. Anatomic abnormalities (intraprostatic ductal reflux into prostate, phimosis)
3. Dysfunctional voiding
4. Iatrogenic (indwelling catheters, transurethral surgery, prostate biopsy)

CLASSIFICATION AND DIAGNOSIS

Prostatitis is a term that encompasses several clinical syndromes, which differ by acuity of inflammation and presence of a bacterial source. They each have different risk factors, differential diagnosis criteria, and treatment modality. The National Institute of Diabetes and Digestive and Kidney Diseases has created the following classification of these clinical syndromes:

Category I: Acute bacterial prostatitis
Category II: Chronic bacterial prostatitis
Category IIIA/IIIB: Chronic nonbacterial prostatitis/chronic pelvic pain syndrome
Category IV: Asymptomatic inflammatory prostatitis

The gold standard for diagnosis is the Meares-Stamey "four-glass test," designed to locate the origin of a lower UTI. The first 10 mL is collected and represents a urethral culture. After voiding 200 mL, the second glass collects midstream urine and represents a bladder culture. At this point, a prostatic massage is performed, and the third glass collects the expressed secretions. The fourth glass collects the next 10 mL of urine after prostate massage, and represents a prostatic culture. In this way, the localization of bacterial flora differentiates an infection as urethritis, cystitis, or prostatitis. However, the Meares-Stamey test has been largely replaced in clinical practice with the pre- and postmassage test (PPMT), or "two-glass test," in which urine is taken before and after prostatic massage. This two-glass test has been shown to have higher sensitivity and specificity than the Meares-Stamey test.

Category I: Acute Bacterial Prostatitis

Many cases of acute bacterial prostatitis occur via spread from the bladder. Therefore, the risk factors, symptoms, and common pathogens for acute bacterial prostatitis overlap significantly with those of bacterial cystitis including indwelling Foley catheters, bladder neck or prostatic urethral obstruction, and instrumentation. Acute bacterial prostatitis less commonly can result from hematogenous or lymphatic spread from distant sources such as the oropharynx, gastrointestinal tract, or respiratory system. Intraprostatic urinary reflux into the ejaculatory and prostatic ducts can also be a risk factor for acute bacterial prostatitis.

Patients often present with dysuria, frequency/urgency, and nocturia, as well as systemic symptoms such as fever/chills and malaise. There may be associated suprapubic, groin, perineal or possibly low back pain. On physical exam, the prostate is enlarged, warm, and boggy, with acute tenderness to palpation. However, the use of digital rectal examination (DRE) should be limited and gentle, as it may increase the risk of bacteremia.

Urinalysis and culture are typically positive and diagnostic in patients with acute bacterial prostatitis. Transrectal ultrasound or cross-sectional imaging can also help with diagnosis and management, especially if prostatic abscess is suspected.

The treatment for acute bacterial prostatitis is antibiotic therapy and supportive care. A 3- to 4-week course of oral fluoroquinolones or TMP-SMX is most commonly used for outpatient therapy, based on sensitivities from the urine culture. Increased hydration should be encouraged. If urinary retention occurs, caution should be used in the decision to insert a urethral catheter; consider placement of a suprapubic cystotomy tube. Acutely ill patients should be admitted for inpatient care with hydration and IV antibiotics.

One rare type of acute infectious prostatitis is granulomatous prostatitis, which may occur in tuberculosis or systemic mycosis, but is more commonly related to use of intravesical bacillus Calmette-Guérin (BCG) therapy for urothelial carcinoma. Typically, urine culture in granulomatous prostatitis will be negative for bacterial pathogens. Tuberculous and mycotic prostatitis should be treated with antitubercular and antifungal therapies, respectively.

PROSTATIC ABSCESS

Clinicians should maintain a high index of suspicion for the possibility of prostate abscess, and consider computed tomography (CT) or magnetic resonance imaging (MRI) of the pelvis in patients who do not respond appropriately to antibiotic therapy for prostatitis and febrile UTIs. Once identified, treatment may require abscess drainage via transurethral unroofing, or percutaneous aspiration/possible drain placement. In the CT shown in Fig. 4.1, a large, well-defined area of low attenuation with an enhancing rim reveals a large prostatic abscess.

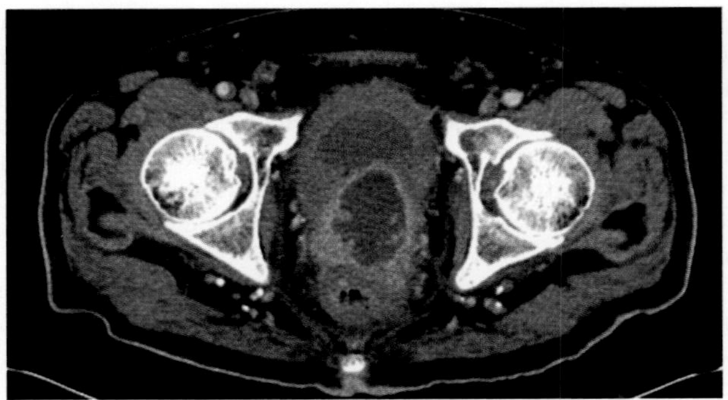

FIGURE 4.1 Axial CT image of large, hypoattenuated prostatic abscess with enhancing rim. *CT*, Computed tomography.

Category II: Chronic Bacterial Prostatitis

The typical presentation for chronic bacterial prostatitis involves recurring episodes of acute UTI with positive urine cultures of the same organism, separated by relatively asymptomatic intervals. This pattern is likely due to persistence of bacteria located deep within the prostate gland, making definitive antibacterial treatment difficult. Bacteria that cause chronic bacterial prostatitis are typically the same as those identified in cases of acute prostatitis.

In contrast to acute infection, diagnosis of chronic bacterial prostatitis requires expression of prostatic fluid, via either the Meares-Stamey "four-glass" test, or the more contemporary PPMT "two-glass" test. The sample is then analyzed for pathogenic bacteria and white blood cells not present in the specimen collected before prostate massage.

Fluoroquinolones are the first-line antibiotic choice for chronic bacterial prostatitis, with a success rate of 50%–75%. Length of treatment should be 4 to 6 weeks if pretreatment cultures are positive, and/or the patient endorses improvement with therapy. The same antibiotic should not be reused if treatment fails. Daily prophylaxis can also be used to prevent recurrent bacteriuria. Alpha blocker therapy should be considered in patients with obstructive voiding symptoms, but evidence supporting its efficacy in the treatment or prevention of prostatitis is mixed.

Category IIIA/IIIB: Chronic Nonbacterial Prostatitis/ Chronic Pelvic Pain Syndrome

The presentation of chronic pelvic pain syndrome (CPPS) differs from chronic bacterial prostatitis (Category II) because symptoms are typically chronic and persistent, compared to the intermittent episodes of acute symptoms seen in chronic bacterial prostatitis. Further, while bacterial prostatitis typically presents with pain as well as symptoms of infection, chronic bacterial prostatitis is characterized by pain alone. Discomfort is nonspecific, and can be described involving the perineum, suprapubic area, penis, groin, and/or testicular area. Lower urinary tract symptoms (LUTS) or sexual dysfunction may also be present, and patients often describe pain during or after ejaculation. The NIH Chronic Prostatitis Symptom Index (NIH-CPSI) was developed to quantify these symptoms and quality of life of patients with CPPS, and is helpful for both accurate diagnosis and tracking response to therapy.

Notably, all of these symptoms are seen in the absence of uropathogenic bacteria. CPPS can then further be divided into the inflammatory subtype (IIIA) and noninflammatory subtype (IIIB), based on the presence or absence of white blood cells in prostate-specific specimens.

The many factors contributing to prostatitis are especially relevant in the pathogenesis of CPPS, but how these factors interact to cause the condition is not fully understood. It is theorized that a bacterial offense may trigger a cascade of inflammatory reactions and immunological responses to lead to a persistence of symptoms. Neurological and psychological factors have also been proposed to impact this multifactorial condition.

In the diagnosis of CPPS, it is critical to rule out other etiologies, such as infection, malignancy, or other reversible causes. Appropriate tests include urine culture and cytology if the patient presents with microscopic or gross hematuria, and urodynamic studies.

Just as the pathogenesis of CPPS is multifactorial, so is the treatment. For patients with the inflammatory subtype (IIIA), treatment can include a 4- to 8-week course of antibiotics, alpha-blockers, antiinflammatory drugs, or immune modulators. For patients with the noninflammatory subtype (IIIB), treatment may include analgesics, muscle relaxants, and alpha-blockers.

Other therapies that can be helpful include biofeedback, relaxation exercises, and pelvic floor physical therapy with myofascial trigger-point release and Thiele massage. Surgical treatment to relieve outlet obstruction, or insertion of neuromodulation devices should be reserved for patients who have an identifiable cause found on urodynamics or cystoscopy.

Category IV: Asymptomatic Inflammatory Prostatitis

This is a diagnosis made when white blood cells are found incidentally on pathology specimens collected for rising prostate specific antigen or abnormal DRE. Because patients are asymptomatic and have no bacterial infection, it requires no treatment.

Epididymitis and Orchitis

EPIDIDYMITIS

Etiology and Risk Factors

Because of the openly connected conduits of the lower urinary tract and genital system, bacteria can migrate in a retrograde manner from the distal urethra, through the ejaculatory duct and vas deferens, and finally to the epididymis, causing acute epididymitis. In patients under the age of 35, the most common pathogens are *Chlamydia trachomatis* and *Neisseria gonorrhoeae*, which are sexually transmitted to the urethra. Enteric bacteria may sometimes also be sexually transmitted in patients who have had anal intercourse. In contrast, coliform bacteria such as *E. coli*, *Klebsiella* species, and *Pseudomonas* are the most common offending pathogens in older patients. In particular, indwelling catheters and urethral instrumentation such as cystoscopy are an important risk factor in the development of epididymitis in elderly patients. Hematogenous spread of bacteria to the epididymis can occur but is rare; also unusual is an inflammatory epididymitis caused by amiodarone, which selectively concentrates in the epididymis and is more often seen when higher doses of the medication are administered.

Diagnosis

Acute epididymitis presents with a tender hemiscrotum and induration on palpation of the epididymis, usually associated with significant swelling. Fever/chills, flank pain, and voiding symptoms may also be associated with acute epididymitis. In addition, inflammation may lead to a reactive hydrocele.

Physical exam findings are notable for pain upon palpation of the testicle (and occasionally the spermatic cord), and relief of pain upon elevation of the testicle (Prehn's sign). The urethral meatus should be inspected for discharge, and the scrotum for presence of an abscess. Urinalysis, urine culture, and urethral swab test or urine-based screening for chlamydia and gonococcus are recommended if sexual transmission is suspected.

Scrotal ultrasound with Doppler should be obtained to rule out other causes of acute scrotal pain, including testicular torsion. Compared to the decreased or absent blood flow to the testicle seen in torsion, Doppler interrogation in acute epididymitis will typically reveal hyperemia of the epididymis and spermatic cord (see Fig. 4.2).

Treatment

Management of acute epididymitis includes antiinflammatory medication, ice and scrotal elevation, as well as appropriate

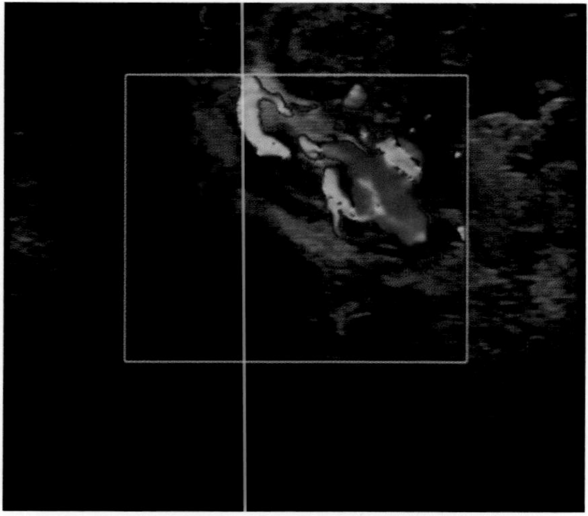

FIGURE 4.2 Acute epididymitis. Doppler ultrasound interrogation of the epididymis shows marked hypervascular appearance.

antibiotic therapy. If a urinary tract pathogen is suspected, a 10- to 14-day course of TMP-SMX or fluoroquinolone is recommended. For *C. trachomatis* or *N. gonorrhoeae* infection, patients should be treated for both with doxycycline (200 mg dose initially, then 100 mg twice daily for 10 days), as well as ceftriaxone (single 250 mg IM injection) or ciprofloxacin (500 mg single dose).

ORCHITIS

Prolonged acute epididymitis may progress to epididymo-orchitis as the infection spreads to the testicle (see Fig. 4.3). Because it is a complication of epididymitis, orchitis has the same presentation, evaluation, and treatment. Progression to orchitis may be more common in patients who are immunocompromised. Surgical intervention, including orchiectomy, may be required if the infected testicle becomes necrotic or develops an abscess.

Pure isolated orchitis without epididymitis is rare, and usually of a viral etiology, such as mumps orchitis. Other infectious causes include mononucleosis, mycobacterium, or fungal sources. These pathogens spread hematogenously to the testicle. Treatment of viral orchitis is supportive, with antiinflammatory medication and analgesics. While mumps orchitis is rare in children under age 10, it can be seen in 20% to 30% of postpubertal men who contract the disease, and can be bilateral. Testicular atrophy may result as a late sequela in adults with mumps orchitis.

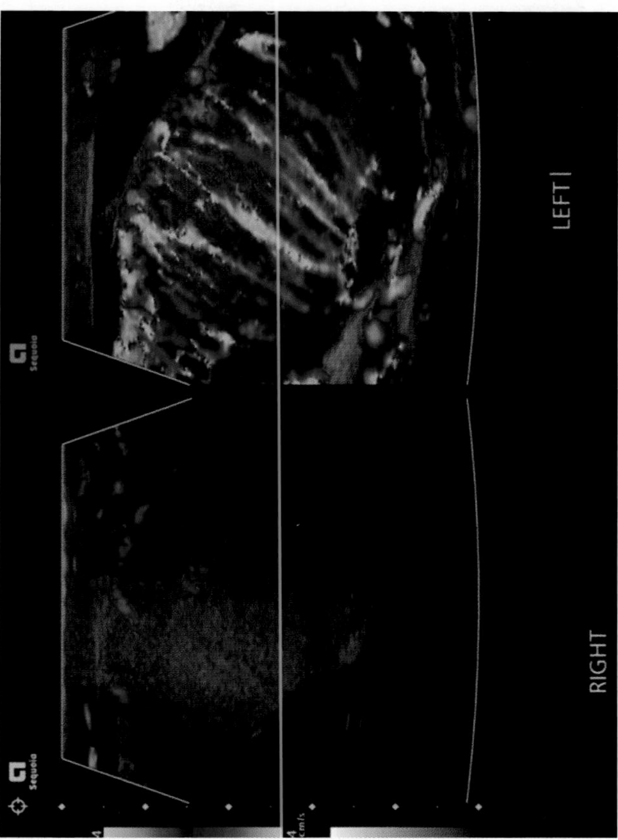

FIGURE 4.3 Orchitis. Hypervascular appearance of left testicle on ultrasound shows progression of epididymitis to include inflammation of the testicle.

Antibiotic Addendum

Antibiotic	Coverage	Indication	Complications
Fluoroquinolones (ciprofloxacin, levofloxacin)	• GNRs (including *Pseudomonas*) • Some GPC	Bacterial cystitis Acute bacterial prostatitis Chronic bacterial prostatitis	• QT prolongation • Tendonitis
TMP-SMX	GPC (including MRSA, Strep)	Bacterial cystitis Acute bacterial prostatitis	• Rash • Stevens-Johnson syndrome (SJS)
Doxycycline	*Chlamydia*	Epididymitis/orchitis	
Ceftriaxone	*Neisseria Gonorrhoeae*	Epididymitis/orchitis	
Rifampin	Active TB treatment regimen		ARV therapy interference
Isoniazid			B6 deficiency
Pyrazinamide			
Ethambutol			• Optic neuritis • Hepatotoxicity
Praziquantel	*Schistosoma haematobium*	Schistosomiasis	
Fluconazole	Antifungal	Fungal UTI	
Amphotericin B	Antifungal	Fungal UTI	
Albendazole	• *Echinococcus granulosus* • *Wuchereria bancrofti*	Hydatid disease Genital filariasis	
Metronidazole	*Entamoeba histolytica*	Amebiasis	

ARV, Antiretroviral; *GRNs*, gram-negative rods; *GPC*, gram-positive cocci; *MRSA*, methicillin-resistant *Staphylococcus aureus*; *TB*, tuberculosis; *TMP-SMX*, trimethoprim-sulfamethoxazole; *UTI*, urinary tract infection.

Specific Infections of the Genitourinary Tract

Joseph F. Harryhill, MD, MSEd, Aseem Malhotra, MD, and Hanna Jia, BA

Genitourinary Tuberculosis

EPIDEMIOLOGY

Tuberculosis (TB), most commonly caused by *Mycobacterium tuberculosis*, is one of mankind's oldest known infections, with signs of TB found in mummies dating back to 3000 BCE. Once known as consumption, the disease reached epidemic proportions in 18th-century Europe. However, it is not just a disease of the past: TB is still a major cause of mortality worldwide. In 2019, the World Health Organization reported 10 million new cases of TB and 1.4 million deaths due to TB. Recently, the global incidence of TB has fallen at a rate of 2% per year since 2015.

Genitourinary tuberculosis (GUTB) is the third most common extrapulmonary site of involvement, comprising 20% of extrapulmonary TB. Active GUTB presents 5 to 25 years after initial infection in 2% to 20% of patients.

PATHOGENESIS

TB spreads very effectively via aerosolized droplets, requiring only a few inhaled bacilli to transmit the disease. Once inhaled, host immunity determines whether the bacteria is eliminated early; if not, the bacilli reside within alveolar macrophages and can then spread hematogenously within a few weeks. Among individuals exposed to TB, 5%–10% will develop active disease, and immunocompromised patients are at increased risk. In fact, human immunodeficiency virus (HIV) is the greatest identifiable risk factor for progression to active disease from latent infection, with TB causing one-quarter of deaths globally in patients with HIV.

During primary infection, lymphocytes and fibroblasts aggregate to form a granuloma around the bacilli and prevent further spread of infection. However, organisms may remain viable and become dormant within the tubercle, resulting in latent disease. These sites may then reactivate due to weakening of host immunity, which can be caused by diabetes, HIV, malignancy, chemotherapy, or immunosuppressant medications. TB can then spread by caseation and cavitation, sometimes after many years of dormancy.

One common primary site of hematogenous spread is the kidney, particularly the renal cortex, due to the high oxygen availability. Tubercles in the glomeruli can cause parenchymal destruction, allowing bacilli to spread into the medulla, which has a hypertonic environment that impairs phagocytic function. Papillary necrosis then allows infection to spread into the urine and travel down the ureters to the bladder. Fibrosis caused by infection can result in ureteropelvic junction obstruction, ureteral stricture, and bladder inflammation and contracture.

Other genitourinary structures (prostate, seminal vesicles, vas deferens, epididymis, testicle) may then become infected via direct extension, with passage of infected urine into the genital ducts, or even by direct hematogenous seeding.

Of note, use of intravesical bacillus Calmette-Guérin (BCG) therapy for urothelial carcinoma, which involves instillation of live attenuated bacilli, has been shown to cause granulomatous prostatitis and, rarely, miliary TB. Patients with granulomatous prostatitis secondary to intravesical BCG may present with a rise in serum prostate specific antigen (PSA) level, or palpable nodularity of the prostate on digital rectal examination.

PRESENTATION AND DIAGNOSIS

GUTB has varied presentations, but patients most commonly report irritative voiding symptoms (50%), which can persist despite antibiotic therapy. Up to one-third of patients may experience either hematuria or flank pain.

Symptomatic GUTB is more common in men (2:1), with the earliest signs of infection typically tuberculous epididymitis or cystitis. However, female GUTB can present as infertility, nonspecific pelvic pain, or menstrual alterations. Ninety-five percent of these women have fallopian tube involvement, from which TB can spread to the peritoneum.

Definitive diagnosis requires demonstration of mycobacterial organisms in urine culture or histopathologic examination of a biopsied granulomatous lesion. Because excretion of the TB organisms can be sporadic, a majority of those infected will have sterile pyuria; 20% of patients may have superimposed bacterial infections. Therefore, three to six early-morning urine specimens are preferred for acid-fast staining and culture. While acid-fast staining is 97% specific, the gold standard is incubation of urine cultures that require up to 6 to 8 weeks for definitive diagnosis and antibiotic sensitivity.

While awaiting culture results, polymerase chain reaction (PCR)–based nucleic acid amplification test (NAAT) of the urine provides rapid results that are reliable and specific, with a 10% false negative rate. However, these results should be correlated with clinical symptoms and confirmed by culture for definitive diagnosis. The Mantoux PPD (purified protein derivative) tuberculin skin test is also a helpful test when positive, while a negative TB tine test makes the diagnosis unlikely.

Imaging in GUTB shows nonspecific findings, but is important to evaluate the extent of disease. Plain radiographs may show calcification in the urinary tract, and 50%–75% of chest x-rays will indicate evidence of pulmonary disease. In addition, intravenous pyelogram (IVP) or computed tomography (CT) urography can show renal parenchymal destruction and obstruction. CT imaging can also identify adrenal involvement, which occurs in 5% of active TB cases.

Cystoscopy yields nonspecific findings, but is useful to rule out malignancy. However, bladder biopsy should be considered carefully as this can cause dissemination of TB if the patient is not on antituberculous therapy.

MANAGEMENT

If there is suspicion for GUTB, an infectious disease consult and notification of the Department of Public Health should be considered during the diagnostic workup.

After GUTB is confirmed, chemotherapy should be started promptly. Early intervention with antituberculosis chemotherapy offers the best prognosis for successful treatment. Standard chemotherapy involves 1 to 2 months of four antimicrobial agents, typically isoniazid, rifampin, pyrazinamide, and ethambutol, followed by another 7 months of rifampin and isoniazid.

Knowledge of side effects related to antituberculosis therapy is essential. Isoniazid should be taken with pyridoxine (vitamin B6, 10–50 mg daily) to prevent central nervous system (CNS) effects and peripheral neuropathy. In HIV patients, rifampin may interfere with antiretroviral therapy, and can be replaced with rifabutin. Because ethambutol can cause optic neuritis, patients should receive a baseline ophthalmology evaluation before treatment.

Alternatively, multidrug-resistant TB is treated with second-line agents, including aminoglycosides, cycloserine, ethionamide, fluoroquinolones, aminosalicylic acid, and prothionamide.

The use of multiple drugs has been shown to provide synergistic benefit and prevent drug resistance. Due to the importance of medication compliance, supervised administration of medications is recommended.

At 3, 6, and 12 months after completion of chemotherapy, reevaluation with cultures and appropriate imaging studies is recommended. Surgery may be necessary for treatment of obstruction or resection of infected, nonfunctioning tissue, but should be deferred for 4 to 6 weeks after starting chemotherapy.

Genitourinary Schistosomiasis

EPIDEMIOLOGY

Schistosomiasis (also known as *bilharzia disease*), caused by the parasitic trematode *Schistosoma*, affects an estimated 300 million people worldwide. While there are four species of *Schistosoma* that can cause infection in humans, genitourinary schistosomiasis is caused by *Schistosoma hematobium*, with paired adult worms residing in the perivesical venules.

The *Schistosoma* trematodes use freshwater snails as intermediate hosts, which then release the trematodes into fresh water. These snails are not found in the United States; genitourinary schistosomiasis is endemic to Africa and the Middle East.

PATHOGENESIS

Schistosoma larvae in fresh water penetrate the skin or mucous membranes, then travel through the venous and lymphatic vessels and settle into the pelvic perivesical veins as pairs of adult male and female worms, of about 1 to 2 cm in length. The female worm then releases 200 to 300 eggs per day into the submucosa of the bladder, causing an intense inflammatory reaction. The bladder develops

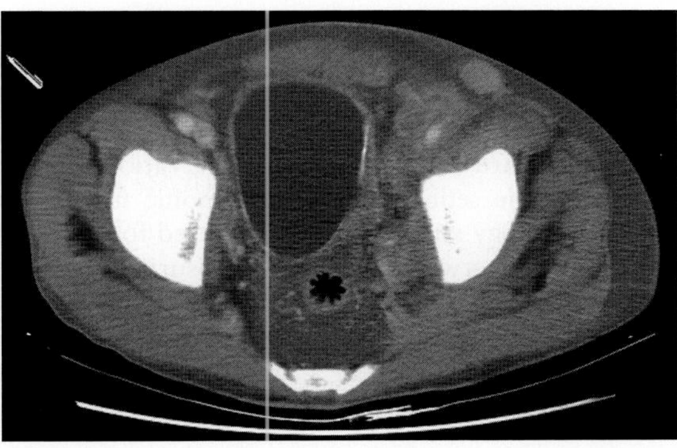

FIGURE 5.1 Submucosal bladder calcification seen on CT in patient with known history of urinary schistosomiasis. *CT,* Computed tomography. (Courtesy Parvati Ramchandani, MD, University of Pennsylvania.)

sandy "patches" of eggs, some of which are excreted in the urine, thus completing the *Schistosoma* life cycle by returning to fresh water and the intermediate snail host. Over the course of years of active infection, these patches can become calcified (see Fig. 5.1).

PRESENTATION AND DIAGNOSIS

Initial contact with *Schistosoma* can produce an intense pruritus due to an allergic reaction to the larval trematode. If the larvae are able to penetrate the skin and enter the circulation, patients may experience systemic symptoms such as fever, cough, malaise, myalgia, and rarely a serum sickness–like syndrome that can be fatal.

Most of the initial genitourinary symptoms occur due to the inflammatory response of eggs laid in the bladder submucosa and typically begin 10 to 12 weeks after infection. These initial symptoms may include terminal hematuria, dysuria, hematospermia, and frequency/urgency. Affected women may also have cervicitis and vaginitis. Urinary tract calcification may occur, and polypoid lesions in the bladder can result in recurrent gross hematuria. Late complications include fibrosis of the bladder that can lead to severely reduced capacity and upper tract deterioration. Women with long-term infection may experience infertility and ectopic pregnancy.

Bilharzial bladder cancer is an important complication of genitourinary schistosomiasis, with earlier age of onset (40–50) compared to typical urothelial malignancy. Histology is usually squamous cell carcinoma (60%–90%) or adenocarcinoma (5%–15%). Prognosis of these tumors is fairly good following surgery and treatment of underlying infection, as nearly half of these tumors are superficial and exophytic.

The gold standard for diagnosis is observation of terminally spined ova in urine sediment, pathognomonic for *S. haematobium*. ELISA serology studies can also be used for diagnosis, but cannot distinguish between previous exposure, acute infection, or chronic disease. Rectal or bladder biopsy may also be used for diagnosis. Imaging studies may reveal evidence of obstruction, and KUB or CT may also reveal a calcified bladder that is diagnostic for chronic schistosomiasis.

MANAGEMENT

The treatment of choice for schistosomiasis is praziquantel (40 mg/kg given in one day), which kills the adult worm by causing contractions of its muscles and detachment from the vein. Praziquantel is highly active in all stages, results in high cure rates, and is well tolerated with few side effects. Alternatively, metrifonate can be also be used for *S. haematobium*.

Medical therapy should be administered before surgery. Obstructive uropathy may require bladder augmentation, urinary diversion, or ureteral dilation or reimplantation.

Genitourinary Fungal Infections

GENERAL CONSIDERATIONS

Mycotic (fungal) infections of the urinary tract have become increasingly common, partly due to the widespread use of broad-spectrum antibiotics. They often arise as opportunistic infections in immunocompromised hosts, such as transplant recipients or patients with HIV/AIDS, and also occur with prolonged use of urinary drainage catheters.

CANDIDIASIS

Candidiasis, caused by *Candida albicans*, is the most common cause of fungal urinary tract infection (UTI). Candida yeast is found on urine culture in the setting of clinical infection, but may also represent colonization. The latter scenario is frequently associated with an indwelling catheter, especially in hospitalized patients being treated with broad-spectrum antibiotics. The rate of progression from candiduria to candemia is quite low, at less than 3%, though patients with concurrent obstructive uropathy are at increased risk.

However, for high-risk patients in ICU, neutropenic patients, or neonates, funguria can be a sign of invasive candidiasis. Candidemia makes up 10% of all nosocomial bloodstream infections with a mortality of 50% in adults, and therefore, special attention should be given to candiduria in high-risk populations. Hematogenous seeding of the upper urinary tract from candidemia can occur in immunocompromised subjects. In addition, newborns with candiduria are at risk for developing obstructing fungus balls in the collecting system.

There are no definitive diagnostic guidelines for candida UTI, but blood and urine cultures are used in conjunction with overall clinical assessment. Upper tract imaging is recommended to rule out obstruction, abscess, or fungal bezoar in susceptible patients.

Management depends most on the clinical scenario. Asymptomatic candiduria need not be treated, and should resolve with discontinuation of predisposing factors (antibiotics, indwelling catheters). High-risk patients and symptomatic patients with fever should be given antifungal treatment. If the patient has symptomatic involvement of the bladder, intravesical amphotericin B or miconazole irrigation (50 mg/1000 mL continuous bladder infusions), or oral flucytosine (50–75 mg/kg/day) is appropriate. If the patient has pyelonephritis or disseminated candidiasis, fluconazole, intravenous capsofungin, or amphotericin B should be used.

ASPERGILLOSIS

Aspergillosis is caused by *Aspergillus* fungus, which can be found on decaying vegetation, compost piles, and marijuana leaves. When *Aspergillus* spores are inhaled, pulmonary infection may occur; if there is compromised host immunity, infection can then spread systemically to other organs, including the genitourinary tract. Pyelonephritis and renal abscess may occur (see Fig. 5.2), or fungal bezoars in the collecting system can cause obstruction. Rarely, *Aspergillus* infection of the prostate can occur, causing bladder outlet obstruction.

Management involves medical therapy with voriconazole, amphotericin B, or capsofungin, with a combination of multiple drugs used for immunocompromised patients.

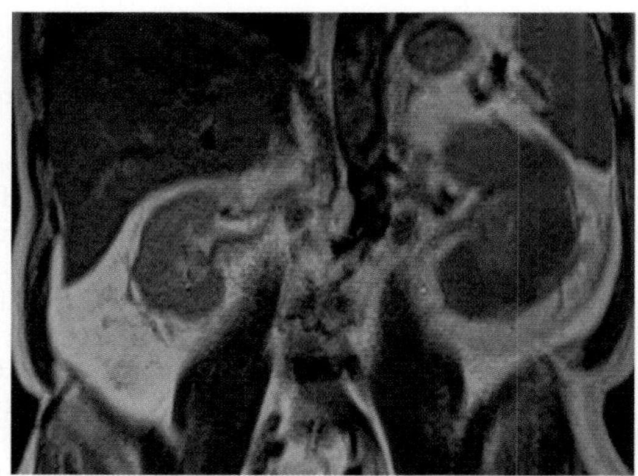

FIGURE 5.2 MRI in patient with fever and flank pain shows left nephromegaly, perinephric stranding, retroperitoneal adenopathy, and hypoattenuated appearance involving the parenchyma of the left kidney with relative sparing of the upper pole. Given its infiltrative appearance, biopsy was required to rule out renal lymphoma. Branched hyphae were identified on histopathology, consistent with the diagnosis of fungal pyelonephritis, possible aspergillosis.

CRYPTOCOCCOSIS

Cryptococcosis is caused by the soil-based fungus *Cryptococcus neoformans*, which most commonly affects the lungs and CNS (cryptococcal meningitis), though it can also rarely involve the genitourinary tract and cause pyelonephritis, focal renal abscess, or prostatitis. It is one of the most common opportunistic infections in HIV patients, and can also occur with other comorbidities such as diabetes mellitus or systemic lupus erythematosus.

Treatment involves systemic antifungal therapy, usually amphotericin B followed by fluconazole. However, cryptococcosis can be fatal even with appropriate treatment, with a mortality rate of more than 50% in patients with disseminated disease.

Rare Parasitic Genitourinary Infections

HYDATID DISEASE (ECHINOCOCCUS)

Hydatid disease is caused by *Echinococcus granulosus*, a canine intestinal tapeworm. Human infection can occur by ingestion of food contaminated by the parasite's eggs, and is thus endemic to sheepherding regions. The larvae then penetrate the intestinal mucosa, enter the portal system, and implant in the liver. Later, pulmonary or systemic spread can occur. Renal involvement is rare, accounting for only 2% of hydatid disease cases.

Patients may present with abdominal mass or flank pain caused by pressure from cyst formation. These hydatid cysts can slowly increase in size up to 20 cm or more, but rarely rupture; rather, they often involute and calcify.

On CT imaging, hydatid cysts are seen as thick-walled, septate cystic lesions in the kidney with a diagnostic rosette or honeycomb pattern. Similarly, ultrasound shows a hypoechoic, septate lesion, while a calcified hydatid cyst will appear on plain film imaging as a curvilinear calcification.

Medical therapy with mebendazole or albendazole has been used with limited success, but is associated with significant hepatotoxicity. Percutaneous aspiration of hydatid cysts in confirmed cases is not recommended due to risk of rupture and spillage of cyst fluid, which can cause an anaphylactic reaction and metastatic seeding. Because of this, surgical intervention should take great care to prevent spillage by avoiding cyst rupture and protection of surrounding structures with saline-soaked pads or towels. Partial nephrectomy may be required to assure cyst removal without rupture. Patients should be treated preoperatively with praziquantel and albendazole for 7 to 10 days.

AMEBIASIS

Amebiasis is caused by *Entamoeba histolytica*, a single-cell parasite transmitted via fecal-oral route with consumption of contaminated food or water, and thus occurs in areas with poor sanitary conditions. Amebiasis most commonly affects the liver, but renal abscess may occur. This renal abscess occurs more frequently in the right kidney, and usually occurs in association with liver abscess.

Diagnosis involves identification of *Entamoeba histolytica* amoebas in stool samples, but serum antigen and PCR tests are available when systemic infection is suspected. Treatment involves medical therapy with metronidazole or tinidazole. Surgical management of abscess should be delayed until after medical therapy has been initiated.

Other Genitourinary Infections

GENITAL FILARIASIS

Genital filariasis is most commonly caused by *Wuchereria bancrofti*, a human parasitic nematode transmitted via mosquito bite. When a host is infected, larvae migrate to periaortic, iliac, and scrotal lymphatics where paired male and female worms mate and release new larvae into the bloodstream diurnally. Patients initially present with lymphangitis and lymphadenitis, then inflammation will result in lymphatic obstruction, causing hydrocele and scrotal/penile elephantiasis. Of the 120 million people estimated to have *Wuchereria bancrofti* infection, over 25 million men have genital disease.

Diagnosis is based on detection of microfilariae in peripheral blood samples. Antihelminthic therapy options include diethylcarbamazine (6 mg/kg/day in 1-day or 12-day course) or albendazole (single dose of 400 mg), which kill both microfilariae and adult worms; ivermectin (single dose of 200–400 μg/kg), kills microfilariae only, and doxycycline (4- to 6-week course, 200 mg/day), kills adult worms. Patients with chronic filarial lymphedema may benefit from compression stockings and leg elevation, but in severe cases may require surgical excision of edematous tissue of the scrotum and penis.

FOURNIER'S GANGRENE

Fournier's gangrene is a potentially fatal necrotizing soft tissue infection involving the male genitalia and perineum with mortality rates up to 20%. The infection may rapidly travel along Colles' and Scarpa's fascial planes into the torso and thighs. This polymicrobial infection can include gram-positive cocci, gram-negative rods, and anaerobes such as *Bacteroides* and *Clostridia*.

Patients often present with scrotal discomfort, swelling, and systemic toxicity out of proportion to local findings. Examination may be notable for crepitus, dusky tissue, and foul-smelling discharge (Fig. 5.3). For diagnosis, urine, tissue, and blood cultures should be sent. KUB or CT imaging may reveal soft tissue gas and help assess extent of soft tissue involvement.

Because Fournier's gangrene can progress rapidly, early diagnosis and treatment is crucial. Antibiotic treatment typically consists of ampicillin/sulbactam or a third-generation cephalosporin plus gentamicin, as well as clindamycin or metronidazole for anaerobic coverage. Urgent surgical debridement of infected and necrotic tissue is imperative.

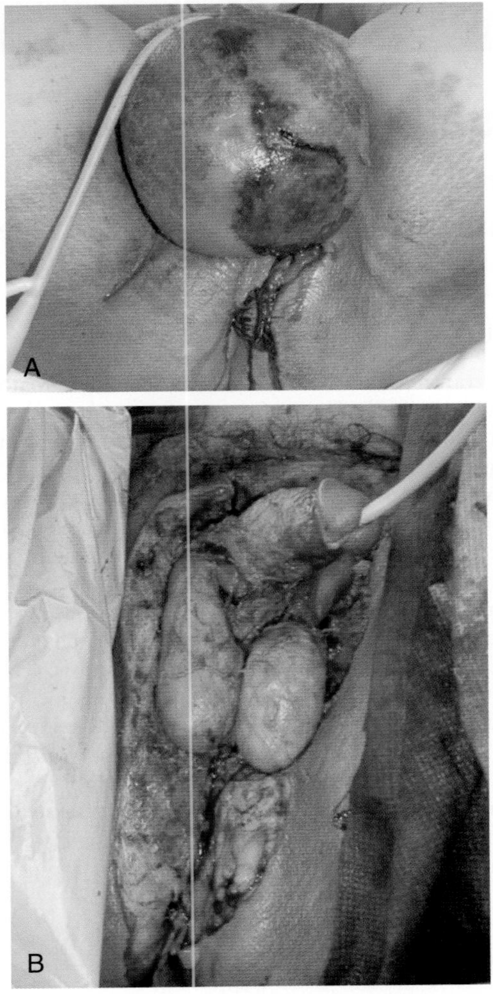

FIGURE 5.3 **Fournier gangrene of the scrotum. (A) Surface appearance of scrotum and perineum showing area of frank necrosis. (B) Extent of soft tissue debridement required to achieve margins of viable tissue. Note that the testes within their tunica vaginalis compartment are spared.** (From Link RE. Cutaneous diseases of the external genitalia. In: Wein AJ, Kavoussi LR, Novick AC, et al., eds. *Campbell-Walsh Urology*. 10th ed. Philadelphia: Saunders; 2012.)

Sexually Transmitted Infections

Ingride Richardson, MD, and Hyezo Kwun, MD, MPH, BA

Introduction

Sexually transmitted infections (STIs) remain a major public health challenge in the United States, affecting more than 20 million men and women annually, nearly half of whom are young people aged 15 to 24 years. In addition to the physical and psychological consequences of STIs, these diseases exact a tremendous economic toll. Direct medical costs associated with STIs in the United States are estimated at $16 billion annually treating a total of 110 million STIs.

The curable STIs include gonorrhea, chlamydia, mycoplasma, ureaplasmal infections, syphilis, trichomoniasis, chancroid, lymphogranuloma venereum (LGV), and donovanosis. STIs caused by yeast or protozoa are also curable. Viral STIs include human immunodeficiency virus (HIV), human papillomavirus (HPV), hepatitis B/C virus (HBV, HCV), herpes simplex virus (HSV), and the Zika virus; they are preventable but not curable.

This introduction to STIs is organized and presented by pathogens. A focus on diagnosis and treatment with some epidemiology will be the blueprint for this chapter.

Bacterial Urethritis

DIAGNOSIS

Urethritis can be diagnosed if any of the following criteria are met:

- Mucoid, mucopurulent, or purulent discharge on examination
- Gram stain of urethral secretions with ≥2 white blood cells (WBCs) per oil immersion field
- Positive leukocyte esterase from a first AM void

- Greater than 10 WBCs per high-power field (HPF) from a first AM void

Once the diagnosis of urethritis is made, a direct Gram stain may be performed as soon as the specimen is collected to further direct management and differentiate between the different microbial etiologies of urethritis.

GONORRHEA

Gonorrhea, *Neisseria gonorrhoeae*, is one of the most reported infectious diseases in the United States, with 583,405 cases reported in 2018, a steadily rising number since 2009 and a 5.0% increase from the previous year. Gonorrhea is thought to be substantially underdiagnosed and underreported; approximately twice as many new infections are estimated to occur each year as are reported.

Urethral smears from men who have symptomatic gonorrhea usually contain intracellular gram-negative diplococci in polymorphonuclear leukocytes. Endocervical smears from women and rectal specimens require careful interpretation because of colonization with other gram-negative coccobacillary organisms. In addition, the Centers for Disease Control and Prevention (CDC) is now recommending annual screening for sexually active women with risk factors (i.e., multiple sexual partners, communities with high disease rate). Pregnant women at risk should also receive screening at first prenatal visit. Men who engage in sexual intercourse with other men should be screened more frequently. Every 3 to 6 months is recommeded if illicit drug use is found (especially methamphetamine).

The isolation and identification of *N. gonorrhoeae* is still the currently accepted gold standard for the diagnosis of gonococcal infections. It is the recommended method for medicolegal investigations of sexual abuse. Specimens should be inoculated onto selective media, such as modified Thayer-Martin, Martin-Lewis, or New York City agar.

Given the low sensitivity of Gram stains for *N. gonorrhoeae*, a negative stain does not rule out an infection. Other current testing for *N. gonorrhoeae* also includes nucleic acid molecular amplification tests (NAATs) that measure deoxyribonucleic acid (DNA) and ribonucleic acid (RNA) rather than live organisms. Polymerase chain reaction (PCR) (Amplicor, Roche Molecular Diagnostics, Branchburg, N.J.) has been used with sensitivity well above 90% for the detection of *N. gonorrhoeae* in cervical specimens. It is highly accurate with male urine and does not require urethral swabs as Gram stains do. NAATs are now the preferred method of initially detecting urethral *N. gonorrhea* and *Chlamydia trachomatis*, but cultures still remain the appropriate route for diagnosing rectal, oropharyngeal, and conjunctival infections, as well as when following up treatment failures and cases of sexual assault.

Strand displacement amplification (ProbeTec, Becton Dickinson, Sparks, Md.) is approved for detection of gonorrhea in cervical, male urethral, and female and male urine samples and has achieved widespread use in clinical laboratories throughout the United States and Europe. The BD ProbeTec ET system demonstrated a sensitivity of 97.9% for the detection of *N. gonorrhoeae* in urine from 680 male patients.

Because NAATs measure DNA or RNA rather than live organisms, caution should be used in using DNA amplification tests for test-of-cure assays. Residual nucleic acid from cells rendered noninfective by antibiotics may give a positive amplified test for up to 3 weeks after therapy, although the patient may actually be cured of viable organisms.

All patients with confirmed diagnosis of gonorrhea should be tested for other STIs including chlamydia, syphilis, and HIV.

Treatment of Uncomplicated Gonococcal Urethritis

Recommended Regimens

Dual therapy to treat chlamydial infection in addition to gonorrhea is recommended because treating prophylactically is more cost effective than testing for associated chlamydial infection. Given increasing antimicrobial resistance, it is important to consistently consult current literature for updates in treatment. Apps are available from the CDC (www.cdc.gov/mobile/mobileapp.html).

GONOCOCCAL URETHRITIS TREATMENT

First line				
	Ceftriaxone	250 mg	IM	Once
	with			
	Azithromycin	1 g	PO	Once

GONOCOCCAL URETHRITIS TREATMENT—Cont'd

Alternatives			
Cefixime	400 mg	PO	Once
with			
Azithromycin	1 g	PO	Once
Cephalosporin allergy			
Azithromycin	2 g	PO	Once
with			
Gemifloxacin	320 mg	PO	Once
OR			
Gentamicin	240 mg	IM	Once

The CDC no longer recommends quinolones for gonorrhea infections because of new data showing increased resistance. In addition, use of quinolones is inadvisable for treating infections acquired in California and in other areas with increased prevalence of quinolone resistance.

Follow-Up

Patients who have uncomplicated gonorrhea and who are treated with any of the recommended or alternative regimens need not return for a test to confirm that they are cured, excepting patients with pharyngeal gonorrhea treated with alternative regiments who should follow up for a test of cure in 14 days. Patients who have symptoms that persist after treatment should be evaluated by culture for *N. gonorrhoeae,* and any gonococci isolated should be tested for antimicrobial susceptibility. Infections identified after treatment with one of the recommended regimens usually result from reinfection rather than treatment failure, indicating a need for improved patient education and referral of sex partners. Persistent urethritis, cervicitis, or proctitis may indicate infection by another organism, including *C. trachomatis.*

All sexual partners who had contact within 60 days of diagnosis should be evaluated, tested, and treated for both *N. gonorrhoeae* and *C. trachomatis*. Sexual activity should be avoided until treatment is completed and symptoms have resolved in all partners.

Given the high rates of reinfection, patients treated with gonorrhea should be rescreened at 3 months follow-up.

Complications

Complications of *N. gonorrhoeae* may be local or systemic. Locally, male gonococcal urethritis may spread to the posterior urethra, seminal vesicles, and epididymis. This can lead to epididymitis, urethral stricture disease, prostatitis, and even sterility. In women, gonorrhea is a major cause of pelvic inflammatory disease (PID). PID results from the ascent of infection from the endocervix into the fallopian tubes. **Symptoms include vaginal discharge, abdominal pain, dyspareunia, menorrhagia, fever, and cervical motion or adnexal tenderness.** This may lead to scarring of the adnexal structures and fallopian tubes resulting in chronic pelvic pain, ectopic pregnancy, and infertility.

N. gonorrhoeae can also lead to systemic diseases. Gonococcal perihepatitis (Fitz-Hugh-Curtis syndrome) is manifested by sharp supraumbilical pain and right upper quadrant pain. It results from ascending infection from the pelvis into the paracolic gutters and subphrenic spaces in females. "Violin string" adhesions may be noted between the liver and anterior abdominal wall and diaphragm. Disseminated gonococcal infection can occur in up to 3% of mucosal cases and may include arthritis, tenosynovitis, dermatitis, meningitis, myopericarditis, and/or sepsis.

CHLAMYDIA

Chlamydia, *C. trachomatis*, is the most frequently reported STI in the United States, with a total of 1,758,668 cases reported in 2018 (539.9 cases per 100,000 population). National surveys indicate that age-specific rates of chlamydia were highest in females aged 15 to 19 years, at 3,306.8 cases per 100,000 females, increased 1.3% from previously, and 20 to 24 years, at 4,064.6 cases per 100,000 females, increased 0.8%. Even so, most chlamydia cases go undiagnosed, as for both men and women, the infection can be largely asymptomatic. The increases in reported cases and rates likely reflect the continued expansion of screening efforts and increased use of more sensitive diagnostic tests, rather than an actual increase in new infections. The availability of urine tests for chlamydia may be contributing to the increased detection of the disease in men and consequently the rising rates of reported chlamydia in men in recent years.

The CDC recommends annual chlamydia screening for sexually active women under age 25, all pregnant women, and older women with risk factors (i.e., new or multiple sex partners). Screening efforts are critical to preventing the serious health consequences of this infection, particularly infertility. Such efforts are linked to a 60% reduction in the incidence of PID. Screening of men who engage in sexual intercourse with other men should be conducted annually, with more frequent screening (every 3–6 months) for men involved with multiple partners. If illicit drug use is involved, parties are at an even higher risk, and they should receive testing at shorter intervals.

C. trachomatis is an intracellular bacterium with multiple serotypes. Types L1-3 cause LGV. Types D, E, F, G, H, I, J, and K cause urethritis and cervicitis. It is transmitted during vaginal, oral, or anal sexual contact with an infected partner. ***C. trachomatis*** **accounts for 30% to 50% of cases of nongonococcal urethritis (NGU).**

Chlamydial infection in men is generally asymptomatic, but symptoms may include urethritis, epididymitis, and proctitis. Urethritis presents 1 to 3 weeks after infection with a mild to moderate clear urethral discharge and dysuria. Chlamydial urethritis may present as persistent dysuria and/or discharge following a course of treatment for gonorrhea because 15% to 35% of patients with known gonococcal infections are also infected with chlamydia.

Chlamydial epididymitis tends to run a more protracted course than epididymitis due to other organisms; it is also often less severe. Chlamydial proctitis may present with rectal pain and bleeding, but it is often asymptomatic.

Chlamydial infection may disseminate systemically in 1% to 3% of patients. Classically know as Reiter's syndrome, it presents with the classic triad of reactive arthritis, urethritis, and conjunctivitis. The Fitz-Hugh-Curtis syndrome may also be seen in about 20% of women with PID secondary to chlamydial infection.

C. trachomatis was the first organism for which there was a commercially available PCR assay. Now there are many published studies using several different types of NAATs and new technologies that are commercially available for detecting *chlamydia* in urine and urethral, cervical, or vaginal secretions.

Treatment

Treatment should be initiated as soon as possible after diagnosis. Single-dose regimens have the advantage of improved compliance. Meta-analysis studies of 12 randomized control trials of chlamydial treatments using azithromycin versus doxycycline showed both were equally effective, with microbial cure rates of 97% and 98%, respectively.

CHLAMYDIA TRACHOMATIS TREATMENT

First line				
Azithromycin	1 g	PO	Once	
OR				
Doxycycline	100 mg	PO	BID	7 days
Alternatives				
Erythromycin base	500 mg	PO	QID	7 days
OR				
Erythromycin ethylsuccinate	800 mg	PO	QID	7 days
OR				
Levofloxacin	500 mg	PO	daily	7 days
OR				
Ofloxacin	300 mg	PO	BID	7 days

RECURRENT AND PERSISTENT INFECTIONS

Patients who have persistent or recurrent urethritis should be retreated with the initial regimen if they did not comply with the treatment regimen or if they were reexposed to an untreated sex partner. Otherwise, a culture of an intraurethral swab specimen and a first morning void specimen for *Trichomonas vaginalis* should be performed. Some cases of recurrent urethritis following doxycycline treatment may be caused by tetracycline-resistant *Ureaplasma urealyticum*. If the patient is compliant with the initial regimen and reexposure can be excluded, the following regimen is recommended:

- **Metronidazole** 2 g orally in a single dose *PLUS* **erythromycin base** 500 mg orally four times a day for 7 days

  or
- **Erythromycin ethylsuccinate** 800 mg orally four times a day for 7 days

Patients who have NGU and also are infected with HIV should receive the same treatment regimen as those who are HIV negative.

NONCHLAMYDIAL NONGONOCOCCAL URETHRITIS

The etiologies of most cases of nonchlamydial nongonococcal urethritis are unknown. *U. urealyticum* and *Mycoplasma genitalium* have been implicated. Specific diagnostic tests for these organisms are not indicated because the detection of these organisms is often difficult and protracted. As there are no Food and Drug Administration (FDA)-approved diagnostic tests, *M. genitalium* should be suspected in cases of persistent or recurrent urethritis.

***MYCOPLASMA GENITALIUM* TREATMENT**				
First line				
Azithromycin	1 g	PO	Once	
Treatment failure				
Moxifloxacin	400 mg	PO	Daily	7, 10, or 14 days

T. vaginalis and HSV can sometimes cause urethritis. Diagnostic and treatment procedures for these organisms are reserved for situations in which these infections are suspected (e.g., contact with trichomoniasis and genital lesions suggestive of genital herpes) or when unresponsive to therapy.

TRICHOMONAS VAGINALIS			
First line			
Metronidazole	2 g	PO	Once
OR			
Tinidazole	2 g	PO	Once

Epididymitis

DIAGNOSIS

Acute epididymitis presents with unilateral pain, swelling, and inflammation of the epididymis lasting less than 6 weeks. In men younger than 35 years, the microbial etiology of epididymitis is commonly *N. gonorrhea* or *C. trachomatis*. In men who are the insertive partner during anal intercourse, enteric organisms can also be present.

Diagnosis does not often require ultrasound but this may be important in ruling out testicular torsion. Diagnosis can be made with one of the following:

1. Gram stain or methylene blue stain of urethral secretions with ≥2 WBCs per oil immersion field
2. Positive leukocyte esterase on first-void urine
3. > 10 WBCs per HPF on spun first-void urine

All cases should be tested for *C. trachomatis* and *N. gonorrhea* with NAAT and urine cultures sent.

TREATMENT

Empiric therapy should be started prior to laboratory confirmation.

Likely 2/2 STI				
Ceftriaxone	250 mg	IM	once	
with				
Doxycycline	100 mg	PO	BID	10 days
Likely 2/2 STI *and* enteric organisms				
Ceftriaxone	250 mg	IM	once	
with				
Levofloxacin	500 mg	PO	daily	10 days
OR				
Ofloxacin	300 mg	PO	BID	10 days
Likely 2/2 enteric organisms (gonorrhea ruled out)				
Levofloxacin	500 mg	PO	daily	10 days
OR				
Ofloxacin	300 mg	PO	daily	10 days

STI, Sexually transmitted infections.

Genital Lesions

CONDYLOMA ACUMINATA (GENITAL WARTS)

HPV is one of the most common STI with an estimated total of 24 million infected individuals and 5.5 million new cases every year in the United States. The CDC estimate that nearly half of civilians aged 18 to 59 years in the United States may have had HPV in the year 2013. HPV vaccination has decreased prevalence by 56% in females aged 14 to 19. HPV, a small, nonenveloped virus containing double-stranded DNA, infects basal epithelial cells and multiplies in the cell nucleus, causing cell death and perinuclear cavitation or **koilocytosis,** a histologic feature specific to HPV. More than 40 types of HPV can infect the genital tract. Most HPV infections are asymptomatic, unrecognized, or subclinical. **Visible genital warts usually are caused by HPV type 6 or 11 (90%).** Other HPV types in the anogenital region (e.g., types 16, 18, 31, 33, and 35) have been strongly associated with cervical cancer.

Biopsy is recommended under certain clinical conditions:

1. Diagnosis is uncertain.
2. Lesions do not respond to standard therapy.
3. Disease worsens during therapy.
4. Patient is immunocompromised.
5. Warts are pigmented, indurated, fixed, and ulcerated (**suggestive of Buschke-Löwenstein tumor**).

No data support the use of type-specific HPV nucleic acid tests in the routine diagnosis or management of visible genital warts.

In addition to the external genitalia (i.e., the penis, vulva, scrotum, perineum, perianal skin), genital warts can occur on the uterine cervix and in the vagina, urethra, anus, and mouth.

When urethral lesions occur, 80% are located within the distal 3 cm of urethra. Patients present with dysuria, bloody urethral discharge, and changes in urinary stream. **Bladder condyloma are rare.** If meatal condyloma are identified, urethroscopy should be performed to look for other urethral lesions. **To prevent iatrogenic seeding of the prostatic urethra and bladder, a tourniquet should be placed at the penopubic junction, or urethroscopy should stop at the external sphincter.**

Intraanal warts are seen predominantly in patients who have had anal-receptive intercourse; these warts are distinct from perianal warts, which can occur in men and women who do not have a history of anal sex.

HPV types 6 and 11 have been associated with conjunctival, nasal, oral, and laryngeal warts. HPV types 6 and 11 rarely are associated with invasive squamous cell carcinoma of the external genitalia. Depending on the size and anatomic location, **genital warts can be painful, friable, and pruritic, although they are commonly asymptomatic.**

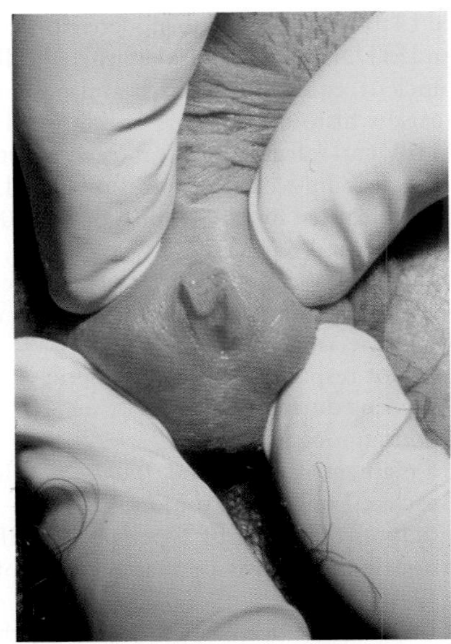

FIGURE 6.1 Meatal wart caused by human papillomavirus. (From Frenkl TL, Potts JM. Sexually transmitted infections. In: Wein AJ, Kavoussi LR, Novick AC, et al., eds. *Campbell-Walsh Urology*. 10th ed. Philadelphia: Saunders; 2012:402-416.)

HPV types 16, 18, 31, 33, and 35 are found occasionally in visible genital warts and have been associated with external genital (i.e., vulvar, penile, anal) squamous intraepithelial neoplasia (i.e., squamous cell carcinoma in situ, bowenoid papulosis, erythroplasia of Queyrat, Bowen disease of the genitalia). These HPV types also have been associated with vaginal, anal, and cervical intraepithelial dysplasia and squamous cell carcinoma. Patients who have visible genital warts can be infected simultaneously with multiple HPV types (Fig. 6.1).

Treatment

The introduction of vaccines has resulted in a shift in focus from treatment of visible lesions to prevention: *Cervarix*, is a bivalent HPV vaccine against types 16 and 18 (approximately 70% of cervical cancers). *Gardasil 4*, is a quadrivalent vaccine against types

16, 18, 6, and 11 (90% of genital warts), Most recently developed, *Gardasil 9*, a 9-valent vaccine covering types 16, 18, 31, 33, 45, 52, and 58, carries an efficacy of 96.7% against incidence of HPV 31, 33, 45, 42, and 58. Gardasil 9 has, since 2016, been the only HPV vaccine used in the United States.

Gardasil 9 is routinely recommended for 11- and 12-year-old girls and boys and can be started as early as 9 years of age and administered until 26 years, ideally prior to initial sexual contact. In 2018, the FDA approved extension of vaccine administration to both men and women aged 27 to 45 years. When administered under the age of 15, a two-dose regimen is sufficient (6–12 months apart), but those who begin the vaccine later should continue with the three-dose schedule (at 0, 2, and 6 months). Vaccination is also routinely recommended for gay and bisexual men and patients with compromised immune systems (including HIV) aged 22 to 26. In the vaccinated population, the percentage of cervical precancers caused by HPV has dropped by 40%; infections in young women with HPV types that cause cancers and genitals warts have dropped by 71%; and infections in teens with HPV types that cause cancers and genital warts have dropped by 86%. However, vaccinations do not replace other prevention strategies.

The primary goal of treating visible genital warts is the removal of symptomatic warts. In most patients, treatment can induce wart-free periods. If left untreated, visible genital warts can resolve spontaneously, remain unchanged, or increase in size or number. Existing data indicate that currently available therapies for genital warts may reduce but probably do not eliminate infectivity.

Most patients have fewer than 10 genital warts, with a total wart area of 0.5 to 1.0 cm^2. These warts respond to most treatment modalities. Factors that may influence the selection of treatment include wart size, wart number, anatomic site of wart, wart morphology, patient preference, cost of treatment, convenience, adverse effects, and provider experience.

Many patients require a course of therapy rather than a single treatment. In general, warts located on moist surfaces and/or in intertriginous areas respond better to topical treatment than do warts on drier surfaces.

Recommended Regimens for External Genital Warts

PATIENT APPLIED				
	Imiquimod cream 3.75%	Daily at bedtime	16 weeks	Wash off 6–10 hours after application
Or				
	Imiquimod cream 5%	Daily at bedtime, 3 times a week	16 weeks	Wash off 6–10 hours after application
Or				
Podofilox 0.5% solution or gel	BID (max 0.5 mL/ day)	3 days	Hold for 4 days, repeat up to 4 cycles	Contraindicated in pregnancy
Or				
	Sinecatechins 15% ointment	TID	16 weeks	Do not wash off

Provider-directed		
	Cryotherapy	q1–2 weeks
	Or	
	Bichloroacetic acid 80%–90%	Weekly
	Or	
	Trichloroacetic acid 80%–80%	Weekly

Surgical Removal for Very Large Wart Burden

Intralesional interferon: Intralesional injection of interferon alpha 2b increases success of podofilox, but the recurrence rate is the same.

Laser surgery: Carbon dioxide (CO_2) laser vaporizes tissue with a shallow depth of penetration. **Must use laser mask and vacuum because viral DNA has been demonstrated in the smoke plume.** Neodymium:yttrium-aluminum-garnet (Nd:YAG) coagulates tissue and causes less plume. Overall success with laser is 88% to 100%. Recurrence may occur in 2 to 3 months.

GENITAL ULCERS

In the United States, most young, sexually active patients who have genital ulcers have genital herpes, syphilis, or chancroid. Although genital herpes is the most prevalent of these diseases, the relative frequency of each differs by geographic area and patient population. Patients with genital ulcers may have more than one disease. Conversely, not all genital ulcers are caused by STIs. Each disease has been associated with an increased risk for HIV infection.

The differential diagnosis of genital ulcers must include premalignant processes (e.g., erythroplasia of Queyrat); malignant processes such as squamous cell carcinoma of the penis; and nonmalignant processes, including syphilis, chancroid, LGV, and granuloma inguinale (GI). Biopsy of ulcers may be helpful in identifying the cause of unusual ulcers or ulcers that do not respond. Only three ulcer presentations are pathognomonic (Table 6.1):

1. A fixed drug eruption is always triggered by the use of one particular medication.
2. A group of vesicles on an erythematous base that does not follow a neural distribution is pathognomonic for herpes simplex infection.
3. A genital ulcer that develops acutely following sexual activity is diagnostic of trauma.

A diagnosis based only on the patient's medical history and physical examination only is often inaccurate; therefore, specific tests may be needed.

Specific tests for evaluation of genital ulcers include:

1. Serology and either darkfield examination or direct immunofluorescence test for *Treponema pallidum*
2. Culture or antigen test for HSV
3. Culture for *Haemophilus ducreyi* (chancroid)

Genital Herpes

Genital herpes is a recurrent, life-long viral infection. Two serotypes of HSV have been identified: HSV-1 (30%) and HSV-2 (70%). Most cases of recurrent genital herpes are caused by HSV-2, although an increasing number of HSV-1 anogenital cases are being seen. Approximately 24 million persons in the United States have a genital HSV-2 infection, and most are undiagnosed; in addition, 776,000 new cases are reported each year.

TABLE 6.1 Genital Ulcer Disease

Disease	Lesions	Lymphadenopathy	Systemic Symptoms
Primary syphilis	Painless, indurated, with a clean base, usually singular	Nontender, rubbery, nonsuppurative bilateral lymphadenopathy	None
Genital herpes	Painful vesicles, shallow, usually multiple	Tender, bilateral inguinal adenopathy	Present during primary infection
Chancroid	Tender papule, then painful, undermined purulent ulcer, single or multiple	Tender, regional, painful, suppurative nodes	None
Lymphogranuloma	Small, painless vesicle or papule progresses to an ulcer	Painful, matted, large nodes develop, with fistulous tracts	Present after genital lesion heals

(From Frenkl TL, Potts JM. Sexually transmitted infections. In: Wein AJ, Kavoussi LR, Novick AC, et al., eds. *Campbell-Walsh Urology*. 10th ed. Philadelphia: Saunders; 2012:402-416.)

Herpes virus invades the body via breaks in the skin or moist membranes of the penis, vagina, urethra, anus, vulva, or cervix. **Genital lesions appear 2 to 20 days after infection.** The lesions are initially papules, which ulcerate and scab before reepithelializing. Flulike symptoms may develop with the initial infection and are much worse than subsequent episodes or in patients without history of previous oral herpes. Local lesions may persist an average of 10 days following the initial infection. Recurrent lesions last 5 to 7 days. Tender inguinal adenopathy can develop in 2 to 3 weeks. Dysuria is present in 80% of females and 40% of males with genital herpes.

Late complications include mild meningitis (10%–30%) and more serious sacral or autonomic dysfunction (1%), which can result in urinary retention, pneumonitis, and hepatitis. The most serious consequence is neonatal transmission, which carries high rates of morbidity and mortality for the infant.

All types of intercourse may transmit HSV, and HSV may be passed on to the baby during birth. Most genital herpes infections are transmitted by persons who are either unaware of their status or asymptomatic. Rarely does first-episode genital herpes manifest with severe disease requiring hospitalization.

Recurrences are much less frequent for genital HSV-1 infection than genital HSV-2 infection. Making the distinction between HSV serotypes is important in prognosis and counseling. As such, the clinical diagnosis of genital herpes should be confirmed by laboratory testing.

Cell culturing and type analysis by immunofluorescence tests are standard options for diagnosis. Fluorescence tests can be done without viral amplification in the cell culture but with decreased sensitivity. PCR and ligase chain reaction (LCR) amplification of HSV show much better sensitivity, but the techniques are too expensive for routine use. Cytologic detection of cellular changes of herpes virus infection is insensitive and nonspecific, in both genital lesions (Tzanck preparation) and cervical Pap smears, and should not be relied on for diagnosis of HSV infection. Alternatively for serum HSV-2 antibody, glycoprotein G type is available and has a specificity of greater than 96% (Fig. 6.2).

TREATMENT

Systemic antiviral drugs partially control the symptoms and signs of herpes episodes when used to treat first clinical episodes and recurrent episodes or when used as daily suppressive therapy. Nonetheless, these drugs neither eradicate latent virus nor affect the risk, frequency, or severity of recurrences after the drug is discontinued.

Randomized trials indicate that **three antiviral medications provide clinical benefit for genital herpes: acyclovir, valacyclovir, and famciclovir.** Valacyclovir is the valine ester of acyclovir and has enhanced absorption after oral administration. Famciclovir, a prodrug of penciclovir, also has high oral bioavailability. Topical therapy with these drugs often offers minimal clinical benefit.

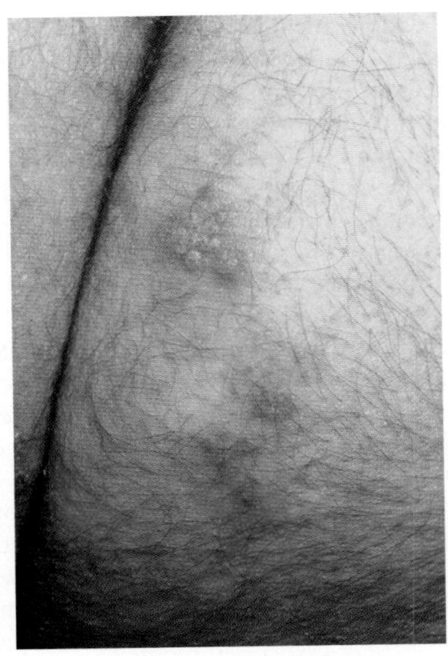

FIGURE 6.2 **Typical vesicular eruption of herpes simplex virus.** (From Frenkl TL, Potts JM. Sexually transmitted infections. In: Wein AJ, Kavoussi LR, Novick AC, et al., eds. *Campbell-Walsh Urology*. 10th ed. Philadelphia: Saunders; 2012:402-416.)

FIRST CLINICAL EPISODE OF GENITAL HERPES

Many patients with first-episode herpes present with mild clinical manifestations. Most first episodes go unnoticed, but later patients can develop severe or prolonged symptoms. Therefore, most patients with initial genital herpes should receive antiviral therapy.

FIRST CLINICAL EPISODE				
Acyclovir	400 mg	PO	TID	7–10 days
OR				
Acyclovir	200 mg	PO	5×/day	7–10 days
OR				
Valacyclovir	1 g	PO	BID	7–10 days
OR				
Famciclovir	250 mg	PO	TID	7–10 days

Episodic Therapy for Recurrent Genital Herpes

Effective episodic treatment of recurrent herpes requires initiation of therapy within 1 day of lesion onset or during the prodrome that precedes some outbreaks. The patient should be provided with a supply of the drug or a prescription for the medication with instructions to self-initiate treatment immediately when symptoms begin.

EPISODIC TREATMENT FOR RECURRENT EPISODES				
Acyclovir	400 mg	PO	TID	5 days
OR				
Acyclovir	800 mg	PO	BID	5 days
OR				
Acyclovir	800 mg	PO	TID	2 days
OR				
Valacyclovir	500 mg	PO	BID	3 days
OR				
Valacyclovir	1 g	PO	daily	5 days
OR				
Famciclovir	125 mg	PO	BID	5 days
OR				
Famciclovir	1 g	PO	BID	1 day
OR				
Famciclovir	500 mg	PO	Once	
followed by				
Famciclovir	250 mg	PO	BID	2 days

Suppressive Therapy for Recurrent Genital Herpes

Suppressive therapy reduces the frequency of genital herpes recurrences by 70% to 80% among patients who have frequent recurrences (i.e., six recurrences per year), and many patients report no symptomatic outbreaks.

The frequency of recurrent outbreaks diminishes over time. Periodically (e.g., once a year), discontinuation of therapy should be discussed with the patient to reassess the need for continued therapy.

Suppressive antiviral therapy reduces but does not eliminate subclinical viral shedding. Therefore, the extent to which suppressive therapy prevents HSV transmission is unknown.

SUPPRESSIVE TREATMENT FOR RECURRENT EPISODESS				
Acyclovir	400 mg	PO	BID	
OR				
Valacyclovir	500 mg	PO	Daily	
OR				
Valacyclovir	1 g	PO	Daily	
OR				
Famciclovir	250 mg	PO	BID	7–10 days

Severe Disease

Intravenous (IV) acyclovir therapy should be provided for patients who have severe disease or complications that necessitate hospitalization, such as disseminated infection, pneumonitis, hepatitis, or complications of the central nervous system (e.g., meningitis, encephalitis). The recommended regimen is acyclovir 5 to 10 mg/kg of body weight IV every 8 hours for 2 to 7 days or until clinical improvement is observed, followed by oral antiviral therapy to complete at least 10 days of total therapy.

Pregnancy and HSV

Given the high vertical transmission rates (30%–50%) for HSV to newborns during vaginal delivery, all expectant mothers should be evaluated for infections or history of infections. Direct exposure is required for transmission; therefore, avoidance of exposure during delivery is the focus of prevention. Cesarean delivery is recommended in the face of active or ongoing infection, thus preventing exposure and decreasing likely transmission at the time of delivery. Acyclovir oral or IV can be administered late in pregnancy and has been documented to decrease the need for cesarean sections. If the neonate is exposed, systemic acyclovir should be administered.

Syphilis

Syphilis is a systemic disease caused by *T. pallidum*, a spirochete bacterium. Patients who have syphilis may seek treatment for signs or symptoms of primary infection, secondary infection, or tertiary infection.

The ulcer in primary syphilis is characteristically **firm, and painless.** In men, the most common area is on the corona of the penis. In women, the most common locations are the labia majora, labia minora, fourchette, and perineum.

The primary mode of transmission is sexual contact. Ten percent of cases are due to transmission via saliva, transfusions, and accidental inoculation. **The disease is most contagious during the secondary stage because of the increased number of lesions present.** The risk of transmission exists during all stages except latent syphilis.

PRIMARY SYPHILIS

The time from transmission to the appearance of primary lesions averages 21 days (the range is 10–90 days). The clinical presentation of syphilis is extremely diverse and may occur decades after initial infection.

The primary chancre appears at the site of initial treponemal invasion of the dermis. It may occur on any skin or mucous membrane surface and is usually situated on the external genitalia. Initial lesions are papular but rapidly ulcerate. They are usually single, but "kissing" lesions may occur on opposing mucocutaneous surfaces. Typically, the ulcers are nontender (unless there is coexisting infection) and indurated and have a clean base and raised edges. There is often surrounding edema, especially with vulval lesions. Nontender, nonsuppurative, rubbery inguinal lymphadenopathy appears 1 week later and usually becomes bilateral after 2 weeks. The chancre usually heals spontaneously within 3 to 6 weeks but leaves a scar (Fig. 6.3).

SECONDARY SYPHILIS

The manifestations of generalized treponemal dissemination first appear about 8 weeks after infection. Constitutional symptoms consist of fever, headache, and bone and joint pains. Physical features are widely diverse. Skin rashes are the most common feature. They are initially macular and become papular by 3 months. Lesions appear initially on the upper trunk, the palms and soles, and flexural surfaces of the extremities.

Generalized lymphadenopathy occurs in 50% of cases of secondary syphilis. It has similar characteristics to the localized lymphadenopathy of primary infection. Other systemic features

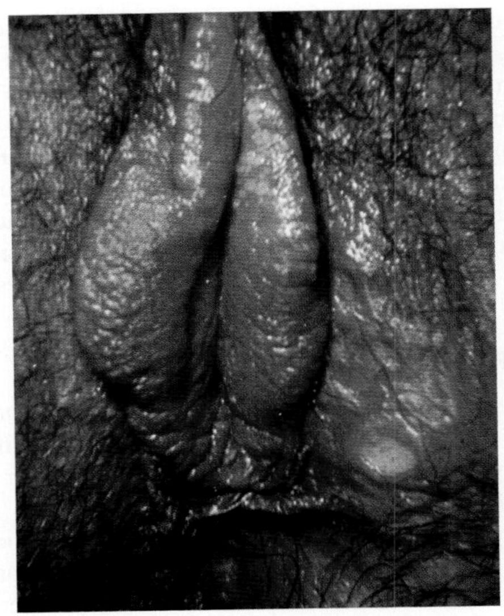

FIGURE 6.3 Syphilis with vulvar chancre. (From Frenkl TL, Potts JM. Sexually transmitted infections. In: Wein AJ, Kavoussi LR, Novick AC, et al., eds. *Campbell-Walsh Urology*. 10th ed. Philadelphia: Saunders; 2012:402-416.)

of secondary syphilis include panuveitis, periostitis and joint effusions, glomerulonephritis, hepatitis, gastritis, myocarditis, and aseptic meningitis.

The lesions of secondary syphilis resolve spontaneously in a variable time period and most patients enter the latency stage within the first year of infection. In some patients, especially the immunocompromised, primary or secondary lesions may recur.

LATENT SYPHILIS

In latent syphilis, no clinical stigmata of active disease are visible, although the disease remains detectable by positive serologic tests. In early latency, within 2 years of infection, vertical transmission of infection may still occur, but sexual transmission is less likely in the absence of mucocutaneous lesions. The late manifestations of syphilis arise, often decades later, in about 25% of those who have latent syphilis.

TERTIARY GUMMATOUS SYPHILIS

The characteristic lesions of tertiary syphilis appear 3 to 10 years after infection and consist of granulomas or gummas. The granulomas appear as cutaneous plaques or nodules of irregular shape and outline and are often single lesions on the arms, back, and face. Gummas can cause painless testicular swelling, which may mimic a tumor. The typical lesion of cardiovascular syphilis is aortitis affecting the ascending aorta and appearing 10 to 30 years after infection. This can result in aortic aneurysms or aortic insufficiency. Symptoms of neurosyphilis include dementia, sensory ataxia, areflexia, paresthesias, auditory abnormalities, and Argyll Robertson pupils (pupils that have accommodation but no pupil response).

Diagnosis

Dark-field examinations and direct fluorescent antibody tests of lesion exudate or tissue are the definitive methods for diagnosing early syphilis. A presumptive diagnosis is possible with the use of two types of serologic tests for syphilis: (1) nontreponemal tests (e.g., Venereal Disease Research Laboratory [VDRL] and rapid plasma reagin [RPR]) and (2) treponemal tests (e.g., fluorescent treponemal antibody absorbed [FTA-ABS] and *T. pallidum* particle agglutination [TP-PA]). The use of only one type of serologic test is insufficient for diagnosis because false-positive nontreponemal test results may occur secondary to various medical conditions.

Nontreponemal test antibody titers usually correlate with disease activity, and results should be reported quantitatively. A fourfold change in titer, equivalent to a change of two dilutions (e.g., from 1:16 to 1:4 or from 1:8 to 1:32), is considered necessary to demonstrate a clinically significant difference between two nontreponemal test results that were obtained using the same serologic test. Nontreponemal tests usually become nonreactive with time after treatment; however, in some patients, nontreponemal antibodies can persist at a low titer for a long period of time, sometimes for the life of the patient. This response is referred to as the *serofast reaction*.

Treatment

Penicillin G, administered parenterally, is the preferred drug for treatment of all stages of syphilis. The preparation(s) used (i.e., benzathine, aqueous procaine, aqueous crystalline), the dosage, and the length of treatment depend on the stage and clinical manifestations of disease. However, neither combinations of benzathine penicillin and procaine penicillin nor oral penicillin preparations are considered appropriate for the treatment of syphilis.

Parenteral penicillin G is the only therapy with documented efficacy for syphilis during pregnancy. Pregnant women with syphilis in any stage who report penicillin allergy should be desensitized and treated with penicillin. Skin testing for penicillin allergy may be useful in pregnant women; such testing also is useful in other patients.

The Jarisch-Herxheimer reaction is an acute febrile reaction frequently accompanied by headache, myalgia, and other symptoms that usually occurs within the first 24 hours after any therapy for syphilis. Patients should be informed about this possible adverse reaction. **It occurs most often among patients who have early syphilis.** Antipyretics may be used, but they have not been proven to prevent this reaction. The Jarisch-Herxheimer reaction may induce early labor or cause fetal distress in pregnant women. This concern should not prevent or delay therapy.

PRIMARY, SECONDARY, AND EARLY LATENT SYPHILIS WITH NO NEUROLOGIC INVOLVEMENT

First line					
	Benzathine penicillin G	2.4 million units	IM	Once	
Penicillin-allergy					
	Doxycycline	100 mg	PO	BID	14 days
	OR				
	Tetracycline	500 mg	PO	QID	14 days

LATE LATENT OR LATENT SYPHILIS, UNKNOWN DURATION, NO NEUROLOGIC INVOLVEMENT

First line					
	Benzathine penicillin G	2.4 million units	IM	Once/week	3 weeks
PCN-allergy					
	Doxycycline	100 mg	PO	BID	28 days
	OR				
	Tetracycline	500 mg	PO	QID	28 days

TERTIARY (LATE) SYPHILIS WITH NO NEUROLOGIC INVOLVEMENT

First line				
Benzathine penicillin G	2.4 million units	IM	Once/week	3 weeks
PCN-allergy				
Consult ID specialist				

NEUROSYPHILIS

First line				
Aqueous crystalline penicillin G	3–4 million units	IV	q4h or continuous for 18–24 million units/day	10–14 days
OR				
Procaine penicillin	2.4 million units	IM	Daily	10–14 days
with				
Probenecid	500 mg	PO	QID	10–14 days

Chancroid

Chancroid is a bacterial disease caused by *Haemophilus ducreyi*, a gram-negative rod, which is transmitted by direct sexual contact. In the United States, chancroid usually occurs in discrete outbreaks, although the disease is endemic in some areas. Chancroid is a cofactor for HIV transmission; high rates of HIV infection occur among patients who have chancroid in the United States and other countries.

An erythematous papule develops where the bacteria entered the body 3 to 14 days after contact. The pustule breaks down into the classic **dirty, painful, nonindurated ulcer.** Fifty percent of patients will have tender inguinal adenopathy, with matting of nodes. The lymph nodes in the groin are filled with pus (buboes).

The combination of a painful ulcer and tender inguinal adenopathy, symptoms occurring in one-third of patients, suggests a diagnosis of chancroid; when accompanied by suppurative inguinal adenopathy, these signs are almost pathognomonic.

DIAGNOSIS

A definitive diagnosis of chancroid requires identification of *H. ducreyi* on special culture media (supplemented gonococcal base and Mueller-Hinton agar) that is not widely available from commercial sources; even when using these media, sensitivity is 80%. No FDA-approved PCR test for *H. ducreyi* is available in the United States.

TREATMENT

Successful treatment for chancroid cures the infection, resolves the clinical symptoms, and prevents transmission to others. In advanced cases, scarring can result despite successful therapy. Resistance to various antibiotics has been a problem in the treatment of chancroid because of plasmid-mediated phenomenon. Those populations with HIV or uncircumcised men will generally not respond to treatment as well as comparative populations (Fig. 6.4).

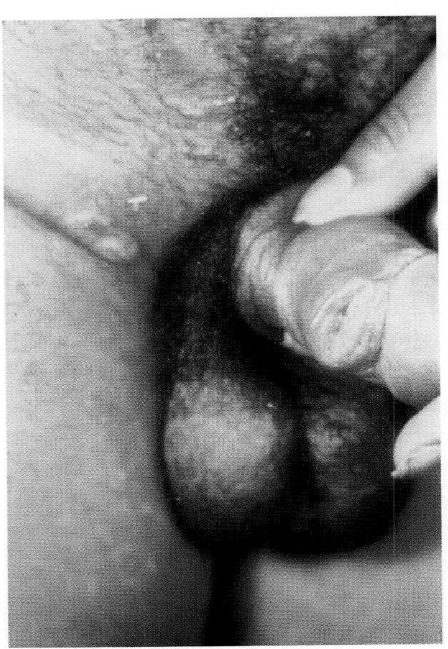

FIGURE 6.4 Chancroid with regional adenopathy. (From Frenkl TL, Potts JM. Sexually transmitted infections. In: Wein AJ, Kavoussi LR, Novick AC, et al., eds. *Campbell-Walsh Urology*. 10th ed. Philadelphia: Saunders; 2012:402-416.)

First line					
	Azithromycin	1 g	PO	Once	
	OR				
	Ceftriaxone	250 mg	IM	Once	
	OR				
	Ciprofloxacin	500 mg	PO	BID	3 days
	OR				
	Erythromycin base	500 mg	PO	TID	7 days

Lymphogranuloma Venereum

LGV is caused by *C. trachomatis* subtype L1, L2, or L3. The disease occurs most commonly in tropical climates and rarely in the United States. The most common clinical manifestation of LGV among heterosexuals is tender inguinal and/or femoral lymphadenopathy that is most commonly unilateral. Women and homosexually active men may have proctocolitis or inflammatory involvement of perirectal or perianal lymphatic tissues resulting in perirectal abscesses, anal fissures, and strictures. A self-limited genital ulcer sometimes occurs at the site of inoculation. The lymphadenopathy occurs 2 to 6 weeks after inoculation. However, by the time patients seek care, the ulcer usually has disappeared (conversely, patients with chancroid have the ulcer and lymphadenopathy concomitantly.)

The diagnosis of LGV is based on clinical suspicion and usually made by exclusion of other causes of inguinal lymphadenopathy or genital ulcers. These chlamydia subtypes must be cultured in special cell cultures (McCoy cells) and can be diagnosed by fluorescence antibody tests. Complement fixation titers 1:64 are consistent with the diagnosis of LGV.

Treatment cures infection and prevents ongoing tissue damage. Aspiration or incision and drainage to prevent formation of inguinal or femoral ulcerations in addition to an appropriate antibiotic regimen may be required.

TREATMENT

First line					
	Doxycycline	100 mg	PO	BID	21 days
Alternative					
	Erythromycin base	500 mg	PO	QID	21 days

Pregnant and lactating women should be treated with erythromycin. Azithromycin may prove useful for treatment of LGV in pregnancy, but no published data are available regarding its safety and efficacy. Doxycycline is contraindicated in pregnant women.

Granuloma Inguinale

GI, also known as *donovanosis*, is a genital ulcerative disease caused by the intracellular gram-negative bacterium *Klebsiella granulomatis* (previously *Calymmatobacterium granulomatis*). The organism is found in vacuolated inclusions within leukocytes known as **Donovan bodies.**

The disease occurs rarely in the United States, although it is endemic in certain tropical and developing areas, including India; Papua, New Guinea; central Australia; and southern Africa. Clinically, the disease commonly presents as painless, progressive ulcerative lesions **without regional lymphadenopathy.** The lesions appear 8 days to 12 weeks after inoculation. They are highly vascular ("beefy red appearance") and bleed easily on contact. However, the clinical presentation can also include hypertrophic, necrotic, or sclerotic variants.

GI is generally diagnosed by visual observation of the external symptoms. Gram-stained samples will show the bacteria, which can be cultured under special conditions only. Donovan bodies are found in macrophages on tissue crush preparation or biopsy.

TREATMENT

Treatment halts progression of lesions, although prolonged therapy may be required to permit granulation and reepithelialization of the ulcers. Relapse can occur 6 to 18 months after apparently effective therapy.

First line				
Azithromycin	1 g	PO	Weekly	3 weeks (until lesions healed)
OR				
Azithromycin	500 mg	PO	Daily	3 weeks (until lesions healed)

Alternative				
Doxycycline	100 mg	PO	BID	3 weeks (until lesions healed)
OR				
Ciprofloxacin	750 mg	PO	BID	3 weeks (until lesions healed)
OR				
Erythromycin base	500 mg	PO	QID	3 weeks (until lesions healed)
OR				
Trimethoprim-sulfamethoxazole DS	160 mg/800 mg	PO	BID	3 weeks (until lesions healed)

Gentamicin (1 mg/kg IV every 8 hours) can be used if lesions do not respond to initial oral therapy in several days or if the patient is HIV positive.

Molluscum Contagiosum

Molluscum contagiosum is a benign dermatologic disease caused by the molluscum contagiosum virus (MCV) (Poxviridae family). MCV may be transmitted by skin-to-skin contact, fomites, or self-inoculation.

The incubation period is 2 to 7 weeks. The lesions caused by MCV typically appear as flesh-colored, pearly pink, umbilicated, raised papules (1–5 mm in diameter) or nodules (6–10 mm), which may be single or multiple. Patients are often asymptomatic.

The diagnosis can be confirmed by light microscopy or electron microscopy of biopsies taken from a blister. Biopsy shows molluscum body, cytoplasmic inclusions containing viral particles. These intracytoplasmic inclusions are also known as Henderson-Paterson bodies and are pathognomonic.

TREATMENT

Blisters will regress spontaneously under the control of the immune system. If not, surgical removal by laser, cryotherapy, electrosurgery, or chemical treatment is recommended.

Vaginitis

Vaginal infection is usually characterized by a vaginal discharge or vulvar itching and irritation; a vaginal odor may be present. The three diseases most frequently associated with vaginal discharge are trichomoniasis (caused by *T. vaginalis*), bacterial vaginosis (BV; caused by a replacement of the normal vaginal flora by an overgrowth of anaerobic microorganisms, mycoplasmas, and *Gardnerella vaginalis*), and candidiasis (usually caused by *Candida albicans*). These infections are often diagnosed in women being evaluated for STIs.

The cause of vaginal infection can be diagnosed by pH and microscopic examination of the discharge. The pH of the vaginal secretions can be determined by narrow-range pH paper for the elevated **pH (greater than 4.5) typical of BV or trichomoniasis.** Discharge can be examined by diluting one sample in one to two drops of 0.9% normal saline solution on one slide and a second sample in 10% potassium hydroxide (KOH) solution. **An amine odor detected before or immediately after applying KOH suggests BV.** The motile *T. vaginalis* or the clue cells of BV usually are identified easily in the saline specimen. The yeast or pseudohyphae of *Candida* species are more easily identified in the KOH specimen.

BACTERIAL VAGINOSIS

BV is a clinical syndrome resulting from replacement of the normal H_2O_2-producing *Lactobacillus* sp. in the vagina with high concentrations of anaerobic bacteria (e.g., *Prevotella* sp., *Mobiluncus* sp.), *Gardnerella vaginalis*, and *Mycoplasma hominis*. BV is the most prevalent cause of vaginal discharge or malodor; however, up to 50% of women with BV may not report symptoms. BV is associated with having multiple sex partners, douching, and lack of vaginal lactobacilli; it is unclear whether BV results from acquisition of a sexually transmitted pathogen. Women who have never been sexually active are rarely affected. Treatment of the male sex partner has not been beneficial in preventing the recurrence of BV.

BV can be diagnosed by the use of clinical or Gram stain criteria. Clinical criteria require three of the following symptoms or signs:

1. A homogenous, white, noninflammatory discharge that smoothly coats the vaginal walls

2. The presence of clue cells on microscopic examination
3. A pH of vaginal fluid greater than 4.5
4. A fishy odor of vaginal discharge before or after addition of 10% KOH (i.e., the whiff test)

Treatment

First line					
	Metronidazole	500 mg	PO	BID	7 days
	OR				
	Metronidazole gel 0.75%	5 g	Intravaginally	Daily	5 days
Alternative					
	Clindamycin cream 2%	5 g	Intravaginally	QH	7 days

TRICHOMONIASIS

Trichomoniasis is caused by the protozoan *T. vaginalis*. Most men who are infected with *T. vaginalis* do not have symptoms. Many infected women present with symptoms characterized by a diffuse, malodorous, yellow-green discharge with vulvar irritation and will typically report similar high-risk behaviors: multiple sex partners, history of STIs, exchange of money for sex, or IV drug use. However, some women have minimal or no symptoms. Diagnosis of vaginal trichomoniasis is usually performed by microscopy of vaginal secretions.

Culture is the most sensitive, commercially available method of diagnosis. No FDA-approved PCR test for *T. vaginalis* is available in the United States.

Treatment

First line					
	Metronidazole	2 g	PO	Once	
	OR				
	Tinidazole	2 g	PO	Once	
	Co-HIV infection				
	Metronidazole	500 mg	PO	BID	7 days

VULVOVAGINAL CANDIDIASIS

Vulvovaginal candidiasis (VVC) usually is caused by *C. albicans* but occasionally is caused by other *Candida* sp. or yeasts. Typical symptoms of VVC include pruritus and vaginal discharge. Other symptoms include vaginal soreness, vulvar burning, dyspareunia, and external dysuria. None of these symptoms is specific for VVC. An estimated 75% of women will have at least one episode of VVC, and 40% to 45% will have two or more episodes.

Treatment

Short-course topical formulations (i.e., single dose, regimens of 1–3 days) effectively treat uncomplicated VVC. The topically applied azole drugs are more effective than nystatin. Treatment with azoles results in relief of symptoms and negative cultures in 80% to 90% of patients who complete therapy.

Over the counter				
	Clotrimazole cream			
	Miconazole cream or intravaginal suppository			
	Tioconazole ointment			
Prescription				
	Butoconazole cream			
	Terconazole cream or intravaginal suppository			
	Nystatin vaginal suppository			
	Prescription, oral			
	Fluconazole	150 mg	PO	Once

Ectoparasites

PHTHIRUS PUBIS

Phthirus pubis (pubic or crab louse) is a tiny insect that infects the pubic hair of its victims and feeds on human blood. They use crablike claws to grasp the hair of their host and can crawl several centimeters per day. Female lice lay two to three eggs daily and affix them to the hairs (nits). During direct sexual contact, the insects can move from one partner to the other. **Itching in the pubic area is a telltale sign.** Microscopic examination of the lice or the nits can confirm this.

First line		
	Permethrin 1% cream rinse	Wash off after 10 minutes
	OR	
	Pyrethrins with piperonyl butoxide	Wash off after 10 minutes
Treatment failure		
	Malathion 0.5% lotion	Wash off after 8–12 hours

Viral Hepatitis

HEPATITIS B

As of 2018, prevalence of hepatitis B infection in the United States stands at 4.3%, with the highest rates in non-Hispanic Asian adults at 21.1% and greater among foreign-born adults than US-born adults. However, that number is on the decline, as infection rates have gone down 1.4% and vaccination rates have increased to 25.2%. HBV is associated with chronic liver disease including cirrhosis and hepatocellular carcinoma, accounting for up to 30% and 45% of cases, respectively.

HBV can be self-limited or chronic, and the risk of developing chronic disease increases with younger age of acquisition.

Diagnosis

Serologic testing is as follows:

	HBcAb IgM	HBcAb IgG	HBsAg	Anti-HBs	HBeAg	Anti-HBe
Susceptible	−	−	−	−	−	−
Immune 2/2 natural infection	−	+	−	+	−	±
Immune 2/2 vaccine	−	−	−	+	−	−
Acutely infected	+	+	+	−	+	−
Chronically infected	−	+	+	−	±	±

Screening

Screening can be done with HBsAg and anti-HBs and is recommended in all those born where HBsAg seroprevalence is ≥2%, in those US-born and not vaccinated as infants whose parents were born in high HBV endemicity (8%), in pregnant women, in the immunosuppressed, and in at-risk groups. Those who screen negative and are anti-HBs should be vaccinated.

Prevention

Vaccination is now recommended for the following:

- Prophylaxis for infants born to HBsAg-positive women
- Universal vaccination for all infants
- Routine vaccination of all previously unvaccinated children under 19 years of age
- Vaccination of adults at risk for HBV infection

Single-antigen and combination HBV vaccines are available: *Engerix-B* and *Recombivax HB* are single-antigen vaccines approved in the United States and administered at birth. In 2017, *Heplisav-B*, a single-antigen HBV vaccine, was approved for 18 years and older. *Pediarix* provides recombinant HBsAg, diphtheria, tetanus toxoids, acellular pertussis adsorbed, and inactivated poliovirus and is administered from 6 weeks to 6 years of age. *Twinrix* contains recombinant HBsAg and inactivated hepatitis A virus and is administered for 18 years and older.

Postexposure

All wounds and skin sites should be washed with soap and water.

Recommendations for postexposure prophylaxis (PEP) in vaccinated health care workers (HCWs) are below:

- If anti-HBs > 10 mIU/mL
  - Do not need to test source patient for HBV
  - No PEP
- If anti-HBs is unknown
  - HCW should be tested for anti-HBs levels
  - Source patient should be tested for HBsAg
- If anti-HBs is < 10 mIU/mL and unknown if source patient is HBsAg-positive
  - Administer one dose of hepatitis B immune globulin (HBIG) and two doses of vaccine
  - Check anti-HBs levels in 1 to 2 months after second vaccine dose

- If anti-HBs is < 10 mIU/mL and source patient is HBsAg-negative
  - Administer one vaccine dose
  - Check anti-HBs in 1 to 2 months after vaccine dose

If a vaccinated HCW continues to have anti-HBs < 10 mIU/mL after two vaccine series, the source patient should be tested. If the source patient is positive, two doses of HBIG should be administered, first at time of exposure and the second 1 month later.

If an exposed HCW is unvaccinated or incompletely vaccinated, the source patient should be tested and if they are HBsAg positive or unknown, the HCW should get one dose of HBIG and one vaccine dose, then complete the remainder of their vaccine series, and follow up with anti-HBs levels 1 to 2 months after the last vaccine. If the source patient is HBsAg negative, the HCW should complete their vaccine series and follow up with anti-HBs levels in 1 to 2 months.

HEPATITIS C

In 2016, the CDC estimated 2.7 to 3.9 million people were living with chronic HCV infections. HCV is predominantly spread through injection drug use, and less commonly through sexual or maternal-fetal transmission.

Diagnosis

One-time testing should be done on individuals born between 1945 and 1965, or in those with risk factors.

Treatment

Current HCV protease inhibitors can cure patients of the viral infection and are curated by genotype and symptomology.

Zika virus

Zika virus is a flavivirus from the same family as dengue, yellow fever, and the West Nile virus. In 2016, the WHO declared it a public health emergency of international concern due to the risks of significant birth defects in pregnant woman. The Zika virus is predominantly transmitted by female mosquito vectors, but can also be spread via maternal-fetal transfer, blood, and sexual contact (both vaginal and anal intercourse), and has been detected in urine, saliva, breast milk, and other bodily fluids.

SYMPTOMS

Most people are asymptomatic. For those who are, symptoms are usually mild and nonspecific, including low-grade fever, conjunctivitis, maculopapular rash, myalgia, and headache. However, Zika has been associated with serious neurologic complications such as microcephaly and Guillain-Barre syndrome, with more severe presentations in infants.

DIAGNOSIS

Testing is recommended for anybody with possible Zika virus exposure and those who are also symptomatic. While any pregnant women with possible exposure should be tested, widespread testing is not recommended for asymptomatic nonpregnant individuals or for general preconception testing.

Testing can be done by Zika virus RNA NAAT of urine or serum samples and Zika virus serum IgM. NAAT is only accurate in samples collected within 14 days of symptom onset. If NAAT is negative, further testing should be followed with IgM serology.

PRECONCEPTION COUNSELING AND PREVENTION

Men with possible Zika exposure should wait 6 months from symptom onset or possible exposure before conception, while women should wait at least 8 weeks.

Human Immunodeficiency Virus

HIV is an RNA virus (retrovirus) that binds to the CD4 molecule on T4 lymphocytes and some other cell types. Viral RNA undergoes reverse transcription to DNA, which is incorporated into the host DNA. Viral replication occurs by transcription of proviral DNA into viral mRNA, which is associated with a decline in the CD4 cell count and defeat of the immune system. HIV has been isolated from blood, semen, vaginal secretions, saliva, tears, urine, amniotic fluid, breast milk, and cerebrospinal fluid. However, **evidence has implicated only blood, semen, and vaginal secretions in the transmission of the virus.**

Both viral load (molecules of viral RNA/mL) and CD4 T-cell count are used to monitor and prognosticate disease progression to acquired immunodeficiency syndrome (AIDS). **CD4 counts of**

fewer than 500 cells/μL are associated with a greater risk of opportunistic infections and progression to AIDS; below 200 cells/μL are at high risk for life-threatening opportunistic infections.

Diagnostic tests for HIV include measurement of anti-HIV antibodies using an enzyme-linked immunosorbent assay (ELISA); antibody-positive specimens are tested using the Western blot assay, which is more specific. Antibodies can be detected on day 21 after initial exposure. Also, after acute infection, HIV RNA can be detected from day 12 through RNA assays. This testing is used in treatment by evaluation of viral load as a response to current therapy.

Treatments include nucleoside analogue reverse-transcriptase inhibitors, nonnucleoside reverse transcriptase inhibitors, and PIs. Indinavir and nelfinavir are associated with renal stones in up to 4% of cases. These stones are not visualized on x-ray or computed tomography. Patients usually improve with hydration and discontinuation of the drug. If necessary, ureteral stenting will usually suffice.

Of concern now with expanding antiviral medication is development of drug resistance. Recommendations include directed viral testing prior to initiation of antiviral therapy.

Epidemiology

According to the CDC estimates, in 2018, 1.2 million people aged 13 and older, in the United States, had a diagnosis of HIV and 37,968 people were newly diagnosed. Worldwide, prevalence of HIV is estimated to be 37.9 million, and the incidence in 2018 was 1.7 million. An estimated 70% of HIV-positive men acquired the virus through vaginal intercourse. HIV is more likely in people who have had sexually transmitted diseases (STDs), especially genital ulcer disease.

Individuals who are infected with STIs are at least two to five times more likely to acquire HIV than uninfected individuals if they are exposed to the virus through sexual contact. In addition, if an HIV-infected individual is also infected with another STD, that person is more likely to transmit HIV through sexual contact than other HIV-infected persons.

STDs likely increase susceptibility to HIV infection by two mechanisms. Genital ulcers (e.g., syphilis, herpes, chancroid) result in breaks in the genital tract lining or skin. These breaks create a portal of entry for HIV. Nonulcerative STDs (e.g., chlamydia, gonorrhea, trichomoniasis) increase the concentration of cells in genital secretions that can serve as targets for HIV (e.g., CD4+ cells).

Studies have shown that when HIV-infected individuals are also infected with other STDs, they are more likely to have HIV in their genital secretions. For example, men who are infected with both gonorrhea and HIV are more than twice as likely to shed HIV in their genital secretions as those who are infected only with HIV. Moreover, the median concentration of HIV in semen is as much as 10 times higher in men who are infected with both gonorrhea and HIV than in men infected only with HIV.

In the HIV-positive patient, genital ulcers are usually caused by STDs such as genital herpes, syphilis, and chancroid, but they may also be part of a systemic illness such as herpes zoster or cytomegalovirus or may be related to drug therapy (e.g., with the antiviral agent foscarnet).

Serologic tests for syphilis may give a false-negative result in the HIV-infected patient, who may have a tendency to delayed appearance of seroreactivity. HIV patients with syphilis are more likely to encounter neurologic complications and have a higher rate of treatment failure. Condyloma acuminatum is very common in HIV-infected patients. Visible genital warts caused by HPV type 6 or 11 are found in 20% of HIV-infected patients, compared with 0.1% of the general population.

MCV infection occurs in 5% to 18% of HIV-positive patients. HIV-positive patients tend to develop giant (greater than 1 cm) lesions or may have clustering of hundreds of small lesions and are at greater risk for secondary inflammation and bacterial infection. MCV lesions in patients with HIV do not resolve quickly, spread easily to other locations, and are refractory to common treatments. Differential diagnosis includes condyloma acuminata for small, and squamous carcinoma for large, solitary lesions. Treatment options for MCV are the same as for genital warts.

Additionally, recent studies support the conclusion that circumcised heterosexual men are at a lower risk for HIV infections. A movement for adult circumcisions has been initiated in HIV-laden populations because this is one of few proven prevention strategies.

MALIGNANCIES

Kaposi sarcoma (KS) is a sarcoma of endothelial origin affecting the feet and lower extremities and (rarely) the genitalia. Prior to 1981 it was seen only in elderly men of Mediterranean descent and ran an indolent course (now called "classic" KS). Development of KS in the HIV population is from a KS-associated herpes virus that is sexually transmitted. Twenty percent of patients with HIV-associated KS will develop lesions on the genitalia. Lesions are subcutaneous, nonpruritic nodules. They can be pigmented, sometimes appearing blue. Lymphedema is common.

Treatment includes local excision, laser fulguration, intralesional injections, radiation, or imiquimod therapy for the small solitary lesion. Larger lesions are treated with radiation therapy with possible side effects of urethral strictures or fistulae. Disseminated KS is treated with highly active antiretroviral therapy (HAART), chemotherapy, and interferon.

Testicular tumors occur in up to 0.2%, or 50 times that of the general population. Seminomatous and extragonadal germ cell cancer are more common, but HIV confers marginally increased risk for nonseminomatous testicular cancer. Testicular lymphoma in HIV patients presents in younger men and with higher-grade tumor than in non-HIV men.

Treatment for these tumors follow the standard treatment guidelines if the patient can tolerate the therapy—three cycles of cisplatin, etoposide, and bleomycin can lower CD4 counts as much as 25%–50%, and thus low-risk nonseminoma patients should be considered for surveillance.

Renal, penile, and cervical cancers are also more common in HIV patients and adopt more aggressive courses.

IMPOTENCE

Erectile and ejaculatory dysfunction are common problems in HIV-infected men. It is estimated that 67% and 33% of men with AIDS have decreased libido and impotence, respectively. Typically, these HIV-positive men have low serum testosterone levels, normal luteinizing hormone but high follicle-stimulating hormone levels, and oligoteratospermia. Testicular atrophy results from the direct cytotoxic effect of HIV on the germinal and Sertoli cells and secondary effects of HIV infection, such as opportunistic infection of the testes, side effects from medication, and effects of cytokines on the hypothalamic-pituitary-gonadal axis.

They may also suffer from psychological depression, AIDS-related dementia, and neurogenic dysfunction, including peripheral neuropathy from viral myelitis and myelopathy. This can occur in 30% to 40% of AIDS patients. Patients can be treated successfully with testosterone supplements, phosphodiesterase-5 (PDE-5) inhibitors, or intracavernosal/intraurethral prostaglandins. However, caution should be taken in patients also taking PIs, as PIs can also inhibit the CYP3A enzyme, causing a 3- to 10-fold increase in serum concentrations of PDE-5 inhibitors; sildenafil should be started at a lower dose.

VOIDING DYSFUNCTION

Impaired micturition becomes more common with disease progression and can occur as part of an overall neurologic dysfunction or through infection. In a series of 39 HIV-positive patients presenting with lower urinary tract symptoms (LUTS) and undergoing urodynamics, a urodynamic abnormality (overactive or underactive detrusor or detrusor sphincter dyssynergia) was identified in 87% of patients. Of these, 61% had AIDS-related neurologic problems, such as cerebral toxoplasmosis, HIV demyelination disorders, and AIDS-related dementia. This heralded a poor prognosis because 43% in this group died after 2 to 24 months (mean 8). Detrusor failure caused by lower motor injury is uncommon and is usually ascribed to malignancy or infection such as herpes. Patients should be taught clean intermittent catheterization (CIC); long-term indwelling catheters are best avoided in HIV-infected patients because of their vulnerability to *Staphylococcus aureus* bacterium.

CLINICAL PEARLS

1. Given the growing rate of microbial resistance to common antibiotics, the Centers for Disease Control and Prevention (CDC) or similar authoritative sources should be periodically consulted for up-to-date therapeutic recommendations.
2. Treatment and education of not only the presenting patient but also their sexual partners is key in treating sexually transmitted infections (STIs) and controlling their spread.
3. Given the asymptomatology of many STIs, screening is key in diagnosing and controlling infections within respective at-risk patient populations.
4. An iPad app about STI is available from the CDC (http://www.cdc.gov/std/std-tx-app.htm).

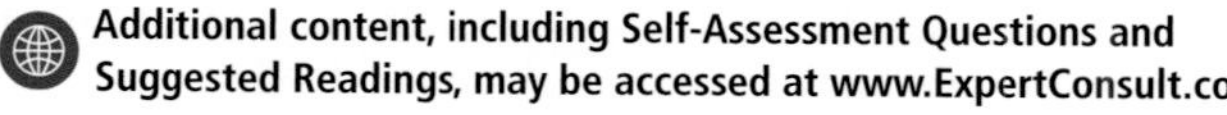
Additional content, including Self-Assessment Questions and Suggested Readings, may be accessed at www.ExpertConsult.com.

Interstitial Cystitis/Bladder Pain Syndrome

Philip M. Hanno, MD, MPH

Originally considered a bladder disease, interstitial cystitis/bladder pain syndrome (IC/BPS) is now positioned in the medical spectrum as a chronic pain syndrome that may begin as a pathologic process in the bladder in many, but not all, patients. In a small percentage of patients, it can progress into a disorder that even cystectomy may not benefit!

IC/BPS encompasses a major portion of the "painful bladder" disease complex, which includes a large group of patients with bladder and/or urethral and/or pelvic pain, irritative voiding symptoms (urgency, frequency, nocturia, dysuria), and sterile urine cultures. Painful bladder conditions with well-understood and established etiologies include radiation cystitis, cystitis caused by microorganisms including some that are not detected by routine culture methodologies, and systemic disorders that affect the bladder. Table 7.1 **IC/BPS is a diagnosis of exclusion.** It may have multiple causes and represent a final common reaction of the bladder to different types of insults. Essentially, one must be confident that the patient with IC/BPS is not actually suffering from any known treatable etiology of bladder pain before making the diagnosis.

Definition

The American Urological Association defines IC/BPS as "An unpleasant sensation (pain, pressure, discomfort) perceived to be related to the urinary bladder, associated with lower urinary tract symptoms of more than six weeks duration, in the absence of infection or other identifiable causes." The term "interstitial cystitis" (IC) has classically been used to describe the clinical

TABLE 7.1 Differential Diagnosis: Some Potential Causes of Frequency and Urgent Desire to Void

- Atrophic urethral changes
- Bacterial urethritis
- Bladder calculus
- Bladder cancer
- Cervicitis
- Chemical irritants: contraceptive foams, douches, diaphragm, obsessive washing
- Chemotherapy
- Diabetes insipidus
- Diabetes mellitus
- Diuretic therapy
- Habit
- Incomplete bladder emptying
- **Interstitial cystitis/bladder pain syndrome**
- Ketamine abuse
- Large fluid intake
- Overactive bladder
- Pelvic mass
- Pelvic radiation
- Periurethral gland infection
- Pregnancy
- Renal impairment
- Upper motor neuron lesion
- Urethral caruncle
- Urethral condyloma
- Urethral diverticulum
- Urinary tract infection
- Vulvar carcinoma

syndrome of urgency/frequency and pain in the bladder and/or pelvis that is unrelated to any defined urologic pathology. When considering IC/BPS, the symptom of pain should be broadened to include "pressure" and "discomfort."

Urgency is left out of the definition of IC/BPS, as it is the cardinal symptom of overactive bladder (OAB) (a confusable disease) and proves to be unnecessary for definition purposes. One can often separate out those patients with the hypersensitivity of IC/BPS from those with the urgency of OAB by doing a cystometrogram. The OAB patient will generally have uninhibited bladder contractions, while the IC/BPS patient will have a stable bladder with hypersensitivity during bladder filling. Simple questions will often suffice to differentiate between the two conditions. "Does your urgency to find a restroom come on suddenly, and is it because you are afraid you will wet yourself, or is it a more gradually appearing sensation of increasing pain and discomfort that you feel in the bladder area?" The former strongly suggests OAB, and the latter is most consistent with IC/BPS. OAB is over 10 times more common in the population than IC/BPS, and the treatment algorithm is very different, making the differential diagnosis critical (Figs. 7.1, 7.2, and 7.3).

The Hunner Lesion

When "interstitial cystitis" was first described over a century ago, the diagnosis was based on symptoms of pain perceived to be related to the bladder with urinary frequency in association with the cystoscopic finding of an isolated inflammatory lesion(s) in

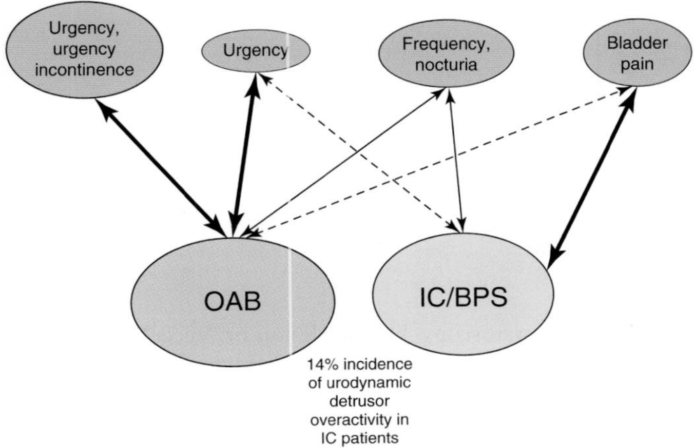

FIGURE 7.1 Relationship of overactive bladder (OAB) and interstitial cystitis/bladder pain syndrome (IC/BPS). (Abrams P, Hanno P, Wein A. Overactive bladder and painful bladder syndrome: there need not be confusion. *Neurourol Urodyn*, 2005;24:149.)

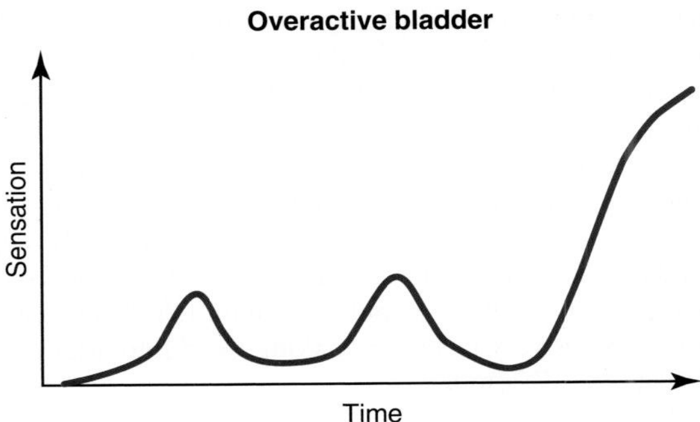

FIGURE 7.2 Undulating onset of true urgency typical of overactive bladder.

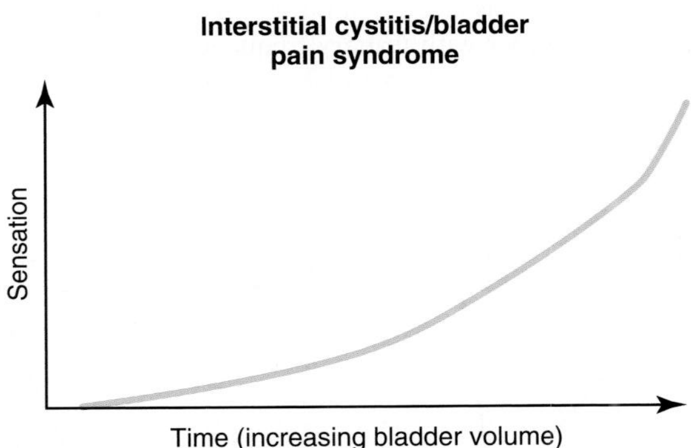

FIGURE 7.3 Steadily increasing pain typical of interstitial cystitis/bladder pain syndrome (IC/BPS).

the bladder at cystoscopy. Hunner lesion or "ulcer" is a distinctive inflammatory lesion presenting a characteristic deep rupture through the mucosa and submucosa provoked by bladder distension (Fig. 7.4). Despite the name that has been commonly used, it is not a true ulcer. Fifty years ago it became apparent that the majority of patients with symptoms consistent with a diagnosis of IC did **not** have Hunner lesions, and many had completely normal bladders on cystoscopic examination. The diagnosis of IC was

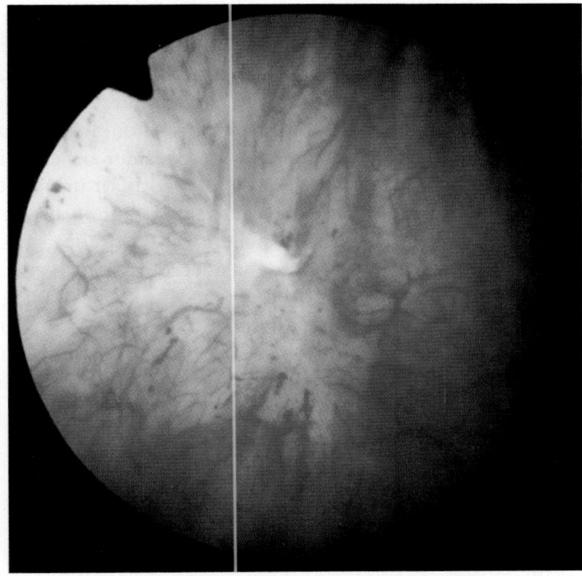

FIGURE 7.4 Typical appearance of Hunner lesion on initial endoscopy and prior to distention, mucosal tearing, and bleeding.

expanded to include these patients, and Hunner lesion was then considered a phenotype within the diagnosis of IC/BPS.

Patients **without** Hunner lesions are younger at diagnosis and symptom onset and have significantly greater bladder capacity under general anesthesia. Patients **with** Hunner lesions tend to void more frequently and have more nocturia and a smaller bladder capacity than those without lesions. Compared to the Hunner group, subjects without lesions report more chronic pain diagnoses and present more often with fibromyalgia, migraines, temporomandibular joint disorders and other non–bladder-centric pain syndromes.

Based on a distinct histopathology, endoscopic findings characteristic of the Hunner lesion, the epidemiologic pattern that distinguishes it from BPS, the clinical response to local treatment of the lesion by resection, fulguration, or steroid injection, the positive response to the immune modulator cyclosporine, and the absence of reports in the literature that non-Hunner patients go on to develop Hunner lesions (i.e., the finding of Hunner lesion does not represent a continuum in the natural history of BPS), it is now widely believed that the presence of a Hunner lesion should be considered a distinct disease. It therefore should drop out of the BPS construct, much like we do not consider other painful conditions like radiation cystitis, ketamine cystitis, or urinary tract infection a part of BPS. While symptoms alone cannot distinguish between the two groups, with the benefit of cystoscopy, it is apparent that Hunner lesion can be considered a disease and BPS a collection of symptoms (syndrome) (Fig. 7.5). The etiology of both of these conditions remains largely unknown. Many of the treatments below are thought to be beneficial for both conditions, but the diagnosis of Hunner lesion allows one to consider direct fulguration of the lesion or steroid injection into the lesion as well as oral cyclosporin as reasonable treatment options as well.

Epidemiology

Epidemiology studies of IC/BPS have suffered from the lack of a universally accepted definition, the absence of a validated diagnostic marker or clinical test that assures the diagnosis is made in a uniform manner by different clinicians in different geographic areas, and the lack of a pathognomonic finding on histologic biopsy of bladder tissue. There is considerable variability in studies on incidence and prevalence not only within the United States, but around the world. The first population-based study included patients with IC in Helsinki, Finland. The prevalence was 18.1 per 100,000 women and 10.6 per 100,000 population. The annual incidence of new female cases was 1.2 per 100,000. Severe cases accounted for 10% of the total. Only 10% of cases were in men.

Another early population study from the United States in 1987 first demonstrated the potential extent of what had been considered a very rare disorder. It concluded that while there were 43,500 to 90,000 diagnosed cases of IC/BPS in the United States (twice the prevalence in Finland), up to half a million people had symptoms of painful bladder and sterile urine, considerably expanding the population of potentially affected individuals. The median age at onset was 40 years and there was a 50% remission rate not clearly related to therapy that lasted a mean of 9 months.

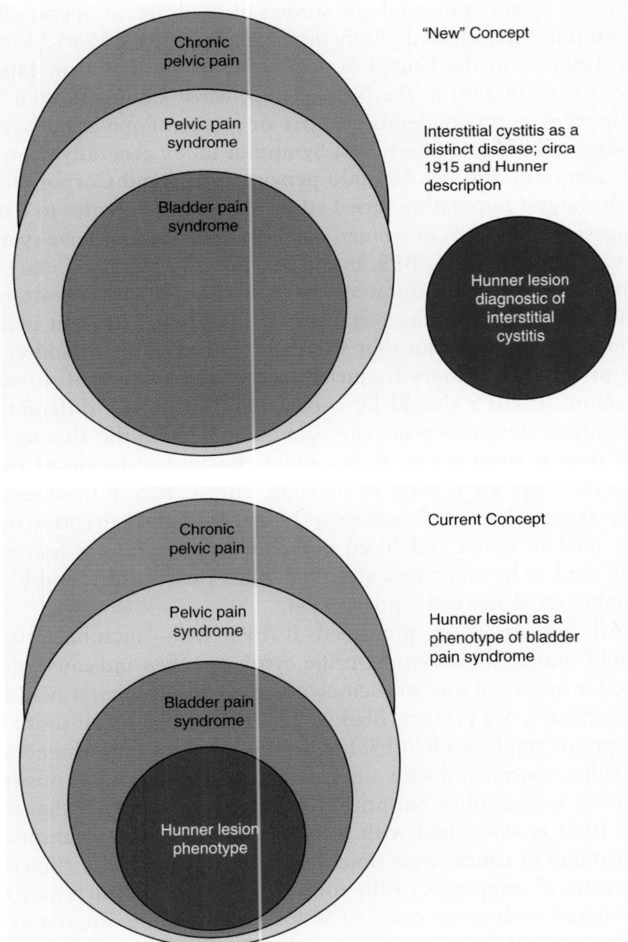

FIGURE 7.5 Evolving concept of Hunner lesion as it relates to bladder pain syndrome. (From Hanno PM, Cervigni M, Dinis P, et al. Bladder pain syndrome. In Abrams P, Cardozo L, Wagg A, Wein A, eds. *Incontinence*. 6th ed. London:ICS and ICUD; 2017:2203-2302. ISBN: 978-0-9569607-3-3.)

More recent epidemiologic studies using different operational definitions have yielded wildly disparate data, from 35 to 24,000 per 100,000 in the United States, to 1.2 per 100,000 in Japan and 7 per 100,000 in the Netherlands. Most studies show a female to male preponderance of 5:1 or greater. Population-based studies using the O'Leary Sant Symptom Index generally show a prevalence of 300 per 100,000 persons. **The Rand Corporation, in the largest population-based study in the United States to date, suggested that 2.7% of women and 1.9% of men may have symptoms suggestive of IC/BPS.** In the absence of a validated marker, it may be difficult to differentiate chronic pelvic pain syndrome (CPPS) in men ("nonbacterial prostatitis") from BPS. **In males who have chronic pain that they associate with the bladder, in the presence of urinary frequency and in the absence of urinary infection, IC/BPS should be considered high in the differential diagnosis.** Men with primarily pain complaints in the absence of any voiding dysfunction fit the more classic description of type 3 CPPS. Only 10%–30% of patients with IC/BPS in most series have true isolated inflammatory bladder lesions on endoscopy that tend to crack and bleed with distention (Hunner lesions). Men tend to be diagnosed at an older age than women and have a higher incidence of Hunner lesion.

All patients with presumed IC/BPS with microhematuria should undergo cystoscopy, urine cytology when indicated, and bladder biopsy of any suspicious lesion to be sure that a bladder carcinoma is not present. Bladder carcinoma in situ can result in symptoms similar to IC/BPS. It would seem that in the absence of microhematuria, and with a negative cytology, the risk of missing a cancer is negligible, but not zero. **There is no evidence that IC/BPS itself is associated with a higher risk of bladder cancer or transitions to cancer over time.** It is important that the clinician be aware of symptoms of the following disorders, which may be associated with some cases of IC/BPS: depression, Sjögren syndrome, irritable bowel syndrome, allergies, fibromyalgia, chronic fatigue syndrome, dyspareunia, and focal vulvitis.

Etiology

It is likely that IC/BPS has a multifactorial etiology. A "leaky epithelium," mast cell activation, neurogenic inflammation, primary pelvic floor dysfunction, and sequelae of bladder infection or pelvic surgery have all been proposed at one time or another. Decades of research from the National Institutes of Health have documented that BPS patients may have changes in neurologic function including brain structure and function, inflammatory response, pain sensitivity and associated comorbid diseases compared to controls. There is little data to support the role of an active infectious etiology, but it is conceivable that a viral or bacterial cystitis could begin the cascade that ultimately leads to a self-perpetuating process resulting in chronic bladder pain and voiding dysfunction.

Associated disorders including irritable bowel syndrome, fibromyalgia, chronic fatigue syndrome, depression, pelvic floor dysfunction, and various other chronic pain disorders may precede or follow the development of IC/BPS in some patients. Patients with Hunner lesions and low bladder capacity under anesthesia are more likely to have bladder-centric disease, while those without Hunner lesions are somewhat more likely to experience associated pain disorders. Whether the etiology of Hunner lesion disease and non-Hunner BPS is similar or distinct is purely speculative at this time (Fig. 7.6). Neural cross talk in the dorsal root ganglia and in the central nervous system and subsequent central sensitization may explain some of the clinical associations of the various chronic pain disorders and why efficacious therapeutic interventions have been relatively few and far between.

Diagnosis

The diagnosis of IC/BPS is the recognition of chronic pain, pressure, and/or discomfort associated with the bladder, usually accompanied by urinary frequency in the absence of any identifiable cause. A high index of suspicion is required on the part of the clinician, as many patients suffer for years in the absence of the correct diagnosis. **Pelvic pain and urinary frequency, lasting more than 6 weeks and unrelated to urinary infection, establish a working diagnosis.** Some patients will not complain of pain, but if the clinician asks them why they void so often, they will admit to a "pressure" or "discomfort" that is relieved, at least momentarily, by emptying the bladder.

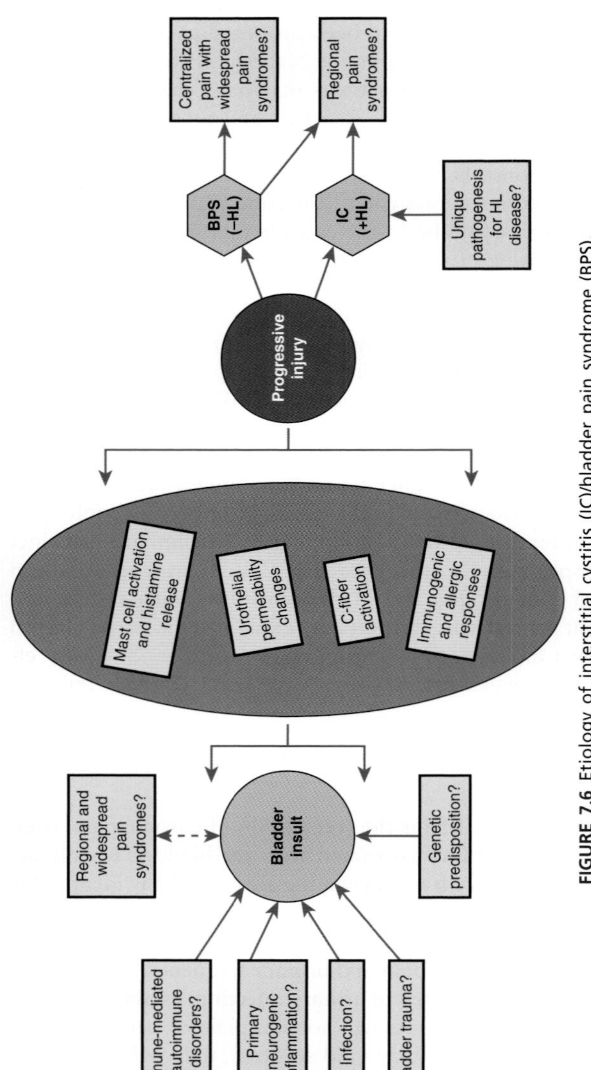

FIGURE 7.6 Etiology of interstitial cystitis (IC)/bladder pain syndrome (BPS). (From Moldwin R, Hanno P. Interstitial cystitis/bladder pain syndrome and related disorders. In: Partin A, Dmochowski R, Kavoussi LR, Peters CA, eds. Campbell-Walsh-Wein *Urology*, 12th ed. Philadelphia:Elsevier, 2021.)

A variety of IC/BPS symptom scales have been developed. They are designed to evaluate the *severity* of symptomatology and monitor disease progression or regression with or without treatment. They have not been validated as diagnostic instruments.

As IC/BPS is a diagnosis of exclusion, one must rule out infection, OAB, and less common conditions including, but not limited to, carcinoma, eosinophilic cystitis, malakoplakia, schistosomiasis, scleroderma, and detrusor endometriosis (Table 7.1). In men under the age of 50, videourodynamics are useful to eliminate other treatable causes of voiding dysfunction. Many drugs including cyclophosphamide, aspirin, nonsteroidal antiinflammatory agents, and allopurinol have caused a nonbacterial cystitis that resolves with drug withdrawal. Illicit use of ketamine can cause a fulminant sterile cystitis, which has now been recognized as a major problem in many parts of Asia.

In the presence of microhematuria, local cystoscopy and upper tract imaging are essential to rule out urothelial cancer or other lesions. Cystoscopy is often completely normal in the non–Hunner lesion majority of patients. Cystoscopy is important, however, in differentiating Hunner lesion disease and this can be done without sedation in the majority of patients. They appear as isolated inflammatory areas of bladder mucosa often with scarring and bleeding with slight distention.

When performed under anesthesia the physician can distend the bladder to 60 cm of water pressure whereupon the fragile mucosa of the Hunner lesion may crack and bleed. Distention can result in symptom relief for weeks to months in some patients even without Hunner lesions, and longer benefit is observed when a Hunner lesion is identified and extensively fulgurated or injected with local steroid. Up to 30% of patients with symptoms of IC/BPS may be Hunner lesion positive in some series. Although recommended by this author in order to differentiate Hunner lesion disease, initial cystoscopy in the office is not mandatory to diagnose the syndrome, and it is certainly justifiable to begin conservative therapy without endoscopy or bladder distention having been performed. If a Hunner lesion is noted, one can move directly to cystoscopy under anesthesia with fulguration or steroid injection of the lesion often resulting in symptom relief for 6 to 12 months. Symptoms generally do recur over time and the procedure will need to be repeated until tachyphylaxis develops.

In patients who do not respond to initial conservative therapy, cystoscopy (if it has not been done previously) is an essential next step in order to diagnose a Hunner lesion. Such a finding will change the treatment algorithm significantly. We recommend cystoscopy be routinely performed early in the diagnosis of the disorder so that patients with Hunner lesion disease can be identified and treated appropriately. Extensive fulguration of a Hunner lesion or intralesional injection of steroid can result in dramatic symptom relief for months to years in some of these patients and can be repeated in the future as needed. **Bladder biopsy is indicated only if necessary, to rule out other disorders that might be suggested by the cystoscopic appearance.** Glomerulations (petechial bleeding points) are not specific for IC/BPS, and their presence or absence should not be a consideration in diagnosis or choice of treatment (Fig. 7.7).

Initial Management

After diagnosis, the first decision the practitioner faces is whether to institute active therapy. If the patient has not had an empiric

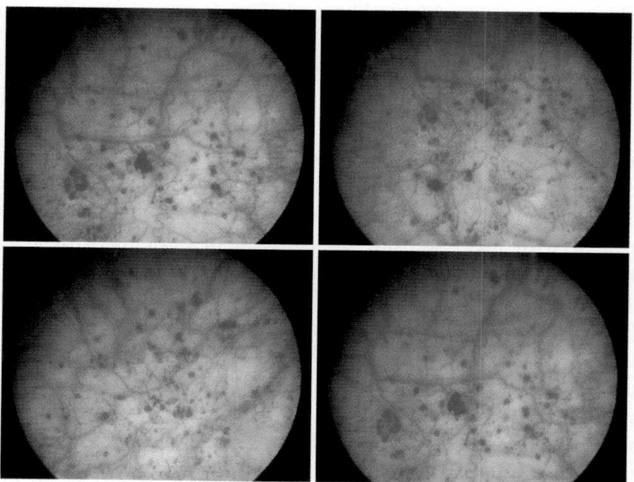

FIGURE 7.7 Typical appearance of glomerulations after bladder distention under anesthesia.

course of antibiotics for their symptoms, such a trial with one course of treatment is not unreasonable. Doxycycline is a good choice. Generally, patients diagnosed with IC/BPS have already been on several courses of antibiotics by the time the diagnosis is even entertained making this decision moot.

If the patient's symptoms are mild to moderate, the withholding of immediate medical treatment is worth considering. Someone who awakens once or twice a night and voids at 2 to 3 hour intervals with minimal pain symptoms is someone active treatment would be unlikely to benefit further. **Data that early intervention affects the natural history or course of the disease are lacking, and an argument for the early institution of therapy cannot be supported on the basis of epidemiologic data or clinical trials.** Patient education and empowerment is an important initial step in therapy. Reassuring the patient that this is not a life-threatening disease; others have similar problems and have learned to live with them; there is a spontaneous remission rate; and symptoms do not invariably progress does much to alleviate the stress that accompanies the diagnosis. The Interstitial Cystitis Association (www.icahelp.org) and the International Painful Bladder Foundation (https://www.painful-bladder.org/) are important resources for information and support for patients and providers alike.

Timed voiding and behavioral modification can be useful in the short-term, especially in patients in whom frequency rather than pain predominates. Many clinicians believe that stress reduction, exercise, warm tub baths, and efforts by the patients to maintain a normal lifestyle all contribute to quality of life. While elaborate dietary restrictions and an "IC diet" are unsupported by any peer-reviewed literature, many patients do find their symptoms are adversely affected by specific foods and beverages and would do well to avoid them. Often these include caffeine, alcohol, hot spicy foods, and beverages that might acidify the urine like cranberry juice.

As pelvic floor dysfunction is a commonly associated problem and, in some cases, may be the primary trigger of perceived bladder pain, pelvic floor physical therapy with myofascial trigger point release and intravaginal Thiele massage administered by an experienced physical therapist can be an excellent therapeutic approach with little in the way of side effects. Education and conservative therapy help many patients, but often more active intervention is required.

Oral Therapy

While many oral medications have been tried for the treatment of IC/BPS, amitriptyline, sodium pentosan polysulfate, and hydroxyzine remain the only commonly used medications outside of research trials.

Amitriptyline has become one of the most popular oral agents for the treatment of IC/BPS. It is an old, inexpensive tricyclic antidepressant available only in its generic form. This class of medication has at least three main pharmacologic actions: (1) central and peripheral anticholinergic activity; (2) blockage of the active transport system in the presynaptic nerve ending responsible for the reuptake of serotonin and norepinephrine; and (3) sedation that may be central or related to antihistaminic properties. It is believed that amitriptyline has analgesic properties and potentiates the body's own endorphins. It may help to stabilize the mast cells in the bladder and also increase bladder capacity through its effect on the beta-adrenergic receptors in the bladder body. Finally, the sedative effects can help the patient sleep.

The physician prescribing amitriptyline should be very familiar with the drug, as it has many significant side effects. These commonly include daytime sedation, constipation, increased appetite, and dry mouth. It should not be prescribed for potentially suicidal patients, or for those with cardiac problems or arrhythmias. The patient with IC/BPS should be started on a dose of 10 mg before bed. The dose is gradually increased by 10 mg each week to a maximum dose of 50 mg at bedtime at the start of the 5th week. If tolerated, this dose is maintained. Often a lower dose will prove effective.

Parson's suggestion that a defect in the epithelial permeability barrier, the glycosaminoglycan layer, contributes to the pathogenesis of IC/BPS has led to an attempt to correct such a defect with the synthetic sulfated polysaccharide sodium pentosanpolysulfate (PPS). This is a heparin analogue (trade name *Elmiron*), which is sold in an oral formulation. Three to six percent of each dose is excreted into the urine. Two placebo-controlled multicenter trials in the United States served as the pivotal studies for Food and Drug Administration (FDA) approval for the pain of IC. In the initial study, overall improvement of greater than 25% was reported by 28% of the PPS-treated group versus 13% in the placebo group. In the follow-up study, the respective figures were 32% on PPS versus 16% on placebo. Average voided volume on PPS increased by 20 mL. No other objective improvements were documented. An NIDDK study looking at both PPS and hydroxyzine alone and in combination compared to placebo failed to show a statistically significant response to either medication. Two FDA-mandated phase 4 studies have been completed. The first showed no dose response from 300 mg total daily dosage PPS to 900 mg total daily dosage. The second failed to demonstrate any efficacy comparing the 300 mg daily dose to placebo. **At best, Elmiron appears to have a modest beneficial effect in a minority of patients who take it for 3 to 6 months.** There are no convincing data that a longer trial is worthwhile in nonresponders. The dose is 100 mg three times daily. Side effects include a 6% incidence of reversible hair loss, gastrointestinal upset, and skin rash. It is generally well tolerated, though not highly efficacious. With the recent publication of multiple studies indicating significant risk of ophthamologic side effects including pigmentary maculopathy associated with use of PPS, and its questionable efficacy, the risk-benefit ratio suggests it should not be employed in treatment.

Antihistamines have been used for their properties blocking the effects of mast cell activation. Hydroxyzine, an H1 antagonist, was studied in 40 patients treated with 25 mg before bedtime, increasing to 50 mg at night and 25 mg in the morning in those for whom sedation from the medicine was not a problem. The vast majority of patients had symptom improvement, but these good results have not been confirmed in placebo-controlled trials. Cimetidine, an H2 antagonist, has been reported effective in a British trial, but confirmatory studies are lacking, and the mechanism of action is unexplained. It is not commonly used.

While the exact role of autoimmunity in the etiology of IC/BPS remains controversial, Finnish studies have demonstrated good results with low dose cyclosporine, an antirejection medication used in organ transplantation. In a direct comparison with PPS, cyclosporine-treated patients had a 75% response rate compared to a 19% response rate with Elmiron. Significant side effects include hypertension, creatinine elevation, headache, gingival hyperplasia, gastrointestinal pain, gingival pain, increased hair growth, paresthesia, flushing, muscle pain, shaking, emesis and risks of lymphoma. Cyclosporine usage should be limited to patients with Hunner lesions who have not benefitted from periodic local treatment of the lesions with fulguration or lesional steroid injection.

Intravesical Therapy

Dimethylsulfoxide (DMSO) is the only FDA-approved medication for intravesical instillation for the treatment of BPS/IC. It recently gained approval for use in Japan based on the results of a double-blind placebo controlled trial in patients with Hunner lesions. It is a by-product of the wood pulp industry and a derivative of lignin. It has exceptional solvent properties and is freely miscible with water, lipids, and organic agents. Pharmacologic properties include membrane penetration, enhanced drug absorption, antiinflammatory, analgesic, collagen dissolution, muscle relaxant, and mast cell histamine release. Intravesical delivery by urethral catheter of 50 mL of a 50% solution (*Rimso-50*^{R}) allowed to remain in the bladder for 15 minutes and repeated at weekly intervals for 6 weeks is effective in ameliorating symptoms in about 60% of patients for a period of several months to over a year. Some patients who respond to an initial 6-week course are treated monthly for 6 months. Patients emit a garlic-like odor for several hours after treatment and may experience a short-term symptom flare after the first instillation. It is often administered as part of a "cocktail" including 10 mg triamcinolone (*Kenalog*), 44 mEq sodium bicarbonate, and 40,000 units heparin.

Heparin, an exogenous glycosaminoglycan, can be administered intravesically in sterile water as a single agent. Forty thousand units in 20 mL of sterile water self-administered via catheter by the patients daily and held for 30 to 60 minutes has been reported beneficial, but no placebo-controlled studies have confirmed efficacy. Intravesical lidocaine solutions may have some short-term therapeutic benefit in some patients.

Intradetrusor injection of 100 units of botulinum toxin type A in 10-unit aliquots in the trigone bladder base seems to be effective in relieving symptoms for 6 to 9 months in some patients. It appears to be a potentially promising addition to the armamentarium, but patients need to be willing to intermittently catheterize for days to weeks if short-term impaired bladder emptying complicates therapy.

Hydrodistention

Hydrodistention under anesthesia is often the first therapeutic modality employed when used as part of the diagnostic evaluation. There is no one "correct" way to do this procedure. Our method is to perform a cystoscopic examination (which is often unremarkable), obtain urine for cytology if carcinoma in situ is suspected, and distend the bladder for 1 to 2 minutes at a pressure of 60 cm H_2O. The bladder is emptied and then refilled to look for Hunner lesions. Biopsy, if indicated, is performed after the distention with the bladder contracted. Little is to be gained by distending the bladder to more than 1 L volume, even if the pressure of 60 cm has not been reached, and the risk of temporary retention seems to increase as the volume infused increases. While over 50% of patients may experience some symptom relief after distention, this is often transitory, and rarely lasts longer than 6 months. In those where relief is prolonged, it is worth considering a repeat distention in the future for therapy. A finding of a bladder capacity of less than 200 mL under anesthesia does not bode well for the success of nonsurgical therapeutic efforts.

Neuromodulation

Sacral nerve stimulation (SNS) involves implanting permanent electrode(s) to stimulate S3 or S4 roots. In 1989, urologists at the University of California San Francisco showed that stimulation of S3 may modulate detrusor and urethral sphincter function. FDA approved the usage of sacral neuromodulation for treating refractory detrusor overactivity in 1997 and for urinary urgency and frequency in 1999. Although the effectiveness of SNS for detrusor overactivity is largely confirmed by a good number of papers, only a relatively few papers report the effect of SNS in treating IC/BPS. It has not been approved by regulatory authorities specifically for this diagnosis. It may be more effective for frequency than for pain.

Surgical Therapy

The surgical therapy of IC/BPS is an option after all trials of conservative treatment have failed. IC/BPS, although a cause of significant morbidity, is a nonmalignant process. **Surgery should be reserved for the motivated and well-informed patient who falls into the category of extremely severe, unresponsive disease, a group which comprises fewer than 10% of patients.** Surgical intervention is aimed at increasing the functional capacity of the bladder or diverting the urine stream. Augmentation (substitution) cystoplasty and urinary diversion with or without cystectomy have been used as a last resort with good results in selected patients.

Philosophy of Management

A reasonable management algorithm developed by an international committee for the International Consultation on Incontinence 2017 publication is presented in Fig. 7.8. While there are many differences of approach to treatment, this author believes that it is best to progress through a variety of treatments. Whereas the shotgun approach of initial multimodal therapy has many adherents, employing or adding one treatment at a time makes the undulating natural history of the disease itself an ally in the treatment process. One should encourage patients to maximize their activity and live as normal a life as possible, not becoming a prisoner of the condition. Although some activities or foods may aggravate symptoms, nothing has been shown to negatively affect the disease process itself. Therefore, patients should feel free to experiment and judge for themselves how to modify their lifestyle without the guilt that comes from feeling they have harmed themselves if symptoms flare. Dogmatic restriction and diet are to be avoided unless they are shown to improve symptoms in a particular patient.

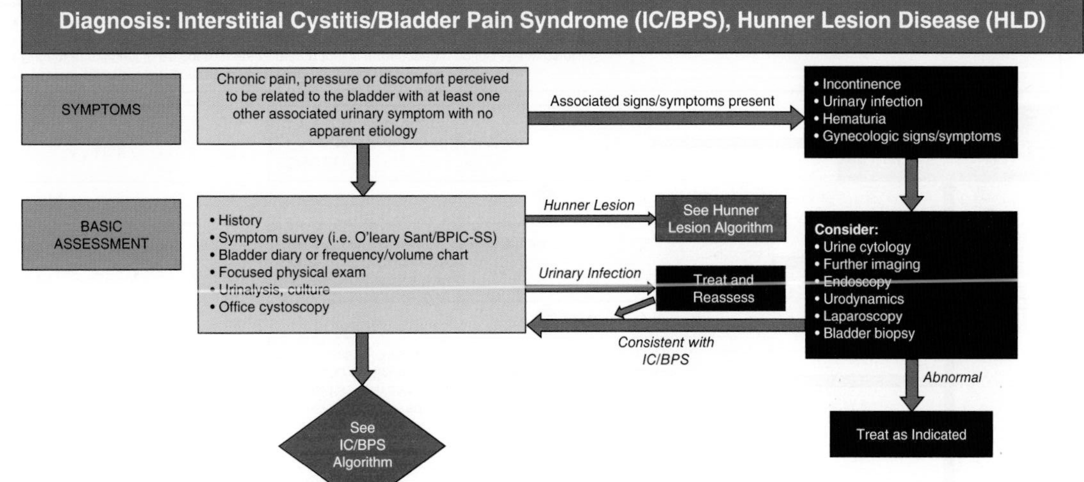

FIGURE 7.8 **Diagnosis and Management of Bladder Pain Syndrome per 2022 International Consultation on Incontinence.** (From Hanno PM, Cervigni M, Choo M, et al. Interstitial Cystitis/Bladder Pain Syndrome. In: Abrams P, Cardozo L, Castro D, et al, eds. Incontinence. 7th ed. 7th international consultation on incontinence recommendations of the international scientific committees. Published by International Continence Society and International Consultation on Urologic Diseases; 2022.)

Continued

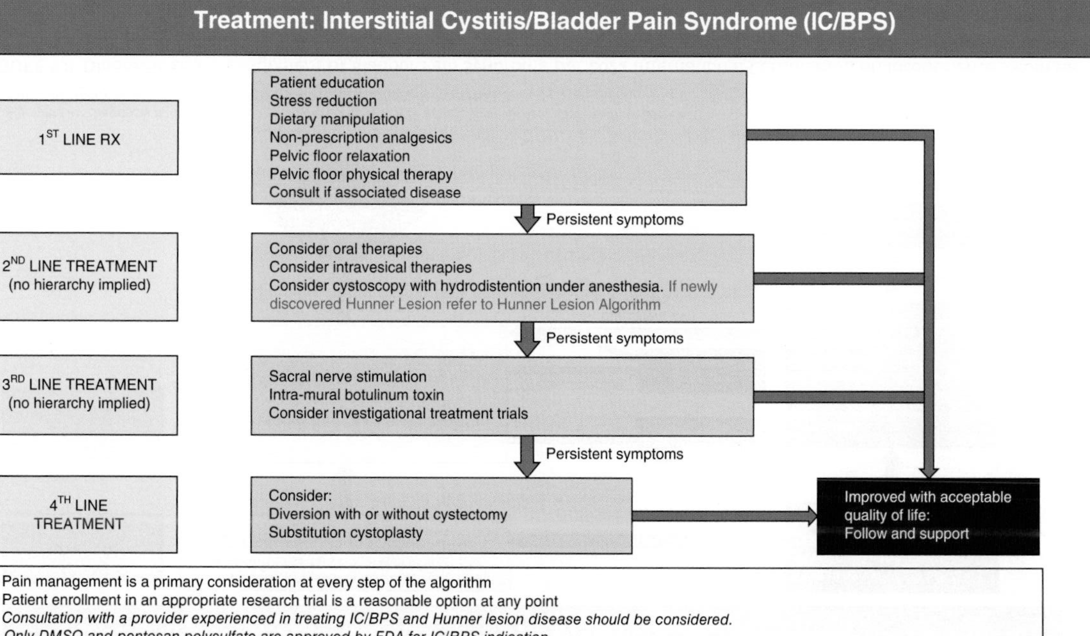
Treatment: Interstitial Cystitis/Bladder Pain Syndrome (IC/BPS)
1ST LINE RX
Patient education
Stress reduction
Dietary manipulation
Non-prescription analgesics
Pelvic floor relaxation
Pelvic floor physical therapy
Consult if associated disease
Persistent symptoms
2ND LINE TREATMENT (no hierarchy implied)
Consider oral therapies
Consider intravesical therapies
Consider cystoscopy with hydrodistention under anesthesia. If newly discovered Hunner Lesion refer to Hunner Lesion Algorithm
Persistent symptoms
3RD LINE TREATMENT (no hierarchy implied)
Sacral nerve stimulation
Intra-mural botulinum toxin
Consider investigational treatment trials
Persistent symptoms
4TH LINE TREATMENT
Consider:
Diversion with or without cystectomy
Substitution cystoplasty
Improved with acceptable quality of life:
Follow and support
• Pain management is a primary consideration at every step of the algorithm
• Patient enrollment in an appropriate research trial is a reasonable option at any point
• Consultation with a provider experienced in treating IC/BPS and Hunner lesion disease should be considered.
• Only DMSO and pentosan polysulfate are approved by FDA for IC/BPS indication

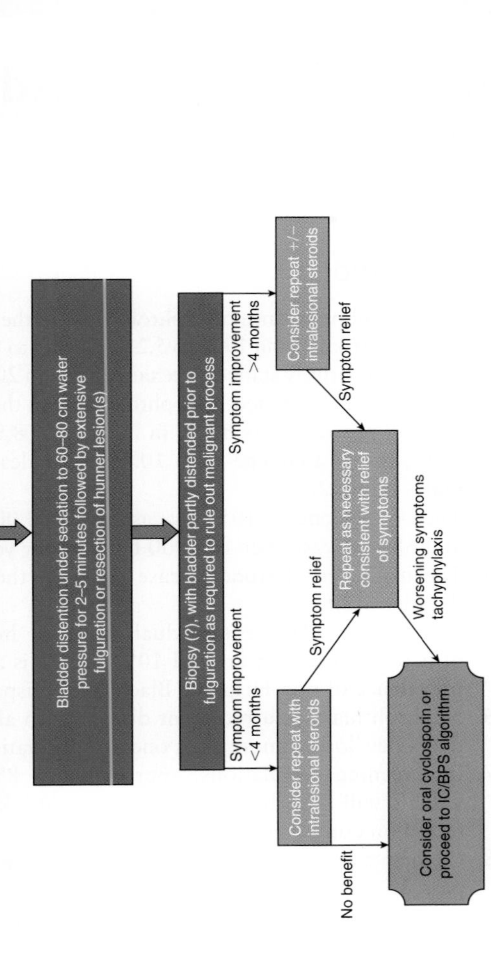
Hunner Lesion Disease
Diagnosis: Patient meeting IC/BPS definition. Cystoscopy local or under sedation–circumscript, reddened mucosal area with small vessels radiating towards a central scar, with a fibrin deposit or coagulum attached to this area. Rupture with increasing bladder distention with oozing of blood.
Bladder distention under sedation to 60–80 cm water pressure for 2–5 minutes followed by extensive fulguration or resection of hunner lesion(s)
Biopsy (?), with bladder partly distended prior to fulguration as required to rule out malignant process
Symptom improvement <4 months
Symptom improvement >4 months
Consider repeat with intralesional steroids
Consider repeat +/− intralesional steroids
Symptom relief
Symptom relief
Symptom relief
Repeat as necessary consistent with relief of symptoms
Worsening symptoms tachyphylaxis
No benefit
Consider oral cyclosporin or proceed to IC/BPS algorithm

Urolithiasis in the Adult

Justin B. Ziemba, MD, MSEd,
and Daniel Roberson, MD

Epidemiology

1. The overall prevalence of nephrolithiasis in the United States has increased from 3% in 1976 to 5.2% in 1994 to 8.8% in 2012 and has been relatively static on reexamination in 2017. One in 11 US persons will be affected by nephrolithiasis in their lifetimes.[1]
2. The US prevalence is 8.1% in males and 8.9% in females in 2017; this is a change from 10.6% in males and 7.1% in females in 2012.[1]
3. The US incidence is 105 new cases per 100,000 males per year and 68 new cases per 100,000 females per year.[1]
4. The incidence of stone disease peaks in the fourth to sixth decades of life.
5. Non-Hispanic White individuals have the highest prevalence of nephrolithiasis at around 10%, which is about double the prevalence of non-Hispanic Blacks and Hispanics.
6. Nephrolithiasis is a recurrent disease with about 40% of patients developing more than one symptomatic stone episode.
7. In screening populations, approximately 8%–10% of individuals will have incidental asymptomatic kidney stones detected on computed tomography (CT).[2]
8. Of these asymptomatic stones, 15% to 20% will spontaneously pass, 15% to 30% will become symptomatic, 30% to 45% will increase in size, and 5% to 25% will require intervention.

Composition of Renal Stones

1. Calcium oxalate (dihydrate and monohydrate): 70%.
2. Calcium phosphate (hydroxyapatite): 20%.
3. Mixed calcium oxalate and calcium phosphate: 11% to 31%.

4. Uric acid: 8%.
5. Magnesium ammonium phosphate (struvite): 6%.
6. Cystine: 2%.
7. Miscellaneous: xanthine, silicates, and drug metabolites, such as indinavir (radiolucent on x-ray and CT scan): <1%.

Pathogenesis and Physiochemical Properties

GENETICS

1. Idiopathic hypercalciuria
   a. Polygenic
   b. Calcium phosphate or calcium oxalate stones
   c. Potential for nephrocalcinosis
   d. Rare risk of end-stage renal disease
2. Primary hyperoxaluria types 1, 2, and 3
   a. Autosomal recessive
   b. Pure monohydrate calcium oxalate stones (whewellite)
   c. Nephrocalcinosis
   d. Risk of end-stage renal and liver disease
3. Distal renal tubular acidosis (RTA)
   a. Autosomal recessive or dominant
   b. Calcium phosphate
   c. Potential for nephrocalcinosis
   d. Risk of end-stage renal disease
4. Cystinuria
   a. Autosomal recessive associated with a defect on chromosome 2 (SLC3A1 and SLC7A9), which is responsible for transporting basic amino acids (cystine, ornithine, lysine, and arginine [COLA])
   b. Cystine stones
   c. No nephrocalcinosis
   d. Risk of end-stage renal disease
5. Lesch-Nyhan syndrome Hypoxanthine-guanine phosphoribosyltransferase (HGPRT deficiency)
   a. X-linked recessive
   b. Uric acid stones
   c. No nephrocalcinosis
   d. Risk of end-stage renal disease

ENVIRONMENTAL

1. Dietary factors
   a. Normal dietary calcium intake is associated with a reduced risk of calcium stones secondary to binding of intestinal oxalate.
   b. Increased calcium and vitamin D supplementation may increase the risk of calcium stones.
   c. Increased dietary sodium intake is associated with an increased risk of urinary sodium excretion, which potentiates urinary calcium, leading to an increased risk of development of calcium-based stones.
   d. Increased dietary animal protein intake may lead to increased uric acid and calcium stones.
   e. Increased water intake is associated with a reduced risk of all types of kidney stones.
2. Obesity
   a. Obesity and weight gain are associated with an increased risk of developing kidney stones.
3. Diabetes
   a. Diabetes is a risk factor for the development of kidney stones.
   b. Insulin resistance may alter renal physiology leading to more acidic urine promoting uric acid stone as well as increased oxalate excretion leading to calcium oxalate stone formation.
4. Geographical factors
   a. The risk of developing kidney stones in the United States increases in a gradient from north to south and west to east. The southeast United States has the highest age-adjusted prevalence of stones, which is why this area is termed the "Stone Belt."
   b. Stone incidence peaks approximately 1 to 2 months after highest annual temperature.
5. Occupational factors
   a. Occupations associated with exposure to excessive heat and other conditions that promote dehydration are associated with an increased risk of kidney stones.
   b. Kidney stones are an occupational hazard in those with jobs who incentivize them to intentionally restrict fluid intake

and void infrequently, such as health care workers and professional drivers.

PHYSICAL AND BIOCHEMICAL PROPERTIES OF STONE FORMATION

1. Supersaturation
   a. Requisite condition for a phase change from a dissolved salt to a solid.
   b. Supersaturation depends on the pH, temperature, and ionic species of the solution.
   c. Thermodynamic solubility product is the concentration at which saturation is reached and crystallization *is possible*.
   d. The formation product is the concentration at which spontaneous crystallization *is inevitable*.
   e. The metastable zone refers to the area between the thermodynamic solubility product and the formation product where no spontaneous crystallization occurs, but existing crystals can grow, and new crystallization can occur on a seed.
2. Crystal formation
   a. Nucleation is the first step in crystal formation and can be either homogenous or heterogeneous.
      1) Homogenous nucleation occurs only in pure solutions (i.e., not urine).
      2) Heterogeneous nucleation, which requires a lower supersaturation value than homogenous nucleation, occurs in urine, and crystallization can begin on cellular components and other crystals.
   b. Epitaxy refers to the ability of one crystalline structure to facilitate the nucleation of another crystalline structure due to similarity in lattice structure.
   c. Once nucleation has occurred, crystals grow via aggregation or agglomeration.
   d. Crystal retention occurs in the renal tubules and is thought to be required for stone formation via two mechanisms, either the free particle or fixed particle hypothesis.
      1) The free particle hypothesis states that nucleation occurs within the renal tubular lumen and that rapid crystal growth traps the stone within the lumen.[3]

    2) The fixed particle hypothesis requires the adherence of the crystals to nearby structures, such as the renal epithelium, which facilitates crystal growth and stone formation.[3]
3. Inhibitors and promoters
    a. Differences in urinary inhibitors and promoters may explain the variability of stone formation in patients with supersaturated urinary components.
    b. Inhibitors can prevent crystal aggregation.
        1) Common inhibitors include citrate, magnesium, Tamm-Horsfall protein, and glycosaminoglycans.
    c. Promoters can enhance crystal aggregation.
        1) Common promoters include cellular matrix, oxalate, low urine volume, and epitaxy.
4. Pathogenesis of stone formation
    a. Crystal-induced renal injury.[3]
        1) Experimental models have demonstrated that hyperoxaluria leads to oxalate deposition within the renal epithelium.
        2) Deposition of oxalate leads to oxidative stress and formation of reactive oxygen species, which injure the renal epithelium.
        3) Stone formation then preferentially develops through crystal adherence to the injured renal epithelium.
    b. Randall plaques.[3]
        1) Calcium phosphate deposits are noted within the basement membrane of the inner medullary collecting duct of the thin loop of Henle presumably caused by abnormal calcium handling.
        2) The calcium phosphate deposits enlarge throughout the interstitium and ultimately erode through the epithelium at the tips of the renal papilla.
        3) This deposit of calcium phosphate serves as a nucleus for secondary calcium oxalate stone formation.
    c. Low urinary inhibitors.
        1) May be thought of as a balance between the supersaturation of the solutes promoting crystallization and urinary inhibitors opposing crystallization.
        2) Urinary citrate is an inhibitor of calcium stone formation by binding to calcium to reduce supersaturation and prevent nucleation.

d. Stasis.
    1) May be a factor in anatomically abnormal kidneys, such as in ureteropelvic junction (UPJ) obstruction or hydronephrosis.
    2) Hypothesis that stasis prevents urinary washout of crystals.

PATHOPHYSIOLOGY OF STONE FORMATION

1. Idiopathic calcium oxalate
    a. Approximately 70% to 80% of incident stones are calcium oxalate.
    b. Initial event is precipitation of calcium phosphate on the renal papilla as Randall plaques, which serve as a nucleus for calcium oxalate precipitation and stone formation.
    c. Calcium oxalate stones preferentially develop in acidic urine (pH less than 6.0).
    d. Development depends on supersaturation of both calcium and oxalate within the urine.
2. Idiopathic hypercalciuria
    a. Identified in 30% to 60% of calcium oxalate stone formers and in 5% to 10% of nonstone formers.
    b. The upper limit of normal for urinary calcium excretion is 250 mg/day for women and 300 mg/day for men.
    c. Need to exclude hypercalcemia, vitamin D excess, hyperthyroidism, sarcoidosis, and neoplasm.
    d. Diagnosed via exclusion in patients with a normal serum calcium but elevated urinary calcium on a random diet.
3. Absorptive hypercalciuria
    a. Increased jejunal absorption of calcium possibly caused by elevated calcitriol (1, 25 dihydroxyvitamin D3) levels and increased vitamin D receptor expression.
    b. Divided into types I, II and III, depending on whether urinary calcium levels can be affected by calcium in the diet (type I and II) or renal phosphate leak leading to increased calcium absorption (type III).
    c. Increased calcium absorption leads to a higher filtered load of calcium delivered to the renal tubule.
    d. The treatment for each subtype is generally the same, so determining which type (often requiring inpatient evaluation) is no longer necessary.
    e. Normal serum calcium.

4. Renal hypercalciuria
   a. Impaired proximal tubular reabsorption of calcium leads to renal calcium wasting.
   b. Normal serum calcium; hypercalciuria persists despite a calcium-restricted diet.
   c. Distinguished from primary hyperparathyroidism by normal serum calcium levels and secondary hyperparathyroidism.
5. Resorptive hypercalciuria
   a. Primary hyperparathyroidism is the underlying mechanism.
   b. Increased parathyroid hormone (PTH) levels cause bone resorption and intestinal calcium absorption, which leads to elevated serum calcium that exceeds the reabsorptive capacity of the renal tubule.
   c. Normal to slightly elevated serum calcium.
6. Hypercalcemic hypercalciuria
   a. Primary hyperparathyroidism, hyperthyroidism, sarcoidosis, vitamin D excess, milk alkali syndrome, immobilization, and malignancy.
7. Hyperoxaluria
   a. The upper limit of normal for urinary oxalate excretion is 45 mg/day in women and 55 mg/day in men.
   b. Acts as a potent promoter of stone formation by complexing with calcium.
   c. Dietary hyperoxaluria is related to increased consumption of oxalate-rich foods, and/or a low-calcium diet, which, by reducing the availability of intestinal calcium to complex to oxalate, allows an increased rate of free oxalate absorption by the gut.
   d. Enteric hyperoxaluria can be caused by small bowel disease or loss, exocrine pancreatic insufficiency, or diarrhea, all of which reduce small bowel fat absorption, leading to an increase in fat complexing with calcium, and thereby facilitating free oxalate absorption by the colon.
   e. Primary hyperoxaluria is a genetic disorder in one of two genes, which results in increased production or urinary excretion of oxalate. In type I, which is an autosomal recessive trait, AGXT (alanine-glyoxylate aminotransferase) is deficient in the liver. This results in increased production of oxalate. These patients develop early oxalosis, stone formation, and ultimate renal failure. In type II, there is a

deficiency in D-glycerate dehydrogenase and glyoxylate reductase, which leads to increased urinary oxalate excretion; this type is extremely rare with only 21 reported cases.

8. Hypocitraturia
   a. The lower limit of normal is less than 500 mg/day for women and 350 mg/day for men.
   b. Acts as an inhibitor of stone formation by complexing with calcium.
   c. Citrate is regulated by tubular reabsorption, and reabsorption varies with urinary pH. In acidic conditions, tubular reabsorption is enhanced, which lowers urinary citrate levels.
   d. Diseases that cause acidosis, such as chronic diarrhea or distal RTA, cause lower urinary citrate levels. Thiazide therapy can also reduce citrate levels via potassium depletion.
   e. In the majority of patients with hypocitraturia, no etiology is identified, and these patients are classified as having idiopathic hypocitraturia.
9. Hyperuricosuria/uric acid stones
   a. Approximately 5% to 10% of incident stones are uric acid.
   b. The upper limit of normal is greater than 750 mg/day for women and 800 mg/day for men.
   c. Uric acid is a promoter for calcium oxalate stone formation by serving as a nucleus for crystal generation and also by reducing the solubility of calcium oxalate.
   d. A low urinary pH is critical for uric acid stone formation. At a urinary pH less than 5.5, uric acid exists in its insoluble undissociated form, which facilitates uric acid stone formation. As the urinary pH increases, the dissociated monosodium urate crystals are predominant and serve as a nucleus for calcium-containing stone formation.
   e. Increased uric acid production is common in patients with a high dietary intake of animal protein, in myeloproliferative disorders, and in gout. However, uric acid stone formation is also common in patients with diabetes and the metabolic syndrome presumably caused by insulin resistance, which impairs renal ammonia excretion necessary for urinary alkalization.

10. Cystinuria
    a. In both men and women, urinary cystine excretion exceeds 350 mg/day.
    b. Caused by autosomal recessive disorder involving the SLC3A1 amino acid transporter gene on chromosome 2.
    c. The dibasic amino acid transporter, which is located within the tubular epithelium, facilitates reabsorption of dibasic amino acids, such as COLA. A defect in this enzyme leads to decreased cystine reabsorption and increased urinary excretion of cystine.
    d. Cystine solubility rises with increasing urinary volume and pH. The solubility of cystine in urine is about 250 mg/L at a pH of 6.5, 500 mg/L at a pH of 7.5, and 750 mg/L at a pH of 8.[4]
    e. Positive urine cyanide-nitroprusside colorimetric reaction is a qualitative screen.
11. Calcium phosphate stones
    a. Approximately 12% to 30% of incident stones are calcium phosphate.
    b. Calcium phosphate stones preferentially develop in alkaline urine (pH greater than 7.5).
    c. Calcium phosphate stones can be present as either apatite or brushite (calcium phosphate monohydrate).
    d. Overalkalization with potassium citrate for hypercalciuria can sometimes lead to calcium phosphate stones.
12. Struvite stones/triple phosphate/infection stones
    a. Approximately 5% of incident stones are struvite.
    b. Struvite stones are composed of magnesium ammonium phosphate and calcium phosphate. They may also contain a nidus of another stone composition.
    c. Often grow to encompass large areas in the collection system or staghorn calculi.
    d. Urinary tract infections (UTIs) with urease splitting organisms, which include *Proteus* spp., *Klebsiella* spp., *Staphylococcus aureus*, *Pseudomonas* spp., and *Ureaplasma* spp., are required to split urea into ammonia, bicarbonate, and carbonate.
    e. A urinary pH greater than 7.2 is required for struvite stone formation.

f. Conditions that predispose to UTIs increase the likelihood of struvite stone formation. Struvite stones are common in patients with spinal cord injuries and neurogenic bladders.

Stone Formation and Vascular Calcification

1. Contemporary work suggests a link between vascular calcification and the formation of idiopathic kidney stones.[3]
2. The exposure of vascular smooth muscle to high levels of calcium and phosphate can cause binding of the calcium phosphate complex with collagen and deposition in the vascular wall.
3. It is believed that the process is mediated by external influence on the vascular smooth muscle cells resulting in them acquiring an osteogenic phenotype.

Clinical Manifestations of Nephrolithiasis

PRESENTATION

1. Asymptomatic kidney stones are found in 8%–10% of screening populations undergoing a CT scan for unrelated reasons.[2]
2. Pain is the most common presenting symptom in the majority of patients.
   a. The stone produces ureteral spasms and obstructs the flow of urine, which causes a resultant distention of the ureter, pyelocalyceal system, and ultimately the renal capsule to produce pain.
   b. Renal colic is characterized by a sudden onset of severe flank pain, which often lasts 20 to 60 minutes. The pain is paroxysmal, and patients are often restless and unable to get comfortable.
   c. Three main sites of anatomic narrowing or obstruction are within the ureter: the UPJ, the lumbar ureter at the crossing of the iliac vessels, and the ureterovesical junction.
   d. The location of pain generally correlates with these sites of anatomic narrowing: the UPJ produces classic flank pain, the midureter at the level of the iliac vessels produces

generalized lower abdominal discomfort, and the uretero-vesical junction produces groin or referred testes/labia majora pain.

3. Associated nausea and vomiting are frequent. Fever and chills are common with concomitant UTI.
4. Dysuria or strangury, which is the desire to void but with urgency, frequency, straining, and small voided volumes, is possible with stones located at the ureterovesical junction.

DIFFERENTIAL DIAGNOSIS

Pyelonephritis: Fever with associated flank pain
Musculoskeletal pain: Pain with movement
Appendicitis: Right lower quadrant tenderness at McBurney point
Cholecystitis: Right upper quadrant tenderness with Murphy sign
Colitis/diverticulitis: Left lower quadrant tenderness with gastrointestinal symptoms
Testicular torsion: Abnormal testicular exam with high-riding testicle
Ovarian torsion/ruptured ovarian cyst: Adnexal tenderness

Evaluation of Patients With Nephrolithiasis (Fig. 8.1)

1. General considerations
   a. All patients in the acute phase of renal colic should have a history and physical, a urinalysis, a urine culture if urinalysis demonstrates bacteriuria or nitrites, and a serum creatinine. If the patient presents with fever or if surgery is being considered, then a complete blood count (CBC) should also be included.
   b. A fever greater than 100° F or tachycardia and hypotension is concerning for obstructive pyelonephritis. Pyuria and leukocytosis are laboratory signs of infection.
   c. All patients with a first stone episode should undergo a basic evaluation with a medical history including family history, dietary history, and medications; physical exam and ultrasound; blood analysis with creatinine, calcium, and uric acid; urinalysis and culture; and stone analysis.[5]
   d. Patients at high risk include those with a family history of nephrolithiasis, recurrent stone formation, large stone

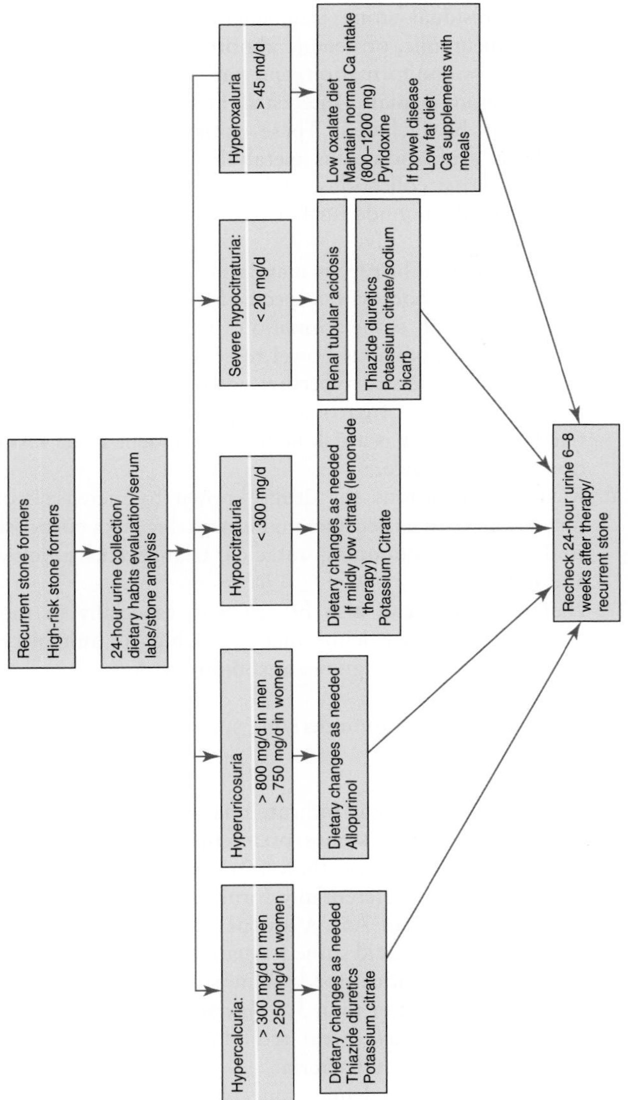

FIGURE 8.1 Treatment algorithm for a patient with recurrent stone disease.

burden, residual stone fragments after therapy, solitary kidney, metabolic, or genetic abnormalities known to predispose to stone formation, and patients with stones other than calcium oxalate. Interested first-time stone formers may also be included. These patients should undergo the basic evaluation, plus metabolic evaluation with two 24-hour urine collections, at least 4 weeks following the acute episode to guide further therapy.[5]

2. Medical history
   a. General medical history is mandatory in all stone formers.
   b. Past medical history with a specific focus on diseases known to contribute to stone formation, including inflammatory bowel disease, previous bowel resection, or gastric bypass, hyperparathyroidism, hyperthyroidism, RTA, and gout.
   c. Family history is of particular importance because a positive family history is a risk factor for incident stone formation and recurrence.
   d. Review medications for drugs known to increase stone formation, such as acetazolamide, ascorbic acid, corticosteroids, calcium-containing antacids, triamterene, acyclovir, and indinavir.
   e. Dietary history can also be relevant, especially in those with high- or low-calcium diets, diets high in animal protein, and diets with significant sodium intake.
3. Physical exam
   a. May provide clues to underlying systemic diseases.
4. Laboratory evaluation
   a. Urinalysis
      1) Specific gravity may indicate relative hydration status.
      2) Calcium oxalate stones preferentially form in a relatively acidic pH (less than 6.0), whereas calcium phosphate stones preferentially form in a relatively alkaline pH (greater than 7.5). A low pH (less than 5.5) is mandatory for uric acid stone formation. A high pH (greater than 7.2) is critical for struvite stone formation. A pH constantly greater than 5.8 may suggest an RTA.
      3) Microscopy may reveal red blood cells, white blood cells (WBCs), and bacteria.
      4) Crystalluria can define stone type: Hexagonal crystals are cystine, coffin lid crystals are struvite, calcium

oxalate crystals can appear as envelop or dumbbell shaped, and rhomboidal crystals are uric acid.

b. Urine culture is mandatory if microscopy reveals bacteriuria or pyuria, if struvite stones are suspected, or if symptoms or signs of infection are present.
c. Electrolytes
   1) Calcium (ionized or calcium with albumin): Elevated calcium may suggest hyperparathyroidism, and a PTH blood test should be done.
   2) Uric acid: Elevated uric acid is common in gout and, in conjunction with a radiolucent on plain x-ray stone, is suggestive of uric acid nephrolithiasis.
d. A CBC may show mild peripheral leukocytosis. WBC counts higher than 15,000/mm^3 may suggest an active infection.
e. Ammonium chloride load test: Identifies distal or Type I RTA. Oral ammonium chloride load (0.1 gm/kg body weight) given over 30 minutes will not raise the urinary pH greater than 5.4 if a Type I RTA is present.
f. Sodium nitroprusside test: Identifies cystinuria. Addition of sodium nitroprusside to urine with cystine concentration higher than 75 mg/L alters the urine color to purple-red.
g. 24-hour urine collection: Typically, one to two 24-hour urine collections are obtained at least 6 weeks after an acute stone event or following initiation of medical therapy or dietary modification. Collection is done to determine total urine volume, pH, creatinine, calcium, oxalate, uric acid, citrate, magnesium, sodium, potassium, phosphorus, sulfate, urea, and ammonia. Cystine is also determined if a cystine screening test is positive. Supersaturation indices are also calculated. An adequate collection is determined by total creatinine, which is 15 to 19 mg/kg for women and 20 to 24 mg/kg for men (Table 8.1).
h. Stone analysis: Performed either with infrared spectroscopy or x-ray diffraction. It provides information about the underlying metabolic, genetic, or dietary abnormality.

5. Imaging considerations
   a. A noncontrast CT scan is the recommended initial imaging modality for an acute stone episode. A noncontrast CT scan has a sensitivity of 98% and a specificity of 97% in

TABLE 8.1 Normal Values of Urinary Excretion of Substances Affecting Stone Formation

Substance	Men (mg/day)	Women (mg/day)
Urinary calcium	< 300	< 250
Urinary uric acid	800	< 750
Urinary citrate	50–600	650–800
Urinary oxalate	45	< 45

detecting ureteral calculi. A low-dose noncontrast CT scan (less than 4 mSv) is preferred in patients with a body mass index (BMI) less than 30.[6] When a ureteral stone is visualized on a noncontrast CT scan, it will be demonstrated 50% of the time on a CT scan scout film.

b. A renal bladder ultrasound is the recommended initial imaging modality in pregnant patients in order to limit ionizing radiation. Ultrasonography has a median sensitivity of 61% and a specificity of 97%. Ultrasonography poorly visualizes stones in the ureter and has limited sensitivity for stones 2 to 3 mm.[6] If ultrasonography is equivocal, and the clinical suspicion is high for nephrolithiasis, then a low-dose noncontrast CT scan may be performed.
c. Plain film of the kidneys, ureters, and bladder (KUB) is also routinely used. Conventional radiography with a KUB has a median sensitivity of 57% and a specificity of 76%.[6] Pure uric acid, cystine, indinavir, and xanthine stones are radiolucent, and are not visible on KUB.
d. Historically, intravenous pyelography (IVP) was commonly utilized for diagnosis of stone disease because it could readily identify radiolucent stones and define calyceal anatomy. It has a median sensitivity of 70% and a specificity of 95%.[6] However, CT has largely replaced IVP.
e. Magnetic resonance imaging is generally not performed for urolithiasis because of cost, low sensitivity, and time needed to acquire images.
f. A combination of ultrasonography and KUB is recommended for monitoring patients with known radiopaque ureteral calculi on medical expulsion therapy because this limits costs and radiation exposure. Those with radiolucent stones will require a low-dose noncontrast CT scan.[5]

g. Following surgical intervention with ureteroscopy (URS) or shock wave lithotripsy, imaging may be performed. If it is to be performed, the recommended imaging modality is ultrasonography because it is inexpensive and has no ionizing radiation. A KUB may also be performed because of low levels of radiation.

h. Limiting radiation exposure is a critical component of modern diagnostic imaging, especially in patients with stone disease and for providers. Imaging modalities with ionizing radiation should conform to the "as low as reasonably achievable" (ALARA) principle. In addition, the use of "last image hold," pulsed fluoroscopy, and strategic shielding are important in the reduction of ionizing radiation exposure. A renal ultrasound has 0 mSv, a KUB has 0.7 mSv, an IVP has 3.0 mSv, a low-dose noncontrast CT scan has 3.0 mSv, and a standard CT scan has 10.0 mSv.[6]

Management of Nephrolithiasis

MEDICAL THERAPY (TABLE 8.2)

1. All stone formers
   a. High fluid intake of 2.5 to 3.0 L/day with urine volume greater than 2.5 L/day.
   b. Normal calcium dietary limit of 1000 to 1200 mg/day. Avoid excess calcium supplementation; however, calcium citrate is preferred if indicated.
   c. Limit sodium to 4 to 5 g/day.
   d. Limit animal protein to 0.8 to 1.0 g/kg per day.
   e. Limit oxalate-rich foods.
   f. Maintain a normal BMI and physical activity.
   g. Targeted therapy depending on underlying metabolic abnormality and/or 24-hour urine collection results.
2. Calcium oxalate stones
   a. Dietary hyperoxaluria: Limit oxalate-rich foods and normalize calcium intake.
   b. Enteric hyperoxaluria: Limit oxalate-rich foods and calcium supplementation at mealtime with greater than 500 mg/day. Potassium citrate and fat restriction have a role in the combination medical therapy of this unique pathology.

TABLE 8.2 Medications for the Medical Management of Urolithiasis

Indication	Drug	Usual Dose	Stone Type
Hypercalciuria (renal leak/absorptive)	Thiazide Hydrochlorthiazide Chlorthalidone Indapamide	25–50 mg BID 50 mg QD 1.25–2.5 mg QD	Calcium oxalate, calcium phosphate
Hypocitraturia, urinary alkalinization, hypokalemia (especially with thiazides)	Potassium citrate	10–20 mEq TID	Calcium oxalate, uric acid, cysteine
Hyperuricosuria	Allopurinol	100–300 mg daily	Uric acid, calcium stones
Cystinuria	D-penicillamine Alpha-mercaptopropionylglycine (tiopronin) Captopril	250–500 mg QID 200–400 mg TID 150 mg QD	Cystine
Absorptive hypercalciuria (second-line agents after thiazides)	Sodium cellulose phosphate Potassium phosphate	5 gm BID/TID 250 mg TID/QID	Calcium oxalate
Urease inhibitor	Acetohydroxamic acid	250 mg TID/QID	Struvite/infection stones

BID, Twice daily; *QD*, once daily; *QID*, four times per day; *TID*, three times per day

c. Primary hyperoxaluria: Pyridoxine (vitamin B6) can decrease endogenous production of oxalate as it serves as a cofactor in the process that diverts the conversion of precursors away from oxalate. The dose is 100 to 800 mg/day. Potassium citrate is also useful in these patients.

d. Hypocitraturia: Potassium citrate both raises the urinary pH out of the stone-forming range and restores the normal urinary citrate concentration. Sodium bicarbonate may also be used, if unable to tolerate potassium supplementation.

e. Hypercalciuria: Thiazide diuretics, which inhibit a sodium-chloride co-transporter, therefore enhancing distal tubular sodium reabsorption via the sodium-calcium co-transporter to promote tubular calcium reabsorption. Thiazides decrease urinary calcium by as much as 150 mg/day.

f. Hyperuricosuria (with or without hyperuricemia): Allopurinol, while primarily used in uric acid stones, has been successful in those with hyperuricosuria and recurrent calcium oxalate stones.
g. Sarcoidosis: Sarcoidosis is associated with hypercalcemia, hypercalciuria, and calcium-based stones. Corticosteroids suppress the production of 1, 25 dihydroxy vitamin D by the granuloma and reduce serum and urinary calcium.

3. Calcium phosphate stones
   a. Primary hyperparathyroidism: Requires parathyroidectomy.
   b. Distal RTA (Type I): Potassium citrate or sodium bicarbonate to restore the natural pH balance.
4. Struvite/infection stones
   a. Total stone removal is paramount as each fragment harbors urease-producing bacteria and serves as a nidus for further stone growth.
   b. Appropriate antibiotic therapy to eradicate the urease-producing bacteria.
   c. Restoration of normal pH with urinary acidification with L-methionine or irreversible inhibition of urease enzyme with acetohydroxamic acid.
5. Uric acid stones
   a. Acidic urine (pH <5.5) is the most common pathophysiologic abnormality. Most patients have normal urinary uric acid.
   b. Low animal protein diet in those with high urinary uric acid.
   c. Specific therapy depends on 24-hour urine collection results.
   d. Alkalization of the urine with potassium citrate or sodium bicarbonate for stone dissolution is possible with a pH of 7.0 to 7.2 and for maintenance of a stone-free state with a pH of 6.2 to 6.8. This increase in urine pH results in conversion of most uric acid into the more soluble urate salt.
   e. Hyperuricosuria (with or without hyperuricemia): Allopurinol at 100 to 300 mg/day, which inhibits xanthine oxidase to reduce uric acid production. It should be reserved

for those who are not able to reduce urinary uric acid through dietary means, such as those with myeloproliferative disorders, hemolytic anemia, or Lesch-Nyhan Syndrome. Allopurinol is rarely beneficial in idiopathic uric acid nephrolithiasis. The drug has been associated with Stevens-Johnson syndrome. Febuxostat is an alternative medication.

6. Cystine stones
   a. Increase daily fluid intake to 3.5 to 4.0 L/day with a goal of >3L of urine volume/day.
   b. Specific therapy depends on 24-hour urine collection results.
   c. Lower sodium intake has been shown to reduce cystine excretion.
   d. Alkalization of the urine with potassium citrate or sodium bicarbonate above a pH of 7.0 to 7.5 to improve solubility of cystine.
   e. D-penicillamine is a chelating agent that forms a disulfide bond with cysteine to produce a more soluble compound, thereby preventing the formation of cysteine into the insoluble, stone-forming, cystine. Alpha-mercaptopropionyl-glycine (tiopronin) is the preferred alternative to D-penicillamine, as it has a better safety and efficacy profile. Alpha-mercaptopropionyl-glycine reduces the disulfide bond of cystine to form the more soluble cysteine, again reducing stone formation. Lastly, captopril is an angiotensin-converting enzyme inhibitor, which can reduce cystine, but its role in therapy is not yet well defined.

ACUTE RENAL COLIC

1. General considerations
   a. Primary considerations include symptomatic control with analgesics, antiemetics, and adequate hydration.
   b. First-line analgesia is generally a nonsteroidal antiinflammatory, such as ketorolac.
   c. Patients should be instructed to sieve their urine for collection of stone fragments.
   d. Spontaneous stone passage occurs in 80% of patients with sizes less than 4 mm. With sizes greater than 10 mm, there is a low probability of spontaneous passage. Location also

influences spontaneous stone passage rates (Table 8.3). When stones are going to pass spontaneously, the majority pass within 6 weeks.

e. Referral to a urologist is necessary with persistent pain, high-grade obstruction, bilateral obstruction, presence of infection, solitary kidney, abnormal anatomy, failure of conservative management, large stone burden, pregnancy, or in children.

2. Medical expulsive therapy (MET)
   a. MET is an option in patients with a good chance of spontaneous passage (distal ureteral calculi less than 10 mm), who have well-controlled pain, no evidence of infection, adequate renal function, and no other contraindications to the therapy.
   b. Alpha-blockers (preferred drug), such as tamsulosin can facilitate stone passage via ureteral smooth muscle relaxation.
   c. Tamsulosin is associated with "intraoperative floppy iris syndrome" and patients should alert their ophthalmologists of its use. The drug should be avoided if cataract surgery is being contemplated.
   d. MET with any agent is an off-label use for the medication and should only be used for 28 to 45 days. The medication should be discontinued after stone passage.
   e. Patients undergoing MET should trial the therapy for 4 to 6 weeks and be reassessed with imaging and undergo treatment if unable to pass the stone.
   f. Significant narcotic support and frequent trips to the emergency room are indications to abandon a MET trial.

SURGICAL THERAPY

1. Shock wave lithotripsy (SWL)
   a. Shock waves are high-energy, focused-pressure waves that can travel in air or water. When passing through two

TABLE 8.3 Spontaneous Passage Rates for Ureteral Stones Based on Location

Location of Stone	Proximal Ureter	Mid Ureter	Distal Ureter
Spontaneous passage rate	25%	45%	70%

different mediums of different acoustic impedance, energy is released, which results in the fragmentation of stones. Shock waves travel harmlessly through substances of the same acoustic density. Because water and body tissues have the same density, shock waves can travel safely through skin and internal tissues. The stone is a different acoustic density and, when the shock waves hit it, they shatter and pulverize it. Urinary stones are thus fragmented, facilitating in their spontaneous passage.

b. Treatment success depends on stone size, location, composition, hardness, patient anatomy, and body habitus. For renal stones, upper or middle polar stones are ideally treated with SWL, whereas lower pole stones have a clearance rate as low as 35%. Stone size is the greatest predictor of SWL success; stone clearance rates decrease with stones greater than 20 mm in size. Stone composition or hardness influences stone fragmentation with the most SWL-resistant stones being cystine and brushite, followed by calcium oxalate monohydrate, struvite, calcium oxalate dihydrate, and uric acid. Furthermore, dense stones, as measured on preoperative CT, with greater than 1000 Hounsfield units (HU), require a greater number of shocks for fragmentation. An acute infundibulopelvic angle, narrow or long infundibula, and multiple infundibula are all thought to be unfavorable factors for stone fragment passage following SWL. Finally, body habitus, as measured by skin-to-stone distance on preoperative CT, also influences success. A decrease in stone-free rates has been observed with skin-to-stone distances of greater than 10 cm.

c. Ideally all stones less than 1 cm in any location in the kidney can be treated with SWL. Stones greater than 1 cm in the lower pole should undergo URS or percutaneous nephrolithotomy (PNL). Stones between 1 and 2 cm in the middle or upper pole with favorable characteristics on noncontrast CT such as a skin-to-stone distance of less than 8 to 10 cm and a density less than 800 to 1000 HU can be successfully treated with SWL.

d. SWL can be offered as first-line therapy for ureteral stones less than 10 mm. The stone-free rates are 82% in the proximal ureter, 73% in the midureter, and 74% in the distal ureter. Placement of a ureteral stent to facilitate stone fragment passage is not recommended with SWL as it does not increase stone-free rates and increases morbidity. For stones less than 10 mm in the mid and distal ureter, SWL can be offered, but higher success rates are achieved with URS. For ureteral stones less than 10 mm, SWL is not recommended. SWL is not recommended to treat cystine stones due to the density and uric acid stones due to location difficulty. If initial SWL fails, endoscopic therapy should be offered.[7,8]

e. Contraindications to SWL include (absolute) pregnancy, bleeding diathesis, and obstruction below the level of the stone and (relative) calcified arteries and/or aneurysms, cardiac pacemaker, and treatment of the mid and distal ureters in women of childbearing age due to potential ovary damage.
f. Other methods to improve SWL success include decreasing the rate of shocks (60 shocks per minute), minimizing air pockets between the patient and coupling head, MET in the form of tamsulosin and nifedipine administered after treatment, percussive therapy, and inversion (for lower pole stones).
g. Complications of SWL include skin bruising, subscapular and perinephric hemorrhage, pancreatitis, urosepsis, and steinstrasse ("street of stone," which may accumulate in the ureter and cause obstruction). Placement of a stent can reduce the complications associated with steinstrasse but does not reduce its occurrence rate. Hypertension has been identified as a possible adverse effect of SWL, with age being a significant modifying factor and those over the age of 60 being at the highest risk of SWL-induced hypertension.

2. Percutaneous nephrolithotomy
   a. It is recommended to obtain a noncontrast CT scan on patients prior to performing PNL to help define disease and anatomy, ultimately lowering the risk of complications.
   b. The technique involves establishment of access at a posterior calyx targeted to provide access to the largest stone burden with rigid instruments, dilation of the tract with a balloon dilator or rigid dilators under fluoroscopy, and stone removal with graspers or its fragmentation using electrohydraulic, ultrasonic, or laser lithotripsy. A nephrostomy

tube or ureteral stent can be left for drainage. Upper pole access is best suited for complete staghorn calculi, complex lower pole stones, stones in a horseshoe kidney, and large proximal ureteral calculi, although it is associated with a higher complication rate and postoperative pain. Percutaneous access under fluoroscopy can be achieved using the eye of the needle or triangulation technique. Dilation should proceed to accommodate the working sheaths, most of which are 30 Fr, but some of which come in sizes as small as 12 to 14 Fr. In the properly selected patient, "tubeless" PNL, meaning no draining nephrostomy tube or ureteral stent is placed, has been shown to be safe. Flexible nephroscopy should be a routine part of PNL. Normal saline must be used as irrigant for PNL.

c. Staghorn calculi are large branched stones that conform to the shape of the calyceal anatomy and fill the collecting system. Partial staghorn calculi are smaller and only fill a portion of the collecting system. Typically, staghorn and partial staghorn calculi are composed of struvite, but uric acid and cystine stones also can form staghorn calculi. Staghorn calculi can lead to recurrent infections, sepsis, renal failure, and possibly death.
d. Treatment for staghorn and partial staghorn calculi is best managed with PNL as well as large (>2 cm) or complex stones, and lower pole renal stones >1 cm. Overall, the stone-free rate with PNL is 78%. Stone-free rates are three times greater with PNL than with SWL, and on average PNL requires a fewer number of overall procedures (1.3 versus 2.8). Furthermore, for lower pole stones greater than 1 cm, PNL has a stone-free rate of greater than 90%, compared to less than 25% for SWL.[3]
e. Additional candidates for PNL include **cystine calculi**, which are large volume and resistant to SWL, and **those with renal anatomic abnormalities**, such as UPJ obstruction, calyceal diverticula, obstructed infundibula (hydrocalyx), ureteral obstruction, malformed kidneys (e.g., horseshoe and pelvic), and obstructive or large adjacent renal cysts.
f. Contraindications to PNL include uncontrolled bleeding diathesis, pregnancy, untreated UTI, and inability to obtain

optimal access for PNL because of obesity, splenomegaly, or interposition of colon.

g. Complications of PNL include hemorrhage (0.4%–11%), perforation, and extravasation (5.4%–26%), damage to adjacent organs (1%), ureteral obstruction (1.7%–4.9%), and infection/urosepsis (0.2%–1.3%).[9] Postoperative hemorrhage that continues more than a few days after surgery is concerning for pseudoaneurysm, AV fistula, or segmental renal artery injury. The most common organs damaged are the pleura, liver, spleen, colon, and duodenum. Pleural violation most commonly occurs when upper pole access is established and hydropneumothorax results in 5% to 16% of cases involving supracostal access. Bacteremia has been reported to occur in up to 37% of patients and postoperative fever in up to 74%, yet fulminant sepsis is much rarer. The American Urological Association (AUA) policy states that all patients undergoing PNL should have a sterile urine culture or have been appropriately treated for >1 week for a positive urine culture and receive appropriate preoperative antibiotics in the form of a first- or second-generation cephalosporin, gentamycin and metronidazole, or clindamycin. If the patient has no internal hardware, antibiotic prophylaxis is not needed past 24 hours.

3. Retrograde intrarenal surgery (URS)
   a. Instrumentation includes both rigid and flexible ureteroscopes. Rigid ureteroscopes are ideally suited for access to the distal ureter but can be utilized up to the proximal ureter. Flexible ureteroscopes are ideally suited for ureteral and intrarenal access. Stones are removed using the stone basket or graspers. Endoscopic lithotripsy devices are used for stone fragmentation (electrohydraulic, ultrasonic, or laser lithotripsy). During URS, as in PNL, only saline should be used as an irrigant, and pressures should be kept as low as will allow good visibility. Ureteral access sheaths are beneficial for decreasing intrarenal pressure and improving stone-free rates, and have not been shown to increase the rate of ureteral stricture.
   b. According to AUA and EAU guidelines, for ureteral stones less than 10 mm, URS can be offered as first-line therapy because URS has higher stone-free rates than SWL (97% versus 86%). Overall, URS has success rates of 93% to 97%

in the distal ureter, 78% to 91% in the midureter, and 79% to 80% in the proximal ureter. Although the clinical guidelines recommend either SWL or PNL for larger intrarenal calculi, URS has become the gold standard for intrarenal stones less than 1.5 cm with stone-free rates of 50% to 80%. Stenting after uncomplicated URS may not be necessary.[7,8]

c. Placement of a ureteral stent prior to URS for nephrolithiasis should not be routinely performed.

d. A stent does not need to be left routinely in URS. Significant ureteral edema or suspicion of ureteral injury is an indication for leaving a ureteral stent. In patients without suspected ureteral injury, without anatomic ureteral abnormalities that would lead to stone impedance, with a normal contralateral kidney, without renal function impairment and in whom a second URS is not planned, leaving a ureteral stent may be omitted.

e. URS may be safely performed in patients with morbid obesity, pregnancy, and bleeding diathesis.

f. Complications include failure to retrieve the stone, mucosal abrasions, false passages, infection/sepsis ureteral perforation, complete ureteral avulsion, and ureteral stricture. Ureteral perforation occurs in 4% of cases as a result of balloon dilation, forceful and misdirected manipulation of the stone, intracorporeal lithotripsy devices, and extraction devices. With perforation that is recognized, the procedure should be immediately terminated, and a stent should be left for 2 to 6 weeks. Avulsion occurs in less than 1% of cases, is almost always secondary to overly forceful extraction of large stone fragments, and most often requires delayed surgical repair. Ureteral stricture occurs in 0.5% to 4% of cases, is associated with a stone that has been impacted for more than 2 months, and is the reason for obtaining postoperative imaging in the form of an ultrasound 4 to 6 weeks following a procedure.[9]

4. Open/laparoscopic/robotic surgery
   a. Since the introduction of minimally invasive techniques such as SWL, URS, and PNL, open surgery has been reduced to rates of 1% to 5%.
   b. Indications for open stone surgery include complex stone burden, treatment failure with endoscopic techniques, anatomic abnormalities, and a nonfunctioning kidney.

c. Laparoscopic or robotic surgery can be used in place of open techniques when appropriate.
d. Nephrectomy or partial nephrectomy is a last line approach to stone disease and is indicated when long-term obstruction has led to partial or total parenchymal and functional loss and the involved segment or kidney is a source of ongoing pain or infection.

Additional Counseling Considerations

FOLLOW-UP

1. If medical therapy was initiated to prevent stone formation, within 6 months of the beginning of therapy patients should obtain a 24-hour urine specimen which should be continued annually thereafter.
2. If medications are prescribed, periodic blood work should also be obtained to assess for adverse effects of medical therapy.

QUALITY OF LIFE

1. Based on validated, self-reported quality of life (QoL) data, stone formers in the United States have a lower QoL than nonstone formers. Female stone formers are reported to have a lower QoL than their male counterparts.
2. Patients with recent stone events (<1 month ago) had lower QoL score than those with remove stone events (>1 month ago).
3. Some studies have shown that cystine stone formers have lower QoL.
4. Studies have shown that kidney stone patients who have undergone surgery have an equal or improved QoL when compared to equivalent patients who opted for conservative management.
5. In terms of differing surgical modality, the best QoL was reported by those undergoing SWL, and those who underwent PNL had the lowest QoL scores.
6. Dietary changes and medical therapy have not been shown to affect QoL with the exception of alkali therapy which has negatively impacted QoL.

RECURRENCE

1. Only 59.3% of patients suffer a single episode, 17.5% of individuals experience two stone events, and 23.2% report three or more episodes of symptomatic kidney stones.[10]
2. For 2, 5, 10, and 15 years following the initial stone event, the respective recurrence risks are 11%, 20%, 31%, and 39%.[10]
3. The Recurrence of Kidney Stone (ROKS) nomogram is a valuable prediction tool that utilizes only factors known at the initial stone event to give patients a relative risk of recurrence of time.

CLINICAL PEARLS

Nephrolithiasis

1. Stone location in the ureter can often be deduced by the distribution of pain or symptoms.
2. Low-dose, noncontrast CT scan is the imaging modality of choice when diagnosing a ureteral stone.
3. Stones less than 1 cm, less than 10 cm skin-to-stone distance, and less than 1000 HU have the highest chance of successful passage after being treated with SWL.
4. URS is rapidly becoming the gold standard surgical treatment modality for all ureteral stones and intrarenal stones <1.5 cm.
5. All stones patients should undergo a basic evaluation and discussion of general prevention strategies. Select and interested patients may benefit from a complete metabolic investigation consisting of, at minimum, one or two 24-hour urine collections.

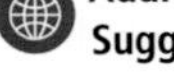

Additional content, including Self-Assessment Questions and Suggested Readings, may be accessed at www.ExpertConsult.com.

REFERENCES

1. Pearle MS, Calhoun EA, Curhan GC, Urologic Diseases of America Project. Urologic diseases in America project: urolithiasis. *J Urol.* 2005;173(3):848-857.
2. Goldsmith ZG, Lipkin ME. When (and how) to surgically treat asymptomatic renal stones. *Nat Rev Urol.* 2012;9(6):315-320.
3. Khan SR, Pearle MS, Robertson WG, et al. Kidney stones. *Nat Rev Dis Primers.* 2016;2:16008.
4. Leslie SW, Sajjad H, Nazzal L. Cystinuria. In: *StatPearls*. Treasure Island, FL: StartPearls Publishing, 2022.
5. Pearle MS, Goldfarb DS, Assimos DG, et al. Medical management of kidney stones: AUA guideline. *J Urol.* 2014;192(2):316-324.

6. Brisbane W, Bailey MR, Sorensen MD. An overview of kidney stone imaging techniques. *Nat Rev Urol.* 2016;13(11):654-662.
7. Assimos D, Krambeck A, Miller NL, et al. Surgical management of stones: American Urological Association/Endourological Society Guideline, PART I. *J Urol.* 2016;196(4):1153-1160.
8. Assimos D, Krambeck A, Miller NL, et al. Surgical management of stones: American Urological Association/Endourological Society Guideline, PART II. *J Urol.* 2016;196(4):1161-1169.
9. Taneja SS, Smith RB, Ehrlich RM. *Complications of Urologic Surgery: Prevention and Management.* 3rd ed. Philadelphia: Saunders; 2001.
10. Rule AD, Lieske JC, Li X, Melton LJ III, Krambeck AE, Bergstralh EJ. The ROKS nomogram for predicting a second symptomatic stone episode. *J Am Soc Nephrol.* 2014;25(12):2878-2886.

Penn Clinical Manual Chapter on Urologic Emergencies

Raju Chelluri, MD, and Robert C. Kovell, MD

Introduction

The purpose of this chapter is to serve as a reference for common urologic consults that the urologist may see on an emergent basis.

Gross Hematuria

Bleeding from anywhere in the urinary tract may manifest via passage of either blood-colored urine and/or urine containing clots. The emergent management concerns are four-fold:

1. Ensuring hemodynamic and patient stability,
2. Establishing urinary drainage,
3. Determining the degree of hematuria,
4. Determining the etiology of hematuria.

Hemodynamic stability: This will tell you the urgency with which you must act.

1. Assess vital signs
2. Serial monitoring of hemoglobin if:
   - signfiicant anemia
   - downtrending Hb levels
   - brisk blood loss
   - clinical instability
3. Transfuse as needed with goal Hb levels based on cardiac status
4. Evaluate and correct any coagulopathy
5. Should the patient be hemodynamically unstable, consider more aggressive imaging and/or intervention strategies based on the presentation to identify and correct the underlying issue

Establish urinary drainage: Determine whether you need to facilitate drainage of the lower or upper tracts.

1. Determine if the patient is urinating, emptying effectively (e.g., postvoid residual [PVR]), and the presence of clots (either in voided urine or in an indwelling Foley's tubing)
   a. If large clots are present or PVRs are elevated in conjunction with symptoms (see later), then intervention may be warranted
   b. Patients with normal urethral anatomy may be able to pass clots easily, but urine pooling in the bladder may promote larger clot formation

NOTE: You will (almost) never be faulted for placing a catheter and irrigating a patient who has significant gross hematuria!

2. If intervention is warranted, then perform the following:
   a. Place a relatively large bore catheter (see later for specifics) to facilitate bladder irrigation
      1) NOTE: Always check whether a patient has an artificial urinary sphincter in place
      2) If so, this should deactivated and may change the size of catheter that can be used safely
   b. Start by hand irrigating the patient using a Toomey or piston-tipped syringe (as discussed later)
      1) In an older male, consider irrigating on tension (inflate the retention balloon and pull with gentle traction) to determine if bleeding is prostatic in origin
      2) In individuals where catheter placement is straightforward, irrigating with the balloon deflated may allow better flow in some catheters
      3) Be sure not to overfill patients who may already have a large volume in their bladder
   c. Should the patient clear their urine and then "pink up" again briskly, consider continuous bladder irrigation (CBI) as they may have ongoing bleeding
   d. Ensure the bladder is cleared of clot burden before starting CBI
3. If a catheter is already in place and the patient develops hematuria
   a. Manipulate the catheter (advance and retract with balloon up) to determine that the Foley is mobile in the bladder
   b. Irrigate the bladder with a Toomey syringe
   c. Consider changing or upsizing the catheter (based on size) to facilitate irrigation and possible CBI as needed

NOTE: In an intubated, sedated, or altered patient, be *extremely careful* about placing the patient on CBI! Their risk of perforation is much higher than the standard patient, as they cannot communicate when pain occurs.

Determine the degree of hematuria: This will tell you the clot burden you are dealing with.

We typically utilize a four-point characterization scheme:

1. "Clear": normal yellow urine, i.e., not red in any way
2. "Urology clear": essentially clear with a slight pink tinge; "pink lemonade"
3. "Light rosae": urine that is mild to moderately red in color without clot. Able to see through to read a newspaper behind Foley tubing; "fruit punch"
4. "Rosae": urine that is dark red, colloid, and unable to be seen clearly through; think tomato juice, port wine, etc.
5. If you are not able to evaluate the patient's urine in person, either have the consulting physician send a picture of the Foley drainage tubing or "rack urine," i.e., save voided specimens to trend the degree of hematuria

Questions to ask of your patient or consulting physician (other **than as noted earlier**):

1. Any recent urologic procedures or history?
2. Has the patient had recent Foley catheter placement attempts before development of hematuria? Details of the Foley attempts should be obtained including the location of difficulty, urine return, balloon inflation, size and type of catheter used, etc.
3. What is the bladder scan? (pertains to Foley in situ or not)
4. Are there any other symptoms (dysuria, suprapubic tenderness, frequency, flank pain, nausea/vomiting [n/v], fevers)? Any lab findings indicative of infection (white blood cell [WBC], urinalysis [U/A], characteristics of the urine)?
5. Any history of bleeding diatheses? Is the patient on anticoagulation or antiplatelet therapy?
6. Other relevant patient history:
   a. Smoker?
   b. Any history of pelvic (i.e., prostatic) radiation?
   c. Occupational exposures?
   d. Any vascular surgery history?
   e. First time hematuria event?

Etiology: Try to think of causes as upper tract (kidney and drainage system) or lower (bladder and urethra). Could also be both.

A classic pneumonic is **Pee Pee ON TTTTHIS**

Period
Prostate
Obstructive uropathy

- (i.e., strictures, UPJ obstruction, etc.)

Nephritis
Tumor
Trauma
Thrombosis

- (i.e., renal vein thrombosis)

Tuberculosis
Hematologic

- (cyclophosphamide exposure, rapid decompression of a chronically retaining bladder, anticoagulation, bleeding diathesis)

Infection
Stones
Specific situations to be aware of:

1. Pseudoaneurysm after partial nephrectomy or percutaneous nephrolithotomy (PCNL)
2. Radiation cystitis
3. Fistula to the arterial system in a vascular surgery patient
4. Patients with artificial urinary sphincters in place

WORKUP

Note that not all of these will be required in every patient and the workup should be individualized based on the presentation

1. History to determine etiology as above
2. Physical exam:
   a. Vital signs
   b. Suprapubic or costovertebral angle (CVA) tenderness
   c. Genital exam: evaluate for trauma, menstruation
   d. Can consider digital rectal exam (DRE) in select patients
   e. Urine: have consulting team “rack urine” or save urine specimens serially for review
3. Laboratory data
   a. Complete blood count (CBC)
   b. Basic metabolic panel (BMP)

   c. Coagulation panel
   d. U/A with micro and culture
      1) Consider having the consulting team send a urine culture (UCx) if it would change management
      2) Try to send the urine before starting antibiotics if possible
4. Imaging
   a. Renal bladder ultrasound (RBUS); can use this to establish baseline bladder clot burden when first called and assure no upper tract dilation
   b. Computed tomography urogram (CTU)
   c. Magnetic resonance (MR) urogram (if renal function precludes CTU)
   d. CT angiogram

MANAGEMENT

1. Hold any anticoagulation if this can be done safely
2. Obtain labs and imaging as earlier
3. Establish drainage, start CBI if needed
4. Address the underlying problem if possible

CATHETER SELECTION RECOMMENDATIONS

- Keep an assortment of catheters in an easily accessible location to use in emergencies in the middle of the night or far off places in the hospital.
- If you suspect heavy bleeding or longstanding large clot burden, start with a 1- or 2-way catheter as they have a larger cross-sectional area for irrigation. You can exchange it to a 3-way and start CBI if needed.
- Good catheters for manual irrigation include *20 Fr hematuria catheter* (which has multiple holes and metal coiling to prevent coaptation) or *22 Fr straight* (or ideally silicone) Foley.
- Consider Coudé' if anatomy issues but have less efficient drainage.
  Coudé catheters usually only have one hole for drainage, limiting irrigation to some degree.
  If there is a large prostate, the hole being angled on the side may help flush around someone with a large median lobe.
- Can also irrigate reasonably well through a 22 or 24 Fr 3-way. Remember that the lumen is smaller than the same size 2-way because there has to be an "in" port.

– Use the smallest possible catheter that will accomplish your goal.

HOW TO IRRIGATE

- Ensure patient comfort with oral (PO) or IV analgesia as needed (a good tip is to have this administered as you are on your way into the hospital).
- Obtain two 1L NS or H_2O bottles, irrigation tray (w/Toomie syringe inside), lube, and a chuck or towel to keep the bed clean.
- Fill irrigation tray with the fluid for flushing in and discard the clots inside the bottles.
- Once you place the Foley catheter, try to let all the urine drain, so that the patient is maximally comfortable.
- Pull back gently on the Toomey before irrigating any fluid in; the bladder may already be distended or filled with clots.
- Try to irrigate with at least two syringe-fulls (~120 cc) if the patient can tolerate this, so the bladder wall is not collapsed, then pull back.
- Flush the bladder with the balloon up or down depending on the situation (usually down to get all the clots sitting at the bladder neck).
- If there is a history of a recent outlet reduction procedure with bleeding, consider a larger Foley balloon (30-cc balloon). Irrigate the patient with the catheter on gentle tension which may help tamponade prostatic or bladder neck bleeding.
- If there is a history of a bladder tumor or unknown pathology, then consider manipulating the catheter back and forth, eventually "parking" the catheter at the bladder neck, as clots tend to pool there.

Escalations in management: if the patient has persistent hematuria after a trial of conservative management, continues to have gross hematuria, or is requiring ongoing transfusion, then management may be escalated to the following steps, depending on which anatomic area is the likely etiology.

1. Prostate/bladder
   a. Cystoscopy, clot evacuation, bladder fulguration
      1) Use the electrocautery cutting loop of a resectoscope to divide and irrigate out any large clots that cannot be cleared with manual irrigation.

2) Inspect mucosa and fulgurate any bleeding areas—this is more effective in the bladder than the prostatic fossa.
3) Manipulation of friable vessels in a radiated or inflamed bladder or prostate can lead to additional bleeding, so this should be undertaken with caution.

b. Aminocaproic acid
c. Intravesical agents (alum, formalin, phenol, silver nitrate)
d. Embolization (bladder or prostate) with interventional radiology (IR)
e. Urinary diversion with nephrostomy tubes
f. Surgery (supratrigonal cystectomy, simple prostatectomy, etc.)

For longer term management

g. If prostatic: consider starting 5-alpha reductase inhibitor
h. If radiation cystitis: may benefit from hyperbaric oxygen after cystoscopy and fulguration; if possible, can begin as an inpatient
i. Consider urinary diversion in refractory cases

2. Renal/ureteral
   a. Angiographic embolization with IR
   b. Surgery (nephrectomy, wall stent, etc.)

Acute Urinary Retention

Establishing urinary drainage in an obstructed patient is a mainstay of general urology. History is critical to determine the likely etiology and thus what intervention to employ, if needed.

HISTORY

1. Age and sex of patient
2. Determine the voiding status of the patient: are they voiding at all? When did they last void?
   a. Determine symptoms. A neurologically intact patient will very likely be having symptoms if truly in retention (i.e., they feel the need to void and cannot).
   b. Determine the PVR or bladder scan.
      1) Be wary of the elevated bladder scan in a patient who has anasarca or edema.
      2) A Foley placed for "elevated PVR" in a fluid overloaded patient may produce no urine return in these patients.

3. What is the urologic history? Any history of congenital urologic issues, benign prostatic hyperplasia (BPH), urethral strictures, urologic procedures, gross hematuria, acute neurologic events (cord injury, MS, CVA, DM), and history of prior catheterizations?
4. How do they void at home? Any clean intermittent catheterization (CIC) history? Any previous PVRs available?

NOTE: An elevated bladder scan or PVR in isolation (e.g., in a voiding or asymptomatic patient) may *not* represent urinary retention in the emergent sense. Not all elevated PVRs will require catheterization and must be evaluated on an individualized basis.

PHYSICAL EXAM

1. Assess the patients' habitus and any degree of contracture.
2. Examine the abdomen to determine if there is a palpable bladder (percuss and palpate).
3. Examine the genitalia to see if there are any urethral (or penile, in a male) abnormalities or any evidence of previous surgeries.
4. In patients with an artificial sphincter (AUS), this should be deactivated before catheter placement.

LABS

1. U/A and reflex UCx
2. BMP (to assess creatinine [Cr], electrolyte elevations)

IMAGING

1. Typically not required in the acute setting other than bladder scan
2. Bilateral hydroureteronephrosis in this scenario is suggestive lower tract obstruction leading to upper tract dilation

DIFFERENTIAL DIAGNOSIS

1. BPH/bladder outlet obstruction (BOO) (especially in an older male)
2. Urethral stricture or bladder neck contracture
3. Urinary tract infection (UTI)/prostatitis
4. Clot obstruction from gross hematuria
5. Neurologic event or condition
6. Constipation
7. Postoperative state

MANAGEMENT

1. If the patient is in acute urinary retention (AUR) and requires drainage, then place a Foley catheter or suprapubic tube (SPT) if possible.
2. In the rare situation that drainage cannot be established from below, consider nephrostomy tubes.

DIFFICULT CATHETERIZATION

Urologic practitioners are often called on to assist with placement of a "difficult Foley" catheter. Typically, consulting physicians or the nursing team may attempt placement of a standard Foley and, depending on the history, one other catheter (e.g., an 18 Fr Coudé) before bringing urologic expertise to Foley placement.

Indications:

Before placing an indwelling catheter, consider indications for placement and the short- and long-term plan for bladder drainage. Assure that a catheter is in fact indicated for the patient before placement given the risks involved.

1. Acute, symptomatic, urinary retention
2. Gross hematuria
3. Accurate monitoring of intake & output (I/O) in a critically ill patient actively undergoing fluid resuscitation
4. In cases of severe UTI (emphysematous cystitis, after a stenting a uroseptic patient who has obstructive pyelonephritis or vesicoureteral reflux, etc.)
5. Surgical or traumatic indications; (intubation with sedation, i.e., in the operating room (OR); bladder trauma, etc.)

HISTORY

1. As earlier in terms of age, sex, etc.
   a. Sex, age, and history will offer a great deal of insight on most likely pathologies and thus, the best approach to catheterization
      1) Elderly male: BPH
      2) Young male: Urethral stricture, inability to relax external sphincter
      3) Male s/p prostatic procedure: BNC, stricture, false passage
      4) Chronic catheter: false passages, stricture
      5) Female: position, habitus

i. Exposure is key in placing Foley catheters
   A. Optimize positioning
      I. Raise legs to allow for better visualization, expose the urethra by spreading the labia
      II. Obtain additional personnel for positioning assistance
ii. Should this fail then you, the urologist, should consider rarer conditions related to stricture, previous surgery, anatomic anomalies, radiation, etc.

2. Take a good "catheterization history" especially regarding recent attempts:
   a. How many attempts were made?
   b. Who made them?
   c. What kind of catheters were attempted?
   d. How far was the catheter advanced?
   e. What happened at maximal advancement?
   f. Was any urine return achieved?

PLANNING

The history and prior attempts will dictate what equipment you need to obtain.

Assure all necessary equipment and personnel are available for the procedure.

Consider collecting the following equipment as a starter set:

1. Coudé catheters (18 or 20 Fr)
2. silicone catheters (12–16 Fr)
3. council-tipped Foley (typically small, 14–18 Fr)
4. hydrophilic glide wires
5. angiocatheters
6. 5 Fr open-ended retrocatheters
7. lubricating jelly or injectable anesthesia jelly
8. sterile field and prep materials

Management: There is a general algorithm to follow that should be modified based on the patient's history.

1. Attempt to place a standard Foley from the kit
   a. In elderly males without known history, consider starting with an 18Fr Coudé ± perineal pressure.
   b. In a younger male with a higher risk of stricture or older male who fails an 18Fr Coudé or has a history of prostatic procedures (BNC), attempt a 12 or 14 Fr silicone.

c. In a female with a recessed urethral meatus, consider passing a 16 Fr silicone or Coudé over a finger placed into the vaginal vault to attempt to guide the catheter into the meatus.
d. If the patient is morbidly obese or diffusely anasarcic, then exposure is key (e.g., having assistants hold a pannus away). Using a stiffer catheter may help.

2. If a standard approach fails, one can consider augmenting your approach with a wire and/or cystoscope.
3. Wire placement
   a. Blind wire placement may be considered with great caution in patients where urethral/prostatic anatomy is unknown.
   b. If the situation is deemed safe for wire placement, pass a hydrated hydrophilic wire into the urethral meatus via a 5 Fr open-ended retrocatheter. Advance the wire until a sufficient amount has passed (remembering the male urethra is ~ 20 cm). If the wire is hitting an obstruction, it should be flexible enough to reverse course and come back out through the meatus.
   c. Advance the open ended over the glide wire into the bladder and withdraw the wire. Urine drip or aspiration of urine confirms placement. While lack of a drip can still occur with the retrocatheter in the bladder, *never* attempt to place a catheter blindly over the wire if this is not confirmed.
   d. The glide wire can be replaced, and over the wire + retrocatheter, you can advance a council-tipped Foley or a modified silicone catheter using an angiocatheter.
   e. Alternatively, you can replace a stiffer wire (such as a Sensor wire) and then advance the catheter without the retrocatheter.
   f. Modifications: sometimes a catheter other than a standard council is needed or council-tipped catheters are not available. In these circumstances you can consider:
      1) Using a large angiocatheter (16g or larger) to puncture the tip to create a passage for a wire—most efficient when using a hydrophilic wire
      2) Cutting the tip with sterile scissors to create a channel, which should be avoided if possible as this creates a blunt edge and the balloon can be damaged

4. Cystoscopy
   a. If a catheter is not passing easily or the patient's current anatomy is not known, cystoscopic evaluation can allow for a better understanding of the problem and can facilitate placement of wires or catheters in a safer manner
   b. In general, you need:
      1) Flexible cystoscope
      2) Light cord and source
      3) Irrigation fluid and tubing
      4) Drape, prep, gauze
      5) Wire (something stiff, not just a glide wire)
      6) Council-tipped Foley (or modified catheter)
   c. After establishing as sterile field, attempt cystoscopy to gain access to the bladder under direct vision
      1) False passages:
         i. Attempt to identify the true lumen into the bladder
         ii. A rule of thumb is that the true lumen is typically anterior (12 o'clock position) if visualization is poor
      2) Stricture:
         i. If a stricture encountered and the patient is not considering definitive repair:
            A. Place a stiff wire under direct vision
            B. Confirm placement in the bladder with a retrocatheter
            C. Dilate with sequential coaxial dilators or a balloon dilator
            D. If placing a urethral catheter, dilate at least 2 Fr over what size you need to pass
         ii. If a stricture is identified in a healthy patient who is considering definitive repair, consider placement of a SPT
5. Suprapubic tube placement
   a. Should all prior maneuvers fail or if considering definitive urethral repair, then consider SPT placement.
   b. Review any imaging and the patients' surgical history to best evaluate any bowel that may intercede between the skin and the bladder in the pelvis.
   c. There are multiple techniques for placement. General principles include:

1) Placing the patient in Trendelenburg position to allow bowel to fall superiorly.
2) Ensuring the bladder is full and pressurized (may consider filling the bladder via a needle just above pubic symphysis if needed).
3) Considering ultrasound for image guidance if needed to confirm location.
4) Ideally, placing the tube in the midline, one to two fingerbreadths above the superior border of the symphysis.

Issues With Indwelling Foley Drainage

An indwelling Foley that stops draining is typically due to displacement of the Foley, obstruction of the catheter lumen, or poor positioning. If gentle manipulation or irrigation of the catheter does not correct the problem, urologic evaluation may become necessary.

HISTORY

1. When was the Foley placed?
2. Was it draining well before?
3. Was there pain at placement or now?
4. Is there hematuria?
5. Is the drainage bag and tubing in a dependent position?

PHYSICAL EXAM

1. Inspect the Foley.
   a. Does it look as though excess is protruding from the meatus?
   b. Is the drainage tubing clear, bloody, or does it have excessive sediment?
2. Palpate the bladder to assess for distension.
3. Evaluate the penis for signs of ventral urethral erosion from indwelling catheters.

DIFFERENTIAL DIAGNOSIS

1. Catheter obstruction (clots, debris, mucus, etc.)
2. Malposition (balloon inflated in the prostate or urethra, positioning in a nondependent place, etc.)
3. Lack of urine output (UOP) due to acute kidney injury (AKI)/ chronic kidney disease (CKD)

MANAGEMENT

1. Manipulate the Foley by gently moving it in and out to assure the catheter is in the bladder with the balloon up.
2. Irrigate the Foley with ~60 to 120 cc of normal saline. Any debris should clear with irrigation if the catheter is of suitable size.
3. Consider bladder ultrasound to confirm Foley placement.
4. Replace the Foley catheter if unable to restore drainage.

Flank Pain and Upper Tract Obstruction

The classic consult for flank pain and upper tract obstruction is for an obstructing ureteral stone, but there is a multitude of etiologies one must consider. However, as with hematuria, assessing stability is the initial concern. Sepsis, renal dysfunction, and symptoms (both pain and inability to tolerate PO) may all be a reason to consider emergent intervention.

Remember, hydronephrosis does not always imply obstruction, and lack of hydronephrosis does not always guarantee lack of obstruction. Further investigation may be warranted depending on the clinical picture.

Is the patient septic?

1. Is the patient febrile, tachycardic, or hypotensive?
2. Determine the WBC and evaluate the U/A (specifically note the status of nitrites, leukocyte esterase, the number of WBC on microscopic U/A, and/or presence of bacteria on gram stain).
3. What is the patient's age?
   a. Older age implies a higher risk.
   b. Some older or younger patients will not manifest a septic response that is to be expected given their degree of illness.
4. Does the patient have other comorbidities that may affect immune function? For example, any history of solitary kidney, diabetes, chronic obstructive pulmonary disease (COPD), immunosuppression, or other high-risk conditions?

What is thcfunction?

1. Does the patient have two kidneys?
   a. Obstruction of a solitary kidney is an emergency
   b. If one kidney is atrophic or compromised, the other may be "functionally solitary," and obstruction also constitutes an emergency
   c. Bilateral obstruction is an emergency

2. Is the patient making urine?
   a. How is the patient voiding?
   b. Is there any evidence of BOO?
3. What is the patient's glomerular filtration rate (GFR)? Are serum Cr, blood urea nitrogen (BUN), and electrolytes normal? Is a baseline GFR available?
4. Has the patient been fluid resuscitated?
   a. Significant pain and nausea/vomiting may lead to poor PO intake and dehydration
   b. Inability to tolerate oral intake may necessitate intervention

DIFFERENTIAL DIAGNOSIS

1. Intrinsic obstruction
   a. Calculus
   b. Ureteral stricture
   c. Tumor or mass
      1) Obstruction can be from upper or lower tract
      2) Ureteral polyps
   d. Hematologic
      1) Blood clot
         i. Can be from a malignant bleed (such as renal cell carcinoma) or from more benign causes such as an angiomyolipoma or ruptured renal cyst
         ii. Spontaneous blood clot should be considered malignant until proven otherwise
      2) Papillary necrosis with obstruction from sloughing
   e. Infection (much rarer)
      1) Fungus ball
      2) Genitourinary (GU) tuberculosis
      3) Bacteriuria with urinary sludging
      4) BK virus
2. Extrinsic obstruction
   a. Abdominal cancer or adenopathy
      1) Colorectal
      2) Gynecologic
      3) Sarcomas or other soft tissue masses
      4) Liquid malignancies with associated adenopathy
   b. Retroperitoneal fibrosis
   c. Trauma

    1) Iatrogenic injury—clipping, suture, unrecognized intra-operative injury
    2) External trauma—gun shot, stabbing, retroperitoneal hematoma
3. Renovascular
   a. Arterial: Thrombosis, trauma, stenosis, emboli
   b. Renal vein thrombosis

SYMPTOMS

1. How bad is the patient's pain? Can it be managed with medications?
   a. Pain is thought to arise secondary to obstruction with peristalsis of the ureter against the obstruction and rise in upstream pressure.
   b. Pain can occur anywhere from flank to the lower abdomen/bladder. Pain can also be referred to the ipsilateral groin or testicle.
2. Do they have nausea and vomiting? When did they last eat?
3. Any urinary symptoms? Gross hematuria, dysuria, cloudy or malodorous urine?

OTHER HISTORY

1. Does the patient have any urologic history?
   a. Any personal or family stone history?
   b. Have they been able to pass stones before?
   c. Stone procedures?
2. Any prior episodes similar to this?
3. How does the patient void at home?
4. Did the patient receive pain medication? Did it help?
5. Do they have baseline renal dysfunction?
6. Do they have any immunocompromising conditions?

PHYSICAL EXAM

1. Vitals; assessment of patient toxicity
2. Abdominal exam
3. CVA tenderness

LABS

1. BMP (Cr, BUN, electrolytes)
2. CBC (WBC, Hgb, platelet count)

   a. WBC may be somewhat elevated in the setting of inflammation from stones.
   b. WBC of < 15 may not be considered elevated in this setting, but should be clinically correlated.
3. UA/Umicro/Gram stain w/UCx (nitrites, leukocyte esterase [LE], blood)
   a. Remember, patients taking pyridium or other urinary tract anesthetics containing this may have false positive nitrites on UA.
4. Coagulation panel
5. Other inflammatory markers such as C-reactive protein (CRP) or ESR can be considered in select cases.

IMAGING

NOTE: If a stone is found on imaging, determine its size, location, and the degree to which it may be causing obstruction. Comparison to previous imaging studies, if available, may be especially helpful.

1. RBUS
   a. Useful as an initial tool as it can provide information regarding hydronephrosis and any bladder issues with minimal radiation
   b. Poor at determining etiology of any hydronephrosis, specifically in the ureter as these are poorly visualized
   c. Can look for ureteral jet in the bladder but not always reliable
   d. No radiation exposure makes this an appealing initial test for patients who may require many studies
2. Abdominal plain film ("KUB")
   a. Can be useful to evaluate for radioopaque stones
   b. May be combined with RBUS or other modalities to pick up ureteral calculi
3. Renal stone protocol CT (abdomen and pelvis)
   a. Low-dose CT specifically designed to evaluate for calculi
   b. Can also provide secondary obstructive information (forniceal rupture, stranding, hydronephrosis, bladder debris, etc.)
4. CT urogram
   a. Can be obtained if calculus is low on the differential but there is evidence of obstruction
   b. Delayed excretory images can help evaluate other etiologies such as strictures, ureteral or pelvic masses, etc.

5. MR urogram
   a. Stones are poorly visualized on MRI—will not be as efficacious in identifying calculi.
   b. Can be obtained instead of a CTU should the patient have contrast allergy or insufficient renal function to tolerate a CT with IV contrast to evaluate for obstruction.
   c. Most institutions can offer this study for almost any range of renal function, but may be less accurate in poorly functional renal units.
6. MAG-3 renal scan (functional nuclear renal scan)
   a. Nuclear medicine study
   b. Can help prove and quantify the amount of obstruction
   c. Less accurate with reduced GFR as the tracer will not be taken up well
   d. Also provides differential renal function
7. Retrograde pyeloureterogram
   a. Requires cystoscopic access to the ureter with dye injected in a retrograde fashion
   b. Fluoroscopic or x-ray images used to look for filling defects in the ureter and for excretion of dye from the upper tract
   c. Can be done at the time of stent placement if intervention needed

INDICATIONS FOR UROLOGIC INTERVENTION

1. Obstruction with urinary infection
2. Renal insufficiency/AKI not responsive to other measures
   a. Obstruction of a solitary system or bilateral obstruction is an absolute indication for intervention
3. Severe, intractable symptoms (pain, nausea/vomiting)

   Infection:
   1. If you have a patient with urinary obstruction and fever, this essentially will force you to act to drain the system emergently
      a. Do not delay as these patients can decompensate rapidly
      b. In these instances, consider Foley catheter placement for maximal drainage
   2. Should the patient be afebrile with equivocal signs of infection (e.g., nitrite positive urine, mild leukocytosis, etc.); some practitioners would argue for immediate stenting

whereas others would monitor for a short period of time to assess clinical course

Renal insufficiency:

1. Significant GFR decrement not responsive to other measures may require intervention
2. Finding a baseline GFR for the patient is extremely helpful if available

NOTE: Obstruction of a solitary functioning kidney is an emergency!

Symptoms or Patient Preference:

1. Intractable symptoms that do not improve with supportive measures
2. Inability to tolerate oral intake
3. Patient profession or situation

MANAGEMENT (SHORT TERM)

General Principles

1. One needs to determine how "sick" the patient is and if drainage is needed immediately or a trial of observation which may allow the situation to resolve is possible
2. Overall, the options in the short term for urinary drainage are cystoscopy with ureteral (JJ) stenting or percutaneous nephrostomy tube placement
3. Urinary drainage
   a. If the patient is unstable, consider IR consultation for percutaneous nephrostomy (PCN) placement as this may be quicker and more reliable than going to the OR for a stent.
   b. Classically, the rate of failure with stenting for extrinsic compression is much higher (~20%–40%) than for intrinsic obstruction.
   c. Ureteral stenting is a reasonable option for many intrinsic obstructive processes.
   d. Other causes to consider PCN or ureteral stenting: pregnant patient, lower tract fistula, severe irritative urinary symptoms, bladder pain syndrome/IC, large burden nephrolithiasis where PCNL is planned, aberrant anatomy that may preclude stent placement (severe BPH, ureteral scarring or stricture, etc.).

   e. If patient follow-up is in question, stents should be placed with great caution due to the risk of encrustation.
4. Observation/medical expulsive therapy
   a. Can be done at home or as a brief admission
   b. Usually entails monitoring of vitals (to see if patient develops a fever), renal function (to trend GFR), IV hydration (to eliminate any prerenal component), straining urine for stone collection, and pain control
   c. In patients with obstructive nephrolithiasis, consider alpha-blocker therapy, increased PO intake, straining the urine, and adequate PO pain control (typically rotating Tylenol and nonsteroidal antiinflammatory drugs (NSAIDs) if renal function allows while reserving narcotics for necessary cases)
      1) If the patient does well clinically, can consider a trial of passage for 2 to 4 weeks to avoid intervention
      2) Alpha blockers have mixed evidence in this setting—may be more useful in patients with smaller, distal ureteral stones
   d. When an obstructing mass causes extrinsic compression, the patient's clinical situation should be discussed with their primary team/oncologist to decide need for drainage to optimize renal function (e.g., plans for chemotherapy/immunotherapy)
5. Further management is typically dictated by the etiology of any obstruction

Postobstructive Diuresis

A sequela of relief of upper tract obstruction (unilateral or bilateral) is the development of postobstructive diuresis (POD). Be mindful of this condition in any patient who has had a relieved obstruction (either upper or lower tract).

DIAGNOSIS

1. Urine output > 200 mL per hour for 2 consecutive hours or producing > 3L of urine in 24 hours
2. No accurate predictive factors for the development of POD
3. If the patient is completely stable (no mental status, vital sign, or laboratory abnormalities and the patient can drink to

thirst), the patient can generally be discharged safely after a period of observation. If not, they will need monitoring

MANAGEMENT

1. Close monitoring
   a. Monitor UOP every 2 hours
   b. Vital signs every 4 hours
   c. Electrolyte monitoring (potassium, sodium, magnesium, phosphate, Cr, BUN) q 12–24 hours
   d. Daily weights
   e. Monitor for mental status changes
2. Fluid repletion
   a. The patient can drink according to their thirst if the patient has intact mental status and can tolerate oral intake
   b. If they cannot tolerate PO fluids or cannot keep up with the UOP, then they should be repleted with half-normal saline at a rate of 0.5 cc normal saline per 1 cc of UOP.
      1) If the patient is at risk for volume overload such as pulmonary edema of CHF exacerbations, consider repletion at a lower amount or rate.
   c. Repletion of electrolytes as needed

Oliguria/Anuria (AKI)

Urologists are often called upon to evaluate decreases in urinary output because of the possibility that an obstruction of either the upper or the lower tract is contributing to AKI. The classic systematic evaluation of prerenal, intrarenal, and postrenal should provide the framework for conceptualizing the differential.

DEFINITIONS

1. Anuria: UOP $<$ 50 mL/24 hours
2. Oliguria: UOP $<$ 500 mL/24 hours

HISTORY

1. What is the urologic history?
2. What is their medical history (cardiac, renal, etc.)?
3. What is the baseline renal function?
4. Are they infected?
5. Is this obstructive uropathy (i.e., a urologic issue)? Why?

a. Stones (with imaging)
b. BPH (with PVR)
c. GU tumors (based on history)
d. Nephrologic history (based on history)

PHYSICAL EXAM

1. Vital sign evaluation
   a. Febrile? May indicate sepsis
   b. Tachycardia/hypotension? May indicate hemorrhage or hypovolemia
2. Inspect for signs of dehydration (skin turgor, dry tongue, sunken eyes)
3. Abdominal exam
   a. Distention, tenderness, mass
   b. Palpably distended bladder
   c. CVA tenderness
   d. Ascites may indicate a medical cause of AKI
4. GU exam
   a. Phimosis, meatal stenosis
   b. DRE to evaluate prostate size
   c. Foley catheter in place? Is this patent?
5. Extremities
   a. Peripheral edema may be indicative of fluid overload.
6. Skin exam
   a. Rash may indicate drug reaction
   b. "Uremic frost"

LABORATORY STUDIES

1. BMP
   a. Cr, BUN, and electrolytes reflect renal function.
   b. AKI can be defined by a variety of scoring systems. The Kidney Disease Improving Global Outcomes (KDIGO) classification of AKI is defined as the rise of serum Cr by 0.3 mL/dL or more in 2 days, rise to at least 1.5-fold from baseline within 7 days, or UOP of < 0.5mL/kg/hour for 6 hours.
   c. If acidotic, check for an anion gap.
2. CBC
   a. WBC to evaluate for possible infection
   b. Hemoglobin to evaluate for possible hemorrhage

3. Urinalysis
   a. Dip
   b. Microscopy
   c. Urine electrolytes to calculate a FeNa
      1) FeNa = (Urine [Na+]/plasma [Na+])/(urine [Cr]/plasma [Cr])
      2) Ratio of < 1 indicates the etiology is likely prerenal
      3) Be careful if the patient is on diuretics as the FeNa will be less reliable

IMAGING

1. Bladder scan
   a. An elevated scan may suggest obstruction or retention
2. RBUS
   a. Can evaluate hydronephrosis and bladder distention
3. CT abdomen/pelvis
   a. Can provide further information on etiology of obstruction found on ultrasound

DIFFERENTIAL DIAGNOSIS

1. Prerenal azotemia
   a. Volume depletion
      1) Hemorrhage
      2) Dehydration
   b. Cardiogenic shock
   c. Septic shock
   d. Other prerenal causes
      1) Neurogenic shock
      2) Renal artery stenosis
      3) Anaphylaxis
      4) Drug overdose; NSAIDS, angiotensin-converting enzyme inhibitor (ACEI)/angiotensin receptor blockers (ARBs)
      5) Cardiorenal syndrome
      6) Hepatorenal syndrome
2. Intrinsic renal disease
   a. Acute tubular necrosis
      1) Specifically in the setting of partial nephrectomy with renal vessel clamping
   b. Acute interstitial nephritis
      1) Typically from medications

   2) Diagnosed with eosinophils on U/A
  c. Glomerulonephritis or other intrinsic nephropathy
   1) Will require nephrology involvement for management
3. Postrenal/obstructive uropathy
  a. Upper tract obstruction
   1) Calculus
   2) Tumor
   3) Stricture
   4) Papillary necrosis
  b. Lower tract obstruction
   1) BPH
   2) Tumor
   3) Urethral stricture
   4) Lower tract calculus
   5) Phimosis
   6) Obstructed catheter
   7) Neurogenic bladder
    i. Spinal cord injury
    ii. Multiple sclerosis
    iii. CVA
    iv. Peripheral denervation
  c. Epidural infusions can cause bladder dysfunction!

MANAGEMENT

1. Determine etiology
2. Prerenal; fluid challenge
   a. A 500-mL crystalloid bolus and close monitoring of urine output afterward to determine response
   b. Defer to medicine expertise unless bleeding
3. Postrenal; evaluate drains
   a. If a Foley is in place, have it irrigated, manipulated.
      1) Can consider imaging to ensure it is in the correct position
   b. If stents are in situ, then obtain a KUB to determine their position.
   c. If drains are not in position, consider need for drainage of the upper or lower tracts based on etiology.
4. Intrinsic renal; likely will require nephrology consultation
5. Avoid nephrotoxic agents, hypotension
6. Closely monitor I/O
7. Serial BMPs to evaluate renal function, electrolytes

Acute Scrotum

Acute scrotal pain has similar management strategies to other acute surgical issues related to end organ ischemia, and the clinical picture gleaned from history and physical exam primarily guides management. Imaging studies may complement, but do not dictate, management.

Unlike other acute conditions, most scrotal pathologies are not life threatening, though management is time sensitive to preserve maximal testicular tissue and function. To that end, when approaching the acute scrotal pain patient, prompt evaluation and diagnosis is key.

DIFFERENTIAL DIAGNOSIS OF ACUTE SCROTAL PAIN

1. Torsion/ischemia (this is the most critical pathology to evaluate acutely!)
   a. Testicular torsion (acute or intermittent)
   b. Torsion of an appendix (testis or epididymis)
   c. Testicular infarction
   NOTE: Time is important in torsion! If the patient is detorsed within 6 hours of developing symptoms, testicular salvage is nearly 100%.
2. Trauma
   a. Traumatic testicular rupture
   b. Scrotal hematoma, hematocele
3. Infection
   a. Fournier's gangrene (see later) is a life-threatening infection
   b. Epididymoorchitis (e/o)
      1) Classically e/o is from sexually transmitted infection (STI) in men over 35 years; GI flora or secondary to obstructed voiding in men under 35
   c. Scrotal skin cellulitis
   d. Scrotal abscess
   e. Pyocele
4. Inguinal hernia
5. Acute or chronic scrotal issues
   a. Hydrocele
   b. Varicocele
   c. Spermatocele
   d. Testicular tumor with rupture

6. Ureteral calculi
   a. Pain can refer to the ipsilateral groin
7. Sexually transmitted diseases
8. Idiopathic inflammatory orchitis or referred musculoskeletal (MSK) pain
9. Nonurologic causes referring pain
   a. Constipation, GI issues
   b. Orthopedic issues (labral tears, hip, knee, pelvis)

HISTORY

1. How old is the patient?
2. Is the pain acute?
3. When did it start? Is it constant or intermittent?
4. Did it wake them from sleep? Any nausea/vomiting, fever, urinary symptoms?
5. Was this preceded by trauma or any event that precipitated the pain?
6. Any history of scrotal or hernia surgery?
7. Any dysuria or lower urinary tract symptoms (LUTS)?
8. Sexually active?

PHYSICAL EXAM

1. Assessment of toxicity (especially if concerned for Fournier's gangrene)
2. Evaluation of vital signs
3. Scrotal examination
   a. Start by examining the contralateral side
   b. Evaluate for scrotal hematoma, evidence of trauma
   c. Evaluate the scrotal skin for signs of infection, crepitus, erythema, signs such a "blue-dot" sign to see if an appendage is torsed (not consistently present)
   d. Evaluate the testes for size, consistency, lie, localizing pain
   e. Evaluate the epididymis for edema or tenderness
   f. Evaluate for Prehn's sign: the painful hemiscrotum is elevated. If the pain improves, this is more likely to be epididymitis; if the pain worsens, this implies torsion
   g. Attempt to elicit a cremasteric reflex: stroking of the inner thigh skin should cause cremasteric contraction and elevation of the testis. Loss of the reflex implies torsion
   h. Evaluate for chronic scrotal pathology (hydroceles, etc.); noting these may be masked by any acute process

LABS

1. U/A, reflex UCx
2. CBC to evaluate WBC

IMAGING

The go-to imaging modality of choice when the diagnosis is in doubt is a scrotal ultrasound ("SCRUS")

1. Color Doppler scrotal ultrasound
   a. Will evaluate, most importantly, for flow to the testis. Compare the vascular waveforms of the normal and affected testis.
   b. One may be able to appreciate a "whirlpool" sign (spiraling and twisting of the spermatic cord).
   c. If the presentation is late into the torsion episode, there may be heterogeneity of the testicular parenchyma (reflecting necrosis).
   d. The epididymis will also have a normal or hyperemic (in the case of infection) appearance.
   e. The technician should be able to evaluate for any large hernia or other masses.
   f. Any evidence of trauma should be evaluated for tunical integrity and hematoma size and complexity.
2. Scintigraphy and MRI have been reported in torsion evaluation or for equivocal diagnosis of testicular rupture.
3. Noncontrast CT scan (including the entirety of the scrotum) can be useful in equivocal cases of Fournier's gangrene.

MANAGEMENT

1. Torsion
   a. If there is a strong clinical suspicion or demonstrated lack of flow on SCRUS, then proceed to scrotal exploration.
      1) Manual detorsion ("open-book maneuver") can be attempted, but this should not delay surgical exploration, as the patient will still require septopexy.
      2) At surgical exploration the affected testicle should be detorsed and evaluated for viability.
         i. If viable, pexy this into place in preferably three locations.
         ii. If questionably viable after detorsion, wrap in warm saline-soaked sponge and reevaluate after

time. Consider incising the tunica albuginea if concern for increased pressure buildup.
3) The contralateral side should be pexied into place given the higher risk of bell-clapper deformity and lateral development of torsion on that side
b. If there is concern for intermittent torsion (clinical presentation highly suspicious for torsion with resolution and demonstration of flow on SCRUS), then one can consider an elective bilateral septopexy with strict return precautions for recrudescence of symptoms
c. Torsion of an appendage does not require further intervention and may be treated conservatively

2. Infection
   a. If concern for a necrotizing infection, see Fournier's section for management
   b. Epididymo-orchitis
      1) STI testing in sexually active men
      2) PVR, U/A, UCx, possible uroflow in older men
      3) Mainstays are antibiotics (fluoroquinolone for 14 days) if bacterial infection is suspected; antiinflammatory medications and analgesics, rest, scrotal elevation, and scrotal support
   c. Cellulitis, scrotal abscess, and pyocele management are discussed later in this chapter
3. Trauma
   a. Penetrating
      1) All penetrating scrotal trauma regardless of mechanism (gunshot wound [GSW], bite, etc.) require surgical exploration and debridement.
   b. Blunt
      1) Testicular rupture/fracture: if this is found on imaging (or, per EAU guidelines, those with equivocal findings) the patient should undergo surgical exploration.
      2) Hematocele: should the hematoma be > 5cm, or expanding, surgical exploration with hematoma evacuation should be considered.
         i. If the hematoma is < 3× the size of the contralateral testis, is < 5cm, and is nonexpanding, then observation and conservative management may be considered.

4. Hernia
   a. The consult should be directed appropriately for hernia management.
   b. Incarcerated hernia can present as scrotal pain and is a surgical emergency.
5. Acute-on-chronic scrotal events
   a. If there is concern for malignancy (i.e., ruptured testicular tumor), the patient should have tumor markers sent and should be scheduled for radical orchiectomy.
   b. Other etiologies (acute symptomatic varicocele, hydrocele, etc.) typically can be managed expectantly with definite management in a performed in a delayed fashion.
   c. If there is concern for an infected collection or hemorrhage, this may push one to consider intervention.
6. Calculi
   a. These may masquerade as scrotal pain if the stone is distal in the ureter.
   b. Management as per the upper tract obstruction section.
7. STI
   a. Generally will be managed by the emergency room (ER) and the patient's primary care physician (PCP).
   b. Test broadly; treat for gonorrhea and chlamydia if high concern.
8. Inflammatory idiopathic orchitis or referred MSK pain
   a. A diagnosis of exclusion
   b. Conservative measures are the mainstay of treatment

Emergent Urologic Infections

Fournier's Gangrene

This disease is a necrotizing soft tissue infection of the genitalia and perineum. It is a true urologic emergency.

DETERMINE STABILITY

1. Given the potential lethality of this disease, it is imperative to establish clinical stability
2. Prompt diagnosis and management is of paramount importance

HISTORY

1. Typical presentation is pain, swelling of the GU area, and fever

2. Age and gender of the patient
   a. Most common in men aged 50 to 79 years
   b. Men > 10-fold increased risk, though it can present in women or children
3. Conditions that lead to impaired circulation or immunosuppression predispose patients to developing Fournier's
   a. *Diabetes is the most commonly associated condition*
   b. Obesity, renal/liver failure, HIV, malignancy, chronic abuse of alcohol or nicotine, COPD, peripheral vascular disease
4. A urologic or anorectal history also can predispose to developing this condition, i.e., chronic Foley catheters, decubitus ulcers, perianal abscess, trauma, urethral strictures, etc.
   a. Also inquire about a history of urologic instrumentation
   b. If so, determine how recently these procedures were performed
5. Determine voiding status
   a. If there is any concern or evidence for retention, then consider early Foley placement or SPT.

PHYSICAL EXAM

1. The pathognomonic finding is *crepitus* (from gas-forming organisms)
2. Evaluate for erythema, overtly necrotic tissue, areas of edema, or tenderness
   a. The superficial fascial planes are typically infected; thus, this can expand from the perineum up the abdominal wall to the clavicles along fascial lines.
   b. Evaluate the genitalia, perineum, perirectal area, thighs, and abdomen.
3. Other findings are pain out of proportion to exam findings, distressed appearance (diaphoretic, anxious).

LABS

1. CBC
2. BMP
3. Hemoglobin A1c (HbA1c)
4. CRP
5. U/A

RISK SCORES

1. Multiple risk scores have been developed to attempt to risk stratify patients with Fournier's gangrene
2. Fournier's Gangrene Severity Index (FGSI): heart rate, temperature, respiratory rate; hematocrit, WBC; Cr, bicarbonate, sodium, potassium levels
   a. Each parameter graded on a 0–4 scale and summed
   b. A score > 9 associated 75% chance of mortality, ≤ 9 with 78% chance of survival
3. Uludag FGSI: adds age and extent of disease
   a. A score > 9 associated 94% chance of mortality, ≤ 9 with 81% chance of survival
4. Laboratory Risk Indicator for Necrotizing Fasciitis (LRINEC): in contrast to the FGSI, this system is intended to distinguish Fournier's from other, less lethal, skin infections
   a. CRP, WBC, Hgb, sodium, Cr, and glucose levels are scored
   b. ≥ 6 is suspicious for Fournier's, ≥ 8 is strongly predictive

IMAGING

1. Imaging is only indicated for the stable patient with borderline findings.
2. The best imaging modality is a CT scan to evaluate for intraparenchymal gas.
   a. Ensure that the scan goes low enough (typically includes the thighs, or down to the knees) to capture the entirety of the scrotum.
   b. Can also show any recent surgical implants (such as an inflatable penile prosthesis).
3. Other options are SCRUS, plain films, etc., but these are more limited in the ability to evaluate for subcutaneous gas.

MANAGEMENT

NOTE: If Fournier's gangrene is suspected, this is a surgical emergency!

1. Broad-spectrum antibiotics are effective against gram-positive and gram-negative, aerobic, and anaerobic organisms
   a. A typical regimen is to go very broad with vancomycin and piperacillin-tazobactam

   b. IV fluid resuscitation and correction of electrolyte disturbances
1. The mainstay of therapy is surgical debridement
   a. Ideally within the first 12 hours of admission—sooner is better to prevent spread of infection and tissue/organ damage.
   b. Usually, there will be an initial, wide, debridement with a planned second look and repeat debridement.
   c. A general goal is to excise tissue until healthy, (i.e., bleeding) is encountered.
   d. A multimodal approach including general surgery (specifically any wound or burn teams) and/or colorectal surgery as the patient may require fecal diversion as well. Plastic surgical expertise may also be required for more complex reconstructions.
   e. The wound should be dressed either wet-to-dry or with wound vacuum-assisted devices.
2. Consideration of hyperbaric oxygen therapy: can be very effective against necrotizing infections but may be logistically difficult in these situations

Pyocele

If Fournier's gangrene is the surgically emergent variant of scrotal cellulitis, then a pyocele is the same for a hydrocele. A pyocele is a purulent collection between the parietal and visceral tunica vaginalis of the testis which typically requires broad-spectrum antibiotics and surgical drainage. This can be difficult to diagnosis on SCRUS alone and requires clinical corroboration.

PRESENTATION

1. Similar to that of the acute scrotal pain; typically will present insidiously over days with pain, swelling, and possibly fever.
2. On exam they may be tachycardic or febrile. They will have the appearance of having scrotal collection on exam (warmth, erythema, tenderness).
3. It is important to determine the voiding status and if there is a concomitant UTI as a pyocele may be a sequela of e/o.
4. The WBC will likely be elevated.
5. A SCRUS will show echogenic fluid collection surrounding the testis.

MANAGEMENT

NOTE: It is important to know that a known sequela of a pyocele is Fournier's gangrene, so this should be managed promptly.

1. As with Fournier's, the principles are IV fluid hydration, correction of electrolyte abnormalities, broad-spectrum antibiotics, and surgical drainage.
2. Evaluation of the ipsilateral testicle—may need to consider orchiectomy if the testicle is heavily involved with infection and deemed not salvageable.

Scrotal abscess

This is a superficial (i.e., not testicular) infected collection in the soft tissues of the scrotum. While it should be managed promptly, it is not typically life threatening.

PRESENTATION

1. Typical infectious symptoms and signs will be present: an area of fluctuance that is tender, erythematous, and warm to touch.
2. The patients will not exhibit systemic signs.
3. There may be concomitant LUTS or evidence of an STI (i.e., penile discharge).
4. As with any abscess, the mainstay is incision and drainage (I&D).
5. SCRUS may be helpful to determine size and depth.
6. Given the association with UTI, would ensure that a UCx is sent.
7. Evaluate for sources such as perianal fistula, Crohn disease, immunocompromised states, etc., that could lead to recurrent abscesses.

MANAGEMENT

1. Typically this can be done with a bedside I&D although based on the size, depth, and patient tolerance, may need to be done in the OR.
   a. Can you feel the abscess as a fluctuant area?
   b. If so proceed, if not, this may require surgical or percutaneous drainage.
2. The authors usually provide topical relief with intradermal analgesia (although these are less effective in the setting of an abscess) as well as PO or IV agents.

3. The area is prepped with betadine and draped.
4. Using an 11-blade, make a cruciate incision over the palpable area of the abscess (size of incision depends on size of abscess).
5. A wound culture should be sent.
6. Using probing Q-Tips, and instrument or the surgeon's finger, probe the area to break up any other areas of infection that may have become septated.
7. Once fully explored and drained, the area should be packed with packing gauze. This should be changed as able, typically BID.
   a. The patient or family members should be taught on wound care.
   b. Proper packing allows the wound to heal from bottom up rather than resealing at the top.
8. Arrange to have the patient seen in 7 to 10 days for a wound check.
9. Antibiotics should be tailored to UCx and wound Cx results.

Emphysematous Cystitis

This is a severe UTI that typically affects diabetic older females or severely immunocompromised individuals. The diagnosis is based on imaging findings showing the presence of gas in the bladder lumen or wall that is not related to urologic instrumentation. The mainstay is Foley catheter drainage and antibiotic coverage.

PRESENTATION

1. Classic patient is a diabetic older female or immunocompromised.
   a. Other risk factors are BOO, chronic UTI, indwelling catheters, neurogenic bladder.
2. Typical presentation will be abdominal pain, LUTS.
3. Pneumaturia may be present.
4. An elevated WBC and hyperglyemia are typical.
5. U/A will show evidence of infection (+ nitrites, blood, etc.).
6. Imaging (CT, ultrasound) will show gas in the bladder and/or bladder wall.

MANAGEMENT

1. Broad-spectrum antibiotics tailored and narrowed to UCx sensitivities as able.

2. Foley catheter drainage
   a. We typically recommend gravity drainage until afebrile or for ~ 7 to 10 days although there is little evidence surrounding this practice.

Emphysematous pyelitis VS Emphysematous pyelonephritis

Gas in the collecting system or renal parenchyma, as is the theme of this section, indicates a more severe infection. However, there is a very important distinction between these two entities. Emphysematous pyelitis reflects a severe UTI with gas in the collecting system but not in the renal parenchyma. Emphysematous pyelonephritis is a necrotizing, suppurative infection of the kidney. Emphysematous pyelonephritis is a medical emergency that requires emergent drainage and possible nephrectomy. It has a high mortality rate (~50%).

PRESENTATION

1. High spiking fever, flank pain, LUTS, and possible hematuria.
2. Risk factors are diabetes, BOO, chronic UTI, indwelling catheters, neurogenic bladder, immunocompromise.
3. An elevated WBC, Cr, and hyperglyemia are typical.
4. U/A will show evidence of infection (+ nitrites, blood, etc.).
5. Imaging (CT, ultrasound) will show gas in the in the collecting system (pyelitis) or renal parenchyma (pyelonephritis).

MANAGEMENT

1. Broad-spectrum antibiotics tailored and narrowed to UCx sensitivities as able.
2. Foley catheter drainage
   a. We typically recommend gravity drainage until afebrile or for ~ 7 to 10 days.
3. Pyelitis will typically not need further intervention other than Foley drainage and antibiotics.
4. Pyelonephritis will require IR drainage/PCN placement, and possible nephrectomy in more severe cases.

Perinephric or renal abscess

This is an infected collection around or within the kidney. It has similar risk factors and presentation as the emphysematous infections described above. Mainstays are broad-spectrum antibiotics and percutaneous drainage for larger or persistent abscesses. Smaller abscesses (< 3 cm) that cannot be drained percutaneously may be managed conservatively with antibiotics and careful observation with periodic reimaging.

Priapism

Priapism is defined as "...a persistent penile erection that continues hours beyond, or is unrelated to, sexual stimulation. Typically, only the corpora cavernoa are affected. For the purposes of this guideline, the definition is restricted to only erections of greater than four hours duration." It is often associated with penile pain. Males in any age group may develop priapism.

Priapism is an emergency. Time is of the essence, as the duration of erectile time correlates with developing ED and penile fibrosis and scarring after the episode.

The history is aimed at determining the classification of priapism (ischemic vs nonischemic), elucidating how long the erection has been present, and trying to elicit inciting factors that may be contributing. The goal of management for ischemic priapism is to achieve detumescence of the penis as soon as possible to preserve erectile function. Once this is achieved, one can further investigate the etiology and discuss preventative management.

CLASSIFICATION

There are three traditional classifications of priapism: ischemic, nonischemic, and stuttering.

Ischemic

This is a failure of venous outflow leading to little or no arterial inflow into the cavernosa. Trapped venous blood creates an acidotic and hypoxic environment within the corpora cavernosa. This leads to a compartment syndrome type of presentation with pain of the penis. If this is not resolved, then end results are penile fibrosis and the development of permanent erectile dysfunction. The development of these sequelae is of a time-dependent manner.

Nonischemic

Nonischemic is defined by unregulated persistent arterial inflow, typically from trauma. In contrast to ischemic it is typically painless and the erection will be softer than that of an ischemic priapism. Also by contrast, this is *not* an emergency and does not need emergent intervention.

Stuttering

Stuttering priapism can be thought of as a subset of ischemic priapism in that it is recurrent ischemic priapism with intervening periods of detumescence. Traditionally this classification is used to prompt the treating physicians to consider preventative measures.

HISTORY

1. Duration of erection
2. Degree of pain
3. Any history of priapism (including acute and chronic treatments)
4. Drug use (recreational and medications)
5. History of genital or perineal trauma
6. History of sickle cell disease or other blood dyscrasias
7. Erectile function prior to the episode
8. Any malignancies in the pelvis (penile cancer, etc.)
9. Previous attempts to manage priapism including aspiration or shunting

PHYSICAL EXAM

1. The corpora should be palpated for rigidity, pain, and tenderness. The glans should be palpated to see if it is soft.
2. Briefly evaluate the perineum and abdomen for trauma, masses/malignancy, or injection marks (e.g., one may note an intercavernosal injection site).

LABORATORY DATA

1. The most critical component of the evaluation is cavernosal blood gas evaluation: In order to initiate appropriate management, you must determine whether the priapism is ischemic or nonischemic.
2. While history and physical will give you clues as to the classification, you must obtain and document a cavernosal blood gas in a patient with new-onset priapism.
3. Cavernosal blood gas is obtained via aspirated blood from the corpora cavernosa.

a. Usually one inserts the needles for aspiration and irrigation and uses this to obtain the blood gas sample.
b. Ischemic: Dark blood, $pO_2 < 30$ mmHg; $pCO_2 >$ 60 mmHg, pH < 7.25.
c. Nonischemic: bright red blood, $pO_2 > 90$ mmHg; pCO_2 < 40 mmHg, pH ~7.4.
   1) Essentially normal arterial blood gas.
4. Other laboratory studies to investigate are CBC, urine and plasma toxicology, and consideration of the workup of sickle cell disease, if appropriate.
   a. Note that obtaining these other studies should not delay management.

IMAGING

1. Typically these studies are not required in the acute setting.
2. Penile color duplex ultrasound can evaluate intracorporeal flow in real time and can help differentiate ischemic vs non-ischemic in the equivocal presentation.
3. MRI can assess smooth muscle viability and any malignant infiltration but has no role in the acute setting.

DIFFERENTIAL DIAGNOSIS OF ETIOLOGY

This does not matter as much in the acute setting but will be useful in determining follow-up management.

1. Approximately 50% of cases are *idiopathic.*
2. *Medications/recreational drugs*
   a. Inappropriate use of intercavernosal injection therapy is a common cause of priapism.
      1) Intraurethral suppositories and oral phosphodiesterase type 5 inhibitor (PDE5i) do not carry such risk.
      2) The type of injection used can be important, as the half-life of these drugs can be longer than those used for injection, and recurrences can occur.
   b. Psychiatric medications for a variety of ailments (antidepressants, antipsychotics)
      1) Classic example is trazodone.
   c. Antihypertensives (hydralazine, prazosin, etc.)
   d. Recreational drugs (cocaine, alcohol, etc.)
   e. Cessation of anticoagulation with rebound hypercoagulability
   f. Total parental nutrition (TPN)

3. *Hematologic issues*
   a. Sickle cell anemia is the classic example where decreased oxygen tension in the corpora predisposes to sickling.
   b. Other hematologic maladies (leukemia, thrombophillic states) can also lead to priapism.
4. *Neoplasm*
   a. Any pelvic malignancy (penile, prostate, bladder) can have metastatic infiltration and blockade of venous outflow.
5. *Neurologic issues*
   a. Any number of neurologic phenomena can lead to priapism.
6. *Trauma*
   a. Any history of penis, perineum, or pelvis can lead to fistulous arteriovenous connections and nonischemic priapism.
   b. The cavernosal artery is the most injured vessel.

TREATMENT

The determination of ischemic vs nonischemic priapism will direct management.

Management of Ischemic Priapism

Ischemic priapism requires prompt management. This is generally undertaken in a stepwise fashion with aspiration/irrigation/injection being the initial management.

While addressing underlying pathology is important (e.g., sickle cell disease), priapism must be managed promptly in most cases to prevent ongoing injury and tissue damage. Risks of ED secondary to the priapism event should be discussed from the outset and well documented.

1. The principles of priapism takedown are aspiration/irrigation and injection of sympathomimetic agents.
2. Aspiration/irrigation protocol
   a. The first step, usually done in conjunction with obtainment of cavernosal blood gas, is aspiration $\pm$ irrigation.
   b. The authors' preference is to obtain the verbal consent of the patient and administer a penile block at the dorsal aspect of the penis at the base with a concurrent ring block. The risk of erectile dysfunction should be explicitly discussed and documented.
   c. Additional IV analgesia should be available as the procedure is performed.

d. The patient should be placed on telemetry as hypertension and bradycardia can occur.
e. The patient will then be prepped and draped.
f. Typically antibiotics to cover skin flora may be considered (i.e., Ancef).
g. A large gauge needle available (12–18 g) is inserted proximally on the penile shaft near the base at the 3 or 9 o'clock position.
   1) Unilateral placement should be sufficient given the fenestration in the septum.
   2) Bilateral placement may be needed if there is extensive clot burden.
h. A variety of techniques is now available to the physician; some will affix a syringe and aspirate blood from the corpora. Others will simply leave the needle in and apply manual pressure to attempt to remove the blood from the corpora.
i. One can use normal saline irrigation in an attempt to break up any old clots.
j. This can be performed until there is detumesence or until the physician feels as though they need further agents.

3. Utilization of sympathomimetics
   a. Sympathomimetics induce contraction of cavernosal smooth muscle and permit venous outflow.
   b. If possible, order injectable phenylephrine to the bedside while you are in route to the hospital as it may take some time to prepare.
      1) Additionally, if the patient is a known sickle cell patient, giving high-flow nasal cannula oxygen and IV fluid hydration is important while you are in route.
   c. The concentration should be 100 to 500 mcg/mL, and this should be given in 1 mL injections every 3 to 5 minutes.
      1) With the needle in place, inject 1 mL and chase this with a few mL of normal saline.
      2) Monitor hemodynamic status. Assess blood pressure for hypertension and heart rate for bradycardia. Have atropine and antihypertensive medications at the bedside.
      3) The authors typically use 500 mcg/mL and give 1 mL injections every 3 to 5 minutes.
   d. Recent literature demonstrated that, in 74 patients, the median dose given was 1,000 mcg; the interquartile range was 500 to 2,000 mcg without HD instability.

1) Thus, one can feel safe to inject up to 2,000 mcg as long as the patient is closely monitored, and the doses given slowly over time.

e. One can aspirate as well between doses.
f. Other agents (ephedrine, epinephrine, norepinephrine, etc.) can be used.
g. Do not give sympathomimetics to those with severe hypertension or those on monoamine oxidase inhibitor (MAOI) medications.
h. The overall attempt to bring someone down should occur for at least 1 hour prior to attempting shunts.
i. Should the erection come down, we typically wrap lightly with Coban and have the patient hold pressure for 5 minutes.
   1) Penile hematoma is inevitable.

4. *Surgical shunting*
   a. The purpose of this is to create a fistulous connection to drain deoxygenated blood.
   b. There are four types of shunts:
      1) Percutaneous distal shunts
         i. Can be attempted in an ER setting
         ii. All other shunts should be done in the OR
      2) Open distal shunts
      3) Open proximal shunts (rarely used)
      4) Vein anastomoses (rarely used)

   NOTE: For the purposes of this chapter, we will only cover percutaneous shunts, as the rest will require a higher level of expertise.

   c. Percutaneous shunts
      1) Wintecopsy gun or a Tru-Cut needle (used for liver biopsies, etc.) is used to puncture the glans distally and connect the glans to the corpora.
         i. The "shunt" is to allow the glans (which is an extension of the corpora spongiosum) to drain the corpora cavernosa.
         ii. Multiple cores of tissue are taken bilaterally.
      2) Ebbehøj shunt: a blade (#10) is used instead of biopsy needles to puncture the glans bilaterally.
      3) T-shunt: an Ebbehøj shunt is performed but the blade is rotated laterally (to avoid the urethra) to create a larger fistula.

i. This can further be dilated using 20-24 Fr urethral sounds to further disrupt any clot.
ii. If dilation is performed, there are data to show that ~50% of patients will recover erectile function.

d. At this point, proximal shunts are rarely used due to lack of efficacy and high rates of subsequent ED.
e. For prolonged priapism episodes or failed shunts:
1) Consider open bilateral corporal decompression through a penoscrotal approach or immediate placement of a penile prosthesis.
2) Patients should be seen back in clinic in a short period of time to assess erectile function and to decide on early prosthesis placement if erectile function is substantially compromised.

Management of Nonischemic Priapism

In contrast to the ischemic priapism, nonischemic is not an emergency.

1. The history, physical, and gas will suggest that the priapism is nonischemic.
   a. The erection will usually be softer, nonpainful, and not fully tumescent.
   b. This is not a surgical emergency, as the penis remains well perfused.
2. Typically at this point the patient should be referred to the outpatient office for close follow-up.
3. For patients with persistent high-flow priapism, consider referral to IR for embolization procedures.

Penile Fracture

Rupture of the corpora cavernosa with a turgid erection, from sheering external blunt trauma usually sustained during sexual activity, merits urgent evaluation and operative repair to decrease the risk of permanent erectile dysfunction.

HISTORY

1. Blunt trauma and bending of a rigid erection
2. Acute penile pain and detumescence
3. May hear or have the sensation of popping or snapping

4. Possible gross hematuria or voiding difficulty signals urethral involvement

PHYSICAL EXAM

1. The classic description is that of the "eggplant sign" or ecchymosis and swelling of the penis in the appearance of an eggplant.
   a. Occasionally a fascial defect will be palpable.
   b. If Buck's fascia is violated, then a hematoma may spread in the "butterfly pattern" along Colles fascia.
   c. The defect is generally on the ventrolateral aspect of the corpora in most cases.
2. Evaluate the meatus and urine; any signal of hematuria mandates urethral evaluation with retrograde urethrography or cystoscopy.
   a. Can be done preoperatively or intraoperatively.
   b. Urethral injuries can occur in 3%–32% of cases.
   c. Have a high degree of suspicion for urethral injuries, with the corporal injury extending bilaterally (and vice versa).

LABORATORY

1. CBC, BMP, and coagulation panel ahead of OR
2. U/A to determine any hematuria

IMAGING

1. Does not typically play a role in emergent management
2. Ultrasound or MRI has been described for borderline cases

MANAGEMENT

While this should be undertaken urgently, the rates of complications such as ED are similar when managed in an early (< 24 h) or late (up to 7 days) fashion in some series

1. Penile exploration with washout and repair of the tunical defect
2. Management of the urethra if injured over a catheter

Foreskin

Phimosis

Phimosis is defined as the inability to retract the foreskin over the glans due to narrowing, constriction, and/or adhesions.

Congenital adhesions usually spontaneously lyse during the early years of life. Poor hygiene may result in chronic infection causing adhesions and fibrosis leading to an inability to retract the foreskin. Complications of phimosis include balanitis, paraphimosis, and voiding dysfunction. Chronic phimosis is a risk factor for developing penile squamous cell carcinoma.

Presentation:

1. Most commonly erythema, itching, discharge, or pain with intercourse
2. Can cause LUTS, UTIs, urinary incontinence/postvoid dribbling

Management:

1. Minor phimosis can be managed with improved genital hygiene and possible topical application of corticosteroid cream.
2. If phimosis is inhibiting the Foley catheter placement in an emergency, one can use a Coudé, catheter guide, a nasal speculum to visualize the meatus, or flexible cystoscopy and wire placement.
    a. Additionally, one could prep and drape the patient and, using clamps dipped in betaine, gently explore the phimosis using the clamp to gently break up any adhesions
    b. This is similar to the method performed in the pediatric setting
3. Mild balanoposthitis can be treated with broad-spectrum PO antibiotics.
4. Severe infection may require an emergent dorsal slit.
5. Elective formal circumcision can be considered for persistent symptoms or recurrent infection.

Paraphimosis

Paraphimosis refers to the retracted foreskin becoming trapped proximal to the glans. This typically occurs when the patient forgets to reduce it or when a clinician unfortunately fails to reduce the foreskin after catheterization.

Presentation:

1. Edema, inflammation, pain, and inability to reduce the foreskin.
2. Left untreated, it can lead to glans ischemia and possibly necrosis.

MANAGEMENT

1. Initially consists of firm compression to decrease edema.
2. Can consider using sugar on the foreskin for 10–15 minutes to help draw out edema.
3. Provide a penile block for pain management.
4. Gripping the glans in a "vice grip" and squeezing for 5 to 10 minutes is commonly taught.
5. A preprocedural penile block should be considered, as this can be quite painful.
6. Once the edema has gone down, place your fingers on the coronal margin and your thumbs on either side of the meatus.
7. Push the meatus/glans proximally while bringing the foreskin around the corona and glans in one maneuver. Rarely will direct incision of the constricting band be required.
8. Elective circumcision may be indicated afterward.

Foreign Bodies

ZIPPER INJURIES

Zipper-associated genital lacerations should be treated conservatively with pressure, cleansing, and topical application of an antibiotic ointment. If there is entrapment of skin, then the zipper must emergently be disassembled. This is accomplished by using a wire cutter to sever the connective metallic assembly of the zipper allowing the teeth of the zipper to separate. A local block may help to control pain control.

EXTERNAL RING INJURIES

The use of various types of constricting bands (rings, washers, etc.) purportedly as "sexual aids" may result in local tissue edema making removal challenging. If not removed, then tissue necrosis may develop. Initially attempt generous lubrication and compression to reduce edema prior to removal. If this fails, a standard ring or bolt cutter can be used to divide the ring. Similarly, a variety of genital piercings, which have recently achieved significant popularity, may serve as a source of inflammation and/or infection necessitating removal.

INTRAURETHRAL FOREIGN BODIES

Various foreign bodies placed into the urethra may become trapped. Pretreatment identification of the foreign body and the extent of migration is advised. This can be evaluated with CT pelvis or kidney ureter bladder (KUB) (if the object is radiopaque). Objects proximal to the external sphincter, densely embedded, or adherent to local tissue, may require open or robotic exploration and removal. Irregularly shaped, sharp, or relatively large objects, especially in the posterior urethra, may be least traumatically extracted by endoscopic relocation into the bladder and then suprapubic cystotomy. In these instances it is advisable to place a Foley catheter postoperatively to decrease stricture risk.

Spinal Cord Compression

A multitude of urologic malignancies, such as prostate cancer, may metastasize to the spine. A high index of suspicion and prompt initiation of treatment may be the difference between functional salvage associated with improved quality of life versus permanent paralysis and the associated morbidity that comes with this condition.

PRESENTATION

1. Acute extremity weakness or numbness
2. Bone pain

EVALUATION

1. MRI spine
2. Bone scan

MANAGEMENT

1. Empiric medical management
    a. Corticosteroids
    b. Spine stabilization
        1) Cervical collar
        2) Thoracolumbar brace/corset
    c. Deep vein thrombosis (DVT) prophylaxis
2. Radiation oncology evaluation to determine candidacy for spot radiation therapy
3. Neurosurgery evaluation to determine if surgical decompression or stabilization is required

4. Ultimately, these patients should be considered for systemic therapy such as androgen deprivation (ADT), chemotherapy, and/or immunotherapy
   a. If ADT is used, start with an antiandrogen for a period of time.
   b. LHRH agonists may cause a "flare phenomenon" with a spike in T levels leading to growth of metastatic lesions and further cord compression—this is blocked by appropriate antiandrogen use.

Additional content, including Self-Assessment Questions and Suggested Readings, may be accessed at www.ExpertConsult.com.

Urinary and Genital Trauma

Alexander J. Skokan, MD, and Hunter Wessells, MD, FACS

Introduction

Trauma remains the leading cause of death among individuals between the ages of 1 and 44 years worldwide, and disability far exceeds mortality. Injuries are responsible for 10% of global mortality and 11% of global disability-adjusted life years. One out of every 12 deaths in the United States is the result of trauma, and genitourinary injuries occur in approximately 10% of all trauma cases. Kidney injuries may result in acute hemorrhage and can be immediately life-threatening, while lower urinary tract and genital injuries may lead to lifelong disability including voiding and sexual dysfunction. While renal injuries predominate in civilian trauma, modern military experiences in Operation Iraqi Freedom and Operation Enduring Freedom have revealed a striking prevalence of external genital injuries among survivors of blast trauma from battlefield improvised explosive devices.

Kidney Injuries

The kidney is the most commonly injured genitourinary organ, with renal injuries occurring in 1% to 5% of all trauma patients. Advances in noninvasive radiologic evaluation, percutaneous interventions, and trauma care have yielded excellent outcomes without the need for surgical intervention in the vast majority of patients with traumatic renal injuries.

INITIAL EVALUATION

Gross inspection of the urine and urinalysis should be performed early after stabilization, since hematuria is often an early sign of underlying renal trauma. **Any blunt trauma patient presenting**

with gross hematuria or microscopic hematuria and hypotension (systolic blood pressure less than 90 mmHg in the field or at any subsequent point) must be evaluated for renal injury (Fig. 10.1). A dipstick urinalysis positive for blood is an adequate surrogate for microscopic hematuria in the setting of trauma. Of note, the degree of hematuria does not reflect the severity of underlying renal injuries. Patients with severe injuries including renal artery thrombosis, ureteropelvic junction (UPJ) disruption, or renal pedicle avulsion may actually have no evidence of hematuria on initial evaluation. Providers must maintain a high degree of suspicion for renal trauma in patients presenting after a high-energy mechanism of injury (fall from height, high-speed road traffic accident, direct blow to the flank) even in the absence of hematuria. Patients with preexisting renal abnormalities are also at higher risk for traumatic renal injury. In general, patients with penetrating trauma to the torso also require a timely evaluation for renal injury.

Prompt imaging is the mainstay of early diagnostic evaluation in hemodynamically stable patients, and computed tomography (CT) is recommended according to the American Urologic Association (AUA) Urotrauma Guideline regardless of mechanism of injury. Stable patients after blunt trauma with microscopic hematuria and no reported hypotension can be observed clinically without renal imaging. **CT studies should include a venous phase to identify parenchymal lacerations, hematomas, and vascular contrast extravasation indicative of ongoing bleeding. It is also important to include a delayed excretory phase, performed approximately 10 minutes after contrast administration, to evaluate for evidence of urinary contrast extravasation.** Hemodynamically unstable patients require resuscitation to achieve prompt stabilization, with a low threshold to proceed to emergent laparotomy. In patients requiring immediate laparotomy that precludes a full radiologic evaluation of suspected injuries, providers may perform a one-shot intravenous pyelogram (IVP) on the table to aid with further management (see Management section). Unstable patients with risk factors for continued hemorrhage (perinephric hematoma $>$ 4 cm, vascular contrast extravasation) should undergo prompt intervention via either angiography with selective embolization or surgical exploration. Angioembolization can be useful in cases with concomitant hepatic or splenic lacerations also amenable to embolization.

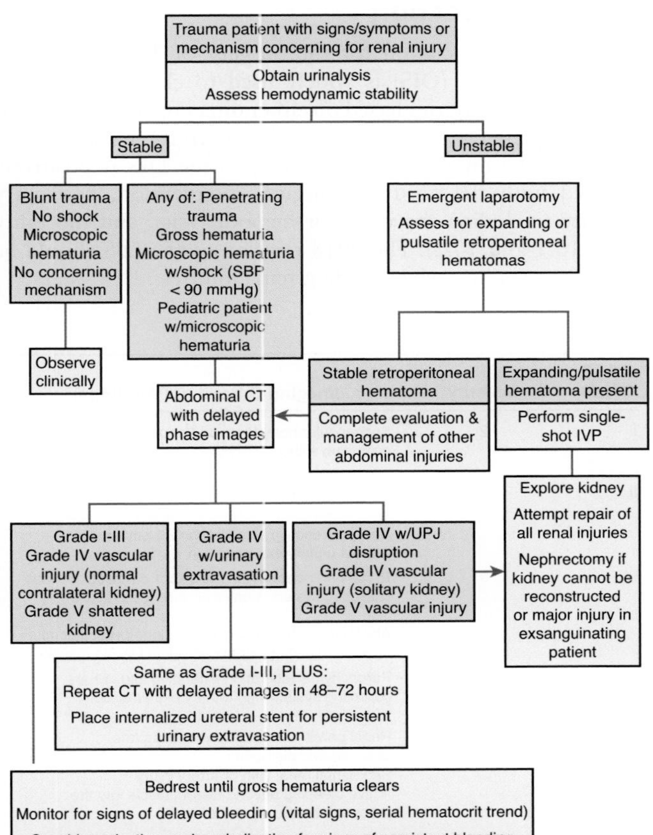

FIGURE 10.1 Algorithm for evaluation and management of renal trauma. ***CT,*** **Computed tomography;** ***IVP,*** **intravenous pyelogram;** ***SBP,*** **systolic blood pressure;** ***UPJ,*** **ureteropelvic junction.** (Modified from Wessells H. Injuries to the urogenital tract. In: Souba WW, Fink MP, Jurkovich GJ, et al., eds: *ACS surgery: principles and practice*, New York: WebMD; 2005; and Brandes SB, Eswara JR. Upper urinary tract trauma. In: Partin AW, et al., eds. *Campbell Walsh Wein Urology*, 12th ed. Philadelphia: Elsevier; 2021.)

INJURY CLASSIFICATION

The American Association for the Surgery of Trauma (AAST) Organ Injury Scale (OIS) is widely used to classify blunt and penetrating renal injuries based on either direct operative exploration or complete CT evaluation (Fig. 10.2). Multiple studies have shown that the injury grade according to the OIS is positively correlated with the need for surgical intervention, postinjury morbidity (including the need for hemodialysis), and mortality (Tables 10.1 and 10.2). The 2018 revision to the OIS should be used as the reference when grading renal injuries.

AAST Grade	AIS Severity	Imaging Criteria (CT Findings)
I	2	– Subcapsular hematoma and/or parenchymal contusion without laceration
II	2	– Perirenal hematoma confined to Gerota fascia – Renal parenchymal laceration ≤ 1 cm depth without urinary extravasation
III	3	– Renal parenchymal laceration > 1 cm depth without collecting system rupture or urinary extravasation – Any injury in the presence of a kidney vascular injury or active bleeding contained within Gerota fascia
IV	4	– Parenchymal laceration extending into urinary collecting system with urinary extravasation – Renal pelvis laceration and/or complete ureteropelvic disruption – Segmental renal vein or artery injury – Active bleeding beyond Gerota fascia into the retroperitoneum or peritoneum – Segmental or complete kidney infarction(s) due to vessel thrombosis without active bleeding
V	5	– Main renal artery or vein laceration or avulsion of hilum – Devascularized kidney with active bleeding – Shattered kidney with loss of identifiable parenchymal renal anatomy

Advance one grade for bilateral injuries up to Grade III.

FIGURE 10.2 AAST organ injury scale for the kidney. *AAST*, American Association for the Surgery of Trauma; *AIS*, Abbreviated Injury Scale; *CT*, computed tomography. (From Kozar RA, Crandall M, Shanmuganathan K, et al. Organ injury scaling 2018 update: Spleen, liver, and kidney. *J Trauma Acute Care Surg.* 2018;85:1119-1122.)

TABLE 10.1 Multivariate Predictors of Morbidity and Mortality After Blunt Renal Trauma*

	Nephrectomy (n = 289)	Dialysis (n = 33)	Death (n = 709)
AAST I	Reference group	Reference group	Reference group
AAST II	2.5 (1.0–6.2)	1.5 (0.41–5.6)	0.95 (0.65–1.4)
AAST III	12 (5.6–25)	1.3 (0.45–4.6)	1.3 (0.90–2.0)
AAST IV	64 (34–120)	3.7 (1.2–11)	1.4 (0.97–2.0)
AAST V	127 (68–236)	4.7 (1.4–16)	1.9 (1.3–2.7)
Bowel surgery	2.3 (1.8–2.9)	3.9 (1.5–10)	
Spleen surgery	2.2 (1.8–2.8)		2.1 (1.4–3.0)
Liver surgery	1.5 (1.2–2.0)		
ISS > 15			2.8 (1.4–5.6)
ISS > 24			3.0 (2.0–4.4)
ISS > 47			1.7 (1.3–2.3)
SBP < 90			2.0 (1.5–2.6)
Abd AIS > 3		5.3 (1.9–15)	
Head AIS > 3			2.5 (1.9–3.4)
Age > 40 years	1.3 (1.0–1.5)	4.0 (2.2–7.3)	2.0 (1.6–2.4)

*Blank cells indicate the parameter was not an independent predictor for that particular outcome.

AAST, American Association for the Surgery of Trauma; *AIS*, Abbreviated Injury Scale; *ISS*, Injury Severity Score; *SBP*, systolic blood pressure.

MANAGEMENT

Over the past several decades, the management of renal trauma has shifted dramatically such that most cases are now approached nonoperatively. There is a low rate of delayed surgical intervention with conservative management, and this approach has achieved a higher rate of renal salvage without an increase in postinjury morbidity or mortality. **The absolute indications for surgical exploration in renal trauma include hemodynamic instability/life-threatening hemorrhage; renal pedicle avulsion; UPJ disruption (discussed in Management of Ureteral Trauma); or an expanding, pulsatile, or uncontained retroperitoneal hematoma.** Many high-grade injuries and complications such as a large or superinfected urinoma previously required open surgery, but these injuries can often be managed via percutaneous or endoscopic interventions. Active arterial bleeding, arterial pseudoaneurysms, and vascular

TABLE 10.2 Multivariate Predictors of Morbidity and Mortality After Penetrating Renal Trauma*

	Nephrectomy (n = 333)	Dialysis (n = 6)	Death (n = 249)
AAST I	Reference group		
AAST II	1.1 (0.3–3.7)		
AAST III	7.7 (3.2–18)		
AAST IV	25 (10–63)		
AAST V	31 (12–82)		
Firearm injury	25 (10–63)		
Bowel surgery	31 (12–82)		
Spleen surgery			0.42 (0.22–0.81)
Liver surgery			0.44 (0.23–0.87)
ISS > 24			4.6 (2.27–9.2)
SBP < 90			2.8 (1.6–4.9)

*Blank cells indicate the parameter was not an independent predictor for that particular outcome. There were too few patients with dialysis (n = 6) for a meaningful prediction model.

AAST, American Association for the Surgery of Trauma; *ISS*, Injury Severity Score; *SBP*, systolic blood pressure.

fistulas are controlled with selective angioembolization, and large urinomas or perinephric abscesses can often be drained percutaneously with consideration for a concomitant indwelling ureteral stent to facilitate antegrade urinary tract drainage. While some patients will benefit from percutaneous drainage of a perinephric collection, primary drainage of the urinary tract can usually be achieved with an indwelling ureteral stent and a percutaneous nephrostomy drain is only rarely required in the acute setting. Recent prospective investigation has led to the development of a nomogram to identify patients likely to require angioembolization or surgical exploration to control bleeding; this nomogram can be a valuable decision support resource for emergency practitioners (Fig. 10.3).

Currently, 20% to 50% of all penetrating renal injuries and fewer than 10% of blunt injuries require operative management. **Grade I–III renal injuries** (Fig. 10.4), **regardless of mechanism, are managed with observation with only rare exceptions. In hemodynamically stable patients, many grade IV** (Fig. 10.5) **and selected grade V injuries can be managed nonoperatively with a high success**

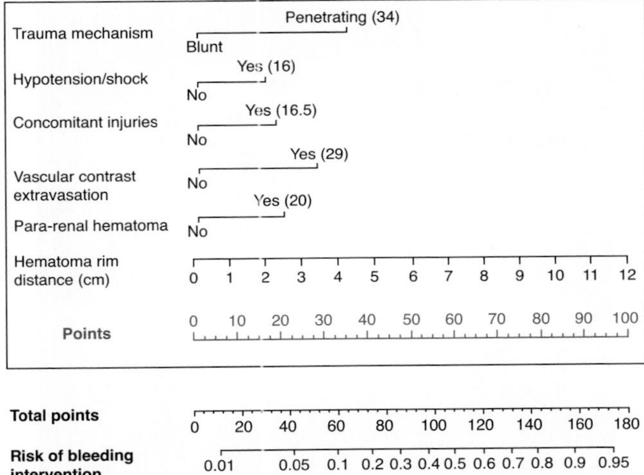

FIGURE 10.3 Nomogram predicting the likelihood of embolization or renal surgery in high-grade renal trauma. (From Keihani S, Rogers DM, Putbrese BE, et al. A nomogram predicting the need for bleeding interventions after high-grade renal trauma. *J Trauma Acute Care Surg.* 2019;86:774-782.)

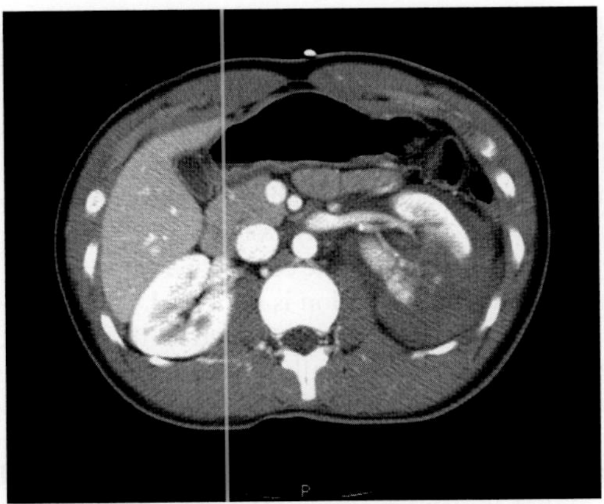

FIGURE 10.4 Grade III or higher left renal injury with deep laceration, extensive parenchymal damage, and large perinephric hematoma. Delayed phase excretory imaging would be needed to further assess the integrity of the collecting system.

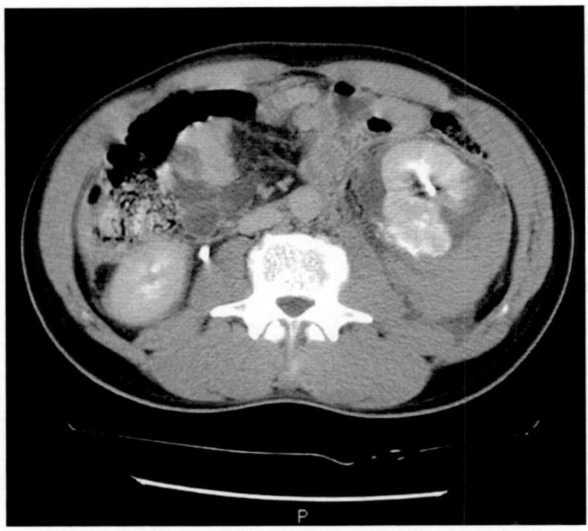

FIGURE 10.5 Grade IV left renal laceration with urinary extravasation and perinephric hematoma.

rate. This entails close monitoring, hydration, serial hematocrit measurements, and repeat imaging in most cases. Patients are kept on bed rest until any ongoing gross hematuria resolves. A Foley catheter is generally not necessary from the standpoint of urinary drainage unless a patient has urinary retention. Thrombosis of the main renal artery or its major segmental branches without active bleeding is treated nonoperatively except in cases of a solitary kidney or severe injury involving the contralateral renal unit, in which case emergency revascularization is indicated.

Open renal exploration is associated with a significant risk of emergent nephrectomy, usually for damage control in an exsanguinating patient or due to exploration by surgeons unfamiliar with the principles and techniques of renal reconstruction. Predictors of nephrectomy after trauma include the OIS grade, patients' global Injury Severity Score (ISS), transfusion requirement, and operations on other intraabdominal organs.

The body of evidence to guide decision-making in children and adolescents with renal trauma is limited. Abdominal CT should be utilized for initial injury diagnosis and staging in stable patients with suspicion for renal injury. The Eastern Association for the Surgery of Trauma (EAST) and Pediatric Trauma Society recommend initial conservative management in stable patients with few exceptions, even in high-grade injuries. When control of persistent or delayed bleeding is necessary, minimally invasive techniques via angioembolization are preferred. Although the sensitivity of renal ultrasound is currently insufficient for initial diagnosis, it may serve a valuable role in follow-up monitoring of high-grade injuries. Since up to 4% of injured children will develop postinjury hypertension, it is critical that pediatric patients undergo interval blood pressure monitoring after recovery.

Operative Management

Some patients with either penetrating or blunt injuries require immediate laparotomy before radiographic evaluation, often for other serious intraabdominal injuries. If a major renal injury is suspected based on the characteristics of a retroperitoneal hematoma, a one-shot intraoperative IVP is recommended before renal exploration to confirm the presence of a contralateral functioning kidney. A 2 mL/kg bolus of contrast material is administered 10 minutes before obtaining a single plain abdominal film. Abnormalities of the affected kidney, including poor visualization, should prompt consideration for operative exploration.

A pulsatile or expanding retroperitoneal hematoma found during laparotomy requires renal exploration, as it suggests ongoing severe and potentially life-threatening bleeding. This primarily arises in the setting of nonelective surgical intervention for critically ill trauma patients, and **in these cases, a rapid nephrectomy is often necessary.** Less severe injuries can be managed with renorrhaphy, partial nephrectomy, perinephric drains, embolization, and damage control techniques described later. In most cases of exploration, renal reconstruction and salvage is technically feasible; however, if the patient is unstable and has a normal contralateral kidney, rapid nephrectomy may be prudent. Selective renal embolization via angiography may be considered in some patients when there is evidence of ongoing segmental vessel bleeding after initial resuscitation. This strategy has demonstrated high success rates with a low incidence of complications for grade IV injuries, although angioembolization often fails in the management of grade V injuries. **When exploring a grade III or IV injury**, surgeons should seek to **first control ongoing hemorrhage, then repair injuries to the collecting system in a watertight fashion, and finally achieve a hemostatic parenchymal closure.** Patients undergoing exploration for a blunt grade V injury will almost always require nephrectomy, with reconstruction reserved for injury involving a solitary kidney or significant bilateral renal injuries.

A midline transabdominal incision permits exploration of either kidney as well as complete evaluation of the other intraabdominal organs. This approach also provides optimal access to the renal hilum. **Renal hilar control via isolation of the renal artery and vein is recommended prior to direct renal exploration, and this can be rapidly achieved by sharply opening the posterior peritoneum medial to the inferior mesenteric vein.** If the surgeon is comfortable reflecting the ipsilateral colon without disrupting Gerota's fascia and the contained perinephric hematoma, this may be considered as an alternative approach to the renal hilum. Early vascular control appears to increase the rate of renal salvage. Once the renal vessels are isolated, Gerota's fascia is opened. If massive bleeding occurs when the hematoma is entered, Rummel tourniquets or vascular clamps are applied to the renal artery and vein to allow controlled exploration and repair of the underlying renal injuries.

The principles of renal reconstruction include complete exposure, debridement of devitalized tissue, achievement of hemostasis, watertight collecting system closure, coverage of the defect, and drainage. Focal areas of bleeding can be controlled with figure-of-eight sutures of fine absorbable monofilament.

Once hemostasis is satisfactory, any open defects in the collecting system are closed with 4-0 absorbable sutures. The defect in the parenchyma can be filled with absorbable hemostatic gelatin sponges, then the capsule is closed over these bolsters. For polar injuries, partial nephrectomy can be considered instead. The addition of hemostatic agents such as Floseal may also be helpful. If the renal capsule has been destroyed, coverage options include an omental or perinephric fat flap, a patch of polyglycolic acid or peritoneum, or a sac of polyglycolic acid wrapped around the kidney. Gerota's fascia is not reapproximated. Closed-suction drainage of the ipsilateral retroperitoneum is utilized to aid with monitoring for surgical site complications postoperatively. Most patients do not require internalized ureteral stents, as these are primarily reserved for complex injuries (e.g., large lacerations of the renal pelvis or the UPJ).

Prompt nephrectomy is generally advised in the rare case of major renovascular injuries because salvage rates after renal vascular reconstruction are low. In unstable patients, damage control with renal packing and planned reevaluation in 24 hours can also be considered in an attempt to avoid nephrectomy.

COMPLICATIONS

The risk of complications increases with the organ injury scale (OIS) grade of renal injury. The most significant early complications are delayed bleeding, infection, and urinary leakage. For some grade IV to V injuries managed nonoperatively, follow-up imaging at 48 to 72 hours after the initial scan may minimize the risk of missed complications. For lower grade injuries and grade IV vascular injuries without evidence of ongoing bleeding, repeat imaging can be safely omitted unless patients develop signs of infection, evidence of continued bleeding, worsening pain, or ileus. Clinical monitoring with reimaging only for symptomatic patients can be cautiously considered even in the setting of urinary extravasation; there is some evidence that this opportunistic reimaging approach may not result in missed complications.

Urinary extravasation on initial imaging can often be managed with systemic antibiotics and close observation. **If an active urine leak persists on follow-up imaging, placement of an internalized ureteral stent is indicated. Early drainage with a ureteral stent should also be considered if there is evidence of urinary obstruction or concern for infection.** The urinary bladder should be drained with a Foley catheter until any extravasation resolves, which can take days to weeks and may require additional interval reimaging. Ultrasonography is useful for following perinephric collections and for reducing the patient's radiation exposure. If a perinephric fluid collection is large enough to cause urinary obstruction or becomes superinfected, percutaneous drainage of the urinoma/hematoma is required. The role for percutaneous urinary tract drainage with a nephrostomy tube is limited in the setting of renal trauma.

Delayed bleeding is a rare, life-threatening complication of major lacerations. Pseudoaneurysm and arteriovenous malformation

(AVM) are the most common causes of delayed bleeding and usually occur within 2 weeks postinjury. **Selective arterial embolization is an effective treatment in most instances of delayed bleeding.**

Hypertension is a rare late complication of renal injuries that is usually renin-mediated and related to an ischemic segment of parenchyma. This occurs in about 5% of adult renal trauma patients. Etiologies include renal arterial injury leading to stenosis and downstream ischemia, extrinsic compression from a perinephric collection (Page kidney), an infarcted parenchymal fragment, or arteriovenous fistula. Angiography, decortication, excision of a nonperfused segment, or nephrectomy may be required in these rare cases. Long-term blood pressure monitoring is often necessary.

Ureteral Injuries

Most ureteral injuries are iatrogenic, primarily resulting from gynecologic, general surgical, or urologic procedures. External ureteral trauma is relatively rare, accounting for approximately 1% of all genitourinary injuries. **Ureteral injuries more commonly occur with penetrating trauma and deceleration injuries in blunt trauma, and patients usually have multiple associated abdominal injuries.** Patients with ureteral injuries from external trauma have a mortality rate of 6% to 10%, primarily due to damage to other organs, as noted earlier. In cases with a plausible mechanism, providers should maintain a high index of suspicion for potential ureteral injury to prevent a delay in diagnosis. Such delays can result in late consequences such as urinoma, sepsis, stricture, and ultimately the need for nephrectomy.

INITIAL EVALUATION

Up to 25%–45% of patients with ureteral injuries may present without hematuria, contributing to the potential for a delay in diagnosis. **Stable patients with suspected ureteral injuries should undergo CT with intravenous contrast and delayed (excretory) phase images to evaluate for urinary extravasation.** If further clinical information is needed, **retrograde pyeloureterography (RPG) can be used** to identify and localize the injury (Fig. 10.6). In the case of delayed identification of an iatrogenic injury, clinicians should also utilize CT imaging and consideration for an RPG,

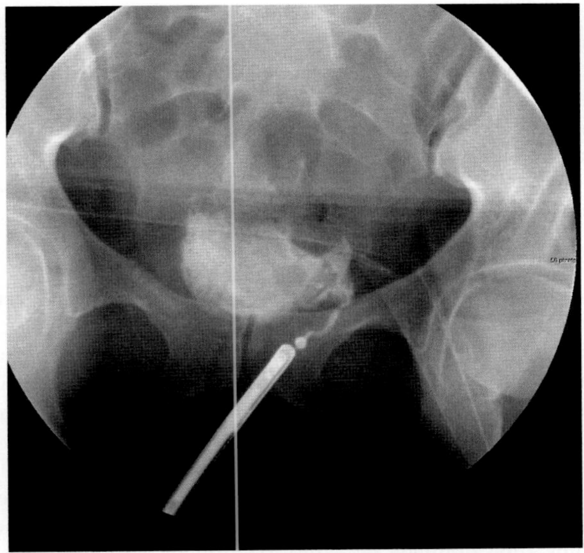

FIGURE 10.6 Left retrograde ureterogram demonstrating a distal ureteral injury. Extensive extravasation of contrast is seen approximately 1 to 2 cm proximal to the left ureterovesical junction. (Courtesy Dr. Parvati Ramchandani, University of Pennsylvania Health System)

as outlined previously. After severe deceleration events (such as ejection from a vehicle in a high-speed collision), UPJ injuries or ureteral injuries near the iliac vessels can occur. UPJ injuries occur disproportionately in children, where it is thought that the hyperextensibility of the spine or underlying congenital urinary tract anomalies can predispose to UPJ avulsion. Clinicians should consider a UPJ injury in cases where a CT scan demonstrates medial or circumrenal contrast extravasation.

When an unstable patient with penetrating trauma is taken emergently for laparotomy without preoperative imaging, **direct inspection of the ureter via retroperitoneal exploration is indicated if the projectile trajectory would place the ureter at risk**, regardless of the presence or absence of retroperitoneal hematoma. A one-shot IVP is of limited utility due to a high rate of false negative or nondiagnostic studies. In a meta-analysis including a series from 16 large trauma centers, **89% of ureteral injuries were identified at the time of exploratory laparotomy.** Gentle instillation of 1 to 2 mL of methylene blue or indigo carmine into the collecting system (or administration of intravenous methylene blue with a period of delay to allow dye excretion) may help to identify sites of laceration or avulsion. In cases with anatomic distortion due to a large retroperitoneal hematoma, an RPG can help to localize injuries to guide surgical exploration and ureteral repair.

MANAGEMENT

Management depends on the etiology and severity of ureteral injury, the location of the injury (Fig. 10.7), the patient's clinical stability, and the time from injury to diagnosis. If recognized intraoperatively in a stable patient, injuries including lacerations, transections, or severe contusions should be debrided and repaired primarily. Stable patients with a limited contusion or equivocal injury findings can be managed with upfront ureteral stent placement. **If a patient is clinically unstable, temporizing measures to achieve safe drainage can include ligation of the ureter and nephrostomy tube drainage or exteriorization of a ureteral stent to allow elective repair in the subsequent few days after clinical stabilization.** If a diagnosis is delayed (especially beyond 5–7 days), initial management should consist of ureteral stenting. If a stent cannot be safely placed, a percutaneous nephrostomy tube should be pursued. Definitive repair is then deferred until 6 to 12 weeks later, which results in a higher rate of ureteral patency and a lower rate of nephrectomy than with early primary repair in this group. **Nephrectomy should be considered in cases where concomitant vascular repair using prosthetic material may be complicated by urine leakage.**

Operative Management

The principles of ureteral reconstruction include debridement of devitalized tissue, preservation of the vascularized ureteral adventitia, creation of a spatulated tension-free anastomosis, watertight closure with absorbable suture, internal stenting, tissue interposition for coverage of the repair, and drainage of the surgical field during early healing. Minor contusions can be managed with stent placement, as noted previously. **Long segment ureteral contusions have a significant risk of stricture or delayed**

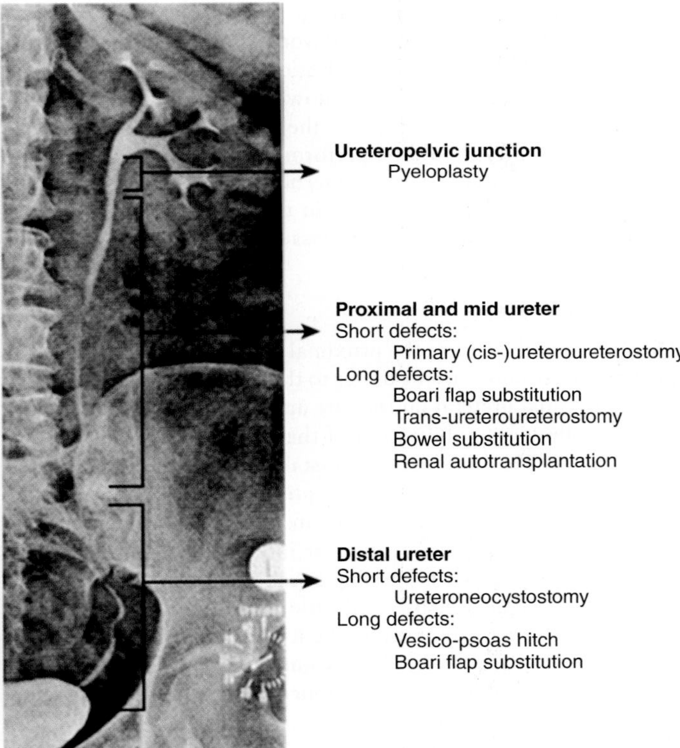

FIGURE 10.7 Management of ureteral injury based on segment of ureter injured. (Modified from Kuan J, Routt ML, Wessells H. Genitourinary and pelvic trauma. In: Mulholland, MW, Lillemoe KD, Doherty GM, et al., eds. *Greenfield's Surgery: Scientific Principles and Practice*. 4th ed. Philadelphia: Lippincott Williams & Wilkins; 2006.)

breakdown with urine leak due to underlying microvascular injury with devitalization of the involved segment. In such cases, excision of the contused segment and primary ureteral repair should be considered. Partial transections not involving the full circumference of the injured segment may be closed primarily. **Gunshot injuries usually require debridement** due to the risk of blast-induced microvascular damage that may not be apparent on visual inspection, **while stab wounds often do not require debridement.** In all cases, mobilization of the ureter should be limited only to the degree that allows a tension-free anastomosis, in order to avoid disrupting the delicate adventitial blood supply. All repairs should be performed with interrupted 5-0 or 6-0 absorbable sutures over an internalized or externalized stent. Closed suction drains are placed in the retroperitoneum, and a Foley catheter is used to decompress the bladder and limit vesicoureteral reflux early after repair.

Proximal Ureter

Disruption of the UPJ or the proximal ureter can be repaired with primary anastomosis of the ureter to the renal pelvis (pyeloplasty). Some proximal ureteral injuries are amenable to cisureteroureterostomy following mobilization of the healthy proximal and distal segments. The proximal and distal ends of healthy ureter are spatulated on opposite sides when preparing for a primary anastomosis. In cases with adjacent organ injuries (colon, duodenum, or pancreas), a flap of omentum or interposition of perinephric fat should be used when possible as an additional layer to cover the ureteral repair. Renal mobilization with a downward nephropexy can aid with shortening the length of a ureteral defect in some cases. **In cases with a long-segment injury, definitive repair should be deferred in favor of temporizing management acutely.**

Mid Ureter

Injuries involving a short segment of the mid ureter can often be repaired primarily via cis-ureteroureterostomy. Alternative approaches include a trans-ureteroureterostomy or Boari flap interposition with creation of a ureteral anastomosis to a tubularized bladder flap. It is important to ensure the bladder has normal or near-normal capacity if considering a Boari flap, since this maneuver will decrease the reconstructed bladder's storage capacity. If a Boari flap is employed, the apex of the flap should be three times the diameter of the ureter and the length of the flap should be no more than three times the width of its base. While repairs more extensive than a primary ureteroureterostomy can be considered in a stable patient, it is reasonable to pursue temporary drainage acutely and formal reconstruction in a delayed manner.

Regardless of the type of repair performed, an internalized ureteral stent should be placed across the anastomosis and into or through the bladder.

Distal Ureter

Injuries below the pelvic brim are often best managed with ureteral reimplantation into the bladder (ureteroneocystostomy). The ureteral stump distal to the site of injury is ligated, and then the spatulated proximal end of the ureter is brought into the bladder through a new hiatus on the posterior wall or dome. This can be achieved intravesically (by opening the anterior bladder wall and making a separate posterior wall cystotomy to mature the ureteral anastomosis) or extravesically (by making a cystotomy only at the site to be used for the ureteral anastomosis) according to surgeon preference. In cases where the ureteral defect is too long for direct reimplantation, the addition of a vesico-psoas hitch can achieve a tension-free anastomosis. This maneuver involves ligating the contralateral bladder pedicle followed by suture fixation of the mobilized bladder to the ipsilateral psoas tendon, shortening the gap between distal ureter and the bladder dome. In rare cases where complex bladder lacerations or pelvic vascular injuries preclude extensive pelvic dissection, a trans-ureteroureterostomy can be considered.

COMPLICATIONS

Fistula formation can rarely occur due to an initially unrecognized ureteral injury, obstruction of the ureter distal to the site of repair, or necrosis of the ureter around the level of repair. Fistulas should be managed with internal drainage via ureteral stent (or alternatively percutaneous nephrostomy if stenting cannot be achieved). Drainage of periureteral fluid collections is essential in these situations to facilitate healing. In the setting of uretero-vaginal fistulas, conservative management with internal stenting can achieve fistula resolution in 64% to 76% of cases. A persistent urine leak can arise occasionally and should be managed in a similar fashion. Stricture can occur after a trial of stenting for ureteral contusions or a primary repair, necessitating ureteral reconstruction in a delayed manner. If recognition of an injury or a complication is delayed, reconstruction should be deferred for at least 12 weeks until all inflammation has subsided.

Bladder Injuries

INITIAL EVALUATION

Traumatic bladder injuries arise most commonly in association with pelvic fractures after blunt trauma. Bladder injury occurs in 4% to 10% of cases with traumatic pelvic fractures, while 70% to 95% of blunt bladder ruptures have associated pelvic fractures. Iatrogenic bladder injury can also occur in the context of gynecologic, urologic, or general surgical procedures.

Fig. 10.8 illustrates an algorithm for the acute evaluation and management of patients with suspected bladder trauma. **CT cystography has become the modality of choice for identifying bladder rupture** (Figs. 10.9 and 10.10). Cystography requires adequate distension of the bladder (generally with greater than 300 mL) to identify or rule out a bladder injury. The sensitivity and specificity of CT cystography at one large trauma center were 95% and 100%, respectively. **Conventional fluoroscopic cystography (85%–100% accuracy) is an acceptable alternative, although its sensitivity and specificity are significantly diminished if scout and postdrainage films are not obtained.** Routine CT urography, even with occlusion of the Foley catheter, has a limited sensitivity for bladder injury. Even if the bladder appears well distended on a delayed phase CT, a bladder injury cannot be reliably excluded and a formal cystogram should be performed.

The indications for cystography after blunt trauma at our institution include gross hematuria, microscopic hematuria (3+ blood on dipstick or > 30 red blood cells per high-power field) in the setting of pelvic fracture (specified later), and free fluid in the abdomen or pelvis on CT following a plausible mechanism. After penetrating trauma, all stable patients with pelvic injury and any hematuria or a projectile trajectory raising concern for bladder injury should undergo cystography. Hematuria occurs in almost all cases of significant bladder injury. Specific fracture patterns have been associated with an increased risk of bladder injury, namely pubic symphyseal diastasis greater than 1 cm and obturator ring fractures with greater than 1 cm displacement.

Bladder injuries are classified as either extraperitoneal or intraperitoneal, with 10% of cases being combined injuries. The distinction can be made on CT or conventional cystography, and accurate classification is critical to determine the appropriate early management strategy in each case.

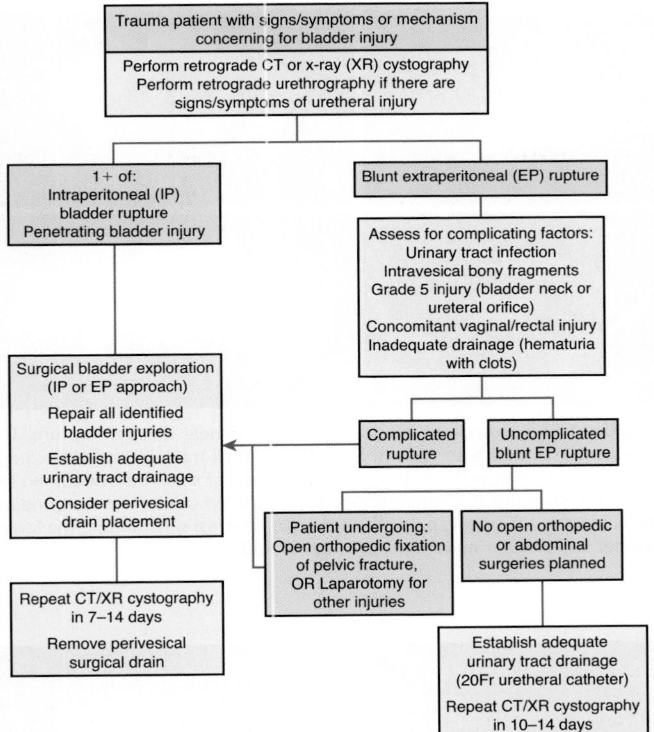
Trauma patient with signs/symptoms or mechanism concerning for bladder injury
Perform retrograde CT or x-ray (XR) cystography
Perform retrograde urethrography if there are signs/symptoms of uretheral injury
1+ of:
Intraperitoneal (IP) bladder rupture
Penetrating bladder injury
Blunt extraperitoneal (EP) rupture
Assess for complicating factors:
Urinary tract infection
Intravesical bony fragments
Grade 5 injury (bladder neck or ureteral orifice)
Concomitant vaginal/rectal injury
Inadequate drainage (hematuria with clots)
Surgical bladder exploration (IP or EP approach)
Repair all identified bladder injuries
Establish adequate urinary tract drainage
Consider perivesical drain placement
Complicated rupture
Uncomplicated blunt EP rupture
Patient undergoing:
Open orthopedic fixation of pelvic fracture,
OR Laparotomy for other injuries
No open orthopedic or abdominal surgeries planned
Repeat CT/XR cystography in 7–14 days
Remove perivesical surgical drain
Establish adequate urinary tract drainage (20Fr uretheral catheter)
Repeat CT/XR cystography in 10–14 days

FIGURE 10.8 Algorithm for evaluation and management of bladder trauma. (Modified from Wessells H. Injuries to the urogenital tract. In: Souba WW, Fink MP, Jurkovich GJ, et al., eds. *ACS Surgery: Principles and Practice*. New York: WebMD; 2005.)

MANAGEMENT

Extraperitoneal Injuries

Blunt extraperitoneal bladder injuries are usually managed nonoperatively, with large-bore (20 French or larger) catheter drainage of the bladder for 10 to 14 days and repeat cystography to confirm interval healing before catheter removal. **Contraindications to this conservative approach include penetrating trauma, urinary tract infection (UTI), the presence of bony fragments or other**

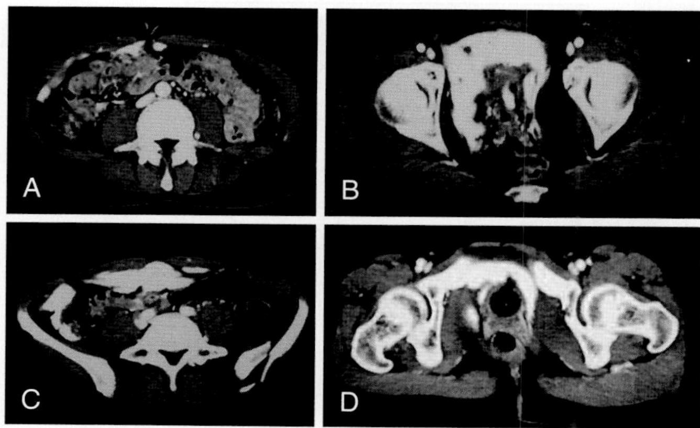

FIGURE 10.9 CT cystogram images of extraperitoneal bladder rupture. (A) Note contrast tracking to the umbilicus. (B) Contrast tracking lateral to colon, not to be confused with contrast outlining loops of small intestine in an intraperitoneal injury. (C) "Molar tooth" configuration of contrast surrounding the bladder in the upper space of Retzius. (D) Contrast surrounding the lower bladder and bladder neck region. *CT*, Computed tomography.

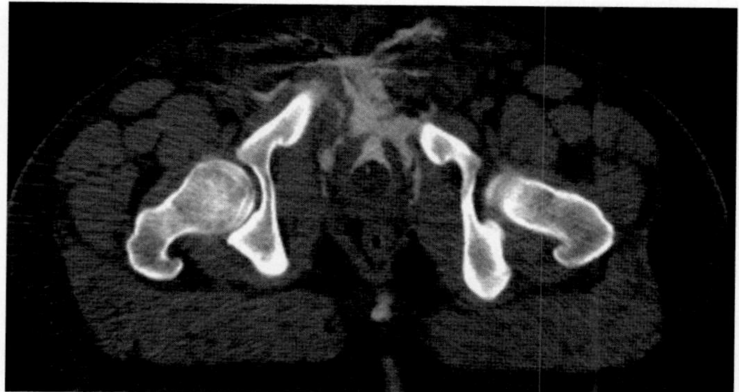

FIGURE 10.10 Traumatic injury to the bladder extending though the bladder neck as seen on CT cystogram. Note contrast extravasation into the extraperitoneal space anterior to the inflated Foley balloon. *CT*, Computed tomography.

foreign body in the bladder, injuries involving the bladder neck or ureteral orifice, and concomitant injuries to the rectum or vagina. Cystorrhaphy can also be considered in stable patients undergoing orthopedic internal fixation of the pubis or laparotomy for other indications. In patients undergoing exploration, the bladder can be approached extraperitoneally by developing the retropubic space if there is not a large pelvic hematoma; this approach allows excellent exposure of the anteriorly located and small lacerations usually associated with pelvic fractures. **Any significant bladder injury following penetrating trauma should be explored.**

Intraperitoneal Injuries

Traumatic intraperitoneal bladder ruptures often result in a large laceration with communication to the peritoneal space, and thus, these injuries generally require surgical exploration with primary repair. **A complete intravesical examination excludes a concomitant extraperitoneal injury, which may occur in up to 25% of patients with an intraperitoneal bladder injury.** The ureteral orifices and bladder neck should be inspected. Additional lacerations found within the bladder are closed with 3-0 absorbable sutures, approximating the detrusor and mucosa in one layer to provide hemostasis during early healing. The primary laceration, usually at the dome, is closed with two layers of continuous 2-0 or 3-0 absorbable sutures; a large-bore (20-French) urethral catheter should be placed to facilitate appropriate bladder drainage. Suprapubic catheters are not indicated unless an unrepaired urethral injury is present or severe hematuria resulting from coagulopathy or extensive injuries necessitates additional access for clot irrigation and sustained bladder decompression. A closed suction drain can be placed near the bladder closure and removed after 2 to 3 days unless an analysis of the drain fluid for creatinine is elevated above the serum creatinine level (suggesting a urine leak) prior to removal.

COMPLICATIONS

After most open repairs and all trials of nonoperative management, cystography should be performed prior to catheter removal. **If extravasation persists, the catheter should be left in place and cystography repeated at appropriate intervals until healing occurs.** Complications of bladder injury are usually related to a delay in diagnosis leading to urinary ascites, complex infections including pelvic abscesses or osteomyelitis, sepsis, and the development of urinary fistulas. Injuries involving the bladder neck can often extend into the proximal urethra, and unidentified or unrepaired bladder neck injuries may result in sphincteric deficiency with long-term urinary incontinence. Persistent leakage after repair is uncommon in the absence of a bladder neck injury, and leaks will usually heal with continued catheter drainage. Persistent extravasation beyond 4 weeks postinjury or postrepair is an indication for cystoscopy to investigate for catheter obstruction or retained intravesical foreign body. Persistent leaks can also be a manifestation of ischemia following the primary injury or early pelvic angioembolization.

Urethral Injuries

Urethral injuries disproportionately affect male patients, occurring in 1.5% to 10% of males and 0.15% to 5% of females with pelvic fractures. In men, traumatic urethral injury usually involves the posterior urethra, primarily at either the bulbomembranous or the prostatomembranous junction. Approximately 10% to 20% of patients will have concomitant bladder injuries. Patients tend to be younger than 40 years of age with mechanisms related to road traffic accidents, higher ISS, and multiple associated injuries (including head, chest, and abdominal trauma). Fig. 10.11 illustrates an algorithm for the evaluation and management of urethral trauma.

MECHANISMS

Pelvic fractures are the most common injury pattern associated with posterior urethral injuries in males. The classic injury is a distraction at the bulbomembranous or prostatomembranous junction. Variations occur, including complete and partial disruption, and the injury can occur above, below, or through the urogenital diaphragm (Fig. 10.12). Displaced fractures of the pubic rami and diastasis of the pubic symphysis are associated with urethral injury in men.

The female urethra is rarely injured, but a review from our institution showed that urethral and bladder neck injuries were always associated with pelvic fracture. Longitudinal tears may

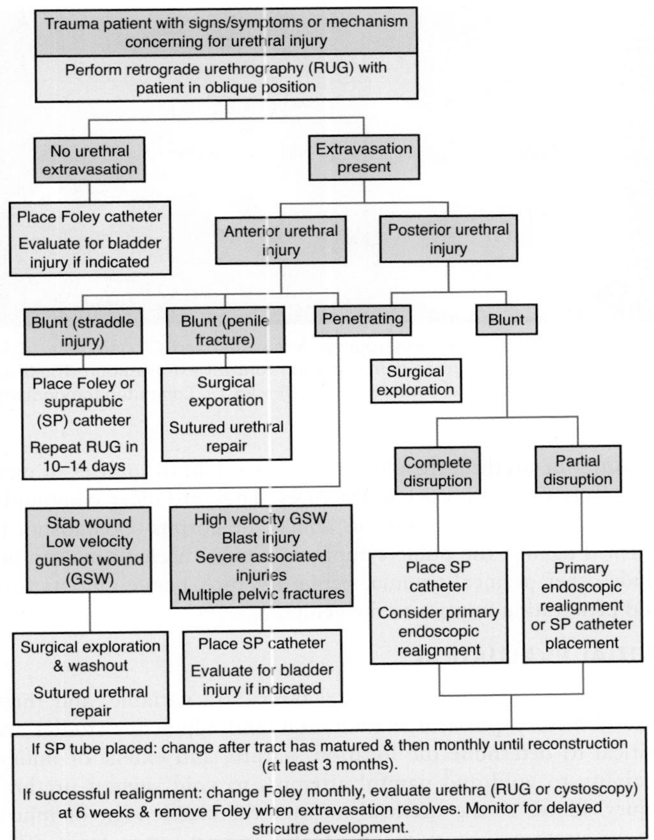

FIGURE 10.11 Algorithm for evaluation and management of urethral trauma. (Modified from Wessells H. Injuries to the urogenital tract. In: Souba WW, Fink MP, Jurkovich GJ, et al., eds. *ACS Surgery: Principles and Practice*. New York: WebMD; 2005.)

originate in the bladder neck, whereas avulsion-type injuries probably share similar mechanisms with distraction injuries around the membranous urethra in males. Vulvar edema or blood at the vaginal introitus should raise suspicion of a urethral injury.

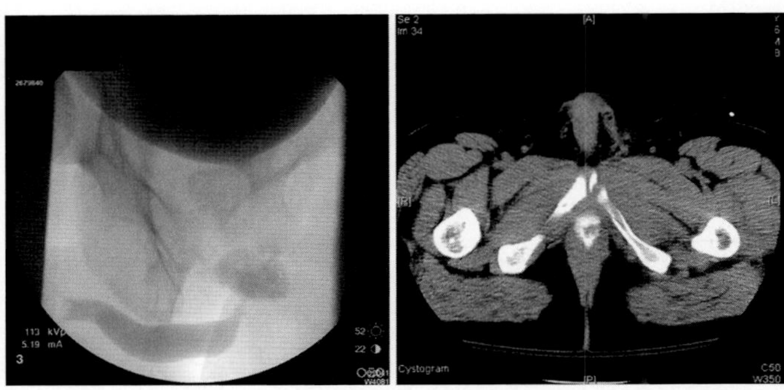

FIGURE 10.12 Retrograde urethrogram (left panel) and CT cystogram (right panel) of urethral disruption demonstrating contrast extravasation. The bladder is full in the left panel because of prior CT scan. *CT*, Computed tomography.

Anterior urethral (penile and bulbar urethral) injuries in men are rarely caused by pelvic fractures. They are most commonly caused by straddle injuries, in which the corpus spongiosum is crushed against the pubic symphysis. Other mechanisms can include other perineal trauma, penile fracture, penile amputation, and penetrating injuries to the genitalia.

INITIAL EVALUATION

Signs and symptoms of urethral injury are variable, and thus, careful history, physical examination, and adjunctive studies are critical to determine the location, nature, and extent of injury. Inability to void and painful attempts to void suggest urethral injury. Blood at the urethral meatus, the classic sign of injury to the urethra, occurs inconsistently (reports vary from 37% to 93%) but is a clear indication for prompt urethral imaging. Other signs include a palpable distended bladder, butterfly perineal hematoma, and a high-riding prostate, although these are significantly less reliable. Gentle attempts to pass a catheter have not been shown to convert partial urethral tears into complete transections, but if a catheter cannot easily be placed, it would be appropriate to avoid repeated attempts until further diagnostic studies are obtained. **Imaging of the urethra with retrograde urethrography is the recommended initial evaluation for suspected urethral injuries in males.**

Urethral and bladder neck injuries can be easily missed in the initial evaluation of female patients, and these injuries are often only detected at the time of operative exploration. Diagnostic urethral imaging is challenging in female patients, so pelvic examination (with cystoscopy if there is concern for a urethral injury) should be considered to facilitate accurate evaluation. The presence of vaginal bleeding or labial swelling should prompt a speculum examination, under anesthesia if necessary, and consideration for imaging or cystoscopy. Bladder neck injuries may be initially evaluated in females with voiding cystourethrography, although this study can miss some injuries and has limited sensitivity for urethral injuries. **For this reason, cystourethroscopy should be pursued in any case of suspected injury not clearly defined on high-quality imaging and bedside pelvic examination.**

MANAGEMENT

Posterior Urethra

Safe and immediate bladder drainage is a priority after pelvic fracture urethral injury (PFUI). This can be achieved with a urethral catheter in some cases, but the standard of care remains suprapubic cystostomy for catheter placement. Percutaneous placement of the tube under fluoroscopic or ultrasound guidance, or open placement through a small infraumbilical incision, allows temporary urinary diversion for initial stabilization and evaluation of the patient. Cystography can be performed via the suprapubic tube to rule out concomitant bladder injury. Suprapubic cystostomy is recommended for penetrating trauma to the urethra if there is extensive tissue loss, there are serious associated injuries, or the urethral injury was caused by a high-velocity weapon.

Primary endoscopic urethral realignment without sutured repair may be considered as an alternative strategy after PFUI. Early endoscopic realignment can be undertaken 2 to 7 days after the initial injury and may decrease stricture rates, allow future endoscopic management, and possibly simplify formal urethroplasty if required. Prolonged attempts at endoscopic realignment should not be attempted because this may increase the risk of pelvic hematoma or infection. Primary endoscopic realignment can be considered in the setting of open reduction and internal fixation of anterior pelvic ring fractures. Realignment allows early removal of suprapubic cystostomy tubes from the orthopedic surgical field, although there is an absence of high-quality evidence to suggest that suprapubic tubes independently increase the risk of infectious complications after internal fixation of the pubis.

Early repair (in females) or realignment (in males) of a urethral injury is necessary in the presence of concomitant bladder neck, vaginal, or rectal injuries. Surgical management should include evacuation of the pelvic hematoma, extensive irrigation, placement of pelvic drains, and primary realignment (men) or sutured repair (women) of the urethra.

Anterior Urethra

Penetrating injuries to the anterior (penile and bulbar) urethra in men are usually best treated with immediate repair. For partial or complete transections without major tissue loss, primary repair is associated with a lower stricture rate than simple realignment over a catheter. **Exceptions to this rule include high-velocity gunshot wounds or injuries associated with extensive tissue destruction**, which should always be treated with urinary diversion and delayed repair. Wounds with major tissue loss and defects longer than 2 cm (e.g., AAST grade V injuries) or complicating associated injuries are best treated with suprapubic diversion and delayed reconstruction at a tertiary referral center. **Prompt urinary drainage is both a priority and the standard of care for acute management of blunt trauma to the anterior urethra (including straddle-type crush injuries).** Drainage can be achieved with suprapubic cystostomy or urethral catheter drainage. **In the case of blunt urethral injury associated with penile fracture, patients should undergo urgent surgical exploration with urethral repair.**

Follow-Up Care

After early realignment of urethral injuries, the urethral catheter is left in place for 6 weeks and a pericatheter retrograde urethrogram (RUG) is obtained to confirm extravasation has resolved before catheter removal. The urethral catheter should remain in place for 1 to 3 weeks after immediate surgical repair of the anterior urethra, and a voiding cystourethrogram (VCUG) should be obtained at the time of catheter removal. If extravasation is present, catheter drainage should be continued for 2 to 3 weeks followed by a repeat fluoroscopic study.

If the patient initially underwent diversion with suprapubic cystostomy, the suprapubic tube should be changed initially after 4 to 6 weeks, then monthly until urethral reconstruction can be performed (usually 3–6 months after the injury). A urethral stricture or stenotic obliteration is expected after most PFUI managed with early suprapubic drainage, and will develop in many patients after straddle injuries. Repeat postinjury radiographic studies will indicate whether secondary endoscopic or open procedures are needed. After PFUI, patients often require months for resorption of pelvic hematoma before urethroplasty can be planned; in addition, they should have external pelvic fixation devices removed and be able to tolerate high lithotomy positioning.

After PFUI, erectile dysfunction (ED) will occur in 20% to 60% of patients and is primarily determined by the severity of the initial injury rather than the method of urinary tract management. ED following trauma is usually neurogenic or vasculogenic in nature and may improve spontaneously up to 2 years posttrauma. After posterior urethral reconstruction, urinary continence is achieved in 95% of all patients. Even patients who do not require delayed reconstruction should be monitored for ED, stricture formation, and urinary incontinence for at least 12 months postinjury.

Injuries to the Male External Genitalia

Genital injuries are significant because of their association with injuries to major pelvic and vascular organs and the potential for chronic disability. In civilians suffering genitourinary gunshot wounds, the scrotum will be affected in 21%, the testes in 12%, and the penis in 8%, with over 90% of these patients sustaining additional nongenital injuries. Combat injuries to the lower genitourinary tract can also affect the scrotum (39%), testis (36%), or penis (20%), with often disfiguring blast injuries accompanied by severe lower extremity or pelvic trauma. **Penetrating injuries to the external genitalia have a high likelihood of damage involving the urinary bladder, urethra, rectum, and vascular structures of the iliac and femoral regions.** General wound care principles include irrigation, debridement, and layered wound closure when feasible. The genital skin has an excellent vascular supply, allowing primary closure of most superficial lacerations. External genital injuries can yield significant transient and potentially permanent changes in urinary, sexual, and reproductive function. In addition to acute injury evaluation and management, clinicians should consider engaging appropriate ancillary resources (mental health, reproductive services, etc.) in all cases of genital trauma for both men and women. In the following sections we discuss the presentation, evaluation, and management of several common injuries to the external genitalia.

MECHANISMS OF PENILE INJURY

The flaccidity of the penis limits the transfer of kinetic energy during trauma. In contrast, the crura of the erectile bodies are relatively fixed to the pubic rami and are prone to blunt trauma from pelvic fracture or straddle injuries. Firearms and missiles have enough kinetic energy to overcome the protective mechanism of penile flaccidity.

PENILE FRACTURE

In the erect state, the penis becomes more prone to blunt injury: missed intromission or manual attempts at detumescence can cause rupture of the tunica albuginea of either corpus cavernosum, known as a penile fracture. Acute bending and a popping sound followed by pain and immediate detumescence of the penis are classic signs of a penile fracture. Swelling is usually limited to the shaft of the penis due to containment of hematoma within Buck's fascia, leading to the commonly described "eggplant deformity." When Buck's fascia has been traumatically ruptured, hematoma can extend onto the perineum in a butterfly pattern or track cranially onto the abdominal wall, as it remains contained by Colles' and Scarpa's fascia. **Urethral injury occurs in 10% to 38% of penile fractures, and evaluation of the integrity of the urethra should be strongly considered in all patients presenting with a penile fracture.**

History and physical examination are usually sufficient to distinguish between subcutaneous hematoma, such as with dorsal vein injury, and penile fracture. In indeterminate cases with a presentation atypical for penile fracture, penile ultrasound or surgical exploration can be considered. Magnetic resonance imaging (MRI) has good sensitivity for tunical disruption, but due to cost and availability, it is generally not recommended except in the case of an indeterminate ultrasound with low or moderate clinical suspicion. **Conservative management of penile fractures is not recommended and has been associated with an increased risk of missed urethral injuries, penile curvature, chronic pain, and ED.**

Operative Management

The deep structures of the penis can be exposed via several skin incisions based upon the anticipated location of injuries and surgeon preference. Wide exposure of the penis can be achieved either with a circumcising subcoronal incision and degloving of the penis or with a ventral longitudinal incision along the penile shaft. For especially proximal injuries, a penoscrotal, infrapubic, or even perineal incision may be necessary. Of note, a circumcising incision can present a unique challenge in uncircumcised patients, as it requires excision of the foreskin to avoid skin necrosis. Tunical injuries are usually 1 to 2 cm in length, ventrolateral, and distal to the suspensory ligament. **Flexible cystoscopy can be performed before catheter placement to evaluate for associated urethral injury.** If urethral injury is discovered, it can be repaired concomitantly with a low incidence of postoperative stricture formation.

If the corporeal tear is difficult to identify at exploration, an artificial erection may be induced to aid with localization of the injury. After clearing clot and hematoma, we close the tunica albuginea with slowly absorbable, interrupted sutures in a transverse fashion to prevent narrowing of the corpora. Urethral injuries are repaired over a catheter with fine slowly absorbable suture in an interrupted fashion. Repaired urethral injuries are managed with Foley drainage for 10 to 14 days, with a VCUG at catheter removal to confirm appropriate healing of the anastomosis.

PENETRATING TRAUMA TO THE PENIS

Up to 83% of patients with penetrating trauma to the penis will have associated injuries. Urethral injury occurs in 11% to 29% of cases. **Retrograde urethrography or cystoscopy should be strongly considered with all penetrating penile injuries**, especially when the clinical picture suggests urethral involvement.

Operative Management

Operative management includes prompt surgical exploration, copious irrigation, removal of any retained foreign material, antibiotic coverage, and closure. Extensive irrigation is appropriate to remove any foreign material, including clothing, missile fragments, or pieces of bone, that may enter the deep structures of the penis and urinary tract. Retained foreign body must be actively sought and removed in order to ensure appropriate healing. Primary closure can be achieved in virtually all cases. We close the tunica albuginea in the same manner as previously described for a penile fracture. Urethral injuries can be managed with standard protocols described earlier. Although rare in civilian trauma centers, injuries in the tunica albuginea may be so large as to preclude primary closure. In such instances, off-the-shelf substitutes including fascia, pericardium, or other collagen matrix-based products may be used as a patch graft to cover the tunical defect.

Defects involving the glans can be salvaged with good cosmetic and functional outcomes. Debridement and trimming of skin edges to create a clean wound allows for closure of even fairly large defects. Although the size of the glans may be reduced, its overall contour can usually be maintained.

PENILE AMPUTATION

A rare cause of penile injury is amputation. Penile amputation may be a manifestation of severe depressive behavior or psychosis, due to either mental illness or substance abuse. In these cases, consultation with psychiatric specialists is an important component of acute and subacute care. Constriction rings can also cause loss of superficial skin, necrosis of the urethra, or uncommonly complete penile loss. When assault is the cause of amputation, appropriate reporting to law enforcement agencies is required.

After penile amputation or self-mutilation, urinary diversion should be established with a suprapubic cystostomy. Immediate management requires attention to two basic goals: resuscitation of the patient and preparation for surgical replantation. The stump is covered with sterile saline-soaked gauze dressings. Transfusion may be required if significant blood loss has occurred. The amputated penis is treated with a double-bag system: the organ is wrapped in sterile saline-soaked gauze and placed in a bag, which is then placed into a second bag containing ice. Appropriate transfer to a tertiary center can be accomplished with **successful reimplantation after up to 16 hours of cold ischemia or 6 hours of warm ischemia.**

Operative Management

Penile amputation requires precise management of urethral, cavernosal, neurovascular, and skin transection in all but the most distal injuries. Simple reapproximation of the urethra and erectile bodies will usually result in survival and function of the organ, although skin loss is unavoidable and glans sensation and accompanying ejaculatory function will be lost. Urethral stricture is also common with this macroscopic approach. Thus, **whenever possible, we advocate complete reimplantation with microvascular and nerve reattachment.** With a clean cut, virtually no preparation is required. However, if the penis has been avulsed, cut with a blunt instrument, or purposefully mutilated by the patient or the assailant, reattachment may be more challenging.

Reapproximation proceeds ventrally to dorsally with anastomosis of the corpus spongiosum and urethral epithelium over a catheter, followed by the tunica albuginea of the bilateral corpora cavernosa. Reanastomosis of the deep arteries of the cavernosum is neither required nor easy, and we routinely favor reanastomosis only of the dorsal arteries. Once the tunica albuginea of the corpus cavernosum has been reapproximated, the ends of the dorsal neurovascular structures are brought into proximity. Microsurgical repair using an operating microscope and fine permanent suture allows reanastomosis of one or both dorsal arteries, the dorsal nerves, and the deep dorsal vein (Fig. 10.13). Failure to reanastomose the deep dorsal vein may lead to glans hyperemia and venous congestion of the shaft skin, which can compromise the reattachment. Postoperative venous congestion is a major problem even with microvascular reattachment. The use of medical leeches is very helpful to reduce swelling and hematoma related to venous congestion and bleeding.

Normal sensation returns in over 80% of microscopic reimplantations but only 10% of macroscopic reconstructions. Erectile function returns to normal in at least 50% of patients repaired by either technique. If the amputated distal penis is not available for reanastomosis, the corpora cavernosa should be closed and a urethral neomeatus spatulated.

TESTICULAR INJURIES

Small hematoceles (less than three times the size of the contralateral testicle) can generally be managed conservatively. Larger

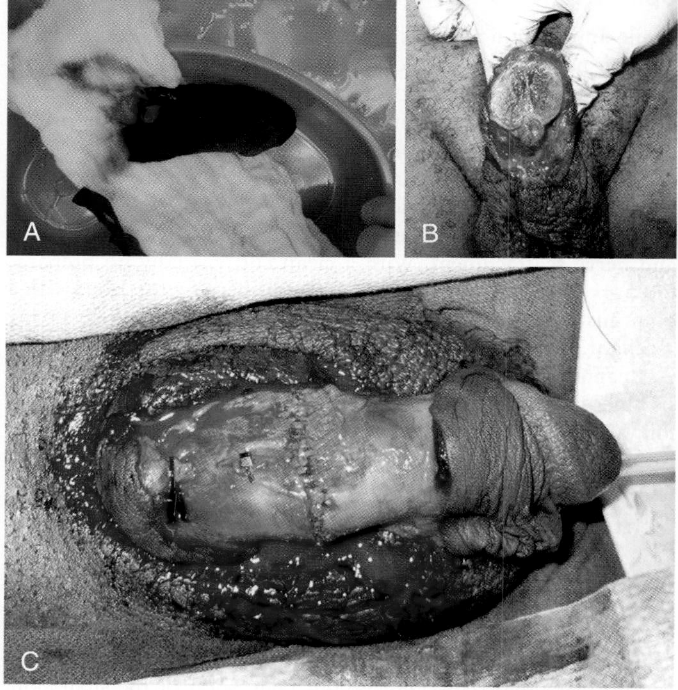

FIGURE 10.13 Penile amputation before and after repair. (A) Detached distal phallus. (B) Proximal penile stump. Note the transected corpora and urethra. (C) Phallus after microscopic reanastomosis.

hematoceles should undergo operative evaluation because they may reflect an underlying testis injury and conservative management often leads to higher rates of complications, a prolonged recovery course, and a higher likelihood of delayed orchiectomy. The testes may also be dislocated outside of the scrotum, which should be considered in any nonpalpable testis in a trauma patient.

Testicular rupture generally presents with pain, nausea, and vomiting associated with an ecchymotic, tender, swollen hemiscrotum. Rupture occurs in up to 50% of blunt scrotal traumas and over 50% of penetrating scrotal injuries. Ultrasound findings suggestive of testis rupture can include an abnormal testis contour, focal heterogeneity of testis parenchyma, and irregularity or disruption of the tunica albuginea. The sensitivity and specificity of ultrasound varies in reported series, and it may be best used to rule out rupture in blunt scrotal trauma with low clinical suspicion. **Prompt scrotal exploration is indicated in cases with a high index of suspicion and should be strongly considered when there is diagnostic uncertainty after a careful exam and diagnostic ultrasound.** Traumatic testicular torsion can also occur and should be considered when patients present with pain out of proportion to exam findings; ultrasonography with color Doppler can help with evaluation of testis perfusion in such cases.

Large traumatic hematoceles should be drained surgically. **Testicular rupture should be managed with immediate exploration, debridement of devitalized seminiferous tubules, and, when possible, primary reapproximation of the tunica albuginea.** Use of a tunica vaginalis flap or graft can allow coverage of larger defects, or can be used in an effort to prevent a testicular compartment syndrome due to evolving postinjury edema. Early repair results in a higher rate of testicular salvage and a greater likelihood of preserved endocrine function and fertility potential.

GENITAL SKIN INJURIES

Scrotal Injuries

Lacerations and avulsions of the scrotum not involving the testis may occur due to blunt trauma, machinery accidents, stab wounds, and occasional firearm injury. Complete avulsion of the scrotal skin is rare and is usually the result of power takeoff, auger, or devastating motor vehicle crashes involving widespread skin loss or degloving.

Scrotal skin lacerations can be closed primarily in the absence of gross infection or heavy contamination. Deficits of up to 50% of the scrotal skin can often be closed primarily with good cosmetic results. Layered closure of the dartos fascia and skin, with a drain brought out dependently, limits postoperative hematoma. Xeroform gauze or other antibacterial dressings and ointments should be placed on the incisions, and the scrotum should be surrounded with loose gauze.

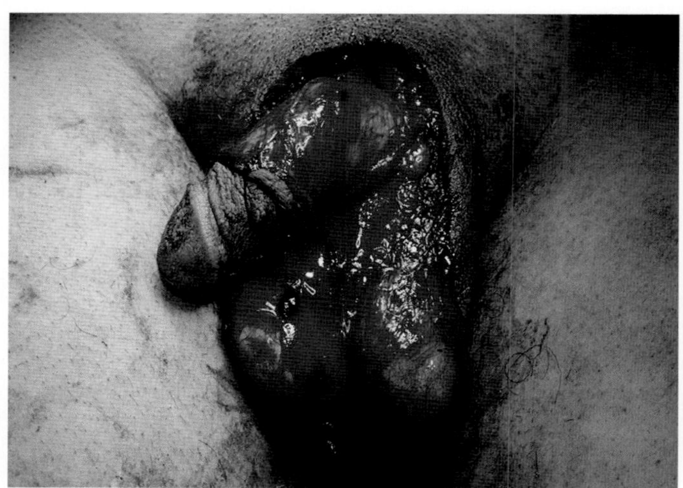

FIGURE 10.14 Scrotal and penile skin avulsion from machinery injury.

Complete scrotal avulsion is a devastating injury (Fig. 10.14). The avulsed skin is not usually suitable for autografting. Immediate grafting should be avoided, and an interval of local wound care should be initiated. This allows the wound bed to granulate, after which very successful results can be obtained with split-thickness skin graft application. Testicular transplantation into subcutaneous thigh pouches can be a temporizing or permanent measure dependent upon patient age, sexual function, patient goals, and overall prioritization of injuries in the setting of polytrauma (Figs. 10.15 and 10.16).

Genital Bite Wounds

Bite injuries by animals or humans require appropriate antibiotic coverage for relevant oral bacterial species and tetanus toxoid administration when needed. Dog and cat bites most commonly lead to pathogenic infection with *Pasteurella*, although anaerobic organisms may also be present. The potential for transmission of rabies must also be considered and appropriate measures taken if the patient is at risk. Human bites are more likely to cause

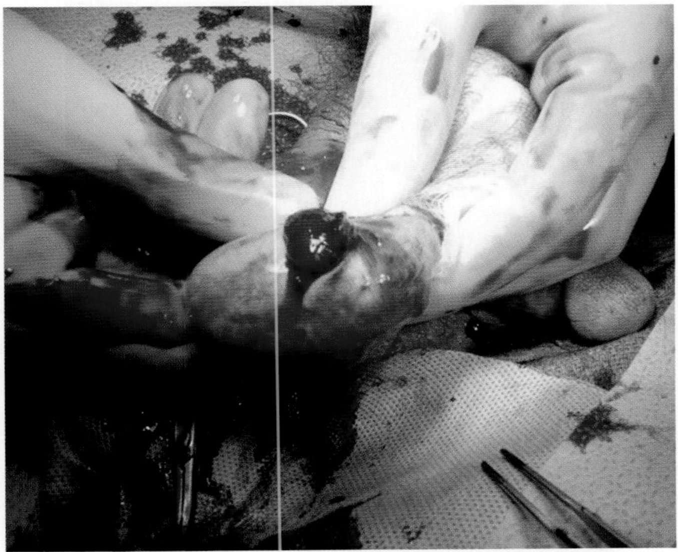

FIGURE 10.15 Intraoperative view of ruptured testis. Note the seminiferous tubules protruding through the tunica albuginea.

complications than dog bites. Transmission of viral infections, including hepatitis and human immunodeficiency virus (HIV), are rare but possible.

Simple uncontaminated bite injuries can be irrigated and closed primarily if appropriate antibiotics are administered, contamination is minimal, and the wound is closed within 6 to 12 hours. Grossly contaminated bite injuries (including most human bites) should be left open and allowed to granulate.

Genital Burns

Genital and perineal burns are present in less than 5% of burn victims. Burns affect the superficial tissues first, and damage progressively spreads into deeper tissues in a manner opposite that of Fournier's gangrene. This allows preservation of some portion of the vascular integrity of the skin in most chemical and thermal

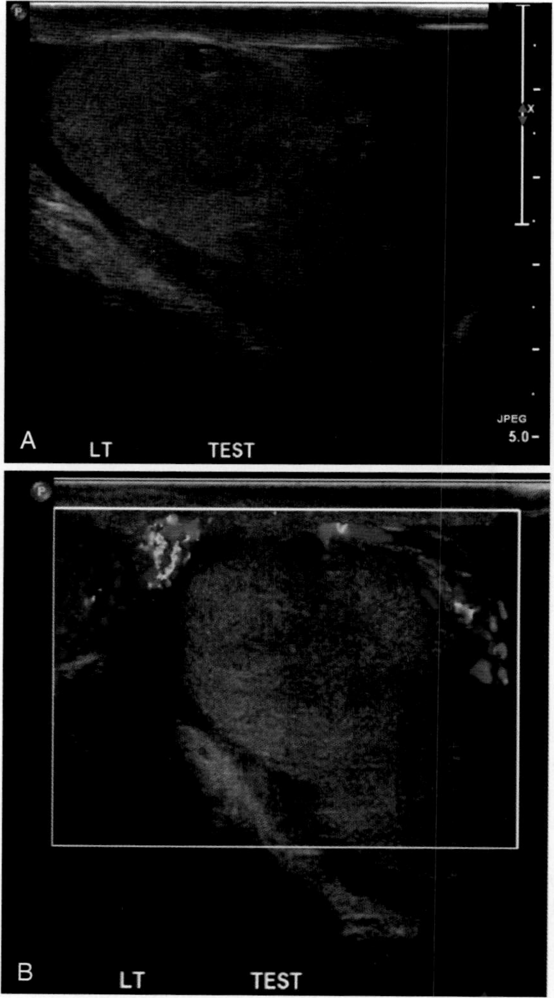

FIGURE 10.16 Ultrasound appearance of a left testicular rupture. (A) Sagittal view showing hemorrhage along the lateral aspect of the left testicle with disruption of the tunica albuginea and parenchymal heterogeneity inferiorly with a small associated hematocele. (B) Transverse color flow view showing absent flow to the left testicle concerning for vascular compromise. (Courtesy Dr. Parvati Ramchandani, University of Pennsylvania Health System.)

injuries. The penile skin is thin, and thus, most burns to the penis are full thickness.

Burns should be covered with appropriate dressings depending on the mechanism; 1% silver sulfadiazine cream is appropriate for thermal injuries. Chemical burns can be irrigated with saline, alkaline burns with dilute acetic acid, and acid burns with sodium bicarbonate.

Early management of burns, electrical injuries, and other injuries to the genital skin should be conservative. The rich vascular supply to genital skin may allow a greater degree of skin preservation than would be expected in other areas of the body. When necessary, early resection of eschar should be undertaken. Complete loss of genital skin usually implies a devastating burn from which patients may be unlikely to survive. In contrast, patients suffering less than complete surface area burns of the genitalia have a remarkable capacity for recovery, and split-thickness skin grafting is the exception rather than the rule.

Injuries to the Female Genitalia

MECHANISMS

Female genital injuries often require careful attention and specialized treatment. These injuries can occur in the setting of severe pelvic fractures or can be related to sexual assault and intimate partner violence. **Although many vulvar lacerations are the result of sports-related straddle-type injuries, genital trauma is reported in 20% to 53% of sexual assault victims. If such history is elicited, appropriate support services and police involvement must be secured.** Informed consent for the patient assessment should be obtained if a history of sexual assault has been identified. This assessment must include history, physical examination, and collection of laboratory and forensic specimens as outlined by the American College of Obstetrics and Gynecologists.

Female patients with external genital injuries should be suspected of having injury to the internal gynecologic organs and the lower urinary tract. Many female urethral injuries are associated with vaginal bleeding. **Female genital injury in the setting of pelvic fracture or impalement injuries should include cystourethrography, proctoscopy, and laparotomy as indicated.** Unrecognized associated urinary tract and gastrointestinal (GI) injuries in the face of vaginal trauma may lead to abscess formation, sepsis, and death. When there is suspicion for a urinary tract injury, lower urinary tract evaluation should be pursued as described in the Bladder Trauma and Urethral Trauma sections.

MANAGEMENT

Perineal and vulvar lacerations can usually be managed in the Emergency Department. Large hematomas should be incised and drained, with ligation of any bleeding vessels. As with the male genital skin, closure with interrupted absorbable sutures is standard. Surgical drains can be used if there is a large cavity or suspected contamination, or if hemostasis is suboptimal.

Internal lacerations of the vagina and cervix can be closed in the Emergency Department if there is no severe bleeding. Large lacerations associated with bleeding and hematomas require a speculum examination under anesthesia to completely assess and repair the injuries. Vaginal lacerations are closed with running absorbable sutures, and vaginal packing is critical for hemostasis.

Complex vaginal and perineal lacerations associated with pelvic fracture, rectal injury, or other adverse features require a more systematic approach. Evaluation under anesthesia is mandatory, including speculum examination, cystoscopy or cystography, and rigid proctoscopy. Diversion of the fecal stream is rarely needed unless perineal injuries extensively involve the rectum, anus, or external sphincter. Bladder ruptures should be repaired if associated vaginal lacerations are present, to prevent deep pelvic infection, abscess, or fistula formation.

Conclusions

Urogenital trauma demands care and attention to prompt diagnosis, selection of an appropriate management modality, integration of the multidisciplinary trauma team, and careful follow-up to monitor for long-term complications and disability.

CLINICAL PEARLS

1. While most renal injuries can be managed nonoperatively, major hemorrhage still poses a risk of clinical instability and death. Clinical judgment and risk stratification of patients are paramount in the acute management of renal trauma.
2. Ureteral injuries often present without specific clinical signs and symptoms. They are frequently associated with significant nonurologic injuries. A high degree of suspicion is required to prevent delayed diagnosis and long-term morbidity.
3. Urethral injury associated with pelvic fracture requires careful evaluation to detect associated bladder neck, rectal, and vaginal injuries that can lead to major complications and lifelong disability if missed.
4. Penile fracture is a diagnosis based on history and physical examination that requires surgical management, and clinicians should maintain a high index of suspicion for associated urethral injuries.

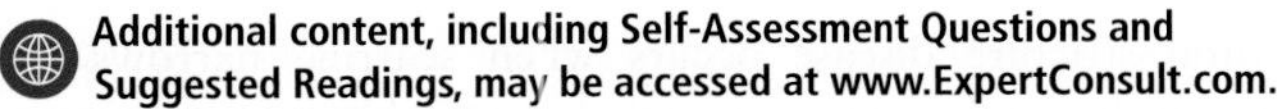

Additional content, including Self-Assessment Questions and Suggested Readings, may be accessed at www.ExpertConsult.com.

Urethral Stricture and Lower Urinary Tract Reconstruction

Esther Nivasch Turner, MD, MBE, and
Robert C. Kovell, MD

Introduction

Urethral stricture disease occurs when scarring narrows the lumen of the urethra with associated spongiofibrosis, often causing bothersome urinary symptoms for those who suffer from it. Stricture disease affects approximately 0.6% of men in the United States. The peak incidence occurs around age 55, but it can affect all ages, races, and socioeconomic groups.

Etiologies

Common causes of urethral stricture disease include pelvic or perineal trauma, urethritis (sexually transmitted infection [STI], urinary tract infection [UTI]), radiation therapy, instrumentation including catheterization, hypospadias, and systemic disease such as lichen sclerosis (LS)/balanitis xerotica obliterans (BXO). For many individuals with stricture, the etiology is idiopathic.

Trauma to the urethra of any type can result in stricture disease. Foley catheters and urologic instrumentation are all-too-common iatrogenic causes of stricture development. While these strictures can be seen anywhere within the urethra, the fossa navicularis, proximal bulbar/membranous urethra, and the distal bulb at the penoscrotal junction tend to be the most common sites. These are the areas of either relative caliber narrowing or angulation of the urethra that can be more affected by tubes and scopes.

Blunt or penetrating external trauma to the urethra can also result in stricture development with straddle injuries and pelvic fracture–related urethra injuries being classic examples. In a straddle injury, the urethra is crushed between the pubic symphysis and the external surface hitting the perineum, resulting in a dense injury at the midbulbar urethra. In a pelvic fracture urethral distraction defect (PFUDD), the fixed membranous urethra is sheared from the bulb or prostate resulting in injury and scar formation. With external trauma, the luminal narrowing is often accompanied by dense scar tissue from the injury.

LS (previously referred to as BXO) is another common etiology of strictures in men. LS is commonly characterized by epithelial thinning, inflammation, plaque formation, and pain/pruritus. The cause remains unknown with some investigations noting an associated genetic predisposition, association with autoimmune diseases, or infectious etiology. The classic dermatological appearance is that of white, atrophic papules that tend to coalesce into plaques starting on the glans and prepuce in men. Strictures tend to start distally, beginning at the meatus. Subsequent development of high-pressure voiding leading to intravasation into the glands of Littre and progressive inflammation/stricture progression proximally from the meatus (Fig. 11.1).

Hypospadias is a relatively prevalent condition encountered by the pediatric urologist that is often associated with stricture formation later in life. It is covered more fully in Chapter 26 of this text. In patients with hypospadias, deficient embryological development of the spongiosum leads to a limited urethral blood supply in these individuals. Multiple surgeries can further reduce

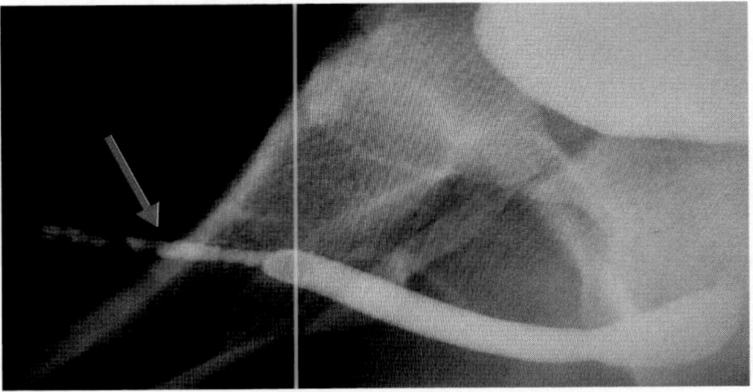

FIGURE 11.1 Retrograde urethrogram with lichen sclerosis–induced stricture. Note intravasation into glands of Littre *(red arrow)*.

health tissue available for later repair if strictures develop, making reconstruction more challenging.

STIs leading to urethritis also can lead to urethral stricture formation. Gonorrhea is the classic example of this with patients developing dense, inflammatory lesions that can form scar and lead to stricture over time if left untreated. These patients can present with strictures, which are often multifocal, anywhere in the urethra. UTIs (cystitis) generally do not lead to urethral stricture formation.

DIFFERENTIAL DIAGNOSIS

Because the presenting symptoms of urethral strictures are typically due to urinary obstruction, a wide differential diagnosis should be maintained. There are many etiologies of urinary obstruction, and the diagnostician must maintain a high degree of suspicion based on the clinical situation. Some of the most common causes of urinary obstruction are as follows:

Causes of obstructive voiding symptoms:

- Benign prostatic hyperplasia (BPH)
- Urethral stricture or stenosis
- Pelvic floor dysfunction
- Detrusor sphincter dyssynergia (DSD)
- Primary bladder neck obstruction (PBNO)
- Detrusor underactivity or acontractility
- Urethral, prostatic, or bladder neck malignancies
- Stones, blood clots, or foreign bodies

Urethral Anatomy

The urethra is typically divided anatomically into the anterior and posterior urethra. The dividing line for these sections generally occurs at the membranous urethra where urethra is fixed, passing through the urogenital diaphragm. Anatomically, these sections are separated by the presence of a layer of surrounding, vascular corpus spongiosum, which covers the anterior urethra but not the posterior urethra (Fig. 11.2).

Anterior

- urethral meatus
- fossa navicularis
- penile urethra
- bulbar (boundaries: urogenital diaphragm to the penoscrotal junction) urethra

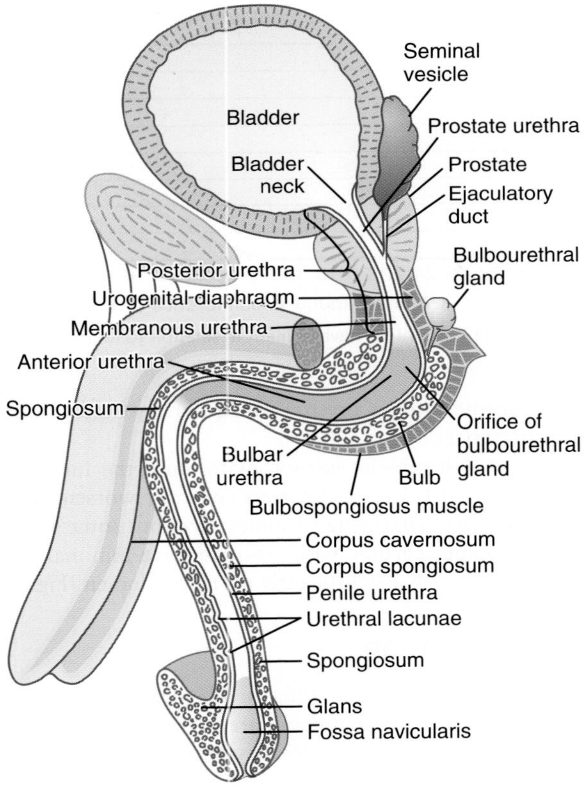

FIGURE 11.2 Anatomy of anterior and posterior urethra.

Posterior
- membranous urethra
- prostatic urethra
- bladder neck

The adult male urethra is typically 20–25 cm long. The lumenal diameter of the urethra varies substantially throughout the different sections of the urethra and from one individual to the next. The normal penile urethra tends to measure 22–26Fr

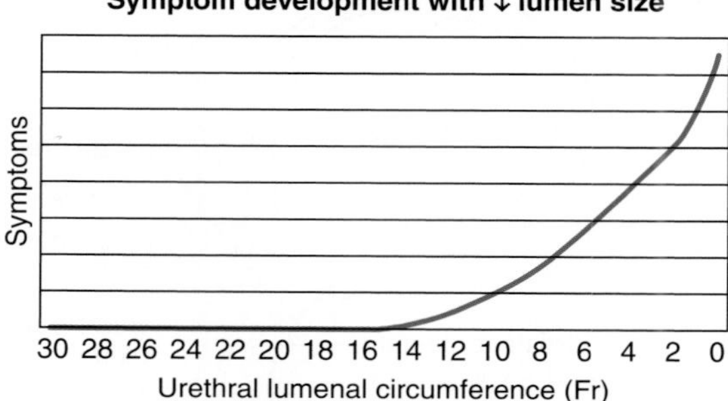

FIGURE 11.3 Symptom development in relation to lumen size.

while the normal bulbar urethra can generally be calibrated to 28–30Fr or above.

Most men will remain asymptomatic until the lumen is decreased to about 14–16Fr. Symptoms generally worsen exponentially with further narrowing of lumen size, but some men with slowly developing, chronic strictures can have minimal voiding complaints even with a significantly narrowed lumen (Fig. 11.3).

Clinical Evaluation

As strictures involve a narrowing of the urethral lumen, most patients with a clinically significant urethral stricture will present with obstructive lower urinary tract symptoms (LUTS) at presentation. As the symptoms and presentations of this condition can mimic many other conditions, a high degree of suspicion must be maintained for other etiologies when evaluating patients. Clinical examination should be tailored toward narrowing the diagnosis and selecting the most appropriate testing to make the correct diagnosis.

HISTORY

Useful questions that indicate urethral obstruction (though they do not identify the anatomical location of the obstruction) include:
- Is your urinary stream weak?
- Do you strain to start to urinate?
- Is there a delay when you start urinating?

- Do you feel like you do not empty completely?
- Do you dribble in between voids?

In symptomatic patients, assessment of the time course and progression of symptoms as well as questions regarding possible etiology can also help narrow the differential. Useful questions include:

- How long have you been experiencing these symptoms?
- Have they gotten better or worse?
- Does anything make them better or worse?
- Have you ever had an injury to your genital region, perineum, or pelvis?
- Have you had several UTIs versus STIs?
- Have you ever had a urologic procedure or pelvic radiation (can specify, for stones, cancer, or blood in the urine as these are likely to lead to ureteroscopy (URS))?
- What other medical problems do you have?

Additionally, it is prudent to inquire whether the patient smokes or uses any tobacco products or other vasoconstrictors, as this could potentially limit surgical healing, especially if graft or flap repairs are utilized. The presence of other comorbidites that may affect the patient's ability to tolerate procedures, such as diabetes and cardiovascular disease, should also be evaluated and optimized.

PHYSICAL EXAMINATION

A complete genital examination should be performed in any patient where a stricture is suspected. Examination of the urethra can reveal the presence of meatal stenosis, hypospadias, previous surgeries, LS changes, or potentially spongiofibrosis/urethral scarring. Evaluation should also note the presence of healthy penile skin, which could be considered in future repairs.

The oral mucosa including the buccal (inner cheek), labial (inner lip), and lingual (tongue) mucosa surfaces, as well as the patients overall dentition and oral hygiene, should also be evaluated if a repair may need to be considered.

Digital rectal examination (DRE) should be considered for any patient with LUTS where the differential diagnosis is unclear and includes BPH. DRE can be potentially useful to identify prostatic hypertrophy (indicated by a large, smooth prostate gland) as the source of obstruction. However, the degree of obstruction does not correlate to prostatic size or hypertrophy; therefore despite a small prostate on DRE, the prostate could be the underlying etiology.

The perineum should be examined for signs of previous surgery, scarring, fistula, or abscess, which could alter management or timing of repair.

DIAGNOSTIC STUDIES

If stricture is considered, further evaluation is warranted. When a patient presents with LUTS, simple, noninvasive testing such as a uroflow and postvoid residual (PVR) may be considered as part of initial office-based work-up that can be suggestive.

While uroflow provides useful information and may signal an existing problem, it does not provide any information about pressures or anatomy. The "classic" uroflow curve for a patient with a narrow urethral stricture would be described as "plateau'd" with a flattened appearance over time due to flow through a constricted lumen. Uroflow may be variable and should be performed with at least 150 cc of voided volume. Additionally, PVR provides somewhat limited information, but an elevated PVR may signal a problem with bladder emptying and suggest potential obstruction or bladder decompensation (Figs. 11.4 and 11.5).

Standardized questionnaires such as the American Urological Association symptom score (AUA-SS) and Sexual Health Inventory

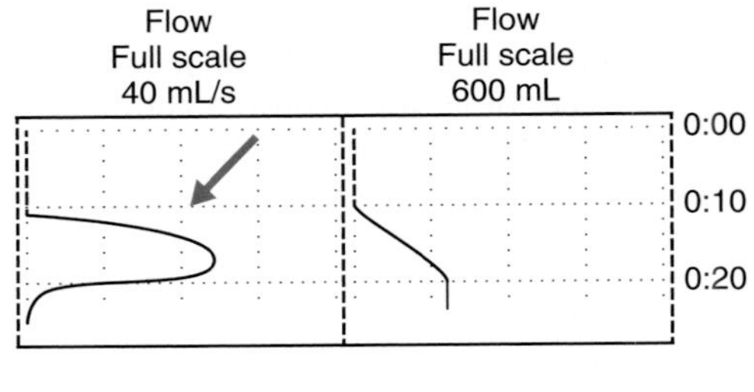

Uroflow summary

	Patient	M%
Maximum flow:	24 mL/s	83
Average flow:	13 mL/s	52
Voiding time:	14 s	32
Flow time:	14 s	
Time to maximum flow:	5 s	50
Voided volume:	187 mL	

FIGURE 11.4 Standard bell-shaped uroflow curve *(red arrow)* seen in normal voiding.

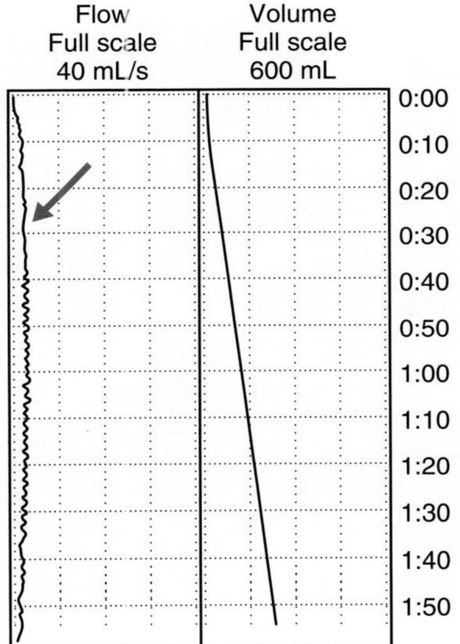

Uroflow summary

	Patient	M%	F%
Maximum flow:	3 mL/s	–79	–83
Average flow:	2 mL/s	–78	–83
Voiding time:	111 s	–402	–535
Flow time:	106 s		
Time to maximum flow:	58 s	–425	–598
Voided volume:	224 mL		

FIGURE 11.5 Classic "plateau'd" uroflow curve *(red arrow)* observed with a urethral stricture.

for Men (SHIM) score can be helpful as a baseline. More specific urethral stricture questionnaires may also be considered.

If urethral stricture is high on the differential diagnosis after history, physical examination, and noninvasive testing, multiple modalities can be considered to confirm the diagnosis and rule out other conditions. Ultimately, the goals of work-up are:

1. Rule in or out the presence of stricture.
2. If stricture is present, further characterize the stricture's location within the urethra, length, caliber, and tissue quality. This

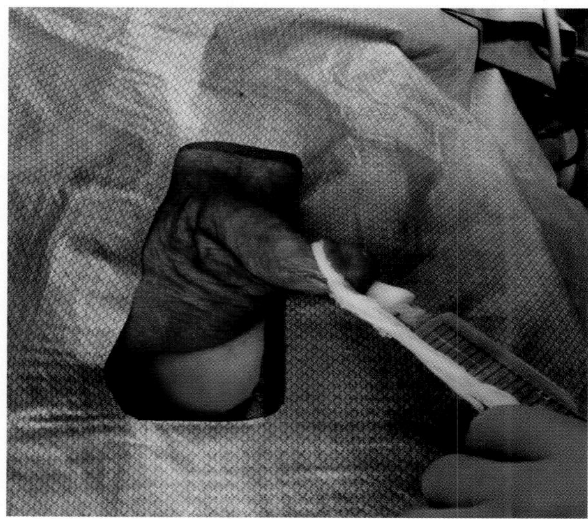

FIGURE 11.6 Positioning for retrograde urethrogram.

is often done through a combination of imaging modalities and direct visual examination.

A retrograde urethrogram (RUG) and voiding cystourethrogram (VCUG) are often the most useful studies for identifying the presence and anatomic location of urethral stricture disease. An RUG gives excellent information about the anterior urethra but often does not accurately visualize the posterior urethra. In men where there is concern for stenosis or narrowing of the posterior urethra (older patients, history of prior prostatic surgery, history of prostatic radiation, etc.) a good VCUG is essential to better define anatomy (Fig. 11.6).

RETROGRADE URETHROGRAM TECHNIQUE

An RUG is performed with a patient in a modified (about 45 degrees oblique) supine position with the lower leg bent and the upper leg straight. This position allows for a more lateral view, which is especially important for the bulbar urethra. This section of the urethra may overlap with itself on anteroposterior (AP) imaging, thus concealing strictures in this area. If both obturator foramina are visible, the patient is likely not rotated sufficiently. The penis must be put on stretch to straighten out the urethra and best show the location of the stricture. We prefer to do this with a thinned, rolled, contrast-soaked gauze wrap, which allows the physician to keep their hands out of the field and to visualize the level of the coronal margin. A tapered adaptor (we prefer a Taylor adaptor, if available) is used to instill fluid into the meatus under very gentle pressure and x-ray images are obtained. Care should be taken not to instrument the stricture as this can limit visualization.

In patients with a meatal stenosis, a calibration with Bougie-a-Boules should be performed first to evaluate the distal urethra before instrumentation is performed (Fig. 11.7). A smaller caliber inserter such as an angiocatheter may be needed in these cases.

A VCUG should be performed in any patient where posterior urethral pathology is a concern. This may include patients who have previously undergone prostate surgery or radiation, recurrent strictures, patients with proximal hypospadias, or pelvic fracture–related injuries. This test may image the entire urethra but is most helpful for the posterior urethra (bladder

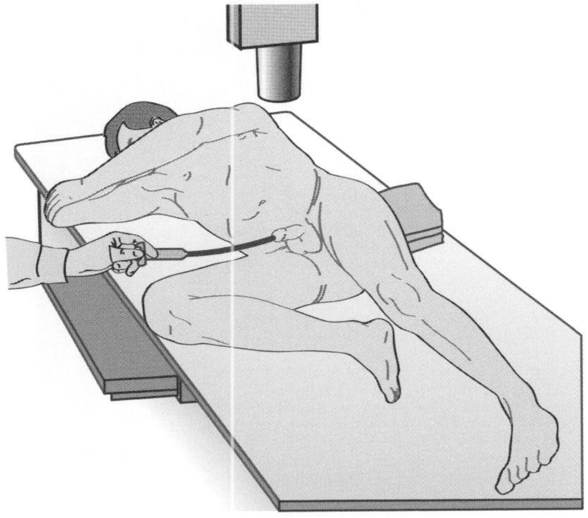

FIGURE 11.7 Positioning for performance of retrograde urethrogram.

neck, prostate, and membranous urethra), which is generally not well seen on an RUG.

This test is performed by filling the bladder with contrast and having the patient urinate. X-ray or fluoroscopic images are taken while the patient voids (Figs. 11.8–11.13).

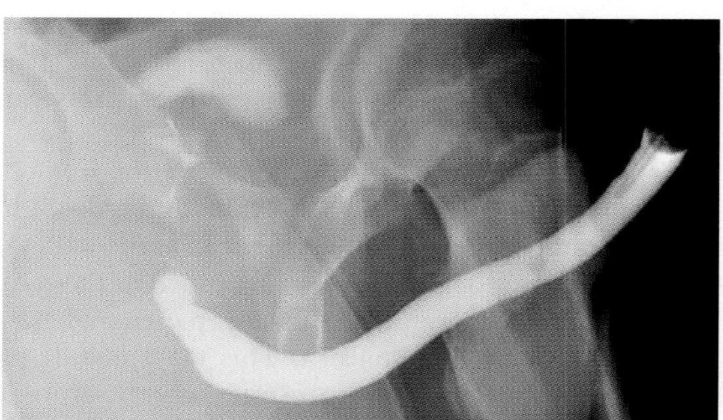

FIGURE 11.8 Normal retrograde urethrogram.

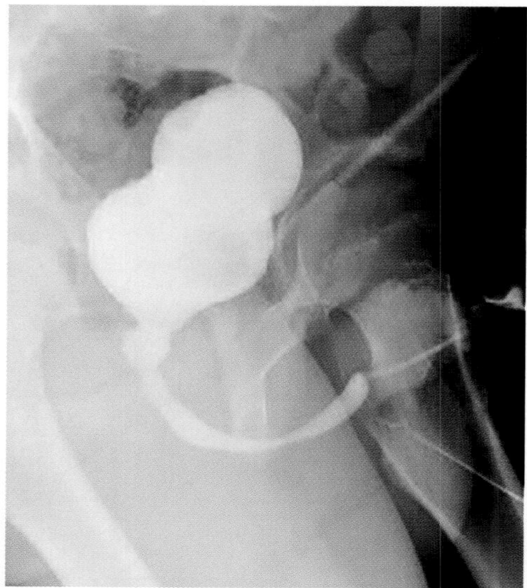

FIGURE 11.9 Normal voiding cystourethrogram.

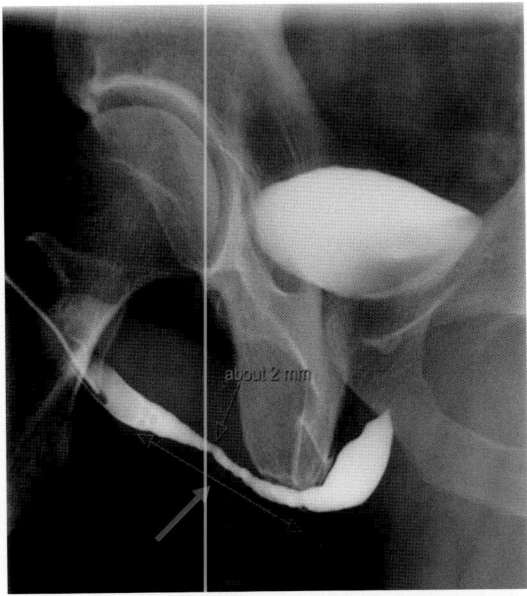

FIGURE 11.10 Retrograde urethrogram—distal bulbar/proximal penile urethral stricture *(red arrow)*.

Fluoroscopic imaging has several limitations. RUG and VCUG do not provide any information on the presence or absence of spongiofibrosis, only evaluating luminal caliber. These studies can often underestimate stricture length especially in the bulbar and posterior urethra. Information on soft tissue and bone location can be somewhat limited. In patients where this information is vital to know preoperatively, other modalities such as ultrasound (US) with intraurethral injection or even magnetic resonance imaging (MRI) can be useful.

Preoperative Evaluation and Optimization

As urethral repairs are generally elective in nature, optimizing nutrition status and comorbidities preoperatively is paramount,

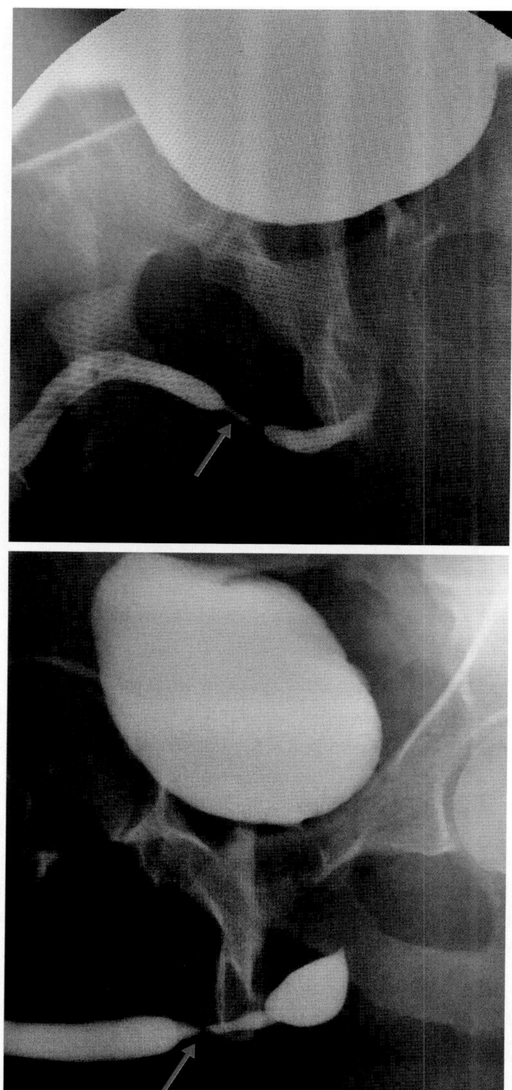

FIGURE 11.11 Midbulbar stricture with near complete obliteration *(red arrow)*.

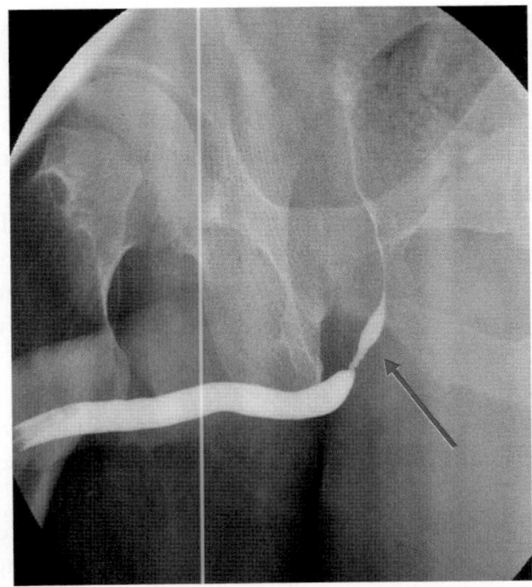

FIGURE 11.12 Retrograde urethrogram—proximal bulbar urethral stricture *(red arrow)*.

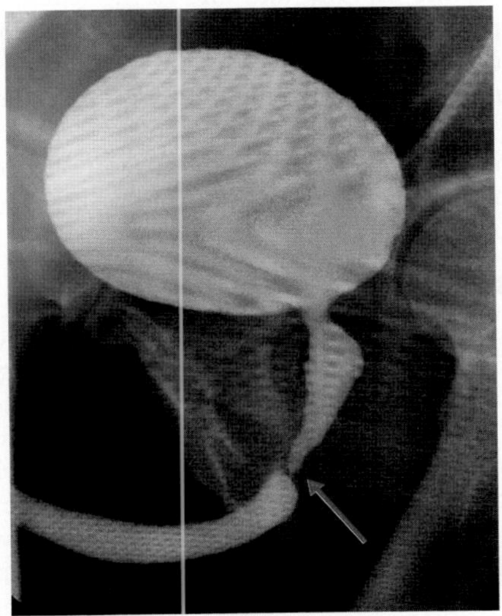

FIGURE 11.13 Voiding cystourethrogram—proximal bulbar stricture *(red arrow)*.

especially in cases where grafts or flaps will be utilized. Consider checking albumin/prealbumin levels in any patient where nutrition is in question. Glucose control should be assessed and managed in patients with diabetes. Smoking cessation is useful for wound healing in general, especially if grafts or flaps may be needed.

Obtain a urinalysis and urine culture. UTIs should be treated prior to urethral stricture intervention whenever possible. In patients with indwelling tubes or where chronic bacteriuria is present, complete eradication of the organisms may not always be possible.

When blood supply is in question, a Doppler US or angiogram can be considered to evaluate. While preoperative revascularization is rarely utilized, this may be useful for counseling about success rates.

A period of "urethral rest" may be considered for patients with stricture disease. Urethral rest involves removing catheters and stopping intermittent catheterization for a period of time before the repair (usually 6–12 weeks if possible). This rest minimizes high-pressure voiding, may decrease trauma/inflammation within the urethra, and allows the extent of the stricture to completely declare itself before definitive repair. In select patients where high-pressure voiding may occur or stricture reformation limits voiding, placing a suprapubic tube (SPT) may be prudent. A suprapubic tract can also be useful for antegrade endoscopic access to better define the stricture. Repeating imaging studies or endoscopic evaluation after a period of rest can be useful for surgical planning.

SUPRAPUBIC TUBE PLACEMENT TECHNIQUE

With the patient supine, mark the superior border of the pubic symphysis. The catheter should be placed two-finger breadths superior to this mark in the midline superior to allow for easy access with a flexible cystoscope at the time of planned repair of more posterior urethral strictures. Under direct vision with a flexible cystoscope or ureteroscope, fill and pressurize the bladder. Place the patient in Trendelenburg position to allow the bowels to fall superiorly. When filling the bladder is challenging, consider temporary needle placement just above the pubic symphysis with instillation via a large syringe until the bladder is pressurized. The tube should be placed percutaneously under direct cystoscopic vision when possible. In complicated cases, US guidance or laparoscopic visualization of the bladder can be helpful.

Operative Management

Management of urethral strictures will depend on a number of factors including the length and location of the urethral stricture, etiology of the stricture, associated scar tissue, patient health and ability to tolerate surgery, previous interventions, availability of graft/flap tissue, and patient preference.

Treatment options include:

- Intermittent self-catheterization
- Long-term catheter (Foley or SPT) placement
- Urethral dilation
  - Serial coaxial dilation
  - Balloon dilation
  - Optilume
- Direct vision internal urethrotomy (DVIU)
- Urethroplasty
  - Excision and primary anastomosis (EPA)
  - Nontransecting repairs
  - Substitution urethroplasty (utilizing grafts or flaps)
  - Augmented anastomotic repair
  - Staged repairs
- Perineal urethrotomy
- Catheterizable channel creation or urinary diversion

Anterior Urethral Strictures

ENDOSCOPIC MANAGEMENT

For short (especially < 2 cm) anterior urethral strictures of the bulbar urethra that have not been treated before, endoscopic procedures can be considered. These techniques attempt to balance the forces of wound contraction with reepithelialization, essentially attempting to break the scar tissue and allow the urethra to heal with a more open scarred configuration. Similar success rates seem to be achieved with dilation and DVIU. For first-time strictures, success rates range from 30%–60% in well-chosen patients, but this drops off precipitously to < 20% long-term success for second-time endoscopic management and approaching 0% for a third attempt at endoscopic management.

In terms of stricture length, success rates generally fall as the stricture length increases:

- < 2 cm: 40% failure rate at 1 year
- 2–4 cm: 50% and 75% failure at 1 and 4 year
- > 4 cm: 80% failure rate at 1 year

Dilation can be performed with serial coaxial dilation, but we prefer to do this with a balloon dilator when possible to avoid the shearing force and injury associated with coaxial dilation. For this, we place a wire under cystoscopic vision and confirm placement into the bladder. A 4 cm × 30Fr balloon is then passed over the wire and inflated to 14–16 atm under direct cystoscopic vision, leaving this inflated for about 2 minutes. A catheter is then generally left in place for 3–5 days. This procedure is generally well tolerated in the office. Long-term success rates are improved if the patient is willing to perform intermittent self-calibration after the procedure. Newer techniques for dilation with coated balloons (Optilume—paclitaxel impregnated) have shown promise as well even for patients with recurrent strictures.

DVIU involves endoscopically incising the strictured tissue with a cold knife or cutting laser. Classically, this is performed at a dorsal (12 o'clock) location in the urethra, but this may not be the optimal location given the thin nature of the spongiosum in this location and proximity to the corpora cavernosa. Some argue for several incisions to "break the ring" of scar tissue more fully. Deep incisions into heavily vascular tissue should be avoided. A catheter is left in place for 3–7 days after the procedure.

URETHROPLASTY AND SURGICAL OPTIONS

Urethroplasty is considered the gold standard for long-term management of urethral strictures. Success rates are generally higher than those of endoscopic management with reasonably low complication rates.

Excision and Primary Anastomosis

This technique involves removal of the scarred segment of urethra with anastomosis of the healthy, spatulated urethral ends. This technique is most commonly considered for shorter strictures in the bulbar urethra, especially when associated with trauma and dense spongiofibrosis or complete occlusions. Generally 2 cm is considered the cutoff for excisional techniques, but this has been extended up to 5 cm in select, healthy patients with proximal bulbar strictures. In select circumstances this can be considered in short pendulous urethral strictures but should be done with care due to risk of penile curvature with erection.

These surgeries have high success rates in both the short and long term (generally quoted as > 85%–90%) in properly selected patients. There is always some concern about the blood and nerve supply when the urethra is transected and this must be carefully assessed before considering these repairs. Concern exists about a potentially higher risk of erectile dysfunction, glans filling, and ejaculatory function with this technique compared to nontransecting techniques, but this has not been demonstrated consistently.

Brief Technique

Position the patient in high lithotomy position. Make a midline perineal incision. Reflect the bulbospongiosus muscle off the urethra. Separate the bulbar urethra from the perineal body. Transect the obliterated segment and excise the scarred area. Spatulate dorsally and ventrally. Free the ends of the urethra to allow a tension-free anastomosis. Bring both ends of the urethra together for a spatulated anastomosis generally with a one-layer closure dorsally and a two-layer closure (1: mucosa and 2: tunica of spongiosum) ventrally (Figs. 11.14 and 11.15).

Substitution Urethroplasty

Substitution urethroplasty involves using nonurethral tissue substitutes to patch or augment the size of the urethral lumen. This is done by using either a graft or a flap. These techniques have a higher long-term stricture recurrence rate than EPA, but part of this could be related to their use on patients with longer, more complex strictures.

Grafts are excised and transferred to a new location without their blood supply; new blood supply is then established via imbibition and inosculation. In urethral reconstruction, oral mucosal tissue tends to be the most commonly used graft material today

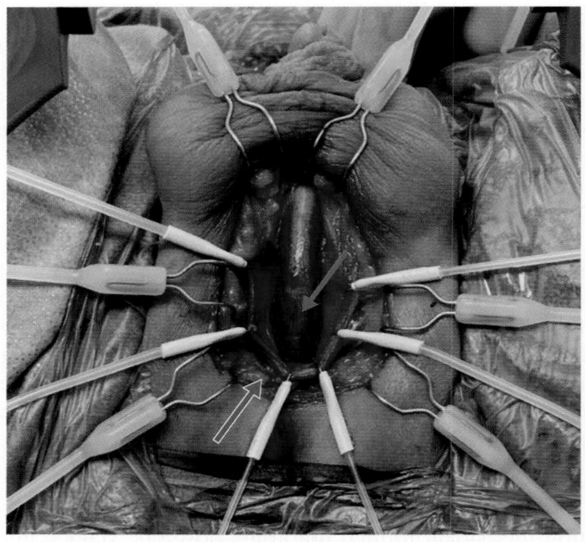

FIGURE 11.14 Exposure of the bulbar urethra *(green arrow)* through a perineal dissection. Note, bulbospongiosus muscle *(red arrow)* retracted downward.

due to its robust nature, favorable characteristics for graft take, availability, and hidden donor site.

Split-thickness grafts carry epidermis and dermal plexus; these do not carry physical characteristics. A full-thickness skin graft carries the epidermis with the superficial dermis layer, along with all the physical characteristics of that layer.

Flaps refer to tissues that are excised with a vascular pedicle or rotated with their blood supply—their vascularity is either intact or it is reestablished after transfer. The most common flap used in urethral reconstruction is a local penile fasciocutaneous flap. Free flaps from the forearm, latissimus dorsi, or anterolateral thigh are often used to create the urethra in gender-affirming surgery.

Flaps and grafts may be sutured dorsally, laterally, or ventrally into the urethra. Debate continues regarding the optimal location for strictures. Flaps/grafts may be fixated as onlay (typically

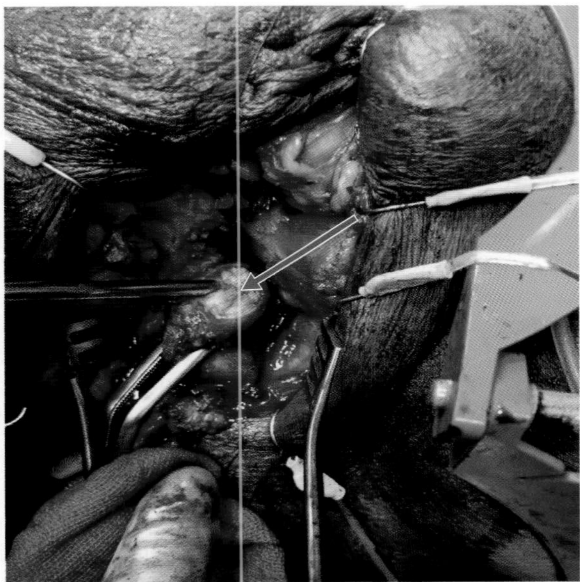

FIGURE 11.15 Transection of urethra during excision and primary anastomosis urethroplasty. Note, full-thickness spongiofibrosis *(red arrow)* at level of stricture.

overlying the defect) or inlay (flap/graft is incorporated directly between the incised urethral edges).

Ventral compared to dorsal approach:

- Limits need for urethral mobilization, better preserves perforating blood supply from corpora
- Technically less challenging dissection
- Avoids dissection of dorsal urethra, which can be scarred from previous procedures
- Requires incising into the more robust ventral spongiosum—increased bleeding/decreased visualization
- Minimal backing of the graft—higher potential for diverticulum formation

Some clinicians prefer the ventral approach when robust sponge is available as it limits urethral mobilization while preserving perforating arteries. It is also less technically challenging. The ventral approach may also be used if the dorsal urethra is scarred down from multiple DVIUs/previous urethral repair. However, a dorsal approach allows spread fixation of grafts to the corpora cavernosa, ensuring a graft bed that remains unaffected by spongiofibrosis. This maximizes contact with the vascular bed and enables optimal graft take. Dorsal urethrotomy requires less dissection through the thick ventral sponge and limits bleeding during the case. Dorsal location may also limit diverticulum formation.

Many techniques exist for more complicated strictures. For some patients, gracilis flaps may be used for backing and to create blood supply to grafts. In others rectal mucosa (harvested transanally) can be used as a substitution material. In rare occasions, a flap of tubularized small bowel or appendix can be considered.

Brief Technique

Expose the urethra throughout the location of the stricture. Create a urethrotomy dorsally, laterally, or ventrally throughout the strictured site into healthy urethra on both ends of the defect. Keep the penis/urethra on some stretch. If dorsal or dorsolateral, spread and fix the graft to the corpora. Suture graft or flap into the defect to augment the size of the lumen. If ventral, close the tunica spongiosum over the graft after sewn into place (Fig. 11.16A,B).

Distal Anterior Urethral Strictures

Strictures in the fossa navicularis are generally repaired with a substitution urethroplasty. For many patients, this can be done with a transurethral ventral inlay buccal mucosal graft placement (Nikolavsky technique) where a wedge of tissue is excised from the ventral wall and a teardrop-shaped oral mucosal tissue is "parachuted" into place. The graft can also be placed as a dorsal inlay with more standard urethroplasty techniques, similar to many hypospadias repairs. For patients with more complex strictures, multistage repairs or local tissue flaps can be used.

For patients seeking a simpler solution, extended meatoplasty/first-stage repair can also be considered although the cosmetic appearance of the phallus and direction of the stream may be more compromised. For those who are unwilling or unable to undergo

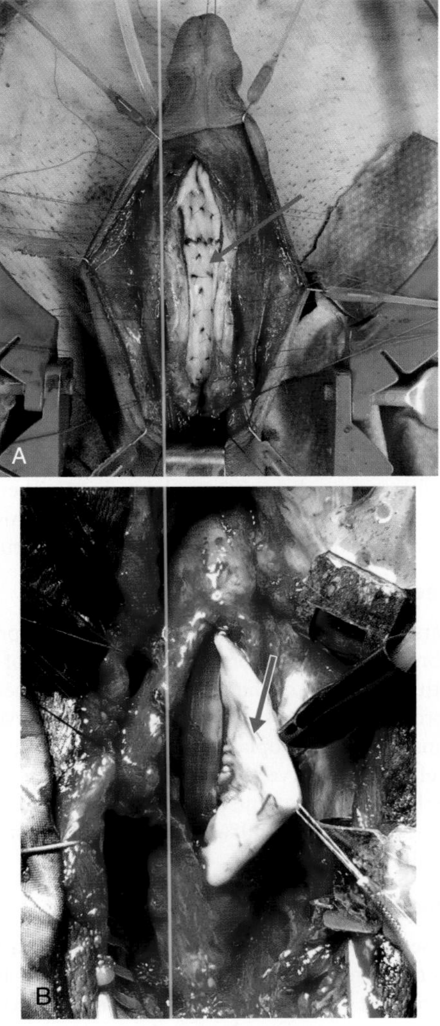

FIGURE 11.16 Substitution urethroplasty. (A) Stricture in the penile urethra—dorsal inlay technique with multiple buccal mucosal grafts *(red arrow)*. (B) Stricture in the bulbar urethra—ventral onlay technique with oral mucosal graft *(red arrow)*.

surgery, self-dilation can be helpful but is generally required in perpetuity to keep the stricture site open.

Augmented Anastomotic Repair

This technique is generally used for longer strictures in which a portion of the stricture is very narrow or obliterated. This necessitates a combined approach where the worst part of the stricture is completely excised with the remaining urethra put back together and then augmented with a graft or flap thus combining the techniques of EPA and substitution repairs.

These types of repairs do have higher recurrence rates, which could reflect the more complex nature of the repair as well as local factors associated with these more complex strictures.

Brief Technique

Follow steps of EPA for removal of the unsalvageable portion of the urethra. Create a urethrotomy through the level of the stricture into healthy tissue. Anastomose the ends on either the ventral surface (preferable) or the dorsal surface. Augment this newly created urethral plate with a graft or flap as in a substitution repair.

Nontransecting Repairs

In recent years, debate has grown around excision and primary anastomotic techniques due to theoretically higher rates of sexual dysfunction with transection of the urethra as well as general concerns about compromising blood supply. This has led to development of the "nontransecting urethroplasty" where the spongiosum is left intact in an effort to preserve as much blood supply as possible.

In properly selected patients, these techniques also yield high short-term success rates (> 90%) although long-term assessment is not yet available.

Brief Technique

Begin by dissecting down to and isolating the urethra through the perineum, similar to the exposure used in an EPA. Rather than transecting the urethra, a dorsal urethrotomy is made through the area of the stricture. For shorter strictures, the dorsal end is closed in a Heineke-Mikulicz fashion to widen the urethral lumen (stricturoplasty). For longer strictures, the ventral mucosa is excised or incised and a graft is inlayed ventrally. The dorsal wall is again closed in Heineke-Mikulicz technique or a dorsal graft is placed as an onlay.

Multistage Urethroplasty

Multistage urethroplasties may be considered when there is excessive urethral scarring severely limiting the caliber of the urethra or poor quality tissue for graft take (such as hypospadias with multiple previous surgeries, severe LS/BXO, or poor tissue with previous attempts at repair). Multistage repair is used in these circumstances as circumferential, tubularized tissue transfer techniques seem to have significantly higher recurrence rates.

During the first stage, graft tissue is transferred onto a well-vascularized tissue bed of the dartos fascia. During the second stage, usually scheduled 6–12 months later after the graft has taken and incorporated, the graft is tubularized and covered. Additional stages may be necessary to lay in additional blood supply, create skin coverage, or further augment grafts/flaps if contraction occurs.

If local tissue is healthy and available, penile fasciocutaneous flaps (penile skin versus prepuce versus deepithelized scrotal skin) can be used to augment the ventral wall of the urethra. Penile skin should not be used in patients with LS (Fig. 11.17).

Perineal Urethrostomy

Perineal urethrostomy is an alternative to urethroplasty for certain patients with urethral stricture disease. A perineal urethrostomy should be at least considered in some of the following situations:

1. Patients who are less medically fit for prolonged procedures
2. Complex urethral stricture disease where success rates may be more limited or multistage procedures may be required
3. Patients who require frequent bladder access for surveillance or resection (e.g., bladder cancer patients)
4. Patients who prefer a simpler (yet less anatomic) procedure to the alternatives for repair

With perineal urethrostomy, the urine is diverted to a new opening on the perineum below the level of the scrotum. As the new urethrostomy is situated distal to the patient's sphincter mechanisms, normal continence should be maintained. Patients do need to sit to urinate after perineal urethrostomy. They will also ejaculate from the urethrostomy site (Fig. 11.18).

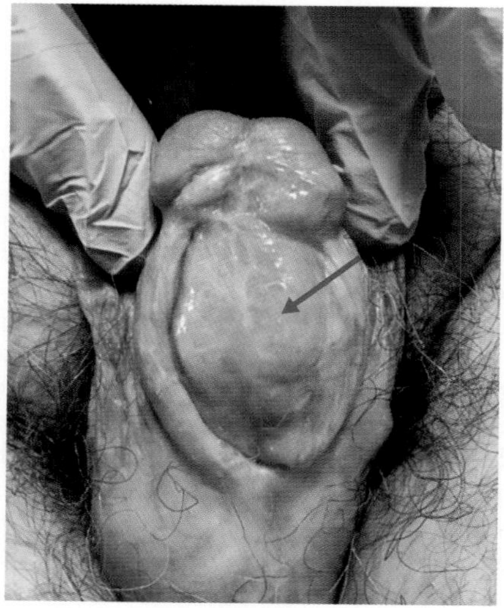

FIGURE 11.17 Appearance after first-stage repair with oral mucosal graft placement and take *(red arrow)*.

Brief Technique

The general dictum in perineal urethrostomy creation is "bring the skin to the urethra" rather than overly mobilizing the urethra and bringing it up to the level of the skin. To accomplish this, skin flaps are often mobilized and advanced to the level of the urethrotomy. The patient is positioned in high lithotomy. An inverted U incision is made, and the bulbospongiosus muscle is identified. The bulbospongiosus is then divided along the midline or retracted downward to expose the corpus spongiosum. A 4- to 5-cm ventral urethrostomy is created at the level of the midbulbar urethra. Lumen calibration is determined with a bougie to 30 Fr proximally. Skin flaps are advanced and fitted to the level of the urethrostomy. The distal urethra can be left in situ to avoid disrupting the blood supply.

Posterior Urethral Stenosis

Stenosis of the posterior urethra generally occurs after traumatic injury or secondary to treatment of prostate cancer or BPH.

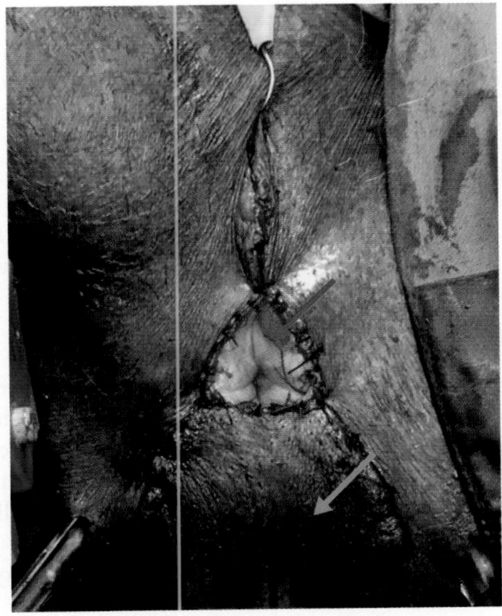

FIGURE 11.18 Appearance of perineal urethrostomy *(red arrow)* at completion of procedure. Note, posterior advancement flap *(green arrow)*.

PELVIC FRACTURE URETHRAL DISTRACTION DEFECTS

Traumatic posterior urethral injuries (otherwise known as PFUDD) generally occur at the bulbomembranous or membranoprostatic junction. These injuries occur due to shearing forces acting on the fixed portion of the urethra (membranous urethra at the urogenital diaphragm). These injuries are highly associated with concomitant pelvic fractures.

Initial management at the time of trauma requires prompt bladder drainage with an SPT or primary realignment with a urethral catheter. Most providers will place an SPT in more significant injuries if a complete transection occurs as the stenosis rate is nearly 100% even if a catheter can be placed across the stenosis. If significant stenosis occurs at the injury site, posterior urethroplasty is the procedure of choice.

VCUG or antegrade cystoscopy coupled with RUG is generally the study of choice to better define the length and location of the stenosis. Antegrade cystoscopy may be a helpful adjuvant to evaluate the bladder neck/posterior urethra in select patients. MRI and contrast-enhanced US can also be used to better define the anatomy in complex situations. In patients with significant pelvic traumas or previous surgery where blood supply is in question, Doppler US and/or angiogram can be considered. In patients with compromised blood supply, preoperative revascularization can also be considered.

Brief Technique

Posterior urethroplasty is generally approached through the perineum with the patient in high lithotomy position with a bump for elevation of the perineum. Scar is completely excised and the healthy ends of the urethra are identified, spatulated, and reanastomosed. In select patients, the bulbar arteries may still be intact and can potentially be spared.

At the time of surgery, additional maneuvers may need to be considered to allow for a tension-free anastomosis as well as proper visualization deep in the perineum. These include:

1. Mobilization of the distal urethral segment
2. Splitting the corpora cavernosa
3. Inferior pubectomy
4. Corporal rerouting

While these can be challenging repairs, the overall success rates are high and generally above 90%. For some patients, robotic techniques may be employed either along with or in lieu of more traditional perineal approaches (Fig. 11.19).

RADIATION-INDUCED STENOSIS

Patients who undergo radiation for prostate cancer or other pelvic malignancies are also prone to stricture disease. These strictures can be anywhere within the urethra, but most commonly tend to occur at the membranous urethra and apical prostatic urethra. These can be challenging stricture to manage due to the diminished blood supply to the area and fibrotic reaction of the surrounding tissue. Urethroplasty success rates are diminished in these cases and generally reported in the 50%–75% success rate.

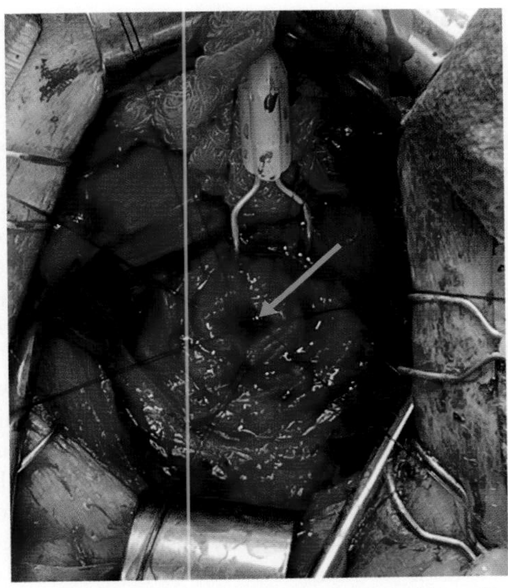

FIGURE 11.19 Posterior urethra exposed *(green arrow)* with urethra transected, scar removed, and circumferential supple edges reached before anastomosis.

Mostly commonly, the surgical technique for these stenoses is similar to that of a PFUDD injury with complete excision of the scar tissue followed by spatulation and primary anastomosis to healthy appearing urethral edges. In some patients where scarring is not dense, substitution urethroplasty with dorsal onlay may be used with good success, and it provides a more robust blood supply to the urethra if artificial sphincter placement is a consideration. Oral mucosal grafts have demonstrated robustness and seem to show a reasonable rate of take even in radiated fields.

For redo cases or in patients who have undergone multiple forms of radiation, a gracilis flap may be interposed into the repair site to try to bring additional vascularity and to fill the defect.

BLADDER NECK CONTRACTURES/VESICOURETHRAL ANASTOMOTIC STENOSIS

Bladder neck contractures (BNCs) generally occur as a result of prostate surgery, generally after BPH procedures and/or radiation therapy. Vesicourethral anastomotic stenoses generally occur at the anastomosis after radical prostatectomy surgeries and are more common in patients who also require adjuvant/salvage radiation.

In general, these contractures are initially managed endoscopically. Dilation can be performed in the office with a balloon dilator and used to dilate to 30Fr under direct vision. Transurethral incision of the BNC can be performed with a hot or cold knife. Incisions are made to "break the ring" of scar in several locations—often at 2, 4, 8, and 10 o'clock or at 3 and 9 o'clock with "crow's feet" extension. Adjuvant agents such as mitomycin C (0.4 mg/cc) can be injected after incision to decrease recurrent rates in refractory BNC. A catheter is left for 3–7 days after the procedure.

Newer techniques such as the transurethral incision with transverse mucosal realignment (TUITMR, Warner technique) has shown promise for BNC. This involves incising the stricture such as a Transurethral incision of bladder neck contracture (TUIBNC) and then using a specialized scope to reapproximate the mucosal edges endoscopically with a catheter left in place after the procedure.

When endoscopic management is unsuccessful, more definitive repair can be undertaken via either a perineal or an abdominal approach. Most abdominal approaches are now being performed robotically with excellent success rates. This can involve excision of the scar with reanastomosis, modified Y-V plasty techniques or substitution repair with graft material to augment the bladder neck lumen.

RECTOURETHRAL FISTULA

Rectourethral fistula is a connection that forms between the urethra and the rectum. Generally, they occur after pelvic surgeries (most commonly prostatectomy or BPH procedures) and/or radiation therapy within the pelvis most commonly at the level of the prostate or the vesicourethral anastomosis. These can be particularly challenging problems to manage, especially in the setting of high-dose radiation therapy.

Work-up is similar to that of urethral stricture in many ways. In most fistula, especially more complex ones involving radiation, patients will need a period of bowel and urinary diversion for at least 3 months before any definitive management. This generally involves an ileostomy or colostomy for gastrointestinal (GI) diversion and an SPT or Foley catheter for urinary diversion. After a period of rest, examination under anesthesia with cystoscopy, RUG, antegrade cystoscopy/cystourethrogram, and sigmoidoscopy is performed to evaluate the tissue quality, size, location, and nature of the fistula. Urodynamics testing may be helpful when lower tract function is in question. Determination is made at this point about moving forward with repair of the bowel and/or urethra or whether permanent diversion should be considered for either of these systems.

Brief Technique

While many techniques are available for small, surgically induced fistula, a perineal approach is the most commonly used in complex fistula. Robotic approaches may be considered if the fistula is relatively proximal and the providers have sufficient expertise in this approach.

For a perineal approach, the patient is positioned in high lithotomy. Cystoscopy is performed and, if possible, retrocatheters are passed through the fistula tract and into the ureters if close to the area. A lambda incision or midline incision is made in the perineum. Dissection is lower than in standard urethroplasty, closer to the anterior rectal wall, with the ischiorectal fossa developed bilaterally until the fistula is identified. The fistula tract is opened and surrounding tissue excised until healthy tissue is identified and able to be sufficiently mobilized. The rectal wall is repaired primarily. In simple repairs, the urethra may be able to be closed primarily as well with interrupted or running suture. In most repairs, oral mucosal graft is used to augment the urethral lumen. The graft is affixed to a gracilis flap, which is transferred into the perineum. The gracilis flap is also used to provide vascular coverage to separate the repairs. A Foley catheter and SPT are maintained until healing is confirmed on imaging (Figs. 11.20 and 11.21).

Devastated Urethras or Outlets

For patients with complicated strictures or BNC that are not amenable to surgical repair with reasonable success rates, alternative options should be considered. These generally include catheterizable channel creation (with or without augmentation cystoplasty and/or bladder neck closure) and/or urinary diversion.

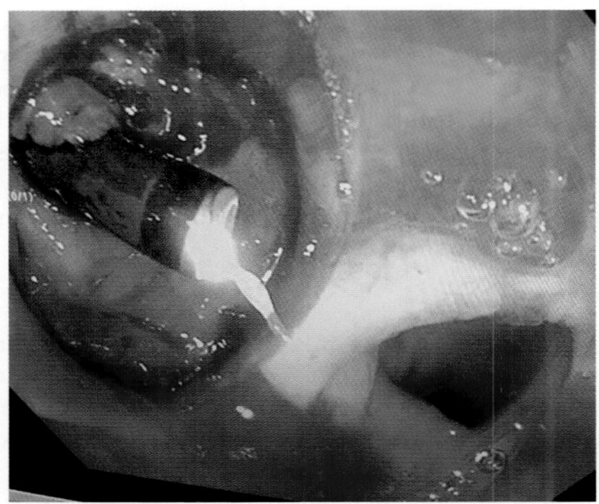

FIGURE 11.20 Rectourethral fistula. Sigmoidoscopy in rectum with cystoscope visualized through prostate in fistula tract.

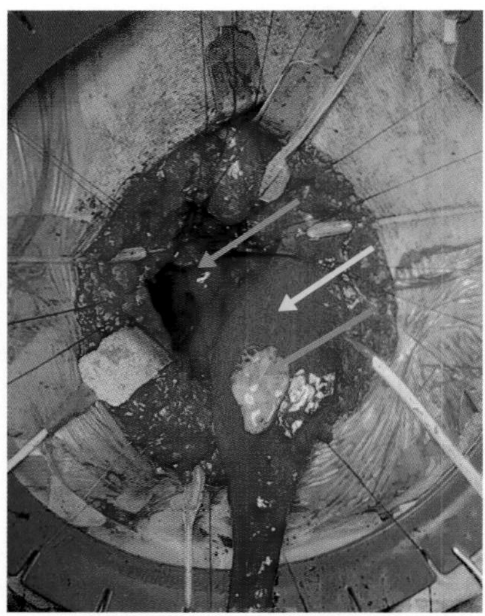

FIGURE 11.21 Rectourethral fistula (RUF). Perineal repair of RUF—fistula tract opened *(green arrow)*, buccal graft *(blue arrow)* quilted to gracilis muscle *(yellow arrow)*.

Urinary diversion should also be considered as an initial management option when there is significant bladder pathology such as refractory radiation cystitis or a small capacity, poorly compliant bladder.

Complications of Urethral Stricture Management

Unfortunately, all of the procedures used to manage urethral strictures carry some degree of risk.

For urethroplasty, common concerns include recurrent urethral stricture, development of a urethral diverticulum or fistula, postvoid dribbling, urinary spraying or splaying, erectile dysfunction, ejaculatory dysfunction, penile curvature, or decreased perineal or penile sensation. (Figs. 11.22 and 11.23).

Female Urethral Strictures

Female urethral stricture disease is quite uncommon, representing less than 1% of females presenting with voiding complaints. Diagnosis can be challenging and a high degree of suspicion is required. Patients typically note decreased force of stream,

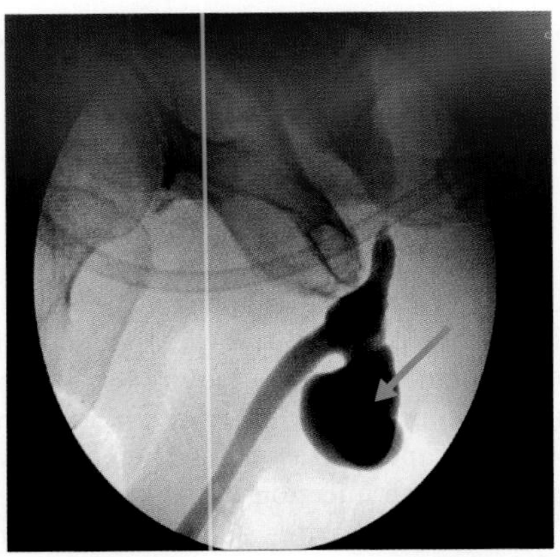

FIGURE 11.22 Retrograde urethrogram with urethral diverticulum *(green arrow)* after previous urethral injury.

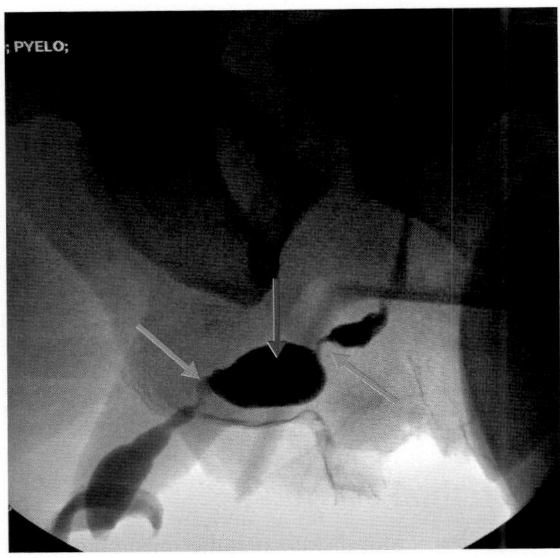

FIGURE 11.23 Voiding cystourethrogram (VCUG)—recurrent strictures *(green arrows)* and diverticulum *(red arrow)* after previous perineal hypospadias repair.

hesitancy, feeling of incomplete emptying, but presentation can be highly variable.

The female urethra is not covered with a robust spongiosum layer, making the blood supply somewhat less robust than in the male.

WORK-UP

RUG and VCUG are technically challenging given the short length of the female urethra but may still yield valuable information. Urethroscopy is essential and may require use of a pediatric cystoscope or ureteroscope to fully evaluate the stricture. Antegrade cystoscopy via a suprapubic tract can be helpful if available.

Transvaginal US with injection of gel-based material into the urethra can be helpful to better define the stricture. MRI can also be a useful adjunct to rule out malignancy or external mass effect.

MANAGEMENT

For some patients, office or operating room (OR)-based endoscopic methods can be considered, generally in the form of urethral dilation or endoscopic incision. This can be combined with self-calibration in some patients to maintain patency. Success rates are widely variable from about 12% to 68%.

Urethroplasty techniques are available for more definitive repair. For more distal strictures, meatoplasty or local mucosal advancement can be used. Substitution repairs with local tissue such as tubularized vaginal flaps, labial flaps, or onlay grafts can be used with reasonably good success rates of 68%–100% at 1 year. Grafts are generally placed dorsally within the urethra although some authors have placed graft material ventrally with success.

Additional content, including Self-Assessment Questions and Suggested Readings, may be accessed at www.ExpertConsult.com.

Urinary Fistula

Eric S. Rovner, MD

Among the most commonly encountered genitourinary (GU) fistulas in the developed world is vesicovaginal fistula (VVF), often at the time of gynecologic surgery, namely hysterectomy.

This chapter will discuss the various fistulae involving the urinary tract, including the presentation, evaluation, and management options.

A fistula represents an extraanatomic communication between two or more epithelial or mesothelial lined body cavities or the skin surface. Although most fistulae in the industrialized world are iatrogenic, they may also occur as a result of congenital anomalies, malignancy, inflammation and infection, radiation therapy, iatrogenic (surgical) or external tissue trauma, ischemia, foreign body, parturition, and a variety of other processes. The potential exists for fistula formation between a portion of the urinary tract (i.e., kidney, ureters, bladder, and urethra) and virtually any other body cavity including the chest (pleural cavity), gastrointestinal (GI) tract, lymphatics, vascular system, genitalia, skin, and reproductive organs. Classification is generally based on the organ of origin in the urinary tract and the termination point of the fistula (i.e., vagina, skin, GI tract, etc.). The presenting symptoms and signs are variable and depend to a large degree on the involved organs, the presence of underlying urinary obstruction or infection, the size of the fistula, and associated medical conditions such as malignancy.

Treatment of urinary fistula depends on several factors including its location, size, and etiology (malignant or benign). Prevention of urinary fistula is, of course, paramount; however proper nutrition, infection, and malignancy are important considerations not only when assessing a patient for the risk of creation of a fistula during any given intervention, but also during an evaluation for the repair of an existing urinary fistula.

Vesicovaginal Fistula

GENERAL CONSIDERATIONS

VVF are the most common acquired fistulae of the urinary tract. As the name suggests, they are an abnormal communication between the bladder and vagina.

1. VVF have been known about since ancient times; however, it was not until 1663 that Hendrik von Roonhuyse first described surgical repair.

ETIOLOGY

The most common cause of VVF differs in various parts of world.

1. In the industrialized world, the most common cause (75%) is injury to the bladder at the time of gynecologic surgery, usually abdominal hysterectomy. Obstetric trauma accounts for very few VVF in the United States and other industrialized nations.
   a. Post-hysterectomy VVF are thought to result most commonly from an incidental unrecognized iatrogenic cystotomy near the vaginal cuff. Additionally, inadvertent suture placement through the bladder may lead to pressure necrosis and tissue loss.
      1) The operative approach to hysterectomy is an important factor as bladder injuries are at least three times more common during abdominal hysterectomy compared to vaginal hysterectomy.
   b. The incidence of fistula after hysterectomy is estimated to be approximately 0.1%–0.2%.
   c. Other causes of VVF in the industrialized world include injuries during stress urinary incontinence surgery and anterior/apical vaginal prolapse repair, malignancy, pelvic radiation, obstetrical trauma including forceps lacerations, and uterine rupture.
   d. Patient risk factors for VVF include large cystotomy, greater tobacco use, larger uterine size, longer surgery time, and greater operative blood loss.
2. In the developing world where routine perinatal obstetrical care may be limited, VVF most commonly occur as a result of

prolonged labor with resulting pressure necrosis to the anterior vaginal wall and underlying trigone of the bladder from the baby. In some instances, VVF may result from the use of forceps or other instrumentation during delivery.

a. Obstetric fistulas tend to be larger, located distally in the vagina, and may involve the proximal urethra.
b. The constellation of problems resulting from obstructed labor is not limited to VVF and has been termed the "obstructed labor injury complex" and includes varying degrees of each of the following: urethral loss, stress incontinence, hydroureteronephrosis, renal failure, rectovaginal fistula, rectal atresia, anal sphincter incompetence, cervical destruction, amenorrhea, pelvic inflammatory disease, secondary infertility, vaginal stenosis, osteitis pubis and foot drop.
c. In sub-Saharan Africa the incidence rate of obstetric VVF has been estimated at 10.3 per 100,000 deliveries.

PRESENTATION

1. The most common complaint is constant urinary drainage per vagina although small fistulas may present with intermittent wetness which is positional in nature.
   a. VVF must be distinguished from urinary incontinence due to other causes including stress (urethral) incontinence, urgency (bladder) incontinence, and overflow incontinence.
   b. Patients may also complain of recurrent cystitis, perineal skin irritation due to constant wetness, vaginal fungal infections, or rarely pelvic pain. When a large VVF is present, patients may not void at all and simply have continuous leakage of urine into the vagina.
   c. VVF following hysterectomy or other surgical procedures may present upon removal of the urethral catheter or may present 1 to 3 weeks later with urinary drainage per vagina.
      1) VVF resulting from hysterectomy are usually located high in the vagina at the level of the vaginal cuff (Fig. 12.1).
   d. VVF resulting from radiation therapy may not present for months to years following completion of radiation. These tend to represent some the most challenging reconstructive cases in Urology due to the size, complexity, and the

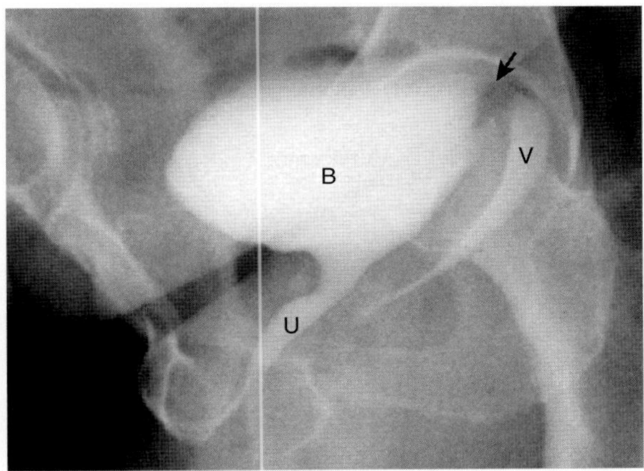

FIGURE 12.1 VCUG demonstrating a VVF high at the level of the vaginal cuff in a patient following hysterectomy. The *arrow* demonstrates the fistula tract (not well seen). *B*, Urinary bladder; *U*, urethra; *V*, vagina; *VCUG*, voiding cystourethrogram; *VVF*, vesicovaginal fistula.

associated voiding dysfunction due to the radiation effects on the urinary bladder. The endarteritis as a result of radiation therapy may involve the surrounding tissues limiting reconstructive options. Fistulas due to prior radiation therapy may be associated with other aspects of radiation injury to the urinary tract including radiation cystitis, diminished bladder capacity, and ureteric stricture.

EVALUATION (FIG. 12.2)

1. History
   a. Symptom assessment, including severity, duration, and onset of urinary drainage
   b. Etiology of VVF
   c. Obstetric history
   d. Prior pelvic surgery or radiation therapy
   e. Sexual function
   f. Prior treatment for VVF
2. Physical Examination
   a. Assessment of health of surrounding local tissues including vaginal depth, vaginal atrophy, and perineal skin.

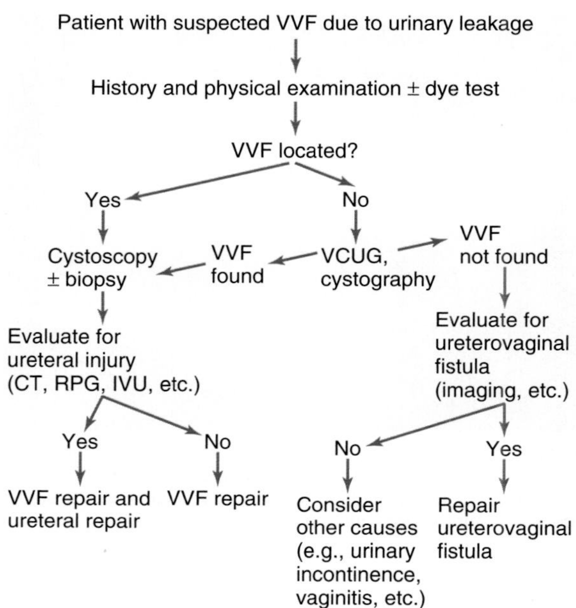

FIGURE 12.2 Algorithm for diagnosis of VVF. *CT*, Computed tomography; *IVU*, intravenous urogram; *RPG*, retrograde pyelogram; *VCUG*, voiding cystourethrogram; *VVF*, vesicovaginal fistula.

b. A pelvic exam with speculum should be performed in an attempt to locate the fistula (located at the anterior/apical segment of the vagina) and assess the size and number of fistulae.
c. Palpate for masses or other pelvic pathology which may need to be addressed at the time of fistula repair.
d. An assessment of inflammation surrounding the fistula is necessary as it may affect timing of the repair.
e. The presence of a VVF may be confirmed by instilling a vital blue dye (e.g., methylene blue) into the bladder per urethra and observing for discolored vaginal drainage.
    1) A double dye test may confirm the diagnosis of urinary fistula as well as suggest the possibility of an associated ureterovaginal or urethrovaginal fistula. A tampon is placed per vagina. Oral phenazopyridine is administered

and vital blue dye is instilled into the bladder. If the tampon is discolored yellow-orange at the top, it is suggestive of a ureterovaginal fistula. Blue discoloration in the midportion of the tampon suggests VVF, whereas blue staining at the bottom suggests a urethrovaginal fistula.

3. Urine culture and urine analysis
4. Cystoscopy and possible biopsy of the fistula tract are performed if malignancy is suspected
   a. Note the location of fistula relative to ureters; repair of the fistula may require reimplantation of ureters if the fistula involves the ureteral orifice.
5. Voiding cystourethrography/computed tomography (CT) cystogram
   a. Some small fistulas may not be seen radiographically unless the bladder is filled to capacity and a detrusor contraction is provoked during filling.
      1) Assess for vesicoureteral reflux.
      2) Examine for multiple fistulae including urethrovaginal fistula.
      3) Assess size and location of fistula as well as bladder capacity.
6. CT urogram, intravenous urography, and/or retrograde pyeloureterography
   a. Assess for concomitant ureteral injury and/or ureterovaginal fistula which has been reported to occur in up to 12% of patients.
7. Cross-sectional pelvic imaging (magnetic resonance imaging [MRI]/CT) if malignancy or other pelvic pathology is suspected

THERAPY

1. Nonsurgical management
   a. Catheter drainage is the initial treatment in most cases when the VVF is recognized early in the clinical course. Antibiotics and topical estrogen creams are adjuvant measures to prevent infection and promote healing. If the patient is not completely dry with an indwelling catheter, then this method of management should be abandoned.
   b. Fulguration of the fistula followed by catheter drainage has been shown to have some efficacy in small (<5 mm), uncomplicated fistulae.

   c. Adjuvant measures such fibrin glue, etc., have been used by some authors in conjunction with fulguration and catheter drainage as a "plug" in the fistula as well as a "scaffolding" to allow the ingrowth of healthy tissue.
2. Surgical management:
   a. Success rates approach 90% to 98% regardless of surgical approach.
   b. Adherence to basic surgical principles is essential in order to achieve success in the repair of all urinary fistulae (Table 12.1).
   c. Choice of the optimal surgical approach to VVF is controversial and there are numerous factors to consider (Table 12.2). No single approach is applicable to all VVF.
      1) Transabdominal approach: Generally performed as described by V.J. O'Conor. Through a midline infraumbilical incision, the bladder is exposed and opened in the sagittal plane down to the level of the fistula. The bladder is separated off the vagina beyond the level of the fistula. The fistulous tract is debrided back to healthy tissue from both bladder and vaginal sides. The bladder and vagina are closed separately. Often, a well-vascularized tissue flap such as omentum is interposed between the vagina

TABLE 12.1 Principles of Vesicovaginal Fistula Repair

1. Adequate exposure of the fistula tract with debridement of devitalized and ischemic tissue
2. Removal of involved foreign bodies or synthetic materials from region of fistula, if applicable
3. Careful dissection and/or anatomic separation of the involved organ cavities
4. Watertight closure
5. Use of well-vascularized, healthy tissue flaps for repair (atraumatic handling of tissue)
6. Multiple layer closure
7. Tension-free, nonoverlapping suture lines
8. Adequate urinary tract drainage and/or stenting after repair
9. Treatment and prevention of infection (appropriate use of antimicrobials)
10. Maintenance of hemostasis

TABLE 12.2 Factors in Approaching the Repair of Vesicovaginal Fistula

	Abdominal: Open	Abdominal: Laparoscopic/ robotic	Transvaginal
Length of hospital-ization	2–5 days	0–2 days	0–1 days
Timing of repair	May be delayed if initial injury was from an abdominal approach and significant in-flammation/ infection remains	Same as open	May be done immediately in the ab-sence of infection
Location of ureters relative to fistula tract	Fistula located near ureteral orifice may ne-cessitate reim-plantation	Same as open	Reimplantation may not be necessary even if fis-tula tract is located near ureteral orifice
Sexual function	Usually no change in vaginal depth	Same as open	Potential risk of vaginal shortening or stenosis
Location of fistula tract/ depth of vagina	Fistula located low on the trigone or near the bladder neck may be difficult to expose	Same as open	Fistula located high at the vaginal cuff may be difficult to expose
Use of adjunc-tive flaps	Omentum, peritoneal flap, intestine	Same as open	Labial fat pad (Martius fat pad), perito-neal flap, gracilis mus-cle, labial myocutane-ous flap

Continued

TABLE 12-2 Factors in Approaching the Repair of Vesicovaginal Fistula—cont'd

	Abdominal: Open	Abdominal: Laparoscopic/ robotic	Transvaginal
Relative indications	Large fistulas, located high in a deep vagina, radiation fistulas, failed transvaginal approach, small capacity bladder requiring augmentation, need for ureteral reimplantation, inability to place patient in the lithotomy position	Minimally invasive approach desired, expertise in lap/robotic surgery, need for shorter recovery time	Uncomplicated fistulas, low fistulas Vaginal exposure may be difficult in some nulliparous patients with narrow introitus and deep vaginal canal

and bladder as an additional layer to promote healing and prevent recurrence.

2) With the advent of robotic laparoscopic surgery, VVF can additionally be repaired via the transabdominal approach using robotic instruments. In this case, it may be helpful to mobilize the omentum laparoscopically prior to placing the patient in steep Trendelenburg and docking the robot to assist in omental placement at the conclusion of the surgery. The same principles apply to robotic fistula surgery as they would in an open approach.
3) Transvaginal approach: Many approaches have been described including Latzko and Raz. Through a vaginal approach, the vaginal wall is mobilized circumferentially about the fistula tract. Either the fistula tract is excised with edges of the debrided tract forming the first layer of closure, or tract is left in situ with fistula edges rolled over forming the primary layer of closure. The

perivesical fascia on either side of the first layer of closure is then imbricated over the primary suture line forming the second layer. A labial fat pad (i.e., Martius flap), peritoneal flap, or gracilis muscle flap may be placed over the suture lines as a well-vascularized flap similar to the omental flap in the transabdominal approach. Finally, a flap of vaginal wall is advanced over the repair forming the final layer of closure.

Regardless of approach, urinary drainage is maintained postoperatively. A cystogram is usually obtained in 2 to 3 weeks following repair to confirm successful closure.

Ureterovaginal Fistula

ETIOLOGY

Most ureterovaginal fistulae are secondary to unrecognized distal ureteral injuries sustained during gynecologic procedures such as abdominal or vaginal hysterectomy, caesarean section, antiincontinence surgery, etc. Occasionally, they may be secondary to endoscopic instrumentation, radiation therapy, pelvic malignancy, penetrating pelvic trauma, or other pelvic surgery (vascular, colonic, etc.).

1. Risk factors for ureteral injuries include a prior history of pelvic surgery, endometriosis, radiation therapy, and Pelvic inflammatory disease (PID).
2. Up to 12% of VVF may have an associated ureterovaginal fistula.

PRESENTATION

May present with clear drainage per vagina or unilateral hydroureteronephrosis and flank pain secondary to partial ureteral obstruction.

Flank pain, nausea, fever, and clear vaginal drainage following pelvic surgery are very suggestive of ureteral injury. Notably, patients will have a normal voiding pattern if the contralateral kidney is unaffected.

EVALUATION

1. CT urogram or intravenous urogram (IVU): A urogram may demonstrate partial obstruction, hydroureteronephrosis, and/or drainage into the vagina.

2. Cystoscopy and retrograde pyelography are performed to evaluate for bladder injury and to visualize the distal ureteral segment if not well seen on the urogram. An attempt at retrograde stenting is reasonable if the imaging demonstrates ureteral continuity. Prolonged internal diversion with ureteral stenting (if possible) may result in resolution of the fistula in select cases.
3. CT/MRI: Cross-sectional imaging may be useful to evaluate for pelvic malignancy when indicated or evaluate for a urinoma in patients with persistent fevers.
4. Cystogram: In cases where a long segment of distal ureter is involved/strictured and a reconstructive procedure such as psoas hitch or Boari flap is being considered, a cystogram may be useful to evaluate the bladder capacity.
5. Percutaneous nephrostomy and antegrade nephrostogram: Percutaneous drainage of the involved kidney followed by antegrade instillation of contrast can provide decompression of a partially obstructed kidney as well as anatomic localization and demonstration of the fistula (Fig. 12.3). An attempt

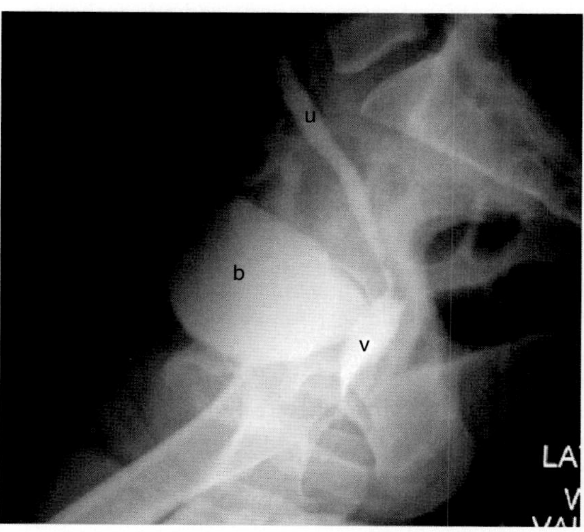

FIGURE 12.3 Antegrade nephrostogram demonstrating ureteral dilation and drainage into the vagina following abdominal hysterectomy. Contrast is seen entering the vagina *(v)* from the ureter *(u)* confirming the diagnosis of ureterovaginal fistula. A simultaneous cystogram demonstrates the bladder *(b)*.

at antegrade ureteral stenting may be successful in treating the fistula if there is ureteral continuity.

THERAPY

1. Percutaneous drainage: If high-grade partial obstruction exists in the setting of sepsis, percutaneous drainage and a course of antibiotic therapy are indicated prior to definitive repair.
2. Ureteral stenting (see previous discussion): Resolution of urinary drainage following placement of a stent suggests that this may be an effective treatment for the fistula. Imaging should be obtained to confirm resolution of the fistula prior to stent removal. Follow-up imaging should also be obtained once the stent is removed to assess for the onset of asymptomatic hydroureteronephrosis due to the development of a ureteric stricture.
3. Surgery: When stenting is unsuccessful, then ureteral reimplantation (with or without psoas hitch/Boari flap) is performed. It is not necessary to excise the distal ureteral segment or even close the fistula unless vesicoureteral reflux is present.
4. Fistulas resulting from advanced pelvic malignancy may best be treated by urinary diversion.

Urethrovaginal Fistula

ETIOLOGY

Usually postsurgical (urethral diverticulectomy, antiincontinence surgery, etc.), although they may occur as a result of trauma, instrumentation (catheterization), radiation, and childbirth (obstetric trauma).

PRESENTATION

Urethrovaginal fistulae are often asymptomatic if located in the distal third of the urethra (beyond the continence mechanism); otherwise, the presentation is similar to VVF. Occasionally, these patients may present with symptoms suggestive of stress or urgency incontinence, and cystourethrography will be necessary to make the diagnosis. Dyspareunia or recurrent urinary tract infection (UTIs) are sometimes seen.

EVALUATION

1. Voiding cystourethrogram (VCUG): Voiding images must be obtained in patients with a competent bladder neck and proximal sphincteric mechanism or the fistula will not be demonstrated.
2. Cystoscopy: Useful to evaluate for concurrent abnormalities of the bladder and urethra.

THERAPY

1. Catheter drainage may be useful in a limited number of cases if the fistula is noted promptly following the causative event.
2. Transvaginal surgical excision with urethral reconstruction, multiple layer closure using periurethral fascia, a labial fat pad (Martius flap), and vaginal wall flaps is usually highly successful.

Enterovesical Fistula

GENERAL CONSIDERATIONS

Enterovesical fistulas may form between any segment of bowel in the pelvis (colon, ileum, etc.) and the bladder.

ETIOLOGY

The most common cause of enterovesical fistula is diverticular disease of the colon (50%–70%). Other common causes include neoplastic disease (colon cancer), inflammatory bowel disease (Crohn disease), radiation therapy, and trauma.

PRESENTATION

1. Enterovesical fistula may present with recurrent UTIs, fecaluria, pneumaturia, and hematuria.
2. Presentation with sepsis or GI symptoms is rare.
3. Gouverneur's syndrome (suprapubic pain, urinary frequency, dysuria and tenesmus) is the hallmark of enterovesical fistula.

EVALUATION

1. Charcoal test: The oral administration of activated charcoal may confirm the diagnosis of enterovesical fistula. Several hours after ingestion, flecks of charcoal may be noted in the urine.

2. Cystoscopy and possible biopsy: Endoscopic visualization has a very high yield for the identification of enterovesical fistula.
   a. 80% to 100% of cases demonstrate bullous edema, erythema, or exudation of feculent material from the fistula site.
   b. Generally, colonic fistulas occur on the left side and dome of the bladder whereas small bowel fistulas occur on the dome and right side of the bladder.
   c. Biopsy of the fistula is indicated in cases where malignancy is suspected.
3. Colonoscopy/barium enema: Although less common than diverticular disease, it is important to exclude primary intestinal malignancy as the cause for the fistula.
4. CT or MRI of the pelvis: Air in the bladder as seen on cross-sectional imaging in the absence of prior lower urinary instrumentation (cystoscopy, catheterization, etc.) or infection is highly suggestive of an enterovesical fistula. CT scan with oral contrast is generally considered to have the best diagnostic yield.
   a. The triad of findings on CT which are suspicious for colovesical fistula consist of:
      1) Bladder wall thickening adjacent to a loop of thickened colon
      2) Air in the bladder (in the absence of previous lower urinary manipulation) and
      3) The presence of colonic diverticula.
5. VCUG may demonstrate the fistulous connection. In some cases, however, the fistula may act as a "flap valve" and contrast will not be seen entering the bowel.
6. Upper tract imaging such as CT urography should be obtained in cases where upper urinary tract involvement is suspected (i.e., malignancy).

THERAPY

1. Bowel rest and hyperalimentation (TPN or total parental nutrition) may allow the spontaneous closure of some enterovesical fistulae.
2. Medical therapy: This is most applicable in enterovesical fistula secondary to Crohn disease. Appropriate use of TPN, corticosteroids, sulfasalazine, and antibiotics may promote spontaneous resolution.

3. Surgery: The application of surgery may involve either one-stage or a multistage approach depending on the presence or absence of inflammation, malignancy, and adjacent organ involvement. In those cases managed with staged procedures, a temporary fecal diversion is performed at the time of fistula repair. Patients with an inflammatory cause of the fistula but without gross contamination can be treated with a one-stage procedure, whereas those with unprepared bowel, gross contamination, or abscess may require a two-stage procedure.
   a. The surgery involves laparotomy, separation of the bladder from the bowel, excision of the fistula tract, primary closure of the urinary tract and either resection and reanastomosis of the involved bowel segment, or a creation of a temporary ostomy.
   b. In some cases partial cystectomy may be necessary.
   c. Interposition of well-vascularized tissue such as omentum between the bowel and bladder may promote healing and prevent recurrence.

Rectourethral Fistula

ETIOLOGY

Rectourethral fistula (RUF) occurs following radical prostatectomy, external beam radiotherapy for pelvic malignancy, pelvic brachytherapy or cryotherapy, inflammatory diseases of the pelvis (e.g., prostatic abscess, Crohn disease), or following penetrating pelvic trauma.

1. During radical prostatectomy, the anterior rectal wall injury may be injured during dissection of the apical portion of the prostate. A postoperative RUF may form from the reconstructed vesicourethral anastomosis to the injured portion of the rectum. In the setting of radical prostatectomy, a prior history of pelvic radiation therapy, rectal surgery, or transurethral resection of the prostate (TURP) is associated with an increased risk of RUF.

PRESENTATION

May present with recurrent UTIs, fecaluria, pneumaturia, or, rarely, urine per rectum. A defect may be palpable at the level of the vesicourethral anastomosis. If a Foley catheter is indwelling, it may be palpable on rectal exam.

EVALUATION

1. Voiding cystourethrography will demonstrate a fistula between the rectum and urethra.
2. CT urogram or intravenous urography may be utilized if there is concern for ureteral injury.
3. Barium enema may be helpful to rule out concurrent colonic malignancy.
4. Cystoscopy and/or colonoscopy.
5. CT or MRI of the pelvis may be utilized to evaluate for inflammatory collections or other pelvic masses (e.g., malignancy).

THERAPY

Many approaches have been advocated for repair of this complex problem. Often however, despite successful repair of the fistula and reconstitution of the GI and GU tracts, the patient may have severe problems with urinary and fecal incontinence postoperatively and should be counseled regarding this possibility prior to attempted repair. Both staged repairs and one-stage repairs have been advocated although most authors would agree that fecal diversion should be performed as an initial measure. In staged repairs, the GI tract is reconstituted only after demonstration of a successful urinary tract repair (usually radiographically). Surgical options include:

1. Colostomy and urethral catheter drainage: an attempt at fecal diversion and urethral drainage is a reasonable option in most patients. With prolonged fecal diversion, the fistula may close over the urethral catheter.
2. Colostomy followed by a combined abdominal and/or perineal approach: the rectum is separated off the urethra and both are closed primarily. Well-vascularized tissue such as omentum or gracilis muscle flap is interposed between the layers.
3. Colostomy followed by a transrectal approach (York-Mason or transphincteric approach): the fistula is exposed using either anal dilation and a speculum, or by transecting the anal sphincters. The fistula is then repaired in multiple layers by advancement and rotation of rectal wall flaps.

Other Urinary Fistula

UROVASCULAR FISTULA

Most commonly these fistulae occur between the ureter and surrounding blood vessels such as the iliacs. Vigorous hematuria in the setting of indwelling stents in a previously irradiated patient or a patient with a history of vascular surgery should alert the physician to the possibility of this type of fistula. If the patient is in extremis (exsanguinating, etc.), immediate surgical or angiographic intervention is indicated. If the patient is stable, imaging studies including CT, MRI, or angiography may be indicated. In some cases, surgery may be avoided with the use of interventional radiological techniques and endovascular stenting.

VESICOUTERINE FISTULA

These rare fistulae most commonly occur following low segment caesarean section. They may present with Youssef syndrome: menouria, apparent amenorrhea, patent cervix, and urinary continence. Treatment is usually surgical and involves either hysterectomy and closure of the bladder (if the patient has completed childbearing) or excision of the fistula tract and separate closure of the bladder and uterus with interposition of omentum. Occasionally, successful treatment has been seen with hormonal induction of amenorrhea and catheter drainage (Figs 12.4a and 4b demonstrating vesicouterine fistula (VUF) on CT with contrast).

Less common urinary fistula include nephropleural, nephrobronchial, vesicocutaneous, ureterocutaneous, urethrocutaneous, pyelocutaneous fistulae.

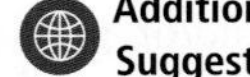

Additional content, including Self-Assessment Questions and Suggested Readings, may be accessed at www.ExpertConsult.com.

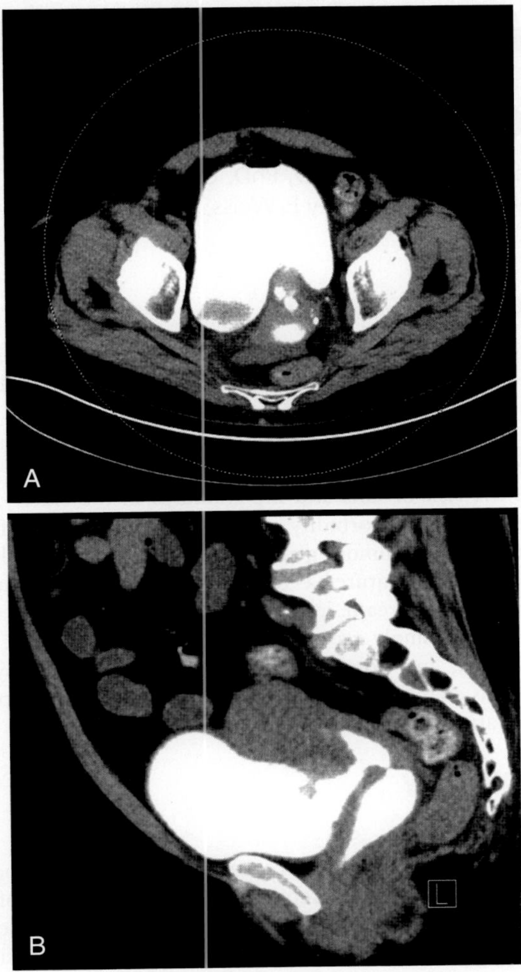

FIGURE 12.4 CT with contrast demonstrating vesicouterine fistula: (A) axial and (B) sagittal. *CT*, Computed tomography.

Nocturia

Thomas F. Monaghan, MD, PhD, Christina W. Augdelo, MD, and Jeffrey P. Weiss, MD, PhD, FACS

Introduction

Nocturia, defined by the International Continence Society as waking to pass urine during the main sleep period, is among the most common and bothersome lower urinary tract symptoms (LUTS) in both men and women of all ages. Nocturia has also been shown to have a direct adverse effect on sleep architecture, as well as increase the risk of falls and hip fractures in the elderly, which lends to significant morbidity and mortality. Although often co-occurring with common genitourinary tract abnormalities, a wealth of recent literature has recognized nocturia as a standalone entity in the mainstream, in large part because nocturnal voiding has been increasingly recognized as a presenting sign, cardinal manifestation, and potential biomarker of underlying systemic disease. This chapter will discuss the epidemiology, pathophysiology, evaluation, and management of nocturia in adults.

Epidemiology

PREVALENCE

Nocturia is one of the most common LUTS in both men and women. The multinational representative Epidemiology of LUTS (EpiLUTS) cross-sectional survey found that nearly 69% of male and 76% of female respondents (age 40 and older) consistently experience one or more nightly voiding episodes. In and of itself, nocturia may constitute the primary urological complaint in both the community and the clinic, but nocturia is also highly interrelated with other voiding abnormalities, identified in upwards of 85% of participants in clinical trials for overactive bladder (OAB). Nocturia is also more common among men with clinically significant benign prostatic hyperplasia (BPH) compared to their community-dwelling counterparts.

The estimated prevalence of nocturia is largely a function of the characteristics of the population at hand. Older age is among the strongest determinants of nocturia, as evidenced by a review on the prevalence of nocturia from Bosch and Weiss, which found nocturia to have been reported by nearly 93% of men and 77% of women aged 70 and older in some community-based populations. Notwithstanding the association between age and nocturia, the aforementioned review found nocturia to also be common among younger cohorts—present in up to 35% of men and 44% of women 20 to 40 years of age. Notably, the Boston Area Community Health (BACH) population-based epidemiologic survey on urologic symptoms and risk factors in adults aged 30 to 79 reported a significantly higher prevalence of nocturia among Black and Hispanic participants compared to White respondents (which persisted even after accounting for differences in socioeconomic status). However, these race-based differences in nocturia prevalence remain poorly understood, and nocturia was nevertheless common across all racial subgroups despite the fact that a majority of BACH respondents were below 50 years of age—ranging from a prevalence of 23% to 38% across racial subgroups.

As will be discussed later in this chapter, many population studies define nocturia as the presence of two or more nocturnal voids because this cutoff has particularly robust associations with morbidity and adverse health-related quality of life outcomes. Even following this higher threshold, Bosch and Weiss found two or more nocturnal voids to have been reported in some studies by nearly one in five community-dwelling younger (aged 20 to 40) men and women, and upwards of 60% of men and women greater than 70 years of age. Taken together, current evidence underscores the pervasive nature of nocturia across multiple criteria in both men and women of all ages and backgrounds.

INCIDENCE

Pesonen and colleagues synthesized current evidence on the incidence, remission, and natural history of nocturia in a recent comprehensive meta-analysis. Pesonen et al. reported a pooled estimate of annual nocturia incidence of 0.4% in adults younger than 40 years of age, 2.8% incidence for those aged 40 to 59 years, and 11.5% in adults 60 years of age and older, with an annual remission rate of 12.1%.

Nocturia and Bother

Nocturia is among the most bothersome LUTS, and LUTS patients with nocturia have been shown to report a significantly greater degree of bother compared to those with only daytime LUTS. Multiple population surveys have identified urinary urgency as the most common reason for nocturnal awakening in adults, and it stands to reason that bother is mediated, in large part, by the direct adverse effect of nocturia on sleep architecture. More specifically, patients reporting a high degree of symptom-related bother are more likely to have **difficulty initiating sleep, as well as difficulty returning to sleep after a nocturnal voiding episode**. Accordingly, sleep quality is an essential component of the initial clinical assessment of nocturia.

Cross-sectional epidemiologic evidence from Tikkinen and colleagues in Finland demonstrates that two or more nocturnal voids is the threshold at which most people begin to report some degree of nocturia-specific bother and impaired quality of life, whereas one void per night does not necessarily confer the adverse effects on quality of life and self-reported health.

Accordingly, nocturia of two or more voids is a highly relevant cutoff in community and clinical nocturia research and used synonymously with "clinically significant nocturia" by some investigators. However, it is important to recognize that **the definition of nocturia does not take into account the degree of bother**. Stated alternatively, individuals who void two or three times per night may report little bother, whereas one void per night may very well be highly bothersome—particularly when it is difficult for the patient to return to sleep. Notably, new multinational observational data from Oelke and colleagues show that most individuals with nocturia live with their symptoms for 1 year or longer before first seeking treatment. Thus, **irrespective of the actual number of nocturnal voids, nocturia which motivates a patient to seek urological care should, by definition, be recognized and treated as "clinically significant."**

Beyond Bother: Nocturia and Quality of Life, Morbidity, and Mortality

Nocturia has been associated with a broad range of adverse effects on health-related quality of life, as well as poor physical and mental health outcomes—the strongest evidence for which stems from the direct adverse effects of nocturia on sleep. Poor sleep has been strongly linked to daytime fatigue, impaired cognition and functional performance, as well as psychiatric disorders, cardiometabolic disease, immune suppression, and other pathologic systemic processes. Multiple epidemiologic studies have identified nocturia as the most common cause of sleep disruption in adults. Importantly, nocturia patients often experience their first nocturnal voiding episode within 2 to 3 hours after going to sleep, which coincides with the time in which slow wave (i.e., N3 or "deep") sleep—the most restorative sleep stage—predominates in the normal sleep cycle. Consistently, a shorter time from sleep onset to the first nocturia episode is associated with lower whole-night sleep quality. Furthermore, a recent pivotal polysomnographic analysis of patients with nocturia from Bliwise and colleagues identified an **independent association between higher nocturnal voiding frequency and loss of slow wave sleep across the *entire* sleep period**. Accordingly, the deleterious effects of nocturia on sleep quality extend far beyond the actual time lost to toileting and trying to fall back asleep.

Nocturia has also been widely implicated as a risk factor for falls and hip fractures in the elderly, which confers a significant risk for morbidity and mortality. Normative aging is associated with decreased functional bladder storage capacity, impaired renal free water conservation, and other physiologic changes which lend to older age being among the strongest predictors of nocturia. Nocturia is not only more prevalent among these patients, but also likely more problematic, given that age also confers and increased risk for disturbances in coordination and gait, decreased muscle strength, cognitive impairment, and vision loss. These factors, compounded by the setting of a dimly lit bedroom, make nocturnal toileting an inherently risky activity for older adults. Notably, a recent landmark meta-analysis from Pesonen and colleagues found nocturia to be associated with a 1.2-fold increased risk of falls and 1.3-fold increased risk of fractures.

Beyond sleep and toileting-related injuries, nocturia is highly relevant to general health and mortality because of its association with several systemic disease states. In recent years, nocturia has been linked to a broad range of cardiovascular diseases, including congestive heart failure, vascular dysfunction, and hypertension, as well as respiratory, renal, hepatic, endocrine, neurologic, psychiatric, and immunologic disease states. Accordingly, nocturnal voiding may be an epiphenomenon of undiagnosed or undermanaged systemic pathology.

The onset of nocturia centers on a mismatch between nocturnal urine production and bladder storage capacity and is highly influenced by sleep-related factors. In patients with congestive heart failure, chronic kidney disease, cirrhosis, and other volume overload states, the recumbency position of sleep has been shown to mobilize fluid sequestered in the third space, culminating in increased nocturnal urine volume. Conversely, cardiometabolic and vascular disease has also been linked to ischemia and oxidative stress to the bladder, likely promoting both overactivity during the filling/storage phase and underactivity during emptying—both of which may contribute to small functional nocturnal bladder storage capacity. Several of the aforementioned comorbidities also contribute to nocturnal voiding via their direct adverse effects on sleep quality. The relationship between nocturia and systemic disorders is further compounded by the fact that medications used to treat the latter, such as diuretics, calcium channel blockers, steroids, and selective serotonin reuptake inhibitors, may promote excess urine volume and sleep impairment.

Taken together, a large body of evidence demonstrates that nocturia is a strong predictor of morbidity and mortality. Most notably, another recent meta-analysis by Pesonen and colleagues reported nocturia to be associated with a 1.3-fold increased risk of mortality. Thus, **the benefits of successful treatment for nocturia are likely far broader than improvement in nocturia-specific bother.**

Causes of Nocturia

Nocturia is highly common in the setting of genitourinary tract abnormalities. As discussed previously, nocturia has also been increasingly recognized as the presenting sign or cardinal manifestation of multiple systemic pathologies, and also highly influenced by concurrent medication utilization and processes related to aging. Additionally, several lifestyle factors, such as excess evening fluid intake, alcohol consumption, and dietary sodium, have been linked to nocturia, and may constitute the primary driving force behind nocturnal voiding, or rather exacerbate predisposing genitourinary tract abnormalities or systemic diseases (Fig. 13.1).

As discussed previously, multiple population surveys have identified urinary urgency as the most common reason for nocturnal awakening in adults. However, a handful of sleep studies involving patients with disordered sleep (and no mention of urinary symptoms) have secondarily identified trips to the bathroom to be a frequent co-occurrence at the time of nocturnal awakening. Taken together, current evidence suggests that the relationship between nocturia and poor sleep quality is likely bidirectional. Thus, the topic of disordered sleep, including dyssomnias (e.g., insomnia disorder, obstructive sleep apnea), parasomnias (e.g., nightmare disorder), as well as impaired sleep secondary to a medical condition (e.g., congestive heart failure,

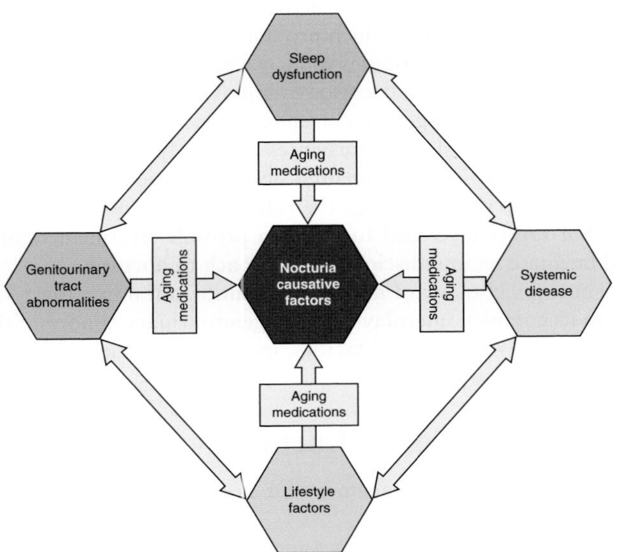

FIGURE 13.1 Causative factors of nocturia.

chronic obstructive pulmonary disease, chronic pain) or psychiatric condition (e.g., depression, anxiety, posttraumatic stress disorder), highly convolutes the pathogenesis of nocturia.

These relationships becomes relevant in view of current International Continence Society terminology, which defines nocturia as the act of awakening during the main sleep period *to pass urine*, and thus may infer that patients with "true" waking *in order to void* must be carefully distinguished from those presenting to the clinic with extraneous causes of nocturnal voiding. Semantics aside, it is essential to recognize that "urinary urgency" varies considerably between individuals, and only modestly correlates with nocturnal urine volume and disease-specific bother in most patients. Furthermore, analyses of urinary urgency based on the robustly validated 5-item urge perception grading scale (commonly incorporated into the standard voiding dairy) have found that self-reported voiding in the absolute absence of urinary urgency (i.e., "convenience voiding") is an exceedingly rare phenomenon in both community and clinical settings. Moreover, primary sleep disturbances may also directly facilitate urge-driven nocturnal voiding. For example, obstructive sleep apnea is well known to cause ventricular strain, which promotes the release of natriuretic peptides and thus contributes to increased urine volume, and also may be associated with detrusor overactivity and urge urinary incontinence. Taken together, current evidence underscores the fact that nocturia and sleep disturbances are highly interrelated, such that **clinical suspicion of impaired sleep in a patient with nocturia should not serve to challenge the validity of their nocturnal voiding, but rather leveraged to broaden possible treatment options and facilitate an interdisciplinary approach to nocturia.**

Thus, the etiology of nocturia is multifactorial in nature, owing to its complex interplay between genitourinary abnormalities, systemic diseases, lifestyle factors, medications, aging, and sleep (Tables 13.1 and 13.2).

Initial Evaluation of Nocturia

The crux of initial management for nocturia is built upon two pillars of care:

1. Comprehensive clinical assessment
2. Voiding diary

TABLE 13.1 Select Etiologies/Causal Factors of Nocturia

Genitourinary Tract Abnormalities	**Systemic Disease Processes**
• Benign prostatic obstruction • Pelvic organ prolapse • Pelvic floor dysfunction/prior surgery (e.g., hysterectomy) • Detrusor overactivity (including idiopathic nocturnal detrusor activity) • Detrusor underactivity • Neurogenic bladder • Prostatitis or cystitis (bacterial, interstitial, tuberculosis, radiation) • Prior bladder surgery/bladder wall fibrosis • Bladder/ureteral calculi • Malignancy of the bladder, prostate, or urethra • Urethral stricture	• Impaired nocturnal arginine vasopressin activity • Congestive heart failure • Metabolic syndrome/obesity • Diabetes mellitus • Chronic kidney disease • Nephrotic syndrome • Liver disease/hypoalbuminemia • Venous insufficiency • Hypertension (especially nocturnal nondipping hypertension) • Primary polydipsia • Central and nephrogenic diabetes insipidus • Hypercalcemia • Hypokalemia • Estrogen deficiency in women
Sleep Disorders	**Lifestyle/Modifiable Factors**
• Insomnia • Obstructive sleep apnea • Periodic leg movements • Arousal disorders • Chronic pain disorders • Impaired sleep secondary to another medical condition • Impaired sleep secondary to a psychiatric condition	• Evening fluid intake • Alcohol • Caffeine • Excess dietary sodium

The comprehensive clinical assessment and voiding diary are equally invaluable, yet individually insufficient, to fully elucidate, characterize, and effectively treat nocturia (Fig. 13.2).

THE CLINICAL ASSESSMENT

The comprehensive clinical assessment of nocturia requires a urological and general medical history, directed review of systems, exploration of relevant lifestyle factors and sleeping

TABLE 13.2 Medications Associated With Nocturia

Increased Urine Output
• Diuretics • Selective serotonin reuptake inhibitors (SSRIs) • Calcium channel blockers • Tetracyclines • Lithium
Insomnia and Central Nervous System (CNS) Effects

• CNS stimulants
  • Dextroamphetamine
  • Methylphenidate
• Antihypertensives
  • α-Blockers
  • β-Blockers
  • Methyldopa
• Respiratory
  • Albuterol
  • Theophylline
• Decongestants
  • Phenylephrine
  • Pseudoephedrine
• Hormones
  • Corticosteroids
  • Thyroid
• Psychotropics
  • Monoamine oxidase inhibitors
  • Selective serotonin reuptake inhibitors
  • Atypical antidepressants
• Dopaminergic agonists (carbidopa)
• Antiepileptics (phenytoin)

Direct Lower Urinary Tract Effects
• Ketamine (direct bladder toxin) • Tiaprofenic acid (Surgam) (toxic cystitis) • Cyclophosphamide

habits, medication reconciliation, and physical examination. Global LUTS and nocturia-specific questionnaires may also be useful in identifying concurrent urinary symptoms and characterizing the impact of nocturia. Altogether, these clinical datapoints can be synthesized to develop a clinical hypothesis as to the potential etiologies contributing to nocturnal voiding. This hypothesis serves as the foundation for subsequent laboratory testing,

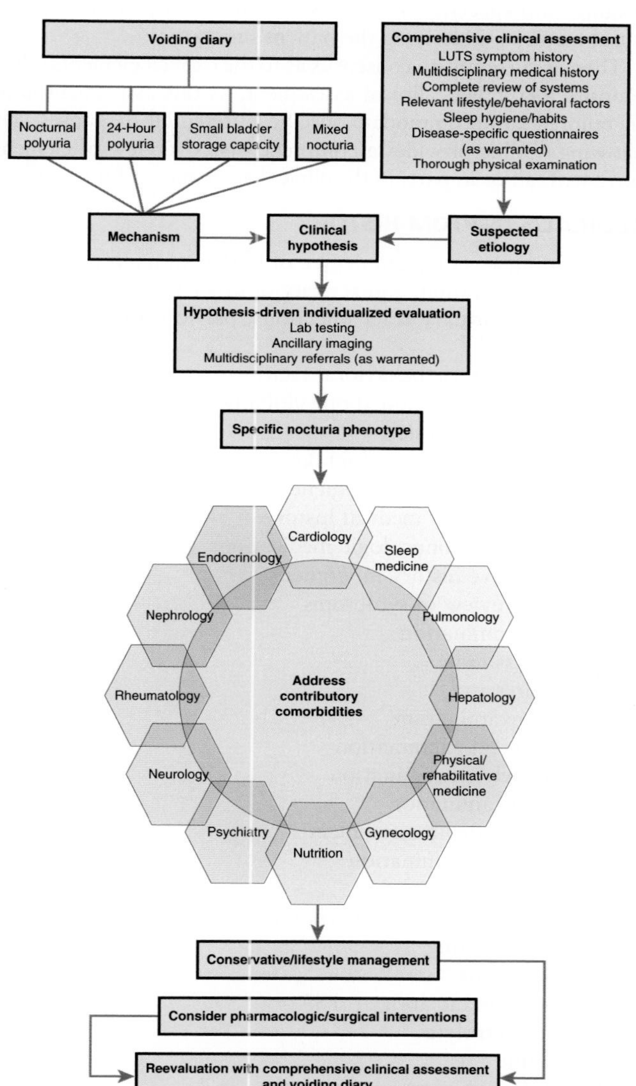

FIGURE 13.2 Algorithm for the evaluation and management of nocturia. *LUTS*, Lower urinary tract symptoms.

imaging, and specialty referral as warranted to establish specific causal factor(s) underlying the patient's nocturia.

There is currently no consensus as to the explicit elements which comprise a complete clinical assessment, as this assessment is often tailored to accommodate specific differential diagnoses. The following outline provides a comprehensive overview of elements warranted (all or in part) in the clinical assessment of nocturia:

MEDICAL/SYMPTOM HISTORY

1. Duration, severity, and degree of bother of nocturia
2. Presence, duration, and severity of other LUTS
3. Recurrent urinary tract infections, pelvic surgery, or radiotherapy
4. Relevant lifestyle/behavioral factors
   a. Fluid consumption (both globally and specifically in the hours prior to sleep)
   b. Caffeine and alcohol intake
   c. Sleeping habits and hygiene
5. Multidisciplinary medical history
6. Urologic and nonurologic medications
7. Reproductive history in women
8. Directed review of symptoms

Physical examination

1. Body mass index
2. Blood pressure
3. Genital examination
4. Digital rectal examination
5. Female pelvic examination
6. Cardiac examination
7. Peripheral edema assessment
8. Respiratory examination
9. Abdominal examination
10. Neurologic examination/reflex testing

Laboratory testing

1. Urine analysis
2. Prostate-specific antigen (PSA)
3. Serum electrolytes
4. Creatinine
5. HbA1c/serum glucose
6. Thyroid hormones

7. Serum lipid profile
8. Brain natriuretic peptide (BNP)

Ancillary testing

1. Postvoid residual volume (PVR)
2. Cystoscopy
3. Electrocardiogram
4. Echocardiogram
5. Fluid/food intake diary
6. Sleep diary/polysomnography
7. Supplemental questionnaires

Nocturia-specific questionnaires

1. Targeting the individual's Aetiology of Nocturia to Guide Outcomes (TANGO)
   a. Nocturia, Nocturnal Enuresis, and Sleep Interruption Questionnaire (NNES-Q)
   b. Nocturia Quality of Life Questionnaire (N-QoL)
2. Global LUTS Questionnaires
   a. Lower Urinary Tract Symptom Score (LUTSS)
   b. International Prostate Symptom Score (IPSS)
   c. Overactive Bladder Symptom Score (OABSS)

THE VOIDING DIARY

It is critically important that the information gleaned through the comprehensive clinical assessment be interpreted in view of the physical mechanism underlying nocturnal voiding, which can only be determined using a voiding diary (Fig. 13.3).

In healthy adults, functional bladder storage capacity is sufficient to hold the volume of urine produced during the hours of sleep. In the absence of primary sleep disturbances, the pathogenesis of nocturia centers on a fundamental mismatch between nocturnal urine production and functional nocturnal bladder storage capacity. In this case, production in excess of capacity gives rise to a sensation of bladder fullness which can overcome the mechanisms maintaining sleep. Accordingly, the majority of cases of nocturia in the clinical setting may be directly attributable to excess urine production and/or insufficient storage capacity.

The voiding diary, which is an objective record of the timing, volume, and urgency accompanying every void across a 24- to 72-hour period, is the main means by which to distinguish the specific mechanism underlying nocturia. Accordingly, the voiding diary is

Voiding diary

Name:____ Date:_______________

Time of day diary started:____________________ ☐ AM ☐ PM

Time you went to bed____________________ Time you got up for the day____________________

Time of urination and / or incontinence episode	Why did you urinate at this time? (see question # (a) for responses)	Amount of urination (measure with a cup in cc, mL or ounces)	Incontinence grade (see question # (b) below for responses)
1			
2			
3			
4			
5			
6			
7			
8			
9			
10			
11			
12			
13			
14			
15			

Please select the number next to your answer and use it for your response to the above questions.

(a) Why did you urinate?

(0) Out of convenience (no urge or desire)
(1) Because I have a mild urge (but can delay urination for over an hour if I have to)
(2) Because I have a moderate urge (but can delay urination for more than 10 but less than 60 minutes if I have to)
(3) Because I have a severe urge (but can delay urination for less than 10 minutes)
(4) Because I have desperate urge (must stop what I am doing and go immediately)

(b) Incontinence grade.

(0) Grade 0 - some drops
(1) Grade 1 - moderate loss (damp underpants)
(2) Grade 2 - extensive loss (wet underpants)
(3) Grade 3 - massive loss (wet outer clothes)

FIGURE 13.3 The voiding diary.

a gold standard in the initial evaluation and management of nocturia, irrespective of the suspected etiology behind the production-storage mismatch.

INTERPRETING THE VOIDING DIARY

Several parameters can be derived from the standard voiding diary and are useful in delineating the mechanisms underlying nocturia and optimizing management (Table 13.3).

TABLE 13.3 Overview of Voiding Diary Parameters

Parameter	Definition
Sleeping hours	The time from when an individual goes to bed with the intention of sleeping until they awaken with the intention of rising
Actual number of nightly voids (ANV)	Number of voids passed during sleeping hours
24-hour total urine volume (TUV)	Total volume of urine passed in a 24-hour period
Nocturnal urine volume (NUV)	Total volume of urine produced during sleeping hours; includes the first morning void volume
Maximum voided volume (MVV)	The single largest voided volume passed in a 24-hour period
Nocturnal maximum voided volume (NMVV)	The single largest voided volume passed during sleeping hours
Nocturia index (Ni)	Nocturnal urine volume/maximum voided volume; a nocturia index >1 indicates that nocturnal urine volume exceeds functional bladder capacity and nocturia or enuresis occurs
Nocturnal urine production (NUP)	Nocturnal urine volume/sleeping hours (mL/hour)
Nocturnal polyuria index (NPi)	Nocturnal urine volume/24-hour total urine volume
Nocturnal bladder capacity index (NBCi)	(Actual number of nightly voids − [nocturia index − 1]); nocturnal bladder capacity index >0 indicates that nocturia occurs at voided volumes less than the maximum voided volume
First uninterrupted sleep period (FUSP)	Time between when the individual goes to bed with the intention of sleeping to the time of first unintended awakening
First nocturnal void volume (FNVV)	Volume of urine passed at the time of first unintended awakening

SPECIFIC VOIDING DIARY–DERIVED DIAGNOSES

Nocturnal Polyuria

1. Excess nocturnal urine production during the main sleep period.
2. Multiple definitions for nocturnal polyuria have been proposed. Irrespective of the exact definition employed, nocturnal polyuria is thought to be the most common cause of nocturia in both men and women of all ages.
3. The most common nocturnal polyuria criterion is a **nocturnal polyuria index (nocturnal urine volume/24-hour total urine volume) >0.33.**
4. Another common cutoff for nocturnal polyuria is **nocturnal urine production >90 mL/hour.** The nocturnal urine production-based threshold for nocturnal polyuria has been shown to be more specific but less sensitive for nocturia in community-based population studies.

Global Polyuria

1. Excess urine production across the 24-hour period.
2. Defined as urine production greater than **40 mL/kg body weight in 24 hours.**

Small Bladder Storage Capacity

1. No consensus exists on a single cutoff for small bladder storage capacity, but values less than **200 to 300 mL are considered abnormal.**
2. Although actual voided volumes *plus* PVRs more accurately describe the true functional bladder capacity, **24-hour maximum voided volumes are used as a readily attainable proxy for small bladder storage capacity assessment.**
3. Small bladder capacity may occur across the 24-hour period or specifically during the hours of sleep.
4. The nocturnal bladder capacity index quantifies the discrepancy between a patient's own maximum voided volume and the volumes at which nocturnal voids actually occur. A nocturnal bladder capacity index >0 indicates that nocturia occurs at voided volumes less than maximum voided volume, and values >2 are strongly associated with severe nocturia.

Abnormalities in the nocturnal bladder capacity index are consistent with decreased nocturnal functional bladder storage capacity.

Mixed Nocturia

1. Nocturnal polyuria, global polyuria, and small bladder capacity are not mutually exclusive, and any combination of these diagnoses may occur.

FURTHER VOIDING DIARY–BASED CHARACTERIZATION OF NOCTURIA

Nocturia Severity

1. The actual number of nocturnal voids is often used to approximate and quantify "nocturia severity."
2. Although limited by the fact that it does not account for the patient's degree of bother, the actual number of nocturnal voids is clinically relevant because the baseline number of voids is directly related to the expected treatment effect across all treatment modalities.

Degree of Production-Storage Mismatch

1. As discussed previously, a mismatch between nocturnal urine production and bladder storage capacity is the fundamental basis for a vast majority of cases of nocturia in the clinical setting.
2. This mismatch is reflected in the nocturia index (nocturnal urine volume divided by maximum voided volume), which considers nocturnal urine production as a function of the patient's own bladder capacity.
3. The nocturia index is the voiding diary parameter most strongly correlated with nocturia severity.

Early Hours of Sleep

1. The first uninterrupted sleep period (time from sleep onset to the first nocturic episode) and accompanying first nocturnal voided volume help to characterize nocturia in the early hours of sleep.
2. Most patients with nocturia experience their first nocturia episode within the first 2 to 3 hours of sleep.

3. The early hours of sleep are particularly meaningful because of the clustering of slow wave sleep during this phase—the most restorative sleep stage.
4. The volume of the first nocturnal void (i.e., urine production in the early hours of sleep) is likely a key mediator of the duration of the first uninterrupted sleep period.
5. Prolongation of the first uninterrupted sleep period improves whole-night sleep quality and may be a target of nocturia treatment.

Treatment

Information gleaned through a comprehensive clinical assessment, coupled with a voiding diary–based mechanistic characterization of the patient's nocturia, can collectively pinpoint the most likely underlying etiology and individualize the treatment plan.

TRENDS IN TREATMENT

General strategy: As nocturia is a cardinal feature of several systemic disease states, best practice management often warrants an interdisciplinary approach, with effective coordination and communication with the primary medical doctor and other specialty services including, but certainly not limited to, sleep medicine, cardiology, pulmonology, hepatology, nephrology, endocrinology, neurology, psychiatry, rheumatology, physical/rehabilitative medicine, pain medicine, gynecology, and nutrition. **By recognizing nocturia as a potential biomarker of systemic disease, the urologist has a unique platform from which to tangibly improve morbidity and overall survival.**

Treat the underlying disease: **Treatment directly targeting congestive heart failure, obstructive sleep apnea, and other serious comorbidities also has a marked effect on improving the severity of nocturia.** In fact, of all treatment modalities, the greatest effect on nocturia is seen with continuous positive airway pressure (CPAP) therapy in sleep apnea patients, consistently reported to improve severe nocturia by two or more voids in multiple studies.

Taken together, current evidence suggests a bidirectional response to treatment, wherein **urologic interventions for nocturia**

are likely to improve sleep, fall risk, and other significant mediators of morbidity and mortality, while those nocturia patients with identifiable comorbidities can expect significant improvement once their other health needs have been addressed.

Conservative measures: Current evidence suggests that conservative management, such as promoting sleep hygiene, evening fluid restriction, bladder and pelvic floor training, emptying the bladder immediately prior to going to bed, limiting dietary sodium intake, physical exercise, weight loss, and cardiovascular risk factor optimization (e.g., blood pressure, glycemic control) are effective across multiple etiologies/mechanisms of nocturia, and **should be considered before primary pharmacologic or surgical interventions in most patients unless otherwise medically contraindicated** (Fig. 13.4).

Pharmacologic strategies: Medications including α-blockers, 5-ARIs, antimuscarinics, and antimuscarinics plus α-blockers have been found to result in statistically significant reduction in nocturia episodes, but are generally less effective than surgical interventions, and **the clinical significance of these existing pharmacologic agents is modest.**

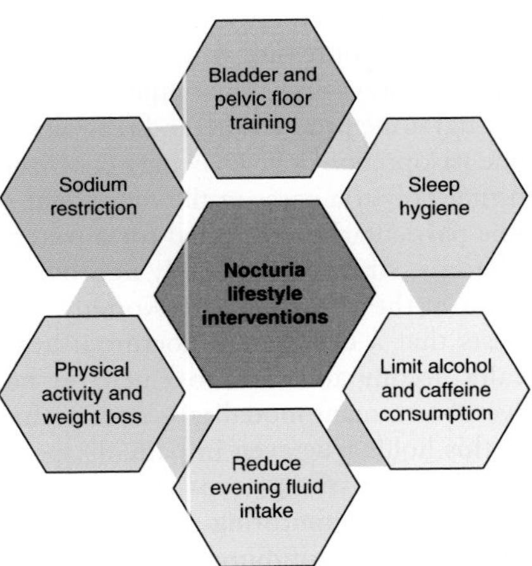

FIGURE 13.4 Evidence-based conservative management strategies for nocturia.

Surgery: Surgical interventions, including transurethral resection of prostate (TURP), transurethral needle ablation (TUNA), high-intensity focused ultrasound (HIFU), visual laser ablation (VLAP), transurethral electrosurgical vaporization (TUVP), and transurethral microwave therapy (TUMT), have been used to address BPH, but very few studies look specifically at these interventions for treatment of nocturia. Procedures that reduce bladder outlet obstruction and lower the PVR volume may increase the amount of time that it takes to reach a volume at which the patient feels the need to void. Regardless, nocturia does not respond as well as daytime LUTS to surgery for relief of bladder outlet obstruction, even though the number of nocturnal micturitions may decline after TURP, TUMT, HIFU, TUNA, and TUVP. **Surgery for relief of bladder outlet obstruction is not indicated for the management of patients with a primary complaint of nocturia unless it is clearly demonstrated that the patient has prostatic obstruction and multiple conservative interventions for nocturia have proven ineffective.** In this regard, preoperative urodynamic investigation may be useful before recommending TURP in men with nocturia as their predominant LUTS.

Recent advancements: In the absence of identifiable contributory comorbidities or lifestyle factors, patients with nocturnal polyuria are thought to have impaired circadian rhythmicity of endogenous arginine vasopressin, which plays a key role in nocturnal free water conservation. This impairment naturally lends to excess nocturnal urine production, and real-world data suggest that an arginine vasopressin deficiency may constitute upwards of 40% of nocturnal polyuria cases in the outpatient setting. These patients may be particularly well suited for a trial of antidiuretic replacement therapy, which was recently approved for the treatment of nocturia in the United States. Notably, however, recent research suggests that a decrease in nocturnal urine production characteristically accompanies improvement in nocturia severity (irrespective of treatment modality)—and, perhaps somewhat paradoxically, this holds true even in patients specifically with a small functional bladder storage capacity. **Careful patient selection and routine sodium monitoring are needed to identify those most likely to respond to antidiuretic replacement therapy and mitigate the risk for clinically significant hyponatremia.**

CLINICAL PEARLS

1. Nocturia is associated with significant morbidity and mortality, owing, in large part, to its adverse effects on sleep architecture, and status as an independent predictor of falls and hip fractures in the elderly.
2. Nocturia has a multifactorial etiology, which may include genitourinary abnormalities, systemic diseases, sleep disorders, lifestyle factors, medications, and processes related to aging—all of which may cause nocturia in of themselves, but often coexist and interact in a complex fashion.
3. The etiology of nocturia must be understood and treated in view of the specific nocturnal urine production-storage mismatch mechanism(s) at play. This assessment can only be accomplished with a **voiding diary—a best practice standard in the evaluation and management of nocturia.**
4. **Because nocturia is often a manifestation of systemic disease, the urologist—both directly and as the catalyst for integrative care—is uniquely positioned to not only ameliorate a highly bothersome symptom, but also tangibly improve morbidity and mortality.**
5. The first step in treatment of nocturia is addressing identifiable contributory comorbidities and lifestyle factors, which will likely improve both nocturia and general health outcomes.
6. Several conservative interventions for nocturia have proven benefits across diverse patient populations and should be favored as first-line interventions unless contraindicated.
7. α-Blockers, 5-alpha reductase inhibitors, antimuscarinics, and antimuscarinics plus α-blockers have a minimal clinical benefit.
8. Surgery is not indicated for the management of patients with a primary complaint of nocturia unless it is clearly demonstrated that the patient has prostatic obstruction and nonsurgical treatment strategies have failed.
9. Antidiuretic replacement therapy, recently approved in the United States for the treatment of nocturia, has a significant benefit in reducing nocturnal urine volume and prolonging the time from sleep onset to the first nocturia episode, but requires careful patient selection to optimize treatment response—particularly in view of the potential risk for clinically significant hyponatremia.

Additional content, including Self-Assessment Questions and Suggested Readings, may be accessed at www.ExpertConsult.com.

Lower Urinary Tract Function and Dysfunction; Urinary Incontinence

Alan J. Wein, MD, PhD (Hon), FACS, Diane K. Newman, DNP, ANP-BC, FAAN, and Ariana L. Smith, MD

Introduction

The lower urinary tract (LUT) functions as a group of interrelated structures with a joint function in the adult to bring about efficient and low-pressure bladder filling, low-pressure urine storage with perfect continence, and periodic complete voluntary urinary expulsion, again at low pressure. Because in the adult the LUT is normally under voluntary neural control, it is clearly different from other visceral organs, which are regulated primarily by involuntary mechanisms.

For description and teaching, the micturition cycle is best divided into two relatively discrete phases: bladder filling/urine storage and bladder emptying/voiding. The micturition cycle normally displays these two modes of operation in a simple on-off fashion. The cycle involves switching from activation of storage reflexes and inhibition of the voiding reflex to inhibition of the storage reflexes and activation of the voiding reflex and back again. In this chapter, we first summarize some relevant facts regarding the anatomy, neuroanatomy, physiology, and pharmacology of the LUT. We then answer certain important functional questions related to the filling/storage phase and the emptying/voiding phase of micturition. Certain "rules" are formulated that must be satisfied for the LUT to function normally. By extrapolation, these "rules" are used as a basis for a very simple functional classification of voiding dysfunction and as a framework to understand urodynamic evaluation and the rationale for all types of treatment. The neurourologic evaluation, classification schemes for voiding dysfunction and the more common types of neurogenic and nonneurogenic voiding dysfunction are considered, followed by a synopsis and summation of pertinent points relative to all types of treatment for filling/storage and for emptying/voiding disorders. Benign prostatic hyperplasia (BPH) and related issues are discussed in Chapter 15.

Relevant Lower Urinary Tract Anatomy, Physiology, Pharmacology, and Terminology

BLADDER, URETHRA, SMOOTH AND STRIATED SPHINCTER

The designation *LUT* includes the bladder, urethra, and periurethral striated muscle. Anatomically and embryologically, the bladder traditionally has been divided into detrusor and trigone regions. The terms *bladder body* and *bladder base* refer to a functional rather than an anatomic division of bladder smooth muscle. This is based on distinct differences in neuromorphology and neuropharmacology between the smooth muscle lying circumferentially above (body) and below (base) the level of the entrance of the ureters posteriorly. The smooth sphincter refers to the smooth muscle of the bladder neck and proximal urethra. This sphincter is not anatomic but physiologic and is not under voluntary control. Others refer to this area as the *internal urethral sphincter*, the *proximal urethral sphincter*, and, simply, the *bladder neck sphincter*. Although most would accept the facts that the proximal urethra is that portion of the LUT between the bladder neck and "urogenital diaphragm" in both sexes and that it contains smooth muscle capable of affecting urethral resistance, there is virtually no physiologic or pharmacologic change that affects the smooth muscle of the bladder urethra without also affecting the smooth muscle of the most proximal urethra and bladder neck. Normally, resistance increases in the area of the smooth sphincter during bladder filling and urine storage and decreases during a normal voluntary emptying bladder contraction. In the human proximal urethra, there is a thick, primarily longitudinal smooth muscle layer and a thinner outer circular layer. The longitudinal layer is believed by many, but not all, clinicians to be continuous with the musculature of the bladder base. Teleologically, this arrangement is consistent with a tonic role of the circular layer in maintaining closure during filling and storage and a phasic role for the longitudinal layer in contributing to the opening of the urethra during voiding. The bladder body does not contain discrete unidirectional layers of smooth muscle as suggested by some older texts. In the bladder base, there is a more-or-less layer-like arrangement of smooth muscle, loosely organized into inner and outer longitudinal and middle circular layers. The superficial and deep layers of the trigone musculature lie on the posterior bladder base smooth muscle.

The classic view of the external urethral sphincter, or external sphincter, is that of a striated muscle within the leaves of a "urogenital diaphragm" that extends horizontally across the pelvis. This view includes the fact that it is responsible for stopping the urinary stream when the command "stop voiding" is obeyed. The striated sphincter concept expands this definition to include intramural and extramural portions. The extramural periurethral portion is under voluntary control and corresponds roughly to the "classic" external urethral sphincter, although there is in reality no unbroken sheet of muscle which extends across the pelvis in either male or female, and thus, no true "urogenital diaphragm" exists. The intramural portion denotes skeletal muscle that is intimately associated with and a part of the urethra in both sexes above the maximal condensation of extramural striated muscle, and which is continuous from that level for a variable distance to the bladder neck in the female and at least to the apex of the prostate in the male, forming an integral part of the outer muscular layer of the urethra. Some call this intramural portion the *intrinsic rhabdosphincter*. Although differences of opinion exist regarding the ultrastructure and physiologic type of striated muscle fibers at various points within the striated sphincter mechanism, there is agreement on the general concept of a gradual increase in activity in the striated sphincter area during bladder filling, maintenance with the potential of increases in this activity during bladder storage, and virtual disappearance of this activity just prior to normal emptying/voiding.

INNERVATION AND RECEPTOR FUNCTION

1. **Autonomic nervous system (ANS):** The physiology and pharmacology of the LUT cannot be separated from those of the

ANS. There are many differences between the ANS and the somatic nervous system (SNS), but the one easiest for clinicians to understand and remember is that the ANS includes all efferent neural pathways having ganglionic synapses outside the central nervous system (CNS). There are no synapses between the CNS and the motor end plates of peripheral structures (striated muscle) in the SNS. Voluntary versus involuntary control is *not* a difference: micturition in the adult human is a voluntary act.

2. **Sympathetic and parasympathetic:** The terms *sympathetic* and *parasympathetic* refer simply to anatomic divisions of the ANS. The sympathetic division consists of those fibers that originate in the thoracic and lumbar regions of the spinal cord, whereas the parasympathetic division refers to those fibers that originate in the cranial and sacral regions.
3. **Innervation and neuronal interaction:** The "classic" older view of the peripheral ANS involves a two-neuron system—preganglionic neurons emanating from the CNS and making synaptic contact with cells within ganglia, from which postganglionic neurons emerge to innervate peripheral organs (Fig. 14.1). This relatively simple concept is still useful for the purposes of discussion but has undergone much expansion and modification. Most autonomic innervation of the LUT actually emanates from peripheral ganglia that are at a short distance from, adjacent to, or within the organs they innervate (the urogenital short neuron system). Additionally, the efferent autonomic pathways frequently do not conform to the classic two-neuron model, as they are often interrupted by more than one synaptic relay. For many years, the only autonomic neurotransmitters recognized were acetylcholine and norepinephrine. It has become obvious that other transmitters are involved in various components of the ANS, and a once relatively simple concept of chemical neurotransmission has been expanded to include synaptic systems that involve modulator transmitter mechanisms, prejunctional inhibition or enhancement of transmitter release, postjunctional modulation of transmitter action, cotransmitter release, and secondary involvement of locally synthesized hormones and other substances. All of these are subject to neuronal and hormonal regulation, desensitization, and hypersensitization. Finally, these relationships

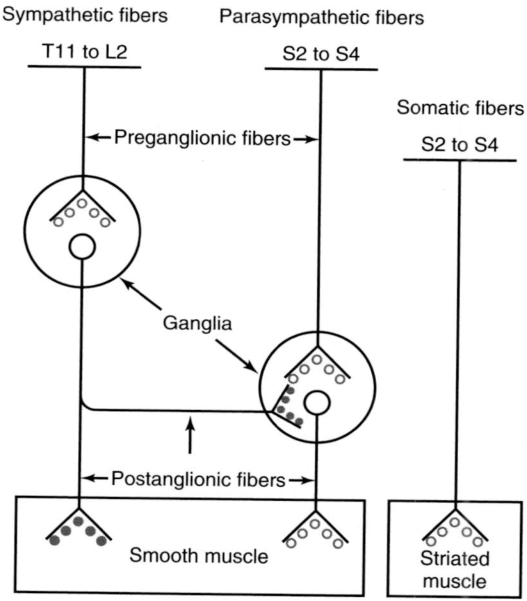

Nature of primary chemical transmitter

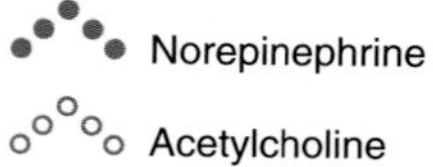

FIGURE 14.1 Classical neuroanatomic and neuropharmacologic description of the innervation of the smooth muscle of the bladder and urethra and the striated muscle of the external urethral sphincter. Note the termination of some postganglionic sympathetic (adrenergic) fibers of parasympathetic ganglion cells, providing the morphologic substrate for sympathetic inhibition of parasympathetic ganglion cell transmission. Note also the lack of ganglia in the somatic innervation. (From Hanno P, Malkowicz SB, Wein A, eds. *Clinical Manual of Urology*, ed. 3. New York: McGraw-Hill; 2001:F14-1, 341.)

may be altered by changes that occur secondary to disease or destruction in the neural axis, obstruction of the LUT, aging, and hormonal status.

4. **Bladder smooth muscle contraction and relaxation:** The classic model of smooth muscle contraction involves synaptic release of neurotransmitters in response to neural stimulation,

with the transmitter agents subsequently combining with a recognition site, or receptor, on the postsynaptic smooth muscle cell membrane. The transmitter-receptor combination then initiates changes (signal transduction) in the postsynaptic effector cell that ultimately results in what we recognize as the characteristic effect of that particular neurotransmitter on that particular smooth muscle.

5. **Excitation contraction coupling:** In bladder smooth muscle, this has been classically described as mediated by mobilization of intracellular calcium via activation of phosphoinositide hydrolysis. The cytosolic calcium binds to calmodulin, initiating the cascade of events necessary to phosphorylate myosin and cause contraction. Relaxation is mediated by a decrease in intracellular calcium. This is accomplished by extrusion extracellularly or reuptake into intracellular stores, generally considered to be the sarcoplasmic reticulum. Smooth muscle relaxation can also be produced by causing intracellular potassium efflux, resulting in membrane hyperpolarization. Both of these latter actions are potential pharmacologic targets for decreasing bladder contractility. Unfortunately, there are no bladder-selective calcium channel blockers or potassium channel openers. It has also been proposed that other pathways for activation or augmentation of bladder contraction include calcium influx through L-type calcium channels and by increased sensitivity to calcium of the contractile machinery by inhibition of myosin light chain phosphatase through activation of Rho kinase.
6. **Neurotransmitter terminology—cholinergic and adrenergic subtypes:** Clinicians are often confused because they assume that the terms *sympathetic* and *parasympathetic* imply particular neurotransmitters. These terms imply only anatomic origin within the ANS. Other adjectives are used to describe the nature of the neurotransmitter involved (see Fig. 14.1). The term *cholinergic* refers to those receptor sites where acetylcholine is a primary neurotransmitter. Peripheral cholinergic fibers include somatic motor fibers, all preganglionic autonomic fibers, and all postganglionic parasympathetic fibers. The cholinergic receptor sites on autonomic effector cells are termed *muscarinic*. Atropine and its congeners competitively inhibit muscarinic receptor sites. Cholinergic receptor sites on

autonomic ganglia and on motor end plates of skeletal muscle are designated *nicotinic*. These are not atropine sensitive. We will not consider these further. The term *adrenergic* is applied to those receptor sites where a catecholamine is the neurotransmitter. Most postganglionic sympathetic fibers terminate on adrenergic receptor sites, including those to LUT smooth muscle, where the catecholamine responsible for neurotransmission is norepinephrine. Adrenergic receptor sites are further classified as alpha (α) or beta (β) on the basis of the differential effects elicited by a series of catecholamines and their antagonists. Classically, the term *α-adrenergic effect* designates vasoconstriction and/or contraction of smooth musculature in response to norepinephrine. These effects are inhibited by phentolamine, phenoxybenzamine, prazosin, and related compounds. The term *β-adrenergic effect* implies smooth muscle relaxation in response to catecholamine stimulation and also includes cardiac stimulation, vasodilation, and bronchodilation. These effects are stimulated most potently by isoproterenol (much more so than by norepinephrine) and antagonized by multiple β-blocker compounds, of which propranolol is a prototype.

7. **Receptor subtyping:** This a relevant concept that explains why some neurotransmitters have differing effects in different organs or anatomic localizations. Subtyping can be based on functional assays, radioligand-binding affinity, or on cloning established genotypes. For instance, there are five different muscarinic receptor subtypes (M_1-M_5). Although it appears that the majority of these in human bladder smooth muscle are of the M_2 subtype, bladder smooth muscle contraction is mediated primarily by the M_3 subtype. There are multiple subtypes of α- and β-adrenergic receptors as well. These are generally tissue specific and explain the selectivity of certain responses. The concept underlies the development of relatively receptor subtype selective drugs for the treatment of BPH and other LUT dysfunctions. Alpha-adrenergic receptors (α-ARs) can be found in the detrusor smooth muscle, the vasculature, afferent and efferent nerve terminals, and intramural ganglia. The predominant receptor subtypes are α_{1D} and α_{1a}, but the total α-$_1$ AR expression is low, and they do not seem to have a significant role in an emptying bladder contraction. Their

density is highest in the bladder base (the area circumferentially below the ureteral entrances posteriorly), bladder neck, and proximal urethra, where they are thought to play a role in the increasing outlet resistance that occurs during bladder filling/storage. There are three subtypes of β-ARs, the most predominant in the bladder being β_3, and the response to activation is detrusor smooth muscle relaxation. These receptors (β-ARs) predominate in the bladder body and are less dense in the base and proximal urethra. Adding to the complexity is the fact that neurotransmitters may have no effect or differing effects at different sites (i.e., brain, pons, spinal cord, efferent ganglia, presynaptic and postsynaptic neural effector junction, sensory afferent fibers, ganglia). In this chapter, we concentrate on peripheral smooth muscle actions.

8. **Other peripheral neurotransmitters:** Other nonadrenergic noncholinergic (NANC) peripheral neurotransmitters exist in the LUT and their roles in normal and abnormal states is the object of much current investigation. These are summarized in Table 14.1. Note, however, that the presence of a potential neurotransmitter and a laboratory tissue response to an agonist or/and antagonist does not necessarily imply physiologic function.
9. **Peripheral innervation:** The pelvic and hypogastric nerves supply the bladder and urethra with efferent parasympathetic and sympathetic innervation, and both convey afferent sensory impulses from these organs to the spinal cord (Fig. 14.2). The parasympathetic efferent supply is classically described as originating in the gray matter of the interomediolateral cell column of sacral spinal cord segments S2-S4. This preganglionic supply is ultimately conveyed by the pelvic nerve. These fibers synapse with cholinergic postganglions in the pelvic plexus or in ganglia within the bladder wall. Efferent sympathetic fibers to the bladder and urethra are thought to originate in the interomediolateral cell column and nucleus intercalatus of spinal cord segments T11-L2 and are carried within the hypogastric nerves. Bilaterally, at a variable distance from the bladder and urethra, the hypogastric and pelvic nerves meet and branch to form the pelvic plexus. Divergent branches of this pelvic plexus innervate the pelvic organs. Efferent innervation of the striated sphincter is classically thought to be somatic and to emanate

TABLE 14.1 Possible Peripheral Transmitters and Modulators in the Lower Urinary Tract

Transmitter (Receptor)	Effect	Site of Action
Acetylcholine (M_3)	Contraction	Bladder smooth muscle
Acetylcholine (M_3, M_2)	Excitation	Peripheral afferents
Acetylcholine (M_2)	Contraction	Bladder smooth muscle
Acetylcholine (M_1, M_3)	Contraction	Prejunctional
Acetylcholine (M_2, M_4)	Relaxation	Prejunctional
Norepinephrine (β_3)	Relaxation	Bladder smooth muscle
Norepinephrine (α_1)	Contraction	Bladder smooth muscle
Adenosine triphosphate ($P2X_1$)	Contraction	Bladder smooth muscle
Adenosine triphosphate ($P2X_3$)	Excitation	Peripheral afferents
Nitric oxide (NO)	Relaxation	Bladder base smooth muscle
Nitric oxide (NO)	Inhibition	Peripheral afferents
Serotonin (5-HT_1, 5-HT_2)	Contraction	Bladder smooth muscle
Prostanoids	Contraction	Bladder smooth muscle
Prostanoids	Excitation	Peripheral afferents
Leukotrienes (LTB_4)	Contraction	Bladder smooth muscle
Angiotensin (AT1)	Contraction	Bladder smooth muscle
Bradykinin (B_2)	Contraction	Bladder smooth muscle
Endothelin (ETa)	Contraction	Bladder smooth muscle
Tachykinins (NK2)	Contraction	Bladder smooth muscle
Vasopressin (V1)	Contraction	Bladder smooth muscle
Vasoactive intestinal peptide ($VPAC_1$/VPC_2)	Relaxation	Bladder smooth muscle
Parathormone	Relaxation	Bladder smooth muscle

(Adapted from Andersson KE, Wein AJ. Pharmacology of the lower urinary tract: basis for current and future treatments of urinary incontinence. *Pharmacol Rev.* 2004;56:581-631; Michel MC, Andersson KE, eds. *Handbook of Experimental Pharmacology: Urinary Tract.* Berlin: Springer; 2011.)

from the Onuf nucleus in sacral spinal cord segments S2-S4, exiting the spinal cord as the pudendal nerve. Some clinicians believe that the striated sphincter, especially the rhabdosphincter, is innervated by branches of the ANS as well.

The afferents traveling in the pelvic nerve are primarily responsible for the initiation of the micturition reflex in the

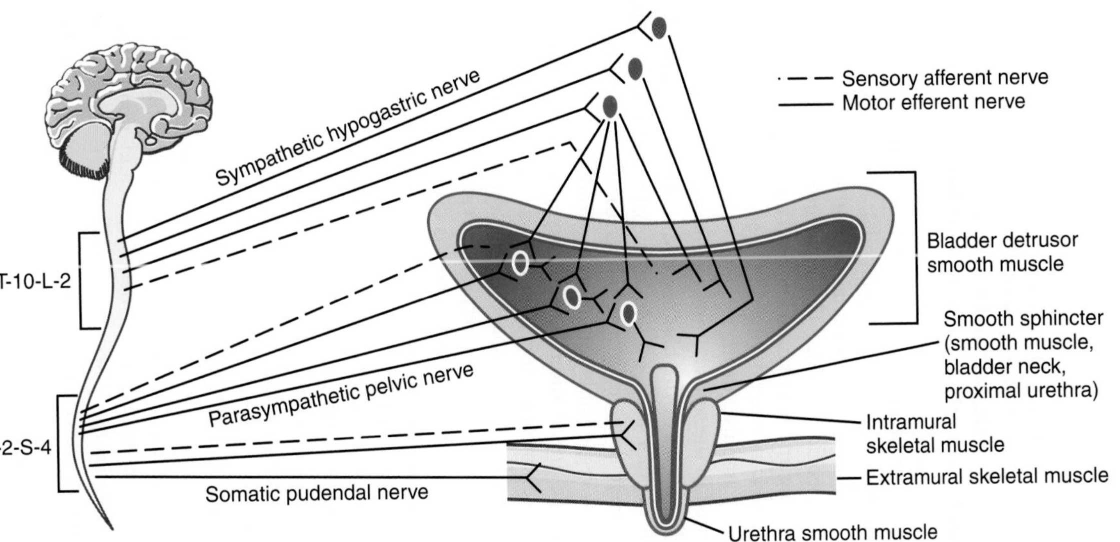

FIGURE 14.2 A current conceptualization of lower urinary tract innervation. (Adapted from Wein AJ. Pharmacologic agents for the treatment of incontinence due to overactive bladder. *Expert Opin Investig Drugs*. 2001;10:65-83.)

normal state. Myelinated A-delta fibers normally subserve this function and convey mechanoreceptor input. Unmyelinated C-fiber afferents are more prevalent but remain relatively silent during normal filling and storage. These become "awakened" and functional under various conditions (i.e., responses to distention after spinal cord injury [SCI], to cold—the "ice water test," to nociceptive stimuli). Myelinated somatic afferents from the striated sphincter travel in the pudendal nerve. Afferents also travel in the hypogastric nerve, but little is known about their specific function. The most important afferents for initiating and maintaining normal micturition are those in the pelvic nerve, relaying to the sacral spinal cord. These convey impulses from tension, volume, and nociceptors located in the serosal, muscle, and urothelial and suburothelial layers of the bladder and urethra. In a neurologically normal adult, the sensations of filling and distention are what develop during filling/storage and initiate the reflexes responsible for emptying/voiding.

10. **Cholinergic innervation and parasympathetic stimulation:** Cholinergic innervation is abundant to all areas of the bladder of animals and humans. Although most researchers agree on the existence of a cholinergic innervation of at least of the proximal urethra in animals, there is disagreement regarding the extent (and in some cases existence) of a similar innervation in humans. It is generally agreed that abundant muscarinic cholinergic receptor sites exist throughout the bladder body and base musculature of various animal species and of humans, and that they are more numerous in the bladder body. A sustained bladder contraction is produced by stimulation of the pelvic nerves, and it is generally agreed that reflex activation of this pelvic nerve excitatory tract is primarily or exclusively responsible for the emptying bladder contraction of normal micturition and for the involuntary bladder contractions seen with various neurologic and nonneurologic diseases/conditions. Whether acetylcholine is the sole neurotransmitter released in a normal human during such stimulation is highly controversial. Atropine resistance refers to the incomplete antagonism produced by atropine of the bladder response to pelvic nerve stimulation or of isolated bladder

strips to electrical field stimulation (producing intramural neural stimulation). This is in contrast to atropine's ability to completely block the response of bladder smooth muscle strips to exogenous acetylcholine. It is generally agreed that atropine resistance occurs in various experimental animal models, and the most logical explanation seems to be release of additional neurotransmitter(s) besides acetylcholine in response to nerve stimulation. Adenosine triphosphate (ATP) is most commonly mentioned as the prime candidate. Normally, atropine resistance does not seem to occur in humans. However, some experts feel that different types of atropine resistance may exist in various types of abnormal bladder overactivity, regardless of the normal state of affairs.

11. **Adrenergic innervation and sympathetic stimulation:** Adrenergic innervation of the bladder and urethral smooth musculature has been extensively demonstrated in animal studies. These studies have shown that the smooth musculature of the bladder base and proximal urethra possesses a rich adrenergic (norepinephrine containing) innervation, whereas the bladder body has a sparse but definite adrenergic innervation. The density of innervation seems, in all areas, to be less than that of the cholinergic systems. Considerable disagreement exists, however, as to the density of postganglionic sympathetic innervation in the human bladder and proximal urethra. There is general agreement that the smooth muscle of the human male bladder neck possesses a dense adrenergic innervation, responsible for the contraction of the bladder neck during ejaculation, but there is little consensus otherwise. Even those who ascribe a significant influence on the micturition cycle to the sympathetic nervous system (SYMPNS) have difficulty demonstrating more than a sparse adrenergic innervation in other areas of the human bladder and urethra. There is general agreement, however, that the smooth muscle of the bladder and proximal urethra in a variety of animals and in humans contains both α- and ß-adrenergic receptors. Alpha-adrenergic contractile responses predominate in the bladder base and proximal urethra, whereas ß-adrenergic relaxation responses predominate in the bladder body. These responses are mediated primarily by the α_{1A} and β-3 receptor subtypes, respectively. Additionally,

there is general agreement that, at least in certain animal models (the cat, primarily), there is a significant inhibitory influence exerted on parasympathetic ganglionic transmission by postganglionic sympathetic fibers (see Figs. 14.1 and 14.2). Those who advocate a major role of the sympathetic nervous system in the micturition cycle summarize the influence as primarily facilitating the filling and storage phase of micturition by three mechanisms:

a. Decreasing bladder contractility via an inhibitory effect on parasympathetic ganglionic transmission
b. Increasing outlet resistance by stimulation of the predominantly α_{1A} adrenergic receptors in the bladder base and proximal urethra
c. Increasing accommodation by stimulation of the predominantly β-3 adrenergic receptors in the bladder body

It should be noted, however, that some researchers are of the opinion that the SYMPNS plays a very minor role in the micturition cycle in the normal human, although acknowledging that the adrenergic receptors can be activated pharmacologically.

CNS INFLUENCES ON MICTURITION

Micturition is basically a function of the peripheral ANS. However, the ultimate control of LUT function obviously resides at higher neurologic levels. There is general consensus that a micturition "center" in the spinal cord is localized to segments S2-S4, with the major portion at S3. Early workers believed that micturition was a simple sacral spinal reflex activity that was modulated by a number of central and peripheral reflexes. It is now acknowledged that the micturition cycle is coordinated in the pontine-mesencephalic reticular formation. Input to this area is derived from the cerebellum, basal ganglia, thalamus, hypothalamus, and cerebral cortex. Bladder contraction elicited by stimulation at or above and through this area seems to occur with a decrease in activity of the periurethral striated musculature, as in normal micturition. The regions of the cerebral hemispheres primarily concerned with bladder function are the superomedial portion of the frontal lobes and the genu of the corpus callosum. In general, the tonic activity of the cerebral cortex and midbrain is inhibitory. There is debate as to whether the cerebral areas controlling bladder and striated sphincter activity are geographically separate.

TABLE 14.2 Potential CNS Neurotransmitters Other than Opioids and Their Effects on the Micturition Reflex

Neurotransmitter	Site	Predominant Action
Glutamate	Brain, SC	+
Glycine	Brain, SC	–
GABA (gamma-amino-butyric acid)	Brain, SC	–
Serotonin	SC	–
Acetylcholine	Brain	±
Dopamine (D-2)	Brain	+
Dopamine (D-1)	Brain	–
Norepinephrine (α-1, α-2)	Brain, SC	±
Tachykinins (NK1, NK2)	Brain, SC	+

CNS, Central nervous system; *SC*, spinal cord.

Evidence exists that endogenous opioid peptides influence micturition by a tonic inhibitory effect on detrusor reflex pathways. These inhibitory effects could be mediated at several levels, including the peripheral bladder ganglia, sacral spinal cord, and brainstem micturition center. Different types of opioid receptors may be responsible at different sites for different types of effects on bladder contractility. Numerous other potential neurotransmitters can be found in various areas of the CNS. A partial list is provided in Table 14.2. It is important that all these components, transmitters, and their connections are potential points of pharmacologic manipulation, allowing for alteration in LUT filling/storage or emptying/voiding.

Normal Lower Urinary Tract Function

WHAT DETERMINES BLADDER RESPONSE DURING FILLING/STORAGE?

The normal adult bladder response to filling at a physiologic rate is an almost imperceptible change in detrusor pressure. During at least the initial stages of bladder filling, this very high compliance (Δ volume/Δ pressure) is due primarily to passive properties of the bladder wall. The elastic and viscoelastic properties of the bladder wall allow it to stretch to a certain degree without any increase in tension exerted on its contents, and at physiologic filling rates, intravesical and detrusor pressure normally remain virtually unchanged. In the usual clinical setting, filling cystometry shows a slight increase in detrusor pressure, but this pressure rise is a function of the fact that cystometry filling is carried out at a greater than normal physiologic rate. Compliance can be decreased clinically by (1) any process that decreases the viscoelasticity or elasticity of the bladder wall components, (2) certain types of neurologic injury or disease, and (3) filling the bladder beyond its limit of distensibility.

The viscoelastic properties of the stroma (bladder wall less smooth muscle and epithelium) and the noncontraction of detrusor muscle account for the passive mechanical properties seen during filling. The main components of stroma are collagen and elastin. When the collagen component increases, compliance generally decreases. This can occur with various types of injury, bladder outlet obstruction (BOO), and neurologic decentralization. Once decreased compliance occurs because of a replacement by collagen or other components of the stroma, it is generally unresponsive to pharmacologic manipulation, hydraulic distention, or nerve section. Under these circumstances, augmentation cystoplasty may be required to achieve satisfactory reservoir function. There may also be an active but nonneurogenic component to the filling/storage properties of the bladder. Some have suggested that an as yet unidentified relaxing factor is released from the urothelium during filling, and others have suggested that urothelium-released nitric oxide (NO) may exert an inhibitory effect on afferent mechanisms during filling.

At a certain level of bladder filling, spinal sympathetic reflexes are clearly evoked in all animals, and there is some indirect evidence to support such a role in humans. An inhibitory effect on bladder contractility is thought to be mediated primarily by sympathetic modulation of cholinergic ganglionic transmission. Through this sympathetic reflex, two other possibilities exist for promoting filling and storage. One is neurally mediated stimulation of the predominantly α_{1A} adrenergic receptors in the area of the smooth sphincter, the net result of which would be to cause an increase in resistance in that area. The other is neurally mediated stimulation of the predominantly ß-3 adrenergic receptors in the bladder body smooth musculature, causing a decrease in tension. Good evidence also seems to support a strong tonic inhibitory effect of endogenous opioids on bladder activity at the level of the spinal cord, the parasympathetic ganglia, and perhaps the brainstem as well. Finally, bladder filling and wall distention may release autocrine-like factors, which themselves influence contractility, either by stimulation or inhibition.

WHAT DETERMINES OUTLET RESPONSE DURING FILLING/STORAGE?

There is a gradual increase in urethral pressure during bladder filling, contributed to by at least the striated sphincter element and perhaps by the smooth sphincter element. The rise in urethral pressure seen during the filling and storage phase of micturition can be correlated with an increase in efferent pudendal nerve impulse frequency. This constitutes the efferent limb of a spinal somatic reflex that is initiated when a certain critical intravesical pressure is reached. This is the so-called *guarding reflex*, which results in an increase in striated sphincter activity (see Fig. 14.8).

Although it seems logical and certainly compatible with neuropharmacologic, neurophysiologic, and neuromorphologic data to assume that the muscular component of the smooth sphincter also contributes to the change in urethral response during bladder filling, it is extremely difficult to prove this either experimentally or clinically. The passive properties of the urethral wall undoubtedly play a large role in the maintenance of continence. Urethral wall tension develops within the outer layers of the urethra; however, it is a product not only of the active characteristics of smooth and striated muscle but also of the passive characteristics of the elastic collagenous tissue that makes up the urethral wall. In addition, this tension must be exerted on a soft, plastic inner layer capable of being compressed to a closed configuration—the "filler material" representing the submucosal portion of the urethra. The softer and more plastic this area is, the less the pressure required by the tension-producing layers to produce continence.

Finally, whatever the compressive forces, the lumen of the urethra must be capable of being obliterated by a watertight seal. This mucosal seal mechanism explains why a very thin-walled rubber tube requires less pressure to close an open end when the inner layer is coated with a fine layer of grease than when it is not—the latter case being analogous to scarred or atrophic urethral mucosa.

WHY DOES VOIDING ENSUE WITH A NORMAL BLADDER CONTRACTION?

Normally, it is increased detrusor pressure or distortion of the bladder wall that produces the sensation of distention that is primarily responsible for the initiation of voluntarily induced emptying of the LUT. Although the origin of the parasympathetic neural outflow to the bladder, the pelvic nerve, is in the sacral spinal cord, the actual organizational center for the micturition reflex in an intact neural axis is in the brainstem (pontine-mesencephalic formation), and the complete neural circuit for normal micturition includes the ascending and descending spinal cord pathways to and from this area and the facilitory and inhibitory influences from other parts of the brain.

The final step in voluntarily induced micturition initially involves centrally mediated inhibition or cessation of activation of the somatic neural efferent activity to the striated sphincter and an inhibition or cessation of activation of all aspects of any spinal sympathetic reflex evoked during filling. Efferent parasympathetic pelvic nerve activity is ultimately what is responsible for a highly coordinated and sustained contraction of the bulk of the bladder smooth musculature. A decrease in outlet resistance occurs with adaptive shaping or funneling of the relaxed bladder outlet. In addition to the inhibition of any continence-promoting reflexes that have occurred during bladder filling, the change in outlet resistance may also involve an active relaxation of the smooth sphincter through a mechanism mediated by local release of NO. The adaptive changes that occur in the outlet are also in part due to the anatomic interrelationships of the smooth muscle of the bladder base and proximal urethra (continuity). Other reflexes elicited by bladder contraction and by the passage of urine through the urethra may reinforce and facilitate complete bladder emptying. Superimposed on these autonomic and somatic reflexes are complex modifying supraspinal inputs from other central neuronal networks. These facilitory and inhibitory impulses, which originate from several areas of the nervous system, allow for the full conscious control of micturition in the adult.

WHY DOES URINARY CONTINENCE PERSIST DURING ABDOMINAL PRESSURE INCREASES?

During voluntarily initiated micturition, the detrusor pressure becomes higher than the outlet pressure and certain adaptive changes occur in the shape of the bladder outlet with consequent passage of urine into and through the proximal urethra. Why do such changes not occur with increases in intravesical pressure that are similar in magnitude but produced only by changes in intraabdominal pressure (IAP), such as straining or coughing? First of all, a coordinated bladder contraction does not occur in response to such stimuli, clearly emphasizing the fact that increases in total intravesical pressure are by no means equivalent to emptying ability. Normally, for urine to flow into the proximal urethra, not only must there be an increase in intravesical pressure but the increase must also be a product of a coordinated bladder contraction, occurring through a neurally mediated reflex mechanism and associated with characteristic conformational and tension changes in the bladder neck and proximal urethral area. Assuming the bladder outlet is competent at rest, a major factor in the prevention of urinary leakage during increases in IAP is the fact that there is normally at least equal pressure transmission to the proximal urethra during such activity. Failure of this mechanism, generally associated with hypermobility of the bladder neck and proximal urethra (another way of describing pathologic descent with abdominal straining), is an almost invariable correlate of effort-related urinary incontinence (UI) in the female. No such hypermobility occurs in the male. The increase in urethral closure pressure that is normally seen with increments in IAP actually exceeds the extrinsic pressure increase. This indicates that active muscular function due to a reflex increase in striated sphincter activity and/or other factors such as midurethral compression that increase urethral resistance are also involved in preventing such leakage. A more complete description of the factors involved in sphincteric incontinence and its prevention can be found in the section on incontinence.

OVERVIEW OF THE MICTURITION CYCLE: SIMPLIFICATION AND SUMMARY

Bladder accommodation during filling is a primarily passive phenomenon. It is dependent on the elastic and viscoelastic properties of the bladder wall and the lack of parasympathetic excitatory input. During bladder filling and urine storage, an increase in outlet resistance occurs via the striated sphincter somatic guarding reflex. In at least some species a sympathetic reflex also contributes to storage by (1) increasing outlet resistance by increasing activity in the smooth sphincter, (2) inhibiting detrusor contractility through an inhibitory effect on parasympathetic ganglia, and (3) by a β_3-induced decrease in tension of bladder body smooth muscle. Continence is maintained during increases in IAP by the intrinsic competence of the bladder outlet and urethral compression against a suburethral supporting layer. A further increase in striated sphincter activity, on a reflex basis, is also contributory during increases in IAP (e.g., by coughing or straining).

Emptying (voiding) can be voluntary or involuntary and involves an inhibition of the spinal somatic and sympathetic reflexes and activation of the vesical parasympathetic pathways, the organizational center for which is in the brainstem. Initially, there is a relaxation of the outlet musculature, mediated not only by the cessation of the somatic and sympathetic spinal reflexes but probably also by a locally released relaxing factor, very possibly NO, released by parasympathetic stimulation or by some other effect on bladder neck smooth muscle.

A highly coordinated parasympathetically induced contraction of the bulk of the bladder smooth musculature occurs, with shaping or funneling of the relaxed outlet, due at least in part to some smooth muscle continuity between the bladder base and proximal urethra. With amplification and facilitation of the bladder contraction from other peripheral reflexes and from spinal cord supraspinal sources, and the absence of anatomic obstruction between the bladder and the urethral meatus, complete emptying will occur.

Whatever disagreements exist regarding the anatomic, morphologic, physiologic, pharmacologic, and mechanical details involved in both the storage and expulsion of urine by the LUT, there is agreement regarding certain points. First, the micturition cycle involves two relatively discrete processes: bladder filling/urine storage and bladder emptying/voiding. Second, whatever the details involved these processes can be summarized succinctly from a conceptual point of view.

Bladder filling/urine storage requires the following:

1. Accommodation of increasing volumes of urine at a low intravesical pressure (normal compliance) and with appropriate sensation

2. A bladder outlet that is closed at rest and remains so during increases in IAP
3. Absence of involuntary bladder contractions (detrusor overactivity [DO])

Bladder emptying/voiding requires the following:

1. A sustained coordinated contraction of the bladder smooth musculature of adequate magnitude and duration
2. A concomitant lowering of resistance at the level of the smooth and striated sphincter (absence of functional obstruction)
3. Absence of anatomic obstruction

Any type of LUT dysfunction must result from an abnormality of one or more of the factors previously listed regardless of the exact pathophysiology involved. This division, with its implied subdivision under each category into causes related to the bladder and the outlet, provides a logical rationale for discussion and classification of all types of LUT dysfunction and disorders as related primarily to bladder filling/urine storage or to bladder emptying/voiding (Table 14.3 and Table 14.4). There are some types

TABLE 14.3 Functional Classification of Lower Urinary Tract Dysfunction

Failure to store
Because of the bladder
Because of the outlet
Failure to empty
Because of the bladder
Because of the outlet

TABLE 14.4 Expanded Functional Classification of Lower Urinary Tract Dysfunction

1. Failure to store
a. Because of the bladder
1) Overactivity
i. Involuntary contractions (detrusor overactivity [DO])
Neurologic disease or injury
Bladder outlet obstruction (BOO; myogenic)
Inflammation
Idiopathic

Continued

TABLE 14.4 Expanded Functional Classification of Lower Urinary Tract Dysfunction—cont'd

ii. Decreased compliance
Neurologic or muscular disease or injury
Fibrosis
Idiopathic
iii. Combination
2) Hypersensitivity
i. Inflammatory/infectious
ii. Neurologic
iii. Psychologic
iv. Idiopathic
3) Underactivity (with retention and overflow incontinence)
b. Because of the outlet
1) Stress urinary incontinence (SUI)
i. Lack of suburethral support
ii. Pelvic floor laxity, hypermobility
2) Intrinsic sphincter deficiency (ISD)
i. Neurologic disease or injury
ii. Fibrosis
3) Combination (SUI and ISD)
c. Combination (bladder and outlet factors)
d. Fistula
2. Failure to empty
a. Because of the bladder (underactivity)
1) Neurogenic
2) Myogenic
3) Psychogenic
4) Idiopathic
b. Because of the outlet
1) Anatomic
i. Prostatic obstruction
ii. Bladder neck contracture
iii. Urethral stricture, fibrosis
iv. Urethral compression
2) Functional
i. Smooth sphincter dyssynergia (bladder neck dysfunction)
ii. Striated sphincter dyssynergia
c. Combination (bladder and outlet factors)

of voiding dysfunction that represent combinations of filling and storage and emptying and voiding abnormalities. Within this scheme, however, these become readily understandable, and their detection and treatment can be logically described. Further, using this scheme, all aspects of urodynamic, radiologic, and video urodynamic evaluation can be conceptualized as to exactly what they evaluate in terms of either bladder or outlet activity during filling and storage or emptying and voiding (see Table 14.6). Treatments for LUT dysfunction can be classified under broad categories according to whether they facilitate filling/storage or emptying/voiding and whether they do so by acting primarily on the bladder or on one or more of the components of the bladder outlet (see Tables 14.7 and 14.8). Finally, the individual disorders produced by various neuromuscular dysfunctions can be considered in terms of whether they produce primarily storage or emptying abnormalities or a combination.

Abnormalities of Filling/Storage and Emptying/Voiding: Overview of Pathophysiology (Tables 14.3 and 14.4)

The pathophysiology of failure of the LUT to fill with or store urine adequately or to empty adequately must logically be secondary to reasons related to the bladder, the outlet, or both.

FILLING/STORAGE FAILURE

Absolute or relative failure of the bladder to fill with and store urine adequately results from bladder overactivity (involuntary contraction and/or decreased compliance), decreased outlet resistance, heightened or altered sensation, or a combination.

1. **Bladder overactivity:** Overactivity of the bladder during filling/storage can be expressed as phasic involuntary contractions, as low compliance, or as a combination. Involuntary contractions are most commonly seen in association with neurologic disease or injury; however, they may be associated with increased afferent input due to inflammation or irritation of the bladder or urethral wall, BOO, stress urinary incontinence (SUI) (perhaps due to sudden entry of urine into the proximal urethra), or aging changes (probably related to neural degeneration), or may be idiopathic. Others have hypothesized that decreased tonic

stimulation from the pelvic floor can contribute to phasic bladder overactivity. Decreased compliance during filling/storage may be secondary to neurologic injury or disease, usually at a sacral or infrasacral level, but may result from any process that destroys the viscoelastic or elastic properties of the bladder wall. Bladder-related storage failure may also occur in the absence of overactivity, due to increased afferent input from inflammation, irritation, other causes of hypersensitivity, and pain. The causes may be chemical, psychologic, or idiopathic. One classic example is bladder pain syndrome, previously and sometimes still known as *interstitial cystitis*.

2. **Outlet underactivity**: Decreased outlet resistance may result from any process that damages the innervation or structural elements of the smooth and/or striated sphincter or support of the bladder outlet. This may occur with neurologic disease or injury, surgical or other mechanical trauma, or aging. Classically, sphincteric incontinence in the female was categorized into relatively discrete entities: (1) so-called genuine stress incontinence (GSI) and (2) intrinsic sphincter deficiency (ISD), originally described as *type III stress incontinence*. GSI in the female was originally described as associated with hypermobility of the bladder outlet because of poor pelvic support and with an outlet that was competent at rest but lost its competence only during increases in IAP. ISD described a nonfunctional or very poorly functional bladder neck and proximal urethra at rest. The implication of classical ISD was that a surgical procedure designed to correct only urethral hypermobility would have a relatively high failure rate, as opposed to one designed to improve urethral coaptation and compression. The contemporary view is that the majority of cases of effort-related incontinence in the female involve varying proportions of support-related factors and ISD. It is possible to have outlet-related incontinence due only to ISD but not due solely to hypermobility or poor support—some ISD must exist.
3. **Stress- or effort-related UI**: This arises primarily from impairment of neural or muscular function and/or nerves and/or connective tissue function within the pelvic floor. Urethral support is important in the female; the urethra normally being supported by the action of the levator ani muscles through their connection to the endopelvic fascia of the anterior vaginal wall.

Damage to the connection between this fascia and this muscle, damage to the nerve supply, or direct muscle damage, can therefore influence effort-related continence Bladder neck and urethral function is likewise important, and loss of normal closure can result in incontinence despite normal urethral support. In older writings, the urethra was sometimes ignored as a factor contributing to continence in the female, and the site of continence was thought to be exclusively the bladder neck. However, in approximately 50% of continent women, urine enters the urethra during increases in abdominal pressure. The continence point in these women (highest point of pressure transmission) is at the midurethra.

4. **Urethral hypermobility**: This implies weakness of the pelvic floor supporting structures. During increases in IAP, there is descent of the bladder neck and proximal urethra. If the outlet opens concomitantly, SUI ensues. In the classic form of urethral hypermobility, there is rotational descent of the bladder neck and urethra. However, the urethra may also descend without rotation (it shortens and widens), or the posterior wall of the urethra may be pulled (sheared) open while the anterior wall remains fixed. However, urethral hypermobility is often present in women who are not incontinent, and thus, the mere presence of urethral hypermobility is not sufficient to make a diagnosis of a sphincter abnormality unless UI is also demonstrated. The "hammock hypothesis" of John DeLancey (1994) proposes that for stress incontinence to occur with hypermobility, there must be a lack of stability of the suburethral supportive layer. This theory proposes that the effect of abdominal pressure increases on the normal bladder outlet, if the suburethral supportive layer is firm, is to compress the urethra rapidly and effectively. If the supportive suburethral layer is lax and/or movable, compression is not as effective. Intrinsic sphincter dysfunction denotes an intrinsic malfunction of the proximal sphincter mechanism itself. In its most overt form, it is characterized by a bladder neck and proximal urethra that are, at rest, incompetent, and a low Valsalva leak point pressure (VLPP) and urethral closure pressure and is usually the result of prior surgery, trauma with scarring, or a neurologic lesion.
5. **Urethral instability**: This refers to the rare phenomenon of episodic decreases in outlet pressure unrelated to increases in

bladder or abdominal pressure. This term may be a misnomer because many believe that the drop in urethral pressure represents simply the urethral component of a micturition reflex in an individual whose bladder does not measurably contract for either myogenic or neurogenic reasons. Little has appeared in the recent literature about this entity. It is sometimes cited as a cause of urgency and urgency incontinence but can be seen in an otherwise asymptomatic individual.

In theory at least, categories of outlet-related incontinence in the male are similar to those in the female. Sphincteric incontinence in the male is not, however, associated with hypermobility of the bladder neck and proximal urethra but is more similar to *ISD* in the female. It is seen most often after radical prostatectomy or in neurologic disease or trauma affecting the sacral spinal cord or pathways distal to this. It is seen occasionally after outlet-reducing surgery as well. There is essentially no information regarding the topic of urethral instability in the male.

The treatment of filling/storage abnormalities is directed toward inhibiting bladder contractility, decreasing sensory output, mechanically increasing bladder capacity, and/or toward increasing outlet resistance, the latter either continuously or just during increases in intraabdominal pressure (IAP).

EMPTYING/VOIDING FAILURE

Absolute or relative failure to empty the bladder results from decreased bladder contractility (a decrease in magnitude, coordination, or duration), increased outlet resistance, or both.

1. **Bladder underactivity (underactive bladder, impaired bladder contractility):** Absolute or relative failure of bladder contractility may result from temporary or permanent alteration in one of the neuromuscular mechanisms necessary for initiating, propagating, and maintaining a normal detrusor contraction. Inhibition of the voiding reflex in a neurologically normal individual may also occur; it may be by a reflex mechanism secondary to increased afferent input, especially from the pelvic and perineal areas, or may be psychogenic. Nonneurogenic causes include impairment of bladder smooth muscle function, which may result from overdistention, ischemia, various centrally or peripherally acting drugs, or fibrosis, the latter most often due to BOO or repeated infection.

2. **Outlet overactivity or obstruction:** Pathologically increased outlet resistance is much more common in men than in women. Although it is most often secondary to anatomic obstruction, it may be secondary to a failure of relaxation or due to active contraction of the striated or smooth sphincter during bladder contraction. Striated sphincter dyssynergia is a common cause of functional or nonanatomic (as opposed to fixed anatomic) obstruction in patients with suprasacral neurologic disease or injury. Anatomic outlet obstruction in the male is most often due to prostatic enlargement, less commonly urethral stricture disease. A cause of outlet obstruction in the female is compression or fibrosis following surgery for sphincteric incontinence. Structure disease can occur but is much less common.

The treatment of emptying failure generally consists of maneuvers to increase intravesical/detrusor pressure, facilitate the micturition reflex, decrease outlet resistance, or a combination. If other means fail or are impractical, intermittent or continuous catheterization is an effective way to circumvent emptying failure.

The Neurourologic Evaluation (Table 14.5)

HISTORY

Symptomatology can be valuable in suggesting whether voiding dysfunction represents an abnormality of storage, emptying, or

TABLE 14.5 Neurourologic Evaluation

History
Bladder diary
Quality-of-life assessment
Physical examination
Neurologic examination
Urine bacteriologic studies
Renal function studies
Radiologic evaluation
Upper tract
Lower tract
Urodynamic/video urodynamic study
Endoscopic examination

both. A complete history of the symptoms and their onset, duration, time course, and relationship to neurologic disease or other neurologic symptoms is essential. Incontinence is generally a primary symptom of filling and storage failure and may be bladder or outlet related; however, it can also result from ureteral ectopy and congenital or acquired urinary fistulas. Leakage that is associated only with increases in IAP implies SUI. Gravitational urethral incontinence that worsens on straining implies ISD. Precipitous incontinence with a more sustained type of leakage similar to voiding is characteristic of involuntary bladder contractions (DO). It can occur with sensation (urgency) or without urgency in the absence of sensation. Incontinence is not always, however, a primary symptom of filling and storage failure. Overflow, or paradoxical incontinence, can develop in a patient with insidious detrusor decompensation with emptying failure. The leakage in this case is generally most prominently associated with changes in position or sudden increases in IAP and can mimic stress incontinence. Urgency is defined in the International Continence Society (ICS) lexicon as a sudden compelling desire to void that is difficult to defer. Previously the definition included "for fear of leaking." A perceived need to void solely because of pain is generally secondary to inflammatory disease.

An increase in daytime urinary frequency can be psychogenic, represent a response to pain on low-volume bladder distention (usually indicative of inflammatory disease), be due to DO, or simply be due to increased fluid intake. Increased frequency can also result from emptying failure with a substantial residual urine volume and therefore a decreased functional bladder capacity. It can also exist in association with outlet obstruction-induced DO. Nocturia usually accompanies nonpsychogenic urinary frequency and can be associated, on the same basis as increased daytime frequency, with either storage or emptying failure. It is most commonly associated with an increased nocturnal urine output (nocturnal polyuria). It is generally considered significant only when it occurs twice or more at night. The time to the first awakening is significant, as the most restful period of sleep occurs within the first 4 hours. The symptom of pressure defies exact definition. It is not quite the urge to void but rather a feeling that the bladder is full or that the urge to void will occur shortly. There is often no discernible urodynamic dysfunction in patients who complain of this, except perhaps for hypersensitivity during filling; however, such dysfunction can be due to an elevated detrusor pressure during filling, but one that is below the level necessary to elicit the sensation of distention or urgency. This symptom also may be representative of an accurate perception of inadequate emptying with a modest or large residual urine volume. A bladder diary is especially useful in accurately portraying symptoms due to a filling/storage abnormality. This should include at least the following: fluid intake, time and amount of voiding, association with urgency (or not), and leakage (or not), including type and amount. The diary will also allow estimation of the functional capacity, which should serve as a guide for filling volume during urodynamics.

Hesitancy, straining to void, and poor or interrupted stream generally may reflect a failure to empty adequately, but they can occur in an individual with frequency and urgency who, on toileting, simply has difficulty initiating a voluntary bladder contraction with a small intravesical urine content.

Pain in the area of the bladder may reflect intrinsic bladder pathology (bladder pain syndrome/interstitial cystitis, malignant or premalignant conditions, infection or inflammation, calculus) or be due to an extrinsic causation (e.g., abscess, compression). A detailed history of prior medical and surgical treatment and the results should always be sought.

PHYSICAL AND NEUROLOGIC EVALUATION

Findings from a general physical examination are nonspecific. There may be cutaneous excoriation secondary to urinary leakage. A focused physical examination may include the lower abdomen, genitalia, and rectum in men and women. Prostate abnormalities should be detected. A careful pelvic examination in women is necessary to detect the presence and degree and type of pelvic organ prolapse. The neurologic examination provides evidence of the presence or absence of a neurologic lesion and, if present, localizes it in an attempt to corroborate and explain a given LUT dysfunction. Mental status is determined by noting the level of consciousness, orientation, speech, comprehension, and memory. Mental status aberrations can be secondary to neurologic diseases that produce LUT dysfunction, such as senile and presenile dementia, Alzheimer disease, brain tumors, and normal pressure hydrocephalus. Cranial nerve dysfunction, except when indicative of a brainstem lesion, has little specific relevance to voiding dysfunction. Careful examination of motor function and coordination and a sensory examination (including touch, pain, temperature, vibration, and position) can have anatomic and etiologic significance. Sensory or motor deficits may suggest specific levels of spinal pathology, either unilateral or bilateral. The abnormalities associated with SCI, Parkinson disease (PD), multiple sclerosis (MS), and cerebrovascular diseases are usually obvious. The presence of lateralizing signs suggests that only one side of the neural axis is affected. Quadriplegia suggests an abnormality of the cervical or high thoracic spinal cord, whereas true paraplegia indicates a cord lesion below the upper thoracic segments. Specific dermatomal sensory alterations or deficits suggest localized pathology at the spinal cord or nerve root level.

Evaluation of the deep tendon reflexes provides an indication of segmental spinal cord function and suprasegmental function. Hypoactivity of the deep tendon reflexes generally is associated with a lower motor neuron (LMN) lesion (in this context, meaning from the anterior horn cells to the periphery), whereas hyperactivity generally indicates an upper motor neuron (UMN) lesion (between the brain and anterior horn cells of the spinal cord). These terms, *UMN* and *LMN*, refer, strictly speaking, only to the SNS. However, by convention, they are often applied by urologists and neurologists to the efferent portions of the ANS innervating the LUT. In this context, the terms are generally understood to mean the following: UMN, between the brain and anterior spinal cord horn cells, and LMN, from anterior horn cells to the periphery, including all preganglionic and postganglionic fibers. Commonly tested deep tendon reflexes include the biceps (C5-C6), triceps (C6-C7), quadriceps or patellar (L2-L4), and Achilles (L5-S2). A pathologic toe sign (Babinski reflex) generally indicates a somatic UMN lesion but can be absent with a complete lesion and marked spasticity. A Babinski reflex may be present contralaterally with a unilateral lesion or may be present unilaterally with a bilateral lesion. The generic term *bulbocavernosus reflex (BCR)* describes contraction of the bulbocavernosus and ischiocavernosus muscles after penile glans or clitoral stimulation, or stimulation of the urethral or bladder mucosa by pulling an indwelling Foley catheter. These reflexes are mediated by pudendal and/or pelvic afferents and by pudendal nerve efferents and, as such, represent a local sacral spinal cord reflex. Most clinicians would agree that the BCR reflects activity in S2-S4, but some believe that this may involve segments as high as L5. Motor control of the external anal sphincter (EAS) is variously described as being served by sacral cord segments S2-S4 or S3-S5. A visible contraction of the EAS after pinprick of the mucocutaneous junction constitutes the anal reflex, and its activity usually parallels that of the BCR. EAS tone, when strong, indicates that activity of the conus medullaris is present, whereas absent anal sphincter tone usually indicates absent conal activity. Volitional control of the EAS indicates intact control by supraspinal centers. The cough reflex (contraction of the EAS with cough) is a spinal reflex that depends on volitional innervation of the abdominal musculature T6-L1. The afferent limb is apparently from muscle receptors in the abdominal wall that enter the spinal cord and ascend. As long as one of these segments remains under volitional control, the cough reflex may be positive. If a lesion above the outflow to the abdominal musculature exists, the cough reflex is generally absent.

In regard to lesions that affect the spinal cord, it must be remembered that the level of the vertebral lesion (such as in SCI or disc disease) usually differs from the spinal cord segmental level. Sacral spinal cord segments S2-S4 are generally at vertebral bone levels L1-L2. Additionally, it must be remembered that after spinal cord trauma, descending degeneration of the cord may occur. In a complete spinal cord lesion above the conus medullaris (otherwise known as *suprasegmental* or *UMN*), there will generally be, after spinal shock has passed, hyperactivity of the deep tendon reflexes, skeletal spasticity, and absent skin sensation below the level of the lesion; pathologic toe signs will exist. Following a complete spinal cord lesion at or below the conus (segmental or infrasegmental or LMN), after spinal shock has passed, there will generally be absent deep tendon reflexes, skeletal flaccidity, and absent skin sensation below the lesion level; pathologic toe signs will be absent.

RADIOLOGIC EVALUATION

1. **Upper tracts** (see Chapter 2): Many urologists believe that contrast imaging (CT urography) is the optimal screening study of the upper tracts (kidneys and ureters) in patients with

significant voiding dysfunction. Ultrasonography (US) can, however, give adequate information about hydronephrosis, the presence of calculi, and occasionally hydroureter. Isotope studies can be useful to evaluate renal blood flow and function and to establish the presence of renal or ureteral obstruction. Dilation of the ureters or renal collecting system or a decrease in function can represent significant complications of LUT dysfunction and as such are often indications for intervention. Upper tract imaging is generally recommended only in specific situations in the evaluation of adult LUT dysfunction: (1) decreased bladder compliance, (2) neurogenic LUT dysfunction, (3) severe urethral obstruction, (4) incontinence associated with significant postvoid residual, (5) coexisting loin and flank pain, (6) severe untreated pelvic organ prolapse, and (7) suspected extraurethral UI.

2. **Lower tracts:** This portion of the chapter considers only basic cystourethrographic patterns that relate directly to LUT dysfunction caused by neuromuscular disease. There are only a few basic cystourethrographic radiologic configurations, but their significance can be fully ascertained only by concomitant urodynamic study. A closed bladder neck is normal in a resting individual whose bladder is undergoing either physiologic or urodynamic filling. However, it can also occur in an individual with an areflexic bladder who is straining to void and in an individual in whom a micturition reflex is occurring but whose smooth sphincter area is dysfunctional or dyssynergic. The closed appearance can sometimes be mimicked to a great degree by significant prostatic enlargement with bladder neck and urethral compression as well. An open bladder neck is normal during voluntarily induced bladder micturition and during most involuntary bladder contractions. However, this appearance during filling/storage may also be due to ISD, seen in some types of neurologic injury or disease, or to endoscopic or open surgical alteration, and it may be seen normally in some women. A closed striated sphincter is normal during physiologic or urodynamic filling and is normally seen with an attempt to stop normal urination or to abort an involuntary bladder contraction. The sphincter also normally remains closed during abdominal straining. During voluntary micturition or during micturition secondary to an involuntary

bladder contraction caused by neurologic disease at or above the brainstem, the striated sphincter should open unless the patient is trying to abort the bladder contractions by voluntary sphincter contraction or detrusor sphincter dyssynergia (DSD) is present. A cystogram in the erect position at rest and during straining may be useful in quantitating the degree of classical SUI (bladder neck closed at rest, open with straining, associated with hypermobility) versus classical ISD (bladder neck open at rest, more leakage with straining, and no hypermobility). Voiding cystourethrography is useful to diagnose the site of obstruction in a patient with proven urodynamic evidence of obstruction.

ENDOSCOPIC EVALUATION

Endoscopy is recommended only in specific situations in the adult with only LUT dysfunction: (1) when initial testing suggests other types of pathology (microscopic or gross hematuria; pain, discomfort, persistent or severe symptoms of bladder overactivity; suspected extraurethral incontinence); (2) in patients who have previously undergone bladder, prostate, or other pelvic surgery; and (3) in men with incontinence. Bladder washings or a voided urine for cytology should be sent if symptoms suggest the possibility of neoplastic or preneoplastic changes in the bladder or urethral epithelium. The presence or absence of trabeculation (which can be compatible with obstruction, involuntary bladder contractions, or neurologic decentralization) can also be determined. Endoscopic examination may be thought to be confirmatory of or exclude anatomic occlusion at a particular site, but it should be recognized that not everything that appears occlusive endoscopically is obstructive urodynamically (all large prostates are not obstructive), and lack of a visually appreciated occlusion does not exclude functional obstruction (striated or smooth sphincter dyssynergia) during bladder emptying and voiding. In describing findings on an endoscopic exam, it is better to use the term *occlusion* because *obstruction* implies urodynamic significance.

URODYNAMIC AND VIDEO URODYNAMIC EVALUATION

The studies that fall under the heading of *LUT urodynamics* consist simply of methods designed to generate quantitative data relevant to events taking place in the bladder and bladder outlet during the two relatively discrete phases of micturition described previously: filling/storage and emptying/voiding. This conceptualization fits nicely with the concept of two phases of micturition and the description of each phase requiring three components to occur normally. Ideally, the evaluation of urodynamic study (UDS) and video urodynamic study (VUDS) should be able to answer the implied questions regarding the normality or abnormality of each of the components of the two phases of micturition. Combined video urodynamic or separate cystourethrographic study (referred to as FLUORO in Table 14.6) also provides information regarding the presence or absence of vesicoureteral reflux (VUR). A simple formulation of the commonly utilized

TABLE 14.6 Urodynamics Simplified

	Bladder	Outlet
Filling/storage phase	Pves[1] Pdet[2] (FCMG[3]) DLPP[4]	UPP[5] VLPP[6] FLUORO[7] MUPP[11]
Emptying phase	Pves[8] Pdet[9] (VCMG)[10]	FLUORO[7] MUPP[11] FLUORO[12] EMG[13]
	FLOW[14] RU[15]	

This functional conceptualization of urodynamics categorizes each study as to whether it examines bladder or outlet activity during the filling/storage or emptying phase of micturition. In this scheme, uroflow and residual urine integrate the activity of the bladder and the outlet during the emptying phase.

[1,2]Total bladder (Pves) and detrusor (Pdet) pressures during a filling cystometrogram (FCMG).

[3]Filling cystometrogram.

[4]Detrusor leak point pressure.

[5]Urethral pressure profilometry.

[6]Valsalva leak point pressure.

[7]Fluoroscopy of outlet during filling/storage.

[8,9]Total bladder and detrusor pressures during a voiding cystometrogram (VCMG).

[10]Voiding cystometrogram.

[11]Micturitional urethral pressure profilometry.

[12]Fluoroscopy of outlet during emptying.

[13]Electromyography of periurethral striated musculature.

[14]Flowmetry.

[15]Residual urine.

urodynamic studies, based on the two phases of micturition concept, is presented in Table 14.6, the individual studies characterized as to whether they evaluate aspects of bladder or outlet activity during filling and storage or emptying. Within this scheme, flowmetry and residual urine are simply ways of integrating bladder and outlet activity during the emptying phase of micturition.

The primary purpose of UDS and VUDS evaluation is threefold: (1) determine the precise etiology(ies) of the LUT symptoms and/or dysfunction, (2) identify urodynamic risk factors for upper and LUT deterioration, and (3) identify factors that might affect the success of a particular therapy. The study should ideally reproduce the patient's symptoms and/or accurately reflect bladder and outlet activity and sensation during filling/storage and emptying/voiding and provide a pathophysiologic basis for management. UDS and VUDS can also be utilized along with symptomatology to assess treatment results. Certain very simple rules aid immeasurably in obtaining the maximum benefit from UDS and VUDS. Although these rules sound obvious, they are often ignored, sometimes even by experienced urodynamicists. The prime directive is that the study must reproduce the clinical symptomatology or clinical abnormality being investigated. If it does not, then insofar as that particular patient is concerned, and despite the fact that the study may be perfectly done and the data beautifully reproduced, it may be worthless. Conversely, the appropriate study done so as to reproduce the symptoms always yields pertinent information. As a corollary, it is not necessary to perform the most complicated type of VDS with every patient. The simplest, most readily reproducible, and least invasive study that gives the information desired is always the best. The subject has become far more complicated than necessary. A large percentage of LUT dysfunction problems can be diagnosed by a logical clinician using relatively simple UDS. As the complexity of the problem and the number of failed prior therapies increase, so does the need for more complicated or combined VDSs. Finally, it must be remembered that urodynamic and video urodynamic evaluation must be an interactive process between the patient and examiner. Information must be constantly exchanged and the study sequence tailored to a given patient and their LUT symptoms and signs.

1. **Flowmetry**: Flowmetry is a way to integrate the activity of the bladder and outlet during the emptying phase of micturition.

The flow rates and pattern represent the recorded variables; if these are both normal, it is unlikely that there is any significant disorder of emptying. A normal flow, however, does not entirely exclude obstruction, which is strictly defined on the basis of a relationship between detrusor pressure and simultaneous flow. Consistently low flow rates with adequate volumes voided generally indicate increased outlet resistance, decreased bladder contractility, or both. Flow rates considerably in excess of normal may indicate decreased outlet resistance. There are only a few abnormal flow patterns. An abnormally broad plateau with a low mean and peak rate generally indicates outlet obstruction or decreased detrusor contractility or both. Intermittent flow is generally secondary to abdominal straining or sphincter dyssynergia, but in rare instances, it can be due to undulating low-amplitude detrusor contractions. An idealized normal flow curve is seen in Fig. 14.3 and flow tracings from individuals with various characteristic abnormalities are seen in Fig. 14.4.

The primary caveat in interpreting uroflow is to make sure that the flow event closely approximates the usual voiding event for that patient. If not, it should be repeated with a comfortably full bladder. In an adult, flow events of 100 mL

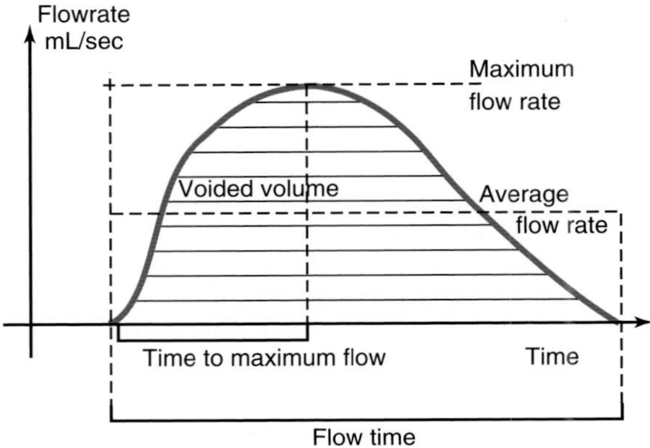

FIGURE 14.3 Terminology of the International Continence Society (ICS) relating to the urodynamic description of urinary flow. (From Wein AJ, English WS, Whitmore KE. Office urodynamics. *Urol Clin North Am*. 1988;15:609-623.)

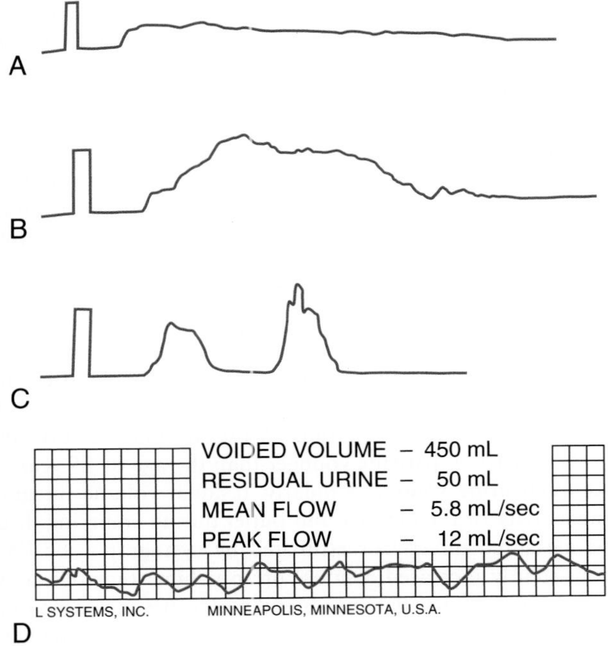

FIGURE 14.4 (A) Flowmetry in the patient with bladder outlet obstruction (BOO). Height of bar represents a flow of 10 mL/sec. Maximum flow is generally established soon after the onset of voiding. Peak and mean flow rates are decreased. Flow time is prolonged. Note that this diagnosis cannot be made from this flow event alone. However, this is most characteristic of BOO in a patient with normal detrusor. (B) Uroflow event from a patient with impaired detrusor contractility. Maximum flow is established near the middle of the flow event. Mean and peak flow rates are decreased. Flow time is somewhat prolonged. To establish this diagnosis beyond a doubt, especially because the therapeutic options differ, a pressure/flow study would be necessary to separate this entity from BOO. (C) Intermittent flow. This type of intermittent flow pattern is most commonly due to abdominal straining. In such a patient with decreased outlet resistance, the peak flow rate is often normal or may even be above normal. (D) Another type of intermittent flow pattern. This can be due either to sphincter dyssynergia or low-amplitude fluctuating detrusor contractions. With sphincter dyssynergia, the changes in flow usually occur faster and are more staccato-like. This is actually from a patient with low-amplitude fluctuating detrusor contraction. (From Wein AJ, English WS, Whitmore KE. Office urodynamics. *Urol Clin North Am*. 1988;15:609-623.)

or less should be interpreted with caution. An overfilled bladder may be accompanied by reduced flow rates probably because of temporary dysfunction introduced by overstretching of detrusor fibers. Measurements of only one flow parameter, such as peak flow, may be misleading because it is possible for patients with decreased outlet resistance to generate very high peak flows with straining. In comparisons of flow rates in a given individual from one time to another, either for the purposes of evaluating treatment or following a given condition, it is very important to standardize the rates to a given volume. Volume/rate nomograms can be useful in this regard. Most data from studies cite norms of 15 and 25 mL/sec for mean and maximum flow rates. However, flow rates should be standardized in terms of the minimum acceptable flow rates for given gender and age groups. Most "normal" data relate to flowmetry in patients younger than the age of 55 years.

2. **Residual urine volume**: Similarly, residual volume integrates the activity of the bladder and outlet during emptying. It can be measured directly or estimated by cystography or US. A consistently increased residual urine volume that reflects the usual status of that patient generally indicates increased outlet resistance, decreased bladder contractility, or both. Negligible residual urine volume is compatible with normal function of the LUT but can also exist with significant disorders of filling and storage (i.e., incontinence) or emptying disorders in which the intravesical pressure is simply sufficient to overcome increases in outlet resistance up to a certain point. Generally, a significant residual urine volume is considered to be indicative of relative detrusor failure, with or without outlet obstruction. Residual urine volume may be expressed as an absolute number (mL) or as a percent of the functional bladder capacity. The amount or percentage that is "normal" or "acceptable" or "pathological" and an indication for treatment is debatable and varies with the clinical circumstances.
3. **Filling cystometry**: Cystometry refers to the method by which changes in bladder pressure are measured. The test was designed originally to evaluate the filling and storage phase of bladder function and to measure changes in bladder pressure with slow progressive increases in volume. Strictly speaking,

this is filling cystometry, as opposed to voiding cystometry. Unless the examiner clearly recognizes the distinction, erroneous conclusions regarding the activity of the bladder during the emptying phase of micturition may be made on the basis of what is commonly called a *cystometrogram* but which, in reality, represents only filling, and not voiding, cystometry. There is no single best method of performing cystometry or any urodynamic study, for that matter. All have their shortcomings. The "experts" often differ significantly in their choice of testing sequences and catheters, but their conclusions about an individual patient are usually remarkably similar. Liquid is used as a medium for filling cystometry. Dilute contrast is required for VUDS.

The first sensation of bladder filling and fullness, the normal urge to void, the sensation of urgency, and the feeling of imminent micturition are important data to record. When a phasic involuntary detrusor contraction occurs, it is important to note whether this coincides with a sensation of urgency and whether suppression is possible. The pressure measured within the bladder is composed of that contributed by the detrusor plus IAP. Thus any pressure increment recorded on a simple cystometrogram may at least partially, and sometimes totally, reflect IAP. To eliminate such artifactual problems, it is desirable to measure IAP simultaneously, as reflected by a catheter-mounted intrarectal pressure balloon, a vaginal catheter, or a catheter inserted next to the bladder. It is true that an experienced operator can very often tell the difference between a true detrusor contraction and an increase in bladder pressure caused by an increase in IAP by the configuration of the curve and by observation of the patient. However, if there is any question about this or if a significant decision is to be based on these data, electronic subtraction of the IAP from the total bladder pressure (yielding detrusor pressure) is desirable.

The normal adult cystometrogram can be divided into four phases (Fig. 14.5).

Phase 1: The initial pressure rise represents the initial response to filling, and the level at which the bladder trace stabilizes is known as the *initial filling pressure*. The first phase of the curve is contributed to by the initial myogenic response

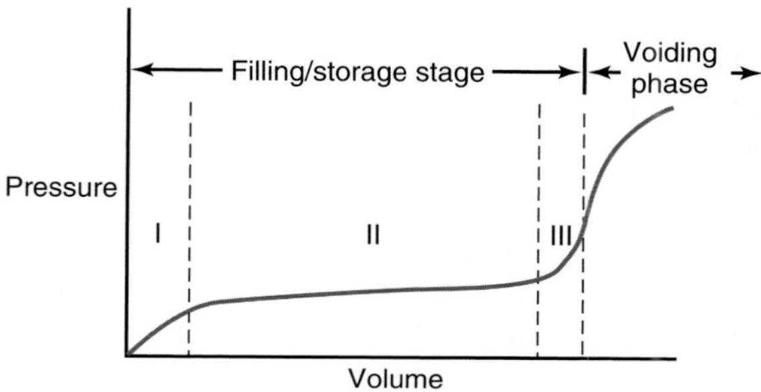

FIGURE 14.5 Idealized normal adult cystometrogram. (From Wein AJ, English WS, Whitmore KE. Office urodynamics. *Urol Clin North Am*. 1988;15:609-623.)

to filling and by the elastic and viscoelastic response of the bladder wall to stretch, factors previously discussed. The initial filling pressure usually develops gradually and levels off between 0 and 8 cm of water in the supine position. With more rapid rates of filling, there may be an initially higher peak, which then levels off. Although this is a detrusor response, its significance is not the same as that of an involuntary bladder contraction during phase 2.

Phase 2: This is called the tonus limb, and compliance (Δ volume/Δ pressure) is normally high and uninterrupted by phasic rises. In practice, the compliance seen in the urodynamic laboratory is always lower than that existing during physiologic bladder filling. It must be remembered that in a normal individual, if the filling rate with liquid is 2.4 times or less than the hourly diuresis rate, phase 2 will be perfectly flat (Bjorn Klemark). Normally, in the urodynamic laboratory, the total rise is less than 6 to 10 cm of water. It is difficult to find agreed upon values for normal compliance.

Phase 3: This is reached when the elastic and viscoelastic properties of the bladder wall have reached their limit. Any further increase in volume generates a substantial increase in pressure. This increase in pressure is not the same as a detrusor contraction. If a voluntary or involuntary contraction occurs, phase 3 can be obscured by the rise in pressure so generated.

Phase 4: Ideally, involuntary bladder contractions do not occur during either phase 2 or 3; phase 4 consists of the initiation of voluntary micturition. Many patients are unable to generate a voluntary detrusor contraction in the testing situation, especially in the supine position. This should not be called detrusor areflexia but simply failure to generate absence of a detrusor contraction during cystometry, a finding that is not considered abnormal unless other clinical or urodynamic findings are present that substantiate the presence of neurologic or myogenic disease.

Involuntary bladder contractions (DO) during filling are always significant. *Detrusor hyperreflexia (neurogenic)* and *detrusor instability (nonneurogenic)* are both terms no longer in use but previously defined by the ICS to relate to the generic term *involuntary bladder contraction*. *Neurogenic DO* (previously *detrusor hyperreflexia*) refers to an involuntary contraction that is the result of associated neurologic disease; *idiopathic DO* (previously *detrusor instability*) refers to an involuntary contraction seen in the absence of neurologic disease. A number of representative adult filling cystometrograms (liquid) are diagrammed in Fig. 14.6.

One of the most important urodynamic concepts to remember is that adequate storage at low intravesical pressure will avoid deleterious upper urinary tract changes in patients with BOO and/or neuromuscular LUT dysfunction. Ed McGuire and coworkers proposed that upper tract deterioration is apt to occur when storage, even though adequate in terms of continence, occurs at sustained urodynamically generated detrusor pressures higher than 40 cm of water. Application of this concept to patients with storage problems and specifically those with decreased compliance and incontinence has resulted in the concept of the detrusor leak point pressure (DLPP) as a very significant piece of urodynamic data. This is to be distinguished from the VLPP described subsequently. The DLPP is also known as the *bladder leak point pressure (BLPP)*. It is important to understand the context in which this test was originally described and the astute intuitive reasoning that went into

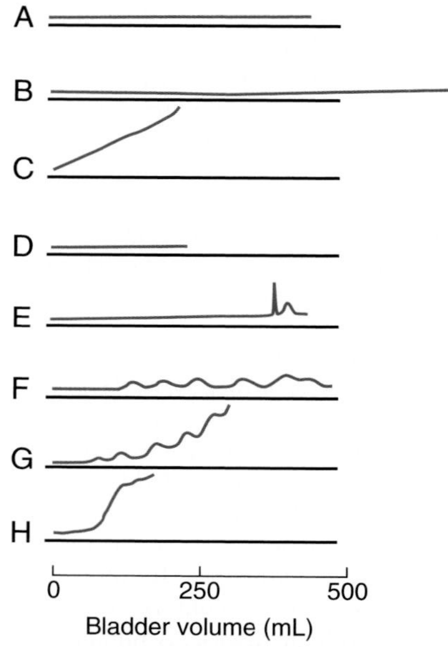

FIGURE 14.6 Various representative adult filling cystometrograms. (A) Normal filling curve in a patient with a bladder capacity of 450 mL, normal compliance, and no involuntary bladder contractions. Nothing can be said about bladder activity during the emptying phase of micturition from this tracing. (B) Large-capacity bladder with increased compliance at medium fill rate. This type of curve is characteristic of an individual with decreased sensation and bladder decompensation. Although most individuals will in fact have no or poor detrusor contraction, that conclusion cannot be made on the basis of this curve. (C) Decreased compliance. (D) Small-capacity bladder secondary to hypersensitivity without decreased compliance or involuntary bladder contraction. (E) Bladder contraction provoked by cough. This particular tracing represents total bladder pressure. To make this diagnosis from this tracing alone, the clinician would need to be either a very astute examiner or review separate recordings of intravesical pressure and intraabdominal pressure (intrarectal pressure). (F) Low-amplitude detrusor contraction. This is a subtracted detrusor pressure, and this type of recording may be seen most characteristically in a patient with suprasacral neurologic disease or idiopathic detrusor overactivity. (G) Decreased compliance and involuntary bladder contractions. (H) High-amplitude early involuntary bladder contraction. (From Wein AJ, English WS, Whitmore KE. Office urodynamics. *Urol Clin North Am.* 1988;15:609-623.)

describing the original concept. In the early 1980s, McGuire and associates studied a group of myelodysplastic children with decreased compliance and incontinence. Those children who did not leak on filling cystometry until their detrusor pressures exceeded 40 cm of water exhibited upper urinary tract deterioration on subsequent follow-up. Classically, the test was performed by passively filling the bladder through a small-caliber urethral catheter with the patient at rest throughout the study, not attempting to volitionally void. The point at which leakage occurs around the catheter is measured as the DLPP. If the DLPP in such an individual with decreased compliance and incontinence is greater than 40 cm of water, the patient is believed to be at risk for upper tract deterioration. Thus this test has become extremely useful in the management of such patients with neurogenic bladder dysfunction. An abnormal test dictates the necessity of reducing storage pressure to a point below which upper tract deterioration will subsequently be seen, even if this means combining measures to decrease bladder contractility and increase bladder capacity with intermittent catheterization. The concept has been extended to cover patients who have decreased compliance and who do not have incontinence, but whose measured detrusor pressure at bladder volumes they often "carry" exceeds 40 cm of water. Some apply the concept also to patients with involuntary bladder contractions whose detrusor pressures frequently exceed 40 cm of water. Whether this concept truly applies to this latter group of patients, except in instances where this occurs extremely frequently, or where the pressure is maintained once contraction has occurred, is unknown.

As a corollary, in patients with decreased compliance and incontinence, one must remember that to accurately measure compliance urodynamically, the bladder outlet must be competent or occluded. This is especially important if there is a plan to correct outlet-related incontinence in an individual with neuromuscular dysfunction associated with decreased compliance (e.g., in the myelomeningocele patient). In other words, one may get a falsely reassuring sense of normal or only slightly decreased compliance in an individual with significant sphincteric insufficiency. Before correcting the sphincteric insufficiency, there needs to be an accurate idea of what bladder compliance will be when the outlet no longer leaks during filling and storage. This can be accomplished very simply by pulling a Foley balloon against the bladder outlet to occlude it during filling.

Cholinergic supersensitivity can be determined during cystometry (bethanechol supersensitivity test). This test is based on Cannon's law of denervation, which implies that when an organ is deprived of its nerve supply, it develops hypersensitivity to a variety of substances, including those that are normally excitatory neurotransmitters for that organ. Originally devised by Jack Lapides and associates, the test has remained virtually unaltered since 1962. It involves controlled liquid cystometry at an infusion rate of 1 mL/sec to a volume of 100 mL, when the bladder pressure is measured. After two or three such infusions, an average value is obtained, and this maneuver is repeated 10, 20, and 30 minutes after subcutaneous injection of 2.5 mg or 0.035 mg/kg of bethanechol chloride. A normal bladder shows a response of less than 15 cm of water pressure above the control value at the 100 mL volume. Under these circumstances, a positive result strongly suggests an interruption in the peripheral neural and/or distal spinal pathways to and from the bladder. The more distal and complete the lesion, the more frequently positive the test seems to be. A negative result in an individual with a normal bladder capacity and no detrusor decompensation (admittedly sometimes hard to judge) and in whom the bethanechol is administered on a weight basis, strongly suggests that there is no such lesion. Known factors that can give a falsely positive test include urinary tract infection (UTI), azotemia, detrusor hypertrophy, and emotional stress. A falsely negative study may result from a decompensated bladder that cannot respond to cholinergic stimulation under any circumstances. False negative results may also be due to an insufficient dose of the cholinergic agonist in a very heavy person, and it is useful to administer bethanechol on a weight basis (0.035 mg/kg) to obviate this. The test is not very useful in individuals with involuntary bladder contractions. Under such circumstances, the cholinergic agonist often simply raises bladder pressure sufficiently to make the involuntary contraction occur at a lower volume than usual. It has never been clear whether this was originally intended to be interpreted as a positive test. If one administers the bethanechol on a weight basis and infection, detrusor hypertrophy, stress, and azotemia have been excluded, there should be few false positive results.

The ice water test was originally described by Bors and Blinn in 1957. Methodology differs among practitioners, but the gist is this: sterile 0°C to 4°C water or saline is rapidly instilled into the bladder (100 mL within 20 seconds or 200 mL/min to a volume of 30% to 50% of a previously determined cystometric capacity). A positive result is considered a detrusor contraction greater than 30 cm of water, with leakage around the catheter, expulsion of the catheter, or emptying immediately after removal of the catheter. The test has been described as a method of demonstrating a segmental reflex that is inhibited centrally in healthy adult subjects without neurologic lesions but which appears when suprasacral lesions are present, but normally occurs in infants and young children. The afferent fibers for the ice water test are thought to be unmyelinated C-fiber afferents, which are normally silent during filling and storage but which become functional with various types of neurologic disease or injury. Thus, a positive test can be considered indicative of a neurologic lesion, even though the neurologic lesion may not become manifest until a subsequent time. However, everyone with such a lesion may not have a positive ice water test.

4. **Voiding cystometry, combined pressure studies, and video urodynamic studies:** Intravesical pressure, IAP (generally reflected by intrarectal pressure), and flow are often measured simultaneously (Fig. 14.7). The purposes of pressure/flow urodynamic studies (PFUDS) are to be able to better define whether obstruction is present and to assess detrusor contractility more precisely. By assessing patterns of detrusor pressure and flow, thereby inferring resistance and patterns of increased resistance, the examiner can often ascertain the exact pathology (e.g., anatomic obstruction versus dyssynergia). The normal

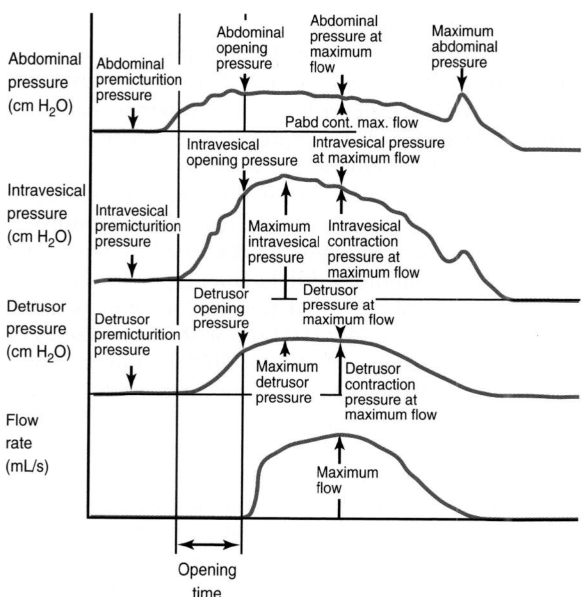

FIGURE 14.7 Recommended International Continence Society (ICS) registration of combined pressure(s) and flow recording. (From Wein AJ, English WS, Whitmore KE. Office urodynamics. *Urol Clin North Am*. 1988;15:609-623.)

adult male generally voids with a detrusor pressure of between 40 and 50 cm of water. The normal adult female voids at a much lower pressure. Indeed, many women void with almost no detectable rise in detrusor pressure. This does not indicate that contraction is not occurring but simply that outlet resistance, lower in the female to begin with, drops to very low levels during voluntary bladder contraction. It should be remembered, however, as Derek Griffiths, a pioneer urodynamicist, has pointed out, that detrusor pressure alone is insufficient to assess the strength of a detrusor contraction. This is because a muscle can use energy to either generate force or shorten its length. With respect to the bladder, a relatively hollow viscus, the force developed contributes to detrusor pressure, whereas the velocity of shortening contributes to flow. With significant obstruction, detrusor pressure can rise to high levels. If resistance is very low, detrusor pressure may be undetectable but the contractility may be equal in the two instances.

Urodynamically, obstruction is generally defined only by the relationship between detrusor pressure and flow (i.e., high pressure and low flow). Pressure-flow studies can be analyzed according to a number of nomograms, a detailed description of which is beyond the scope of this chapter. We find that most often, a detailed visual analysis of the entire study is just as or more helpful. Two easy and useful concepts to remember in this regard are the Abrams-Griffiths (AG) number or bladder outlet obstruction index (BOOI), and the bladder contractility index (BCI). The BOOI relates to whether outlet obstruction is present in the male. It is calculated as [Pdet @ $Q_{MAX} - 2Q_{MAX}$]. A value greater than 40 indicates obstruction, less than 20 indicates no obstruction, and 20 to 40 is considered equivocal. The BCI is calculated in the male as [Pdet @ $Q_{MAX} + 5Q_{MAX}$]. Over 150 indicates a "strong" bladder, 100 to 150 a normal one, and less than 100 a "weak" bladder. There are many other formulas, integrated numbers, and graphs that are designed to assess flow and detrusor contractibility, strength, and work. There are no universal precepts in this regard at this time. The values and studies apply to men only.

Once obstruction is diagnosed, it is necessary to determine the site, and to do this, simultaneous fluoroscopy is often used. This VUDS combines the cystourographic imaging described previously with simultaneous urodynamic studies, permitting a generally accurate determination of the site of obstruction at the time high pressure and low flow coexist. VUDS is also extremely useful in assessing the etiology of complex cases of incontinence because the precise pressure relationships existing in the bladder and urethra can be correlated with the cystourethrographic radiologic patterns, and therefore a judgment can be made of why involuntary leakage occurs at a particular time. In this case, the issue is generally whether the fluoroscopic demonstration of leakage occurs with or without DO or whether the incontinence is due in part to both detrusor and outlet-related causes. VUDS also can demonstrate other bladder pathology (e.g., diverticula, reflux, external compression or displacement, abnormal shape), abnormal activity of the sphincter areas during filling/storage and emptying/voiding, and pathologic descent of the bladder base and proximal urethra.

One of the most difficult problems in urodynamics is the clarification of whether contractile function is adequate, that is, whether it is sustained and coordinated. Phasic DO does not imply normal contractile function. There is a subset of patients with incontinence in whom DO and impaired contractile function coexist—so-called *detrusor hyperactivity with impaired contractility (DHIC)*. The detrusor is overactive in these patients during filling/storage, but empties ineffectively because of diminished detrusor contractile function during emptying and not necessarily because of outlet obstruction. In some patients, obstruction coexists with impaired detrusor contractility, and this diagnosis often cannot be made.

Several very sophisticated resistance formulas exist that attempt to calculate a number for outlet resistance, utilizing data based on intravesical pressure, flow rate, and other mathematical factors. These formulas generally assume that the urethra is a rigid tube with a constant diameter and that the pressure always reflects that generated by a normal bladder, not a decompensated one. If a bladder has normal contractility and the pressure that it generates during contraction is high and if the corresponding flow rate that results is low, one does not need a formula to diagnose obstruction. On the other hand, if the bladder is decompensated and incapable of producing a significant rise in pressure, obstruction cannot be quantitated by these formulas. More sophisticated and innovative methods of defining the relationship between intravesical pressure and uroflow have been devised, and the relative worth of these methods and debates are beyond the scope of this discussion of urodynamics. The global question surrounding all noncomputer-assisted and computer-assisted characterizations and interpretations of pressure-flow data is: What do these add? Is the evaluation of the average older man with LUT symptoms more likely to lead to a better treatment outcome if PFUDS or VUDS is performed, including the analysis of results in various mathematical ways with computer assistance? Do sophisticated or unsophisticated urodynamic studies predict the outcome of various treatments for lower urinary tract symptoms (LUTS), including watchful waiting? Are patients with LUTS in whom outlet ablation fails as treatment the same patients as those in whom detrusor contractility is judged ineffective by the criteria under consideration? Unfortunately, those of us who perform urodynamics have not done a terribly good job of looking into these aspects of outcome analysis. Fig. 14.7 displays the ICS's recommended registration of combined pressure and flow recording. Kinesiologic electromyography is often added as an additional channel, and some investigators record urethral pressure at one or various sites along the urethra simultaneously as well. The typical VUDS configuration includes this and a fluoroscopic lower tract image.

5. **Electromyography**: For the majority of urologists, electromyography is a urodynamic study that permits evaluation of the striated sphincter during the emptying phase of micturition. *Kinesiologic electromyography* is the term that describes this application, that is, the study of the activity of one group of muscles (the striated musculature of the outlet) with respect to another (the bladder). Normally, as the bladder fills with urine, there is a gradual and sustained increase in electromyographic (EMG) activity recruited from the pelvic floor muscles. This reaches a maximum just before voiding. Compositely, this is known as the *guarding reflex*. The lack of a guarding reflex suggests neural pathology, as does the inability to produce a sphincter "flare" when given the command to "stop voiding." Voluntary voiding is normally accompanied by complete electrical silence-relaxation of the striated sphincter. There is a marked increase in EMG activity in response to a number of stimuli, including cough, Credé and Valsalva maneuvers, the BCR, and the request to stop voiding, a maneuver accomplished by most through forceful contraction of the pelvic floor musculature (Fig. 14.8). Kinesiologic electromyography enables the urodynamic examiner to ascertain whether the striated sphincter appropriately increases its

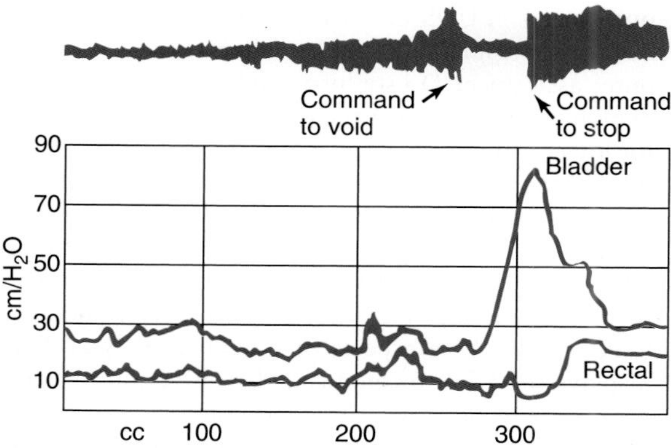

FIGURE 14.8 Normal pressure electromyographic tracing. Note the gradual increase in electromyographic activity during bladder filling (this is called the guarding reflex) with a decrease to control levels just before the onset of what is voluntary bladder contraction. Note that the command to stop voiding evokes a pelvic floor striated muscle contraction reflected by a flare in sphincter electromyography. (From Wein AJ, English WS, Whitmore KE. Office urodynamics. *Urol Clin North Am*. 1988;15:609-623.)

activity in a gradual fashion during bladder filling (whether the guarding reflex is normal) and whether quiescence occurs normally before and during bladder contraction. Kinesiologic electromyography can be performed with either needle electrodes or surface or patch electrodes. Needle electrodes certainly permit more accurate placement and more accurate recording, but in many cases, surface electrodes seem perfectly adequate to obtain the necessary information. When EMG activity gradually increases during filling cystometry and then ceases prior to or at the onset of attempted voiding, this is normal and can be taken as a reflection of what goes on during actual bladder filling and emptying. However, a simultaneous increase of EMG activity with an increase in intravesical pressure during filling cystometry is not always indicative of detrusor-striated sphincter dyssynergia. Abdominal straining or attempted inhibition of a bladder contraction will yield an identical pattern. For a patient with normal sensation, no matter how cooperative, it is extremely difficult to maintain true relaxation during an involuntary bladder contraction. In fact, the appropriate response is to try to suppress such a contraction by voluntary contraction of the anal sphincter, the pelvic floor musculature, or both. All of these circumstances represent types of pseudodyssynergia and are extremely difficult to differentiate from true dyssynergia on the basis of any type of urodynamic study done solely during bladder filling. The term *detrusor-striated sphincter dyssynergia*, generally referred to as just *detrusor sphincter dyssynergia (DSD)*, should refer to obstruction to the outflow of urine during bladder contraction caused by involuntary contraction of the striated sphincter. This is most often seen in patients with discrete neurologic disease, such as suprasacral spinal cord transection after spinal shock has passed. Individuals suspected of having detrusor-striated sphincter dyssynergia but who lack identifiable neurologic disease should always be further investigated with sophisticated video urodynamic evaluation during a full micturition study. True detrusor-striated sphincter dyssynergia is extremely uncommon (some examiners say that it does not exist) in patients without neurologic disease, and such a diagnosis deserves exhaustive study before it is in fact confirmed.

6. **Urethral profilometry**: The term *urethral profilometry* refers to many entities utilized in various settings. The most common usage refers to a static infusion urethral pressure profile. In this study, a small catheter with radially drilled side holes is placed in the bladder and, through it, a medium, usually liquid, is infused. The catheter is then withdrawn at a constant rate, and the pressure required to push the medium through the side holes is recorded from inside the bladder to a site where the pressure becomes essentially isobaric with bladder pressure. The infusion profile curve is thus a result of a number of factors, including urethral wall compliance, resistance to inflow of the medium, resistance to runoff of the medium into the bladder and out the urethral meatus, and artifact generated by the apparatus. Because the study is usually done at rest and not during bladder filling or emptying, it is difficult to associate the recorded events with bladder-urethral interaction during filling or emptying. Specifically with relevance to neuromuscular dysfunction, the static infusion profile has been cited as useful at various times in history in diagnosing stress incontinence, DSD,

and obstruction. In our opinion, it is not very useful for the specific diagnosis of any of these. There is much overlap in maximum urethral pressures and functional urethral lengths between individuals with stress incontinence and normal individuals, especially in the elderly population. The rationale of diagnosing either smooth or striated sphincter dyssynergia on the basis of a static infusion profile is difficult to understand. A high pressure at a given point in the passage of the catheter from the bladder through the urethra can be secondary to a number of phenomena, and this result by no means indicates that there will always be contraction or obstruction in this area during voluntary or involuntary micturition. The static infusion urethral profile is certainly useful for testing the function of an artificial genitourinary sphincter. With specific relevance to neuromuscular dysfunction, it is useful for suspecting intrinsic sphincter dysfunction. In an individual with such an abnormality (Figs. 14.9 and 14.10), the proximal urethra is isobaric or almost isobaric with the bladder, and the striated sphincter peak is generally lower than normal. In men, the static infusion profile can also be used to estimate prostate size, through the length of the prostate "shoulder" that occurs prior to the peak

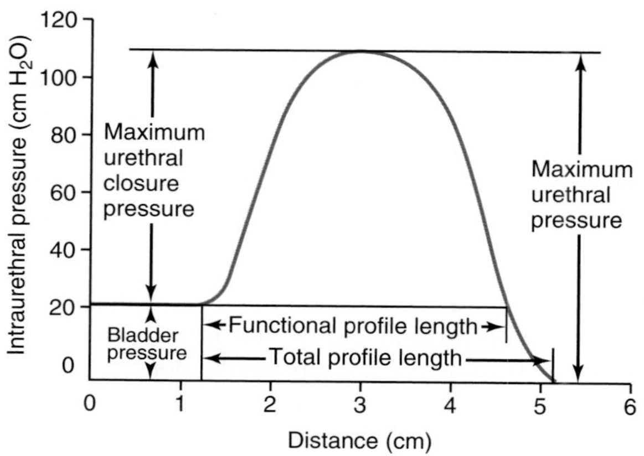

FIGURE 14.9 Idealized static infusion urethral pressure profile utilizing International Continence Society (ICS) nomenclature (female). (From Wein AJ, English WS, Whitmore KE. Office urodynamics. *Urol Clin North Am.* 1988;15:609-623.)

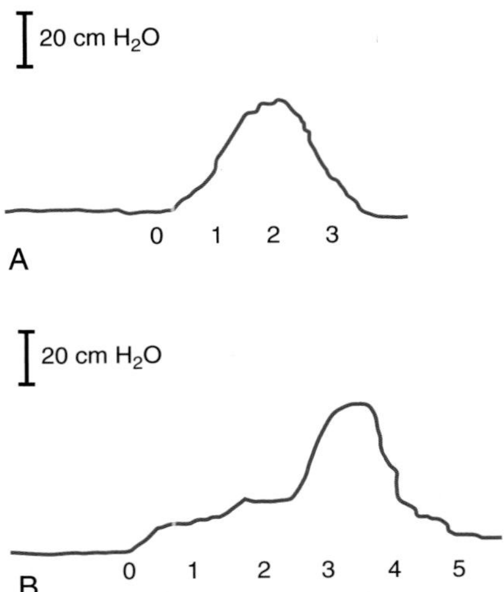

FIGURE 14.10 Actual static infusion urethral pressure profiles from normal female (A) and male (B) subjects. Numbers represent centimeters with 0 representing the level of the bladder neck. The maximum urethral pressure in both males and females is normally at the level of the urogenital diaphragm. The initial portion of the curve in the male, from the bladder neck to the pressure rise culminating at the maximum urethral pressure, is sometimes called *prostatic plateau*. The area under this portion of the curve corresponds roughly to prostatic size. (From Wein AJ, English WS, Whitmore KE. Office urodynamics. *Urol Clin North Am*. 1988;15:609-623.)

pressure (generally taken to represent the site of the maximum consideration of striated sphincter).

Stress urethral profilometry refers to a study done with a catheter with dual sensors, one in the bladder and one in the proximal urethra. With coughing or straining, the change in urethral pressure should always be equal to or greater than the change in bladder pressure. In patients with stress incontinence, along with much of the profile curve, the change in urethral pressure will be less than the change in bladder pressure.

Dynamic urethral profilometry implies the use of a catheter with dual sensors—bladder and proximal urethra—with pressures recorded during bladder filling and emptying. An actual urethral pressure profile is not recorded. The interaction between bladder pressure and pressure in one area of the urethra, generally in the area of maximal closure pressure, usually at the level of the striated sphincter, is recorded.

Micturitional urethral profilometry refers to a study in which a catheter with dual or triple sensors, one of which is in the bladder, is withdrawn during voiding in a patient with known obstruction. In such a patient, the area of the maximal urethral pressure drop is the site of obstruction. Micturitional profilometry generally requires fluoroscopic monitoring to identify the anatomic location of this maximal pressure decrease.

7. **Abdominal leak point pressure:** The abdominal leak point pressure (ALPP) is a measure of the ability of the urethra to resist changes in abdominal pressure as an expulsive force. It has been popularized by Ed McGuire as a clinically useful test, perhaps the most useful one to differentiate the extremes of ISD from hypermobility-related stress incontinence. It is easy to see why the concept of this test appeals to straightforward logic: If straining or increases in IAP produce incontinence, and a filling study shows normal compliance, without DO, there must be a problem with the bladder outlet. The amount of abdominal pressure necessary to cause leakage under such circumstances is inversely proportional to the amount of outlet dysfunction. A pressure catheter is placed in the bladder or rectum or both, and the bladder is filled to a predetermined volume, usually 150 to 200 mL. The patient is then asked to perform a graded Valsalva maneuver until leakage is seen per urethra. If this does not produce leakage, the patient is asked to cough. The pressure at which leakage is first seen is the ALPP. The higher the ALPP, the better the intrinsic sphincter function, and, conversely, the lower the ALPP, the worse the intrinsic sphincter function. There are still problems concerning standardization of technique, specification of variables, optimal location of pressure measurement, size of urethral catheter to be used, and the bladder volume at which the study is to be carried out. There is also disagreement about what "numbers" indicate a significant degree of intrinsic sphincter dysfunction. Originally, an ALPP of less than 60 to 65 cm of water was said to indicate ISD. One caveat to remember is that a large cystocele can invalidate the results, making the ALPP artificially higher.

8. **Ambulatory urodynamics:** An obvious limitation to routine or conventional urodynamic testing is the artificial environment and circumstances in which the test is conducted. Ambulatory urodynamics is an alternative technique in which the pressure-transducing catheters are placed into the bladder and rectum but are attached to portable recording devices. The patient resumes their normal daily routine and cycles of natural bladder filling and storage. Emptying and voiding are recorded, while the patient writes down the time and qualitative nature of relevant subjective sensations. Provocative maneuvers such as coughing, climbing, jumping, and hand washing can be performed in an attempt to reproduce the patient's symptomatology. At the conclusion of the study, the data are downloaded to a computer, compared with the written record of symptomatology, and analyzed. Advocates of this type of study cite the ability to objectively confirm the complaints of many patients in whom nonambulatory urodynamics have been unrevealing. However, limitations of this study include the following: (1) the triggering effect of a catheter in the bladder can cause a higher incidence of involuntary bladder contractions than in standard cystometry; (2) if one is recording urethral pressures as well, small movements of the catheter are unavoidable in an ambulatory patient, often resulting in artificial pressure dips; (3) measurement of actual leakage is difficult or near impossible; (4) the bladder-filling rate depends on many factors that are still not controllable (such as intake, diuretic usage, and congestive failure); (5) different states of rectal filling and rectal catheter stimulation in the ambulatory patient may exert reflex effects on the bladder; (6) it is difficult to simultaneously measure flow during ambulatory urodynamics, and so, at present, the study is more useful in the evaluation of filling and storage abnormalities than emptying/voiding abnormalities; (7) detrusor pressure values for certain parameters are different during ambulatory urodynamics as opposed to laboratory urodynamics (new agreed-on standards for normality and abnormality need to be developed); and (8) a certain percent of records will be unable to be interpreted because of artifacts. At present, ambulatory urodynamics are utilized primarily as a research tool, although the potential range of clinical applications, with some technologic improvements, is numerous.

Classification of Lower Urinary Tract Dysfunction

There are many classification systems for LUT dysfunction, and these are based on neurologic, urodynamic, or functional considerations, or on a combination of these. That there are at least six to eight of these attests to the fact that none is prefect. The purpose of any classification system should be to facilitate understanding and management and to avoid confusion among those who are concerned with the problem for which the system was designed. A good classification should serve as intellectual shorthand and should convey, in a few key words or phrases, the essence of a clinical situation. Most systems of classification for LUT dysfunction were formulated primarily to describe dysfunction secondary to neurologic disease or injury. The ideal system should be applicable to all types of LUT dysfunction.

In this section, we describe the functional type of classification that we have found most useful and also the ICS classification and the Lapides system. A more exhaustive listing can be found in *Campbell-Walsh-Wein Urology*.

THE FUNCTIONAL SYSTEM

Classification of LUT dysfunction can be formulated on a simple functional basis, describing the dysfunction in terms of whether the deficit produced is primarily one of the filling/storage or the emptying/voiding phases of micturition (see Tables 14.3 and 14.4). This simple-minded scheme assumes only that, whatever their differences, "experts" would agree on the two-phase concept of micturition (filling/storage and emptying/voiding) and on the simple overall mechanisms underlying the normality of each phase.

Storage failure results because of either bladder or outlet abnormalities or a combination. The proven bladder abnormalities very simply include only involuntary bladder contractions, low compliance, and heightened or altered sensation. The outlet abnormalities can include only an intermittent or continuous decrease in outlet resistance. Emptying failure, likewise, can occur because of bladder or outlet abnormalities or a combination. The bladder side includes only inadequate, uncoordinated, or unsustained bladder contractility, and the outlet side includes only anatomic obstruction and sphincter(s) dyssynergia (functional obstructions).

Failure in either category generally is not absolute, but more often is relative. There are indeed some types of LUT dysfunction that represent combinations of filling/storage and emptying/voiding abnormalities. Within this scheme, however, these become readily understandable and their detection and treatment can be logically described. Various aspects of physiology and pathophysiology are always related more to one phase of micturition than another. All aspects of urodynamic and video urodynamic evaluation can be conceptualized in this functional manner as to exactly what they evaluate in terms of either bladder or outlet activity during filling/storage and emptying/voiding (see Table 14.6). In addition, one can easily classify all known treatments for LUT dysfunction under the broad categories of whether they facilitate filling/storage and emptying/voiding and whether they do so by an action primarily on the bladder or on one or more of the components of the bladder outlet (Tables 14.7 and 14.8).

TABLE 14.7 Therapy to Facilitate Urine Storage/Bladder Filling

1. Bladder related (inhibiting bladder contractility, decreasing sensory input, and/or increasing bladder capacity)
   a. Behavioral therapy, including any or all of:
      1) Education
      2) Bladder training
      3) Timed bladder emptying or prompted voiding
      4) Fluid restriction
      5) Pelvic floor physiotherapy ± biofeedback
   b. Pharmacologic therapy (oral, intravesical, intradetrusor)
      1) Antimuscarinic agents
      2) Beta-3-adrenergic agonists
      3) Botulinum toxin
      4) Drugs with combined actions
      5) Calcium antagonists
      6) Potassium channel openers
      7) Prostaglandin inhibitors
      8) Alpha-adrenergic antagonists
      9) Tricyclic antidepressants; serotonin and norepinephrine reuptake inhibitors
      10) Dimethyl sulfoxide (DMSO)
      11) Polysynaptic inhibitors
      12) Capsaicin, resiniferatoxin, and similar agents

Continued

TABLE 14.7 Therapy to Facilitate Urine Storage/Bladder Filling—cont'd

- c. Bladder overdistention
- d. Electrical stimulation (sacral neuromodulation, posterior tibial and other peripheral nerve stimulation)
- e. Acupuncture and electroacupuncture
- f. Interruption of innervation
    - 1) Very central (subarachnoid block)
    - 2) Less central (sacral rhizotomy, selective sacral rhizotomy)
    - 3) Peripheral motor or/and sensory
- g. Augmentation cystoplasty (auto, bowel, tissue engineering)

2. Outlet related (increasing outlet resistance)
    - a. Behavioral therapy, including any or all of:
        - 1) Education
        - 2) Bladder training
        - 3) Timed bladder emptying or prompted voiding
        - 4) Fluid restriction
        - 5) Pelvic floor muscle training ± biofeedback
    - b. Electrical stimulation
    - c. Pharmacologic therapy
        - 1) Alpha-adrenergic agonists
        - 2) Tricyclic antidepressants; serotonin and norepinephrine reuptake inhibitors
        - 3) Beta-adrenergic antagonists, agonists
    - d. Vaginal and perineal occlusive and/or supportive devices; urethral plugs
    - e. Nonsurgical periurethral bulking
        - 1) Synthetic bulking agents, tissue engineering
    - f. Retropubic vesicourethral suspension ± prolapse repair (female)
    - g. Sling procedures ± prolapse repair (female)
    - h. Midurethral tapes ± prolapse repair (female)
    - i. Perineal sling procedure (male)
    - j. Artificial urinary sphincter
    - k. Myoplasty (muscle transposition)
    - l. Bladder outlet closure
    - m. Regenerative medicine
3. Circumventing the problem
    - a. Absorbent products
    - b. External collecting devices
    - c. Antidiuretic hormone-like agents
    - d. Short-acting diuretics
    - e. Intermittent catheterization
    - f. Continuous catheterization
    - g. Urinary diversion

TABLE 14.8 Therapy to Facilitate Bladder Emptying/Voiding

1. Bladder related (increasing intravesical pressure or facilitating bladder contractility)
   a. External compression, Valsalva
   b. Promotion or initiation of reflex contraction
      1) Trigger zones or maneuvers
      2) Bladder "training," tidal drainage
   c. Pharmacologic therapy (oral, intravesical)
      1) Parasympathomimetic agents
      2) Prostaglandins
      3) Blockers of inhibition
         i. Alpha-adrenergic antagonists
         ii. Opioid antagonists
   d. Electrical stimulation
      1) Directly to the bladder or spinal cord
      2) Directly to the nerve roots
      3) Intravesical (transurethral)
      4) Sacral neuromodulation
   e. Reduction cystoplasty
   f. Bladder myoplasty (muscle wrap)
2. Outlet related (decreasing outlet resistance)
   a. At a site of anatomic obstruction
      1) Pharmacologic therapy—decrease prostate size or tone
         i. Alpha-adrenergic antagonists
         ii. 5-Alpha-reductase inhibitors
         iii. Luteinizing hormone-releasing hormone agonists/antagonists
         iv. Antiandrogens
      2) Prostatectomy, prostatotomy (diathermy, heat, laser, water jet, dilation of prostatic fossa)
      3) Bladder neck incision or resection
      4) Urethral stricture repair or dilation
      5) Intraurethral stent
      6) Balloon dilation of stricture/contracture
   b. At level of smooth sphincter
      1) Pharmacologic therapy
         i. Alpha-adrenergic antagonists
      2) Transurethral resection or incision
      3) Y-V plasty
   c. At level of striated sphincter
      1) Behavioral therapy ± biofeedback
      2) Pharmacologic therapy
         i. Benzodiazepines

Continued

TABLE 14.8 Therapy to Facilitate Bladder Emptying/Voiding—cont'd

ii. Baclofen
iii. Dantrolene
iv. Alpha-adrenergic antagonists
v. Botulinum toxin (injection)

3) Urethral overdilation
4) Surgical sphincterotomy
5) Urethral stent
6) Pudendal nerve interruption

3. Circumventing the problem
   a. Intermittent catheterization
   b. Continuous catheterization
   c. Urinary diversion (conduit or reservoir)

Such a functional system can easily be "expanded" and made more complicated to include etiologic or specific urodynamic connotations (see Table 14.4). However, the simplified system is perfectly workable and avoids argument in those complex situations in which the exact etiology or urodynamic mechanism for a voiding dysfunction cannot be agreed on.

Proper use of the functional system for a given LUT dysfunction obviously requires a reasonably accurate notion of what the urodynamic data show. However, an exact diagnosis is *not* required for treatment. It should be recognized that some patients do not have only a discrete storage or emptying failure, and the existence of combination deficits must be recognized to properly utilize this system of classification. For instance, the classic T10 paraplegic patient after spinal shock generally exhibits a relative failure to store because of involuntary bladder contraction and a relative failure to empty the bladder because of striated sphincter dyssynergia. With such a combination deficit, to utilize this classification system as a guide to treatment, one must assume that one of the deficits is primary and that significant improvement will result from its treatment alone or that the LUT dysfunction can be converted primarily to a disorder of either storage or emptying by means of nonsurgical or surgical therapy. The resultant deficit can then be treated or circumvented. Using this example, the combined deficit in a T10 paraplegic patient can be converted primarily to a storage failure by procedures directed at the dyssynergic striated sphincter; the resultant incontinence (secondary to involuntary contractions) can be circumvented (in a male) with an external collecting device. Alternatively, the deficit can be converted primarily to an emptying failure by pharmacologic or surgical measures designed to abolish or reduce the involuntary contractions, and the resultant emptying failure can then be circumvented with clean intermittent catheterization (CIC). Other examples of combination deficits include impaired bladder contractility or overactivity with sphincter dysfunction, BOO with DO, BOO with sphincter malfunction, DO during filling/storage with impaired contractility during emptying (DHIC), and sphincteric incontinence with DO or impaired bladder contractibility. One of the advantages of this functional classification is that it allows the clinician the liberty of "playing" with the system to suit their own preferences without an alteration in the basic concept of "keep it simple but accurate and informative." For instance, one could easily substitute the terms *overactive or oversensitive bladder* and *underactive outlet* for *because of the bladder* and *because of the outlet* under "Failure to store" in Table 14.3. One could choose to categorize the bladder reasons for overactivity (see Table 14.4) further in terms of neurogenic, myogenic, or anatomic causes and further subcategorize neurogenic in terms of decreased inhibitory control, increased afferent activity, increased sensitivity to efferent activity, and so on. *The system is flexible and it works.*

INTERNATIONAL CONTINENCE SOCIETY CLASSIFICATION

The classification system proposed by the ICS (Table 14.9) is in essence an extension of a urodynamic classification system. The storage and voiding phases of micturition are described separately, and, within each, various designations are applied to describe bladder and urethral function. Some of the definitions were changed by the standardization subcommittee of the ICS in 2002 and the relevant changes are indicated here. Normal bladder function during filling/storage implies no significant rises in detrusor pressure. Overactive detrusor function indicates the presence of "involuntary detrusor contractions during the filling phase which may be spontaneous or provoked." If caused by neurologic disease, the term *neurogenic DO* (previously *detrusor hyperreflexia*)

TABLE 14.9 International Continence Society Classification

Storage Phase	Voiding Phase
Bladder function	**Bladder function**
Detrusor activity	Detrusor activity
Normal or stable	Normal
Overactive	Underactive
Neurogenic	Acontractile
Idiopathic	Areflexic
Bladder sensation	
Normal	**Urethral function**
Increased or hypersensitive	Normal
Reduced or hyposensitive	Abnormal
Absent	Mechanical obstruction
Bladder capacity	Overactivity
Normal	Dysfunctional voiding
High	Detrusor sphincter dyssynergia (DSD)
Low	Nonrelaxing urethral sphincter dysfunction
Urethral function	
Normal closure mechanism	
Incompetent closure mechanism	

is used; if not, the term *idiopathic DO* (previously *detrusor instability*) is applied. Bladder sensation can be categorized only in qualitative terms as indicated. Bladder capacity and compliance (Δ volume/Δ pressure) are cystometric measurements. Bladder capacity can refer to cystometric capacity, maximum cystometric capacity, or maximum anesthetic cystometric capacity. Normal urethral function during filling/storage indicates a positive urethral closure pressure (urethral pressure minus bladder pressure) even with increases in IAP, although it may be overcome by DO. Incompetent urethral function during filling/storage implies urine leakage in the absence of a detrusor contraction. This may be secondary to classical (hypermobility related) stress incontinence, intrinsic sphincter dysfunction, a combination, or an involuntary fall in urethral pressure in the absence of detrusor contraction (without instability).

During the voiding/emptying phase of micturition, normal detrusor activity implies voiding by a voluntarily initiated sustained contraction that leads to complete bladder emptying within a normal time span. An underactive detrusor defines a contraction of inadequate magnitude and/or duration to empty the bladder within a normal time span. An acontractile detrusor is one that cannot be demonstrated to contract during urodynamic testing. Areflexia is defined as acontractility due to an abnormality of neural control, implying the complete absence of centrally coordinated contraction. Normal urethral function during voiding indicates a urethra that opens and is continuously relaxed to allow bladder emptying at a normal pressure. Abnormal urethra function during voiding may be due to either mechanical obstruction or urethral overactivity. Dysfunctional voiding describes an intermittent or/and fluctuating flow rate due to involuntary intermittent contractions of the periurethral striated muscle in neurologically normal individuals. DSD defines a detrusor contraction concurrent with an involuntary contraction of the urethral or periurethral striated muscle or both. Nonrelaxing urethral sphincter obstruction usually occurs in individuals with a neurologic lesion and is characterized by a nonrelaxing obstructing urethra resulting in reduced urine flow.

LUT dysfunction in a classical T10-level paraplegic patient after spinal shock has passed would be classified in the ICS system as follows:

- Storage phase—overactive neurogenic detrusor function, absent sensation, low capacity, normal compliance, and normal urethral closure function.
- Voiding phase—overactive detrusor function and overactive obstructive urethral function.

The micturition dysfunction of a stroke patient with urgency incontinence would most likely be classified during storage as overactive neurogenic detrusor function, normal sensation, low capacity, normal compliance, and normal urethral closure function. During voiding (this refers to voluntary micturition), the dysfunction would be classified as normal detrusor activity and normal urethral function, assuming that no anatomic obstruction existed.

LAPIDES CLASSIFICATION

Jack Lapides contributed significantly to the classification and care of the patient with neuropathic voiding dysfunction by

TABLE 14.10 Lapides Classification

Sensory neurogenic bladder
Motor paralytic bladder (motor neurogenic bladder)
Uninhibited neurogenic bladder
Reflex neurogenic bladder
Autonomous neurogenic bladder

slightly modifying and popularizing a system originally proposed by McLellan in 1939 (Table 14.10). Lapides classification differs from that of McLellan in only one respect, and that is the division of the group of "atonic neurogenic bladder" into sensory neurogenic and motor neurogenic bladder. This remains one of the most familiar systems to urologists and others because it describes in recognizable shorthand the clinical and cystometric conditions of many (but not all) types of neurogenic voiding dysfunction.

A sensory neurogenic bladder results from disease that selectively interrupts the sensory fibers between the bladder and the spinal cord or the afferent tracts to the brain. Diabetes mellitus, tabes dorsalis, and pernicious anemia were cited as most commonly responsible. The first clinical changes are described as those of impaired sensation of bladder distention. Unless voiding is initiated on a timed basis, varying degrees of bladder overdistention can result with resultant hypotonicity. If bladder decompensation occurs, significant amounts of residual urine result, and at that time, the cystometric curve generally demonstrates a large-capacity bladder with a flat, high-compliance, low-pressure filling curve.

A motor paralytic bladder results from disease processes that destroy the parasympathetic motor innervation of the bladder. Extensive pelvic surgery or trauma may produce this. Herpes zoster has been listed as a cause as well, but recent evidence suggests that the voiding dysfunction seen with herpes may be more related to a problem with afferent input. The early symptoms of a motor paralytic bladder may vary from painful urinary retention to only a relative inability to initiate and maintain normal micturition. Early cystometric filling is normal but without a voluntary bladder contraction at capacity. Chronic overdistention and decompensation may occur, resulting in a large-capacity bladder with a flat, low-pressure filling curve; a large residual of urine may result.

An uninhibited neurogenic bladder was described originally as resulting from injury or disease to the "corticoregulatory tract." The sacral spinal cord was presumed to be the micturition reflex center, and the corticoregulatory tract was believed to normally exert an inhibitory influence on the sacral micturition reflex center. A destructive lesion in this tract would then result in overfacilitation of the micturition reflex. Cerebrovascular accident (CVA), brain or spinal cord tumor, PD, and demyelinating disease were listed as the most common causes in this category. The LUT dysfunction is most often characterized symptomatically by frequency, urgency, and urge incontinence and urodynamically by normal sensation with involuntary contraction at low filling volumes. Residual urine is characteristically low unless anatomic outlet obstruction or true smooth or striated sphincter dyssynergia occurs. The patient generally can initiate a bladder contraction voluntarily but is often unable to do so during cystometry because sufficient urine storage cannot occur before involuntary contraction is stimulated.

Reflex neurogenic bladder described the postspinal shock condition that exists after complete interruption of the sensory and motor pathways between the sacral spinal cord and the brain stem. Most commonly, this occurs in traumatic SCI and transverse myelitis, but it may occur with extensive demyelinating disease or any process that produces significant spinal cord destruction. Typically, there is no bladder sensation, and there is inability to initiate voluntary micturition. Incontinence without sensation generally results because of low-volume involuntary contractions. Striated sphincter dyssynergia is the rule.

An autonomous neurogenic bladder results from complete motor and sensory separation of the bladder from the sacral spinal cord. This may be caused by any disease that destroys the sacral cord or causes extensive damage to the sacral roots or pelvic nerves. There is inability to voluntarily initiate micturition, no bladder reflex activity, and no specific bladder sensation. This is the type of dysfunction seen in patients with spinal shock. The characteristic cystometric pattern is initially similar to the late stages of the motor or sensory paralytic bladder, with a marked shift to the right of the cystometric filling curve and a large bladder capacity at low intravesical pressure. However, decreased compliance may develop secondary either to chronic inflammatory change or to the effects of denervation/decentralization with secondary neuromorphologic and neuropharmacologic reorganizational changes. Emptying capacity may vary widely, depending on the ability of the patient to increase intravesical pressure and on the resistance offered during this increase by the smooth and striated sphincters.

These classic categories in their usual settings are generally easily understood and remembered, and this is why this system provides a good framework for teaching some fundamentals of neurogenic LUT dysfunction to students and others. Unfortunately, many patients do not exactly "fit" into one or another category. Gradations of sensory, motor, and mixed lesions occur, and the patterns produced after different types of peripheral denervation/decentralization may vary widely from those that are classically described. The system is applicable only to neuropathic dysfunction.

Neurogenic Lower Urinary Tract Dysfunction

GENERAL PATTERNS

Discrete neurologic lesions generally affect the filling/storage and emptying/voiding phases of LUT function in a relatively consistent fashion. The abnormalities depend on: (1) the area(s) of the nervous system affected, and whether the area is completely or incompletely involved, (2) the normal physiologic function(s) and the contents and location of the area(s) affected, and (3) whether the lesion or process is destructive or irritative. The acute dysfunction produced may differ from the chronic one for a variety of reasons.

Table 14.11 summarizes many of these dysfunctions on the basis of the most common type of abnormal pattern that results from a given disease or injury, insofar as the parameters just listed are concerned. This abbreviated classification is not meant to be all inclusive, but to simply indicate that, for the most part, an individual with a specific neurologic abnormality, and LUT dysfunction because of it, will, in general, have the type of dysfunction shown.

1. **Lesions above the brainstem:** Neurologic lesions above the brainstem that affect micturition generally result in involuntary

TABLE 14.11 Most Common Patterns of Typical Voiding Dysfunctions Seen with Types of Neurologic Disease or Injury

Disorder	Detrusor Activity	Compliance	Smooth Sphincter	Striated Sphincter	Other
Cerebrovascular accident	O	N	S	S ± VC	There may be decreased sensation of lower urinary tract (LUT) events.
Brain tumor	O	N	S	S	There may be decreased sensation of LUT events.
Cerebral palsy	O	N	S	S D (25% of those with DO) ± VC	
Parkinson disease	O I	N	S	S Bradykinesia	
Multiple system atrophy	O I	N †	O	S	Striated sphincter may exhibit denervation.
Multiple sclerosis	O	N	S	S D (30%–65%)	Dyssynergia figures refer to percentage of those with detrusor overactivity (DO).
Spinal cord injury Suprasacral	O	N	S	D	Smooth sphincter may be dyssynergic if lesion is above T7.
Sacral	A	N † (may develop)	CNR O (may develop)	F	
Autonomic hyperreflexia	O	N	D	D	

Continued

TABLE 14.11 Most Common Patterns of Typical Voiding Dysfunctions Seen with Types of Neurologic Disease or Injury—cont'd

Disorder	Detrusor Activity	Compliance	Smooth Sphincter	Striated Sphincter	Other
Myelodysplasia	A	N O	O †(MA)	F	Findings vary widely in different series. Striated sphincter commonly shows some evidence of denervation.
Tabes, pernicious anemia	I A	N ‡	S	S	Primary problem is loss of sensation. Detrusor may become decompensated secondary to overdistention.
Disk disease	A	N	CNR	S	Striated sphincter may show evidence of denervation and fixed tone.
Radical pelvic surgery	I A	† N	O	F	
Diabetes	I A O	N ‡	S	S	Sensory loss contributes, but there is a motor neuropathy as well.

Detrusor activity: *I*, impaired; *O*, overactive; *A*, areflexia.
Compliance: *N*, normal; †, decreased; ‡, increased.
Smooth sphincter: *S*, synergic; *D*, dyssynergic; *O*, open, incompetent at rest; *CNR*, competent, nonrelaxing.
Striated sphincter: *S*, synergic; *D*, dyssynergic; ± *VC*, voluntary control may be impaired; *F*, fixed tone.

bladder contractions with coordinated sphincter function (smooth and striated sphincter synergy). Sensation and voluntary striated sphincter function are generally preserved, but sensation may be deficient or delayed. Detrusor areflexia may, however, occur either initially or as a permanent dysfunction. UI may occur due to the DO.

2. **Complete spinal cord lesions above the sacral spinal cord:** Such patients, after they recover from spinal shock, generally exhibit involuntary bladder contractions without sensation, smooth sphincter synergy, and striated sphincter dyssynergia. Those with lesions above T6 also may experience smooth sphincter dyssynergia and autonomic hyperreflexia (AH). Incontinence may occur due to DO, but the outlet obstruction can also cause urinary retention.
3. **Complete or incomplete lesions at the sacral spinal cord or root level:** Such patients generally do not manifest involuntary bladder contractions per se. Detrusor areflexia is initially the rule after spinal shock, and, depending on the type and extent of neurologic injury, various forms of decreased compliance during filling may occur. An open smooth sphincter area may result, but whether this is caused by sympathetic or parasympathetic decentralization or defunctionalization (or both or neither) has never been determined. Various types of striated sphincter dysfunction may occur, but commonly, the area retains a residual fixed sphincter tone (not the same as dyssynergia) and is not under voluntary control.
4. **Interruption of peripheral reflex arc:** The dysfunctions that occur with interruption of the peripheral reflex arc may be very similar to those of distal spinal cord or nerve root injury. Detrusor areflexia often develops, low compliance may result, the smooth sphincter area may be relatively incompetent, and the striated sphincter area may exhibit fixed residual tone not amenable to voluntary relaxation. True peripheral neuropathy can be motor or sensory, with the usual expected sequelae, at least initially.
5. **Cerebrovascular disease:** Thrombus, occlusion, and hemorrhage are the most common causes of stroke, cerebrovascular accident (CVA) leading to ischemia and infarction of variably sized areas in the brain, usually around the internal capsule.

After the initial acute episode, urinary retention from detrusor areflexia may occur. The neurophysiology of this "cerebral shock" is unclear. After a variable degree of recovery from the neurologic lesion, a fixed deficit may become apparent over a few weeks or months. The most common long-term expression of LUT dysfunction after CVA is phasic DO. Sensation is variable but is classically described as generally intact, and thus, the patient has urgency and frequency with DO. The appropriate response is to try to inhibit the involuntary bladder contraction by forceful voluntary contraction of the striated sphincter. If this can be accomplished, only urgency and frequency result; if not, urgency with incontinence results.

The exact acute and chronic incidence of any LUT dysfunction after CVA, and specifically of incontinence, is not readily discernible. Cited prevalences of UI on hospital admission for stroke generally range from 30% to 80%, on discharge from 20% to 30%, and some months later from 10% to 20%. Previous descriptions of the voiding dysfunction after CVA have all cited the preponderance of DO with coordinated sphincter activity when the bladder does contract. It is difficult to reconcile this with the relatively high incontinence rate that occurs, even considering the probability that a percentage of these patients had an incontinence problem before the CVA. There are two possible mechanisms: (1) impaired sphincter control and (2) lack of appreciation of bladder filling and of impending bladder contraction. It has been reported that the majority of patients with involvement of the cerebral cortex and/or internal capsule are unable to forcefully contract their striated sphincter when an impending involuntary bladder contraction is sensed. Reduced bladder sensation has been reported in patients with global underperfusion of the cerebral cortex, especially the frontal areas.

Detrusor underactivity (DU) or areflexia can also exist after CVA. True detrusor-striated sphincter dyssynergia does not occur following a CVA. Pseudodyssynergia may occur during urodynamic testing. Smooth sphincter function is generally unaffected by CVA. Poor flow rates and high residual urine volumes in a male with pre-CVA symptoms of prostatism generally indicate prostatic obstruction. A urodynamic evaluation may be advisable before committing such a patient to mechanical outlet reduction to exclude DHIC as a cause of symptoms.

In the functional system of classification, the most common type of LUT dysfunction after stroke would then be characterized as a failure to store secondary to bladder overactivity, specifically involuntary bladder contractions.

In the ICS Classification System, the dysfunction would most likely be classified as overactive neurogenic detrusor function, normal sensation, low capacity, normal compliance, and normal urethral closure function during storage; during voiding the description would be normal detrusor activity and normal urethral function assuming that no anatomic obstruction existed. Treatment, in the absence of coexisting significant bladder obstruction or significantly impaired contractility, is directed at decreasing bladder contractility and increasing bladder capacity (see Table 14.7).

6. **Dementia:** Dementia is a poorly understood disease complex involving atrophy and the loss of gray and white matter of the brain, particularly the frontal lobes. When LUT dysfunction occurs, the result is generally incontinence. It is difficult to ascertain whether this is due to DO with the type of disorder of voluntary striated sphincter control mentioned with CVA or whether it is a type of situation in which the individual has simply lost the awareness of the desirability of voluntary urinary control and all it implies.
7. **Cerebral palsy (CP):** This is the rubric applied to a nonprogressive injury of the brain in the prenatal or perinatal period (some say up to 3 years) producing neuromuscular disability and/or specific symptom complexes of cerebral dysfunction. The etiology is generally infection or a period of hypoxia. Most children and adults with only CP have urinary control and what seems to be normal filling and storage and normal emptying. The incidence of LUT dysfunction is vague because the few available series report mostly subcategorizations of those who present with LUT symptoms. In those individuals with CP who exhibit significant dysfunction, the type of damage that one would suspect from the most common urodynamic abnormalities seems to be localized anatomically above the brainstem. This is commonly reflected by phasic DO and

coordinated sphincters. However, spinal cord damage can occur, and perhaps this accounts for those individuals with CP who seem to have evidence of striated sphincter dyssynergia or of a more distal type of neural axis lesion.

8. **Parkinson disease:** This neurodegenerative disorder of unknown cause affects primarily the dopaminergic neurons of the substantia nigra, the origin of the dopaminergic nigrostriatal tract to the caudate nucleus and putamen. Dopamine deficiency in the nigrostriatal pathway accounts for most of the classic clinical motor features of PD. The classic major signs of PD consist of tremor, skeletal rigidity, and bradykinesia, a symptom complex often referred to as parkinsonism. There are causes of parkinsonism other than PD. The combination of asymmetry of symptoms and signs, the presence of a resting tremor, and a good response to levodopa best differentiates PD from parkinsonism produced by other causes, although none of these is individually specific for PD. Multiple system atrophy (MSA; see next section) is the entity most commonly confused with PD.

   LUT dysfunction occurs in 35% to 70% of patients with PD. Preexisting detrusor or outlet abnormalities may be present, and the symptomatology may be affected by various types of treatment for the primary disease. When voiding dysfunction occurs, symptoms generally (50%–75%) consist of urgency, frequency, nocturia, and urge incontinence. The remainder of patients have "obstructive" symptoms or a combination. The most common urodynamic finding is DO. The smooth sphincter is synergic. There is some confusion regarding EMG interpretation. Sporadic involuntary activity in the striated sphincter during involuntary bladder contraction has been reported in as many as 60% of patients; however, this does not cause obstruction and cannot be termed *true dyssynergia*, which generally does not occur. True. Pseudodyssynergia may occur, as well as a delay in striated sphincter relaxation (bradykinesia) at the onset of voluntary micturition, both of which can be urodynamically misinterpreted as true dyssynergia. A delay in the ability to initiate a voluntary striated sphincter contraction to prevent incontinence due to DO can also occur. Impaired detrusor contractility may also occur, either in the form of low amplitude or poorly sustained contractions or a combination.

Detrusor areflexia is relatively uncommon in PD. Many cases of PD in the older literature may actually have been MSA, and citations regarding symptoms and urodynamic findings may not therefore be accurate. An example of this is the inference that transurethral resection of the prostate (TURP) in the patient with PD is associated with a high incidence of UI (because of poor striated sphincter tone and control). Retrospective interpretation of case studies has concluded that these were patients with MSA and not PD and that TURP should not be contraindicated in patients with PD because striated sphincter denervation and hyopfunction are rare in PD patients. However, one must be cautious with such patients, and a complete urodynamic or video urodynamic evaluation is advisable. Poorly sustained bladder contractions, sometimes with slow sphincter relaxation, should make one less optimistic regarding the results of outlet reduction in the male with PD. LUT dysfunction secondary to PD defies "routine" classification within any system. It is most manifest by storage failure secondary to bladder overactivity, but detailed urodynamic evaluation is mandatory before any but the simplest and most reversible therapy. The therapeutic menus (see Tables 14.7 and 14.8) are perfectly applicable, but the disease itself may impose certain limitations on the use of certain treatments (e.g., limited mobility for rapid toilet access, hand control insufficient for CIC).

9. **Multiple system atrophy**: MSA is a progressive neurodegenerative disease of unknown etiology. The symptoms encompass parkinsonism and cerebellar, autonomic (including urinary and erectile problems), and pyramidal cortical dysfunction in a multitude of combinations. The clinical features are separable from PD.

   The neurologic lesions of MSA consist of cell loss and gliosis in widespread areas, much more so than with PD, and this more diffuse nature of cell loss probably explains why LUT symptoms generally occur earlier than in PD and be more severe, and why erection is commonly affected as well. Affected areas have been identified in the cerebellum, substantia nigra, globus pallidus, caudate, putamen, inferior olives, intermediolateral columns of the spinal cord, and Onuf nucleus. Males and females are equally affected, with the onset in middle age. MSA is generally progressive and associated with a poor prognosis. Shy-Drager syndrome, an older initially utilized rubric, has been described in the past as characterized clinically by orthostatic hypotension, anhidrosis, and varying degrees of cerebellar and parkinsonian dysfunction. Voiding and erectile dysfunction (ED) are common. Some consider this as late-stage MSA.

Clinical urogenital criteria favoring a diagnosis of MSA are as follows: (1) urinary symptoms precede or present with parkinsonism, (2) male ED precedes or presents with parkinsonism, (3) UI, (4) significant postvoid residual, and (5) worsening LUT dysfunction after urologic surgery. The initial urinary symptoms of MSA are urgency, frequency, and urge incontinence, occurring up to 4 years before the diagnosis is made, as does erectile failure. DO is frequently found, as one would expect from the CNS areas affected, but decreased compliance may occur, reflecting distal spinal involvement of the locations of the cell bodies of autonomic neurons innervating the LUT. As the disease progresses, difficulty in initiating and maintaining voiding may occur, probably from pontine and sacral cord lesions, and this generally is associated with a poor prognosis. Cystourethrography or video urodynamic studies may reveal an open bladder neck (ISD), and many patients exhibit evidence of striated sphincter denervation on motor unit electromyography. The smooth and striated sphincter abnormalities predispose women to sphincteric incontinence and make prostatectomy hazardous in men. The treatment of significant voiding LUT caused by MSA is difficult and seldom satisfactory. Treatment of DO during filling may worsen problems initiating voluntary micturition or worsen impaired contractility during emptying. Patients generally have sphincteric insufficiency, and rarely is an outlet-reducing procedure indicated. Drug treatment for sphincteric incontinence may further worsen emptying problems. Generally, the goal in these patients is to facilitate storage, and CIC would often be desirable. Unfortunately, patients with advanced disease often are not candidates for CIC.

10. **Multiple sclerosis:** MS is believed to be immune mediated and is characterized by neural demyelination, generally characterized by axonal sparing in the spinal cord and brain. The demyelinating process most commonly involves the lateral corticospinal (pyramidal) and reticulospinal columns of the cervical spinal cord, but involvement of the lumbar and sacral cord occurs to a lesser extent. Lesions may also occur in the optic nerve and in the cerebral cortex and midbrain, the latter accounting for the intellectual deterioration and/or euphoria that may be seen as well. The incidence of LUT dysfunction in MS is related to the overall disability status. Of patients with MS, 50% to 90% complain of voiding symptoms at some time; the prevalence of incontinence is cited as 35% to 70%. LUT involvement may constitute the sole initial complaint or be part of the presenting symptom complex in up to 15% of patients, usually in the form of acute urinary retention of "unknown" etiology or as an acute onset of urgency and frequency, secondary to overactivity.

    DO is the most common urodynamic abnormality detected, occurring in 35% to 95% of cases in reported series. Of the patients with overactivity, 30% to 65% have coexistent striated sphincter dyssynergia. Impaired detrusor contractility or areflexia may also exist, a phenomenon that can considerably complicate treatment efforts. Generally, the smooth sphincter is synergic. It is also possible to see relative degrees of striated sphincteric flaccidity caused by MS, which could predispose and contribute to sphincteric incontinence.

    Because sensation is frequently intact in MS patients, one must be careful to distinguish urodynamic pseudodyssynergia from true striated sphincter dyssynergia. Jerry Blaivas was the first to subcategorize true striated sphincter dyssynergia in patients with MS and identify some varieties that are more worrisome than others. For instance, in a female with MS, a brief period of striated sphincter dyssynergia during detrusor contraction, but one that does not result in excessive intravesical pressure during voiding, substantial residual urine volume, or secondary detrusor hypertrophy may be relatively inconsequential, whereas those varieties that are more sustained—resulting in high bladder pressures of long duration—are most associated with urologic complications. A significant proportion of patients with MS with and without new symptoms will develop changes in their detrusor compliance and urodynamic pattern during the course of their disease. Caution should therefore be exercised in recommending irreversible therapeutic options.

The most common functional classification applicable to patients with LUT dysfunction secondary to MS would thus be storage failure secondary to DO. This is commonly complicated by striated sphincter dyssynergia, with varying effects on the ability to empty completely at acceptable pressures. Other abnormalities and other combined deficits are obviously possible, however. Once the dysfunction is broadly characterized, the treatment options should be obvious from the therapeutic menus (see Tables 14.7 and 14.8).

11. **Spinal cord injury**: Altered LUT and sexual function occur frequently secondary to SCI and significantly affect quality of life; SCI patients are at risk urologically for UTI, sepsis, upper and LUT deterioration, upper and LUT calculi, AH (dysreflexia), skin complications, and depression. Failure to properly address the LUT dysfunction can lead to significant morbidity and mortality. The changes after severe acute trauma generally occur in stages.
    a. **Spinal shock:** Following a significant SCI, a period of decreased excitability of spinal cord segments at and below the level of the lesion occurs, referred to as *spinal shock*. There is absent somatic reflex activity and flaccid muscle paralysis below this level. Spinal shock includes a suppression of autonomic and somatic activity, and the bladder is acontractile and areflexic with a closed bladder neck. The smooth sphincter mechanism seems competent but nonrelaxing, except in some cases of thoracolumbar injury. Some EMG activity can generally be recorded from the striated sphincter, and the maximum urethral closure pressure is still maintained at the level of the external sphincter zone; however, the normal guarding reflex is absent. Because sphincter tone exists, UI generally does not result unless there is gross overdistention with overflow.

Urinary retention is the rule, and catheterization is necessary to circumvent this problem. Intermittent catheterization is an excellent method of management during this period. If the distal spinal cord is intact but is simply isolated from higher centers, there is generally a gradual return of detrusor contractility. At first, such reflex activity is poorly sustained and produces only low pressure changes, but the strength and duration of such involuntary contractions increase, producing involuntary voiding, usually with incomplete bladder emptying. Spinal shock generally lasts 6 to 12 weeks in complete suprasacral spinal cord lesions but can last for as long as a year or two. It can last for a shorter period of time in incomplete suprasacral lesions and only a few days in some patients. In evolving lesions, every attempt should be made to preserve as low a bladder storage pressure as possible.

b. **Suprasacral SCI:** The characteristic pattern that results when a patient has a complete lesion above the sacral spinal cord is DO, smooth sphincter synergia (with lesions below the sympathetic outflow), and striated sphincter dyssynergia. Neurologic examination shows spasticity of skeletal muscle distal to the lesion, hyperreflexic deep tendon reflexes, and abnormal plantar responses. There is impairment of superficial and deep sensation. The guarding reflex is absent or weak in most patients with a complete suprasacral SCI. In incomplete lesions the reflex is often preserved but very variable.

The striated sphincter dyssynergia causes a functional obstruction with poor emptying and high detrusor pressure. Incomplete bladder emptying may be compounded by what seems to be a poorly sustained or absent detrusor contraction. The urodynamic and upper tract consequences of the striated sphincter dyssynergia vary with severity (generally worse in complete lesions than in incomplete ones), duration (continuous contraction during detrusor activity is worse than intermittent contraction), and anatomy (is worse in men than women). Once reflex voiding is established, it can be initiated or reinforced by the stimulation of certain dermatomes, such as by tapping the suprapubic area.

From a functional standpoint the voiding dysfunction most commonly seen in suprasacral SCI represents both a filling/storage and an emptying failure. Although the urodynamics are "safe" enough in some individuals to allow only periodic stimulation of bladder reflex activity, many will require some treatment. If detrusor pressures are suitably low or if they can be made suitably low with nonsurgical or surgical management, the problem can be treated primarily as an emptying failure, and CIC can be continued, when practical, as a safe and effective way of satisfying many of the goals of treatment. Alternatively, sphincterotomy, stenting, or intrasphincteric injection of botulinum toxin can be used in males to lower the detrusor leak point to an acceptable level, thus treating the dysfunction primarily as one of emptying. The resultant storage failure can be obviated either by timed stimulation or with an external collecting device. In the dexterous SCI patient, the former approach using CIC is common. Electrical stimulation (ES) of the anterior sacral roots with some form of deafferentation is also now a distinct reality.

As with all patients with neurologic impairment, a careful initial evaluation and periodic follow-up evaluation must be performed to identify and correct the following risk factors and potential complications: bladder overdistention, high-pressure storage, high DLPP, VUR, stone formation (lower and upper tracts), and complicating infection, especially in association with reflux.

c. **Sacral SCI**: Following recovery from spinal shock, there is usually a depression of deep tendon reflexes below the level of the lesion with varying degrees of flaccid paralysis. Sensation is generally absent below the lesion level. Detrusor areflexia with high or normal compliance is the common initial result. Decreased compliance may develop, a change often seen with neurologic lesions at or distal to the sacral spinal cord and most likely representing a response to neurologic decentralization.

The classical outlet findings are described as a competent but nonrelaxing smooth sphincter and a striated sphincter that retains some fixed tone but is not under voluntary control. Closure pressures are decreased in both areas. However, the late appearance of the bladder neck may be open. Attempted voiding by straining or Credé results in obstruction at the bladder neck (if closed) or at the distal sphincter area by fixed sphincter tone. Potential risk factors are those previously described, with particular emphasis on storage pressure, which can result in silent upper tract decompensation and deterioration in the absence of VUR. The treatment of such a patient is generally directed toward producing or maintaining low-pressure storage while circumventing emptying failure with CIC when possible.

12. **Neurologic and urodynamic correlation in SCI:** Although generally correct, the correlation between somatic neurologic findings and urodynamic findings in suprasacral and sacral SCI patients is not exact. A number of factors should be considered in this regard. First, whether a lesion is complete or incomplete is sometimes a matter of definition. A complete lesion, somatically speaking, may not translate into a complete lesion autonomically, and vice versa. Multiple injuries may actually exist at different levels, even though what is seen somatically may reflect a single level of injury. Even considering these situations, however, all such discrepancies are not explained. Management of the urinary tract in such patients must be based on urodynamic principles and findings rather than inferences from the neurologic history and evaluation. Similarly, although the information regarding "classic" complete lesions is for the most part valid, neurologic conclusions should not be made solely on the basis of urodynamic findings.
13. **Autonomic hyperreflexia (dysreflexia [AH]):** AH is a potentially fatal emergency unique to the SCI patient. AH represents an acute massive disordered autonomic (primarily sympathetic) response to specific stimuli in patients with SCI above the level of T6 to T8 (the sympathetic outflow). It is more common in cervical (60%) than thoracic (20%) injuries. Onset after injury is variable, usually soon after spinal shock but may be up to years after injury. Distal cord viability is a prerequisite. Symptomatically, AH is a syndrome of

exaggerated sympathetic activity in response to stimuli below the level of the lesion. The symptoms are pounding headache, hypertension, and flushing of the face and body above the level of the lesion with sweating. Bradycardia is a usual accompaniment, although tachycardia or arrhythmia may be present. Hypertension may be of varying severity, from causing a mild headache before the occurrence of voiding to life-threatening cerebral hemorrhage or seizure. The stimuli for this exaggerated response commonly arise from the bladder or rectum and generally involve distention, although other stimuli from these areas can be precipitating. Precipitation of AH may be the result of simple LUT instrumentation, tube change, catheter obstruction, or clot retention; in such cases, the symptoms resolve quickly if the stimulus is withdrawn. Other causes or exacerbating factors may include other upper or LUT pathology (e.g., calculi), gastrointestinal (GI) pathology, long bone fracture, sexual activity, electrocoagulation, and decubiti. DO and striated sphincter dyssynergia invariably occurs, and smooth sphincter dyssynergia is generally a part of the syndrome as well, at least in males.

The pathophysiology of AH is that of a nociceptive stimulation via afferent impulses that ascend through the cord and elicit reflex motor outflow, causing arteriolar, pilomotor, and pelvic visceral spasm below the level of the lesion, especially in the large splanchnic bed. This results in hypertension. Normally, these reflexes would be countered by secondary output from the medulla via parasympathetic output, but this does not occur below the lesion level—thus, the flushing and sweating above the level of the lesion.

Ideally, any endoscopic procedure in susceptible patients should be done under spinal anesthesia or carefully monitored general anesthesia. Acutely, the hemodynamic effects of this syndrome may be managed with α-adrenergic blocking agents, nitrates, calcium channel blockers, or angiotensin-1-converting enzyme inhibitors (ACEIs). Ganglionic blockers had previously been the mainstay of treatment, but their usage has mostly been abandoned. Various prophylactic regimens using vasodilators prior to hazardous procedures (e.g., cystoscopy and urodynamics) are utilized and are generally institution specific. Chronic prophylaxis against AH with an α-1 adrenergic blocker has been recommended and found useful by some authorities. Such prophylaxis may be particularly important in view of the fact that significant elevations in blood pressure can occur without other symptoms of AH. Prophylaxis, however, does not eliminate the need for careful monitoring during provocative procedures. There are patients with severe AH that is intractable to any pharmacologic treatment and correction by urologic procedures. For these unfortunate individuals, a number of neurologic ablative procedures have been used—sympathectomy, sacral neurectomy, sacral rhizotomy, cordectomy, and dorsal root ganglionectomy.

14. **Neurospinal dysraphism:** Although primarily a pediatric problem, certain considerations regarding the adult with these abnormalities should be mentioned. Secondary to progress in the overall care of children with myelodysplasia, urologic dysfunction often becomes a problem of the adult with this disease (transitional urology). The "typical" myelodysplastic patient shows an areflexic bladder with an open bladder neck. Decreased compliance may be present. The bladder generally fills until the resting residual fixed external sphincter pressure is reached, and then leakage occurs. Stress incontinence often occurs also. A small percentage of patients demonstrate DO and striated sphincter dyssynergia.

    After puberty, most male myelodysplastic patients note an improvement in continence probably due to prostatic enlargement. In adult patients, the problems encountered in myelodysplastic children still exist, but are often compounded by prior surgery, upper tract dysfunction, and one form of urinary diversion or another. In adult females, the goal is to increase urethral sphincter efficiency without causing an undue increase in urethral closing pressure, which might result in a change in bladder compliance. Periurethral injection therapy to achieve continence may give as good a result as a pubovaginal sling or artificial sphincter in this circumstance. Continence in adult male myelodysplastic individuals follows the same general rules as in females, and injectable materials may give good results in this group as well, unless the outlet is widely dilated. Dry individuals, of course, will be on intermittent self-catheterization. Nowhere is the failure of a neurologic examination to predict urodynamic behavior more obvious than in patients with myelomeningocele. The prime directive of therapy remains the avoidance of high storage pressures.

Tethered cord syndrome: This is defined as a stretch-induced functional disorder of the spinal cord with its caudal part anchored by inelastic structures. Vertical movement is restricted. The anchoring structures can include a scar from prior surgery, fibrous or fibroadipose filum terminale, a bony septum, or tumor. Adults with tethered cord syndrome (TCS) can be divided into those with a prior history of spinal dysraphism with a previously stabilized neurologic status who present with subtle progression in adulthood, and those without associated spinal dysraphism who present with new subtle neurologic symptoms. Symptoms can include back pain, leg weakness, foot deformity, scoliosis, sensory loss, and bowel or LUT dysfunction. TCS is reported to occur in 3% to 15% of patients with myelomeningocele. There is no typical dysfunction in TCS, and treatment must be based on contemporary urodynamic evaluation.

15. **Disc disease, cauda equina syndrome, and spinal stenosis**
    a. **Disc protrusions:** These compress the spinal roots in the L4-L5 or L5-S1 interspaces. LUT dysfunction may occur as a result, and when present, generally occurs with the usual clinical manifestations of low back pain radiating in a girdle-like fashion along the involved spinal root areas. Examination may reveal reflex and sensory loss consistent with nerve root compression. The most characteristic findings on physical exam are sensory loss in the S2-4 dermatomes (perineum or perianal areas), S1-2 dermatomes (lateral foot), or both. The incidence of LUT dysfunction in disc prolapse ranges from 1% to 18%. The most consistent urodynamic finding is a normally compliant acontractile bladder associated with normal innervation or incomplete denervation of the perineal floor muscles. There is a lower incidence of decreased compliance in root

damage secondary to disk prolapse, as opposed to myelomeningocele. Occasionally, patients may show DO, attributed to irritation of the nerve roots. Patients with LUT dysfunction generally present with difficulty voiding, straining, or urinary retention. It should be noted that laminectomy may not improve bladder function, and prelaminectomy urodynamic evaluation is desirable, because it may be difficult postoperatively to separate causation of voiding dysfunction due to the disc sequelae alone from changes secondary to the surgery.

b. **Cauda equina syndrome:** This is a term applied to the clinical picture of perineal sensory loss with loss of voluntary control of both anal and urethral sphincter and of sexual responsiveness. This can occur not only secondary to disc disease (severe central posterior disk protrusion) but to other spinal canal pathologies as well. It can also be an unfortunate result of distal spinal surgery. Typically, patients have an acontractile detrusor with decreased or absent bladder sensation. The findings are variable, however, and depend on the extent and location of nerve root or cord damage.

c. **Spinal stenosis:** This is a term applied to any narrowing of the spinal canal, nerve root canals, or intervertebral foramina. It may be congenital, developmental, or acquired. Compression of the nerve roots or cord by such a problem may lead to neuronal damage, ischemia, or edema. Spinal stenosis may occur without disc prolapse. Symptoms may range from those consequent to cervical spinal cord compression to a cauda equina syndrome with corresponding urodynamic findings. Back and lower extremity pain, cramping, and paresthesias related to exercise and relieved by rest are the classic symptoms of lumbar stenosis caused by lumbar spondylosis and are believed to result from a sacral nerve root ischemia. The urodynamic findings are dependent on the level and the amount of spinal cord or nerve root damage.

16. **Radical pelvic surgery:** LUT dysfunction after pelvic plexus injury occurs most commonly after abdominoperineal resection and radical hysterectomy. The incidence has been estimated in older literature to range from 20% to 68% of

patients after abdominoperineal resection, 16% to 80% after radical hysterectomy, 20% to 25% after anterior resection, and 10% to 20% after proctocolectomy. Current incidence is generally reported as significantly lower because of the use of nerve-sparing techniques during these types of pelvic surgery. It has been estimated, however, that in 15% to 20% of affected individuals, the LUT dysfunction is permanent. The injury may occur consequent to denervation or neurologic decentralization, tethering of the nerves or encasement in scar, direct bladder or urethral trauma, or bladder devascularization. Adjuvant treatment, such as chemotherapy or radiation, may play a role as well. The type of LUT dysfunction that occurs is dependent on the specific nerves involved, the degree of injury, and any pattern of reinnervation or altered innervation that results over time. When permanent voiding dysfunction occurs after radical pelvic surgery, the pattern is generally one of a failure of voluntary bladder contraction, or impaired bladder contractility, with obstruction by what seems urodynamically to be residual fixed striated sphincter tone, which is not subject to voluntarily induced relaxation. Often, the smooth sphincter area is open and nonfunctional. Whether this appearance of the bladder neck-proximal urethra is caused by parasympathetic damage or terminal sympathetic damage or whether it results from the hydrodynamic effects of obstruction at the level of the striated sphincter is debated and unknown. Decreased compliance is common in these patients, and this, with the "obstruction" caused by fixed residual striated sphincter tone, results in both storage and emptying failure. These patients often experience leaking across the distal sphincter area but are unable to empty the bladder because, although intravesical pressure may be increased, nothing occurs which approximates a true bladder contraction. The patient often presents with UI that is characteristically most manifest with increases in IAP. This is usually most obvious in females because the prostatic bulk in males often masks an equivalent deficit in urethral closure function. Alternatively, patients may present with variable degrees of urinary retention. Urodynamic studies may show decreased compliance, poor proximal urethral closure function, loss of voluntary control of the striated sphincter, and a positive bethanechol supersensitivity test. Upper tract risk factors are related to intravesical pressure and the DLPP, and the therapeutic goal is always low-pressure storage with periodic emptying. The temptation to perform a prostatectomy should be avoided unless a clear demonstration of outlet obstruction at this level is possible. Otherwise, prostatectomy may simply further decrease urethral sphincter function and thereby may result in the occurrence or worsening of sphincteric UI. Most of these dysfunctions will be transient, and the temptation to "do something" other than perform CIC initially after surgery in these patients, especially in those with little or no preexistent history of LUT dysfunction, cannot be too strongly discouraged.

17. **Diabetes mellitus:** If specifically questioned, anywhere from 5% to 60% of patients with diabetes report symptoms of LUT dysfunction. However, the symptoms may or may not be caused by just the diabetes. In trying to come to conclusions regarding the incidence and types of voiding dysfunction specifically from diabetes, one has to carefully discriminate between articles that consider patients referred for LUT symptoms versus those that have evaluated patients from a population known to have diabetes. Cai Frimodt-Moller coined the term *diabetic cystopathy* to describe the involvement of the LUT in this disease. The classic description of LUT dysfunction secondary to diabetes is that of a peripheral autonomic neuropathy that first affects sensory afferent pathways, causing the insidious onset of impaired bladder sensation. As the classic description continues, a gradual increase in the time interval between voiding results, which may progress to the point at which the patient voids only once or twice a day without ever sensing any real urgency. If this continues, detrusor distention, overdistention, and decompensation ultimately occur. Detrusor contractility, therefore, is classically described as being decreased in the end-stage diabetic bladder.

    Current evidence points to both a sensory and a motor neuropathy as being involved in the pathogenesis, the motor aspect per se contributing to the impaired detrusor contractility. The typically described classic urodynamic findings include impaired bladder sensation, increased cystometric capacity, decreased bladder contractility, impaired uroflow, and, later, increased residual urine volume. The main differential diagnosis, at least in men, is generally BOO because both conditions commonly produce a low flow rate. PFUDS easily differentiate the two. Smooth or striated sphincter dyssynergia generally is not seen in classic diabetic cystopathy, but these diagnoses can easily be erroneously made on a poor or incomplete urodynamic study—voiding may involve abdominal straining, which will produce an interference EMG pattern (pseudodyssynergia), and abdominal straining alone will not open the bladder neck area.

Recent articles, however, seem to show that DO and not this "classic" diabetic cystopathy is the predominant finding of LUT dysfunction. Although it is obvious that some (or even many) of the patients with diabetes who exhibited involuntary bladder contractions may have had factors other than diabetes to account for their bladder overactivity, the importance of urodynamic study in diabetic patients before institution of therapy cannot be overemphasized.

18. **Tabes dorsalis and pernicious anemia:** Although syphilitic myelopathy is disappearing as a major neurologic problem, involvement of the spinal cord dorsal columns and posterior sacral roots can result in a loss of bladder sensation and large residual urine volumes and therefore be a cause of "sensory neurogenic bladder." Another spinal cord cause of the classic "sensory bladder" is the now uncommon pernicious anemia that produced this disorder by virtue of subacute combined degeneration of the dorsolateral columns of the spinal cord.

COMMON NONNEUROGENIC LOWER URINARY TRACT DYSFUNCTIONS

Outlet obstruction secondary to BPH: This is probably the most common LUT dysfunction seen by the urologist (see Chapter 15). Classically, the patient complains of hesitancy and straining to void, with the urodynamic correlates of low flow and high detrusor pressure during attempted voiding. This situation can represent a pure failure to empty, but approximately 50% to 80% of the time, the patient with significant prostatic obstruction develops DO, with resultant urgency, frequency, and, if the overactivity cannot be inhibited, urgency incontinence. Under such circumstances, the dysfunction becomes a combined emptying and filling and storage problem. Treatment is relief of the obstruction either by reduction of prostatic bulk or tone. Relief of the outlet obstruction will result in the eventual disappearance of DO, where present, in approximately 50% to 70% of cases, but this may take 6 to 12 months. However, the DO may return years later and be unrelated to outlet obstruction.

Bladder neck dysfunction: Bladder neck dysfunction is characterized by an incomplete opening of the bladder neck during voluntary or involuntary voiding. It has also been referred to as *smooth sphincter dyssynergia, proximal urethral obstruction, primary bladder neck obstruction,* and *dysfunctional bladder neck*. The term *smooth sphincter dyssynergia* or *proximal sphincter dyssynergia* is generally used when referring to this urodynamic finding in an individual with AH. The term *bladder neck dysfunction* more often refers to a poorly understood nonneurogenic condition first described over a century ago but first fully characterized by Richard Turner-Warwick and associates in 1973. The dysfunction is found almost exclusively in young and middle-aged men, and characteristically they complain of long-standing voiding/emptying (obstructive) and filling/storage (irritative) symptoms. These patients have often been seen by many urologists and have been diagnosed as having psychogenic voiding dysfunction because of a normal prostate on rectal examination, a negligible residual urine volume, and a normal endoscopic prostate and bladder appearance. The differential diagnosis also includes anatomic bladder neck contracture, BPH, dysfunctional voiding, prostatitis or prostatosis, neurogenic dysfunction, and low pressure/low flow. Objective evidence of outlet obstruction in these patients is easily obtainable by urodynamic study. Once obstruction is diagnosed, it can be localized at the level of the bladder neck by VUDS, cystourethrography during a bladder contraction, or micturitional urethral profilometry. The diagnosis may also be made indirectly by the urodynamic findings of outlet obstruction in the typical clinical situation and in the absence of urethral stricture, prostatic enlargement, and striated sphincter dyssynergia. Involuntary bladder contractions or decreased compliance may occur. When prostatic enlargement develops in individuals with this problem, an augmented obstruction results, and Turner-Warwick applied the term *trapped prostate* to this entity. The lobes of the prostate cannot expand into or through the bladder neck and therefore expand into the urethra. A patient so affected generally has a lifelong history of voiding dysfunction that has gone relatively unnoticed because he has always accepted this as normal, and exacerbation of these symptoms occurs during a relatively short and early period of prostatic enlargement. Although α-adrenergic blocking agents may provide mild improvement in some patients with bladder neck dysfunction, definitive relief in the male is best achieved by bladder neck incision. In patients with this and a trapped prostate, marked relief is generally effected by a "small" prostatic resection or ablation that includes the bladder neck or a transurethral incision of the bladder neck and prostate with resection of a small amount of prolapsing prostate tissue. Such patients often note afterward that they have never voided as well as after their treatment.

Bladder outlet obstruction in women: The female counterpart of nonneurogenic bladder neck dysfunction in men does exist, although it is unusual. Definitions and diagnostic criteria vary. Victor Nitti best defines BOO as radiographic evidence of obstruction between the bladder neck and the distal urethra in the presence of a sustained detrusor contraction of any magnitude, which is usually associated with a reduced or delayed urinary flow rate. Obstruction at the level of the bladder neck is diagnosed when the bladder neck is closed or narrowed during voiding. Strict pressure-flow criteria are used by some to classify cases in women as obstructed or not. Jerry Blaivas' group defines obstruction in the woman as a persistent low, noninvasive maximum flow rate less than 12 mL/sec on repeated study combined with a detrusor pressure at maximum measured flow rate of more than 20 cm of water in a pressure-flow study. Most authors would agree that surgical treatment of this problem in women (incision of the bladder neck) should be approached with caution because sphincteric incontinence is a significant risk.

Low-pressure/low-flow voiding in younger men – the Bashful Bladder: Low-pressure/low-flow voiding can be the result of a number of causes, most notably a decompensating detrusor (generally from BOO) or as a part of the syndrome known as DHIC. When this occurs in a young man, it is generally symptomatically characterized by frequency, hesitancy, and a poor stream. The entity is readily demonstrated on urodynamic assessment and with no coexisting endoscopic abnormality. The patient generally notes marked hesitancy when attempting to initiate micturition in the presence of others, and some have therefore described this condition as an "anxious bladder" or a "bashful bladder." Our experience has been similar to that of others who have stated that, in the younger unobstructed male with this condition, neither empirical pharmacologic treatment nor transurethral surgery has had any consistent beneficial effect.

Dysfunctional voiding: This syndrome, also sometimes known as *nonneurogenic/neurogenic bladder, occult voiding dysfunction*, or *Hinman syndrome*, presents the unusual circumstance of what appears urodynamically to be involuntary obstruction at the striated sphincter level existing in the absence of demonstrable neurologic disease. It is very difficult to prove urodynamically that an individual has this entity. This requires simultaneous pressure/flow EMG evidence of bladder emptying occurring simultaneously with involuntary striated sphincter contraction in the absence of any element of abdominal straining component, either in an attempt to augment bladder contraction or as a response to discomfort during urination. The etiology is uncertain and may represent a persistent transitional phase in the development of micturitional control or persistence of a reaction phase to the stimulus of LUT discomfort during voiding, long after the initial problem that caused this has disappeared. The preferred treatment is behavioral modification with biofeedback. Intermittent catheterization may be useful, both as therapy and as an aid to facilitating teaching the ability to voluntarily relax the striated sphincter.

The underactive bladder (DU): DU is defined by ICS as a contraction of reduced strength or duration resulting in prolonged bladder emptying and/or a failure to achieve complete bladder emptying within a normal time span. It is readily acknowledged, however, that no exact definition or description exists for any of these terms. It may exist by itself or in combination with DO during filling, outlet obstruction, or both. The symptoms are indistinguishable from those of BOO. The etiology can be neurologic or myogenic, and the pathophysiology generally involves increased connective tissue and fibrosis in the detrusor. This situation may occur after long-standing BOO or as a chronic response to overdistention due to any cause or due to neurologic injury or disease. Attempts to produce emptying pharmacologically with a cholinergic agonist and an α-adrenergic antagonist have been generally unsuccessful, and the best treatment, when necessary, is intermittent catheterization. There is always a temptation to surgically decrease bladder outlet resistance, especially in men, in the hopes of "tipping the balance" in favor of emptying. Although seasoned clinical judgment plays a role here, there are contradicting data for and against such an approach. The BCI (see section on UDS) may be of help in men, but there is a wide variability for potential emptying with outlet reduction between a BCI of 90 and one of 30. Similarly, the BOOI may be deceptively low in individuals with DU. In evaluating such individuals, one must think of what the BOOI would be if the BCI was normal or close to normal.

Postoperative retention: Urinary retention can occur postoperatively for a number of reasons. Nociceptive impulses can inhibit the initiation of reflex bladder contraction, perhaps through an opioid-mediated mechanism or sympathetic-mediated inhibition. Transient overdistention of the bladder can occur under anesthesia or under the influence of analgesic medication. Purely neurologic injury during abdominal and pelvic surgery can also occur. Generally, in the absence of neurologic injury and with proper decompression, a patient's voiding status will return pretty much to what it was prior to the surgery and anesthesia. Therefore, the optimal treatment is intermittent catheterization. Return of bladder function may be facilitated by the use of an α-adrenergic antagonist. Treatment with cholinergic agonists alone has been generally unsuccessful. A male with BPH-induced BOO on the borderline of having significant voiding dysfunction may have his previously tenuous and abnormal ability to empty compromised. In these cases, outlet reduction may be justified.

Urinary retention, the Fowler syndrome in young women: The Fowler syndrome refers particularly to a syndrome of urinary retention in young women in the absence of overt neurologic disease or anatomic obstruction. The typical history is that of a woman younger than 30 years who has found herself unable to void for a day or more with no urinary urgency but increasing lower abdominal discomfort. A bladder capacity of more than 1 L with no sensation of urgency is necessary for the diagnosis. There are no neurologic or laboratory features to support a diagnosis of any neurologic disease. MRI of the brain and the entire spinal cord is normal. The urodynamic problem is detrusor acontractility. On concentric needle electrode examination of the striated muscle of the urethral sphincter, however, Fowler and associates described a unique EMG abnormality that impairs sphincter relaxation. This may not be specific to those with this disorder. These patients often have polycystic ovaries. Efforts to treat this condition by hormonal manipulation, pharmacologic therapy, or injection of botulinum toxin into the striated sphincter have been relatively unsuccessful. This condition is frequently responsive to sacral neuromodulation (SNM).

Urinary Incontinence

UI is defined as the involuntary loss of urine. The term is used in various ways. It may denote a symptom, a sign, or a condition. The symptom is generally thought of as the patient's complaint of involuntary urine loss. The sign is the objective demonstration of urine loss. The condition is the underlying cause (pathophysiology). A simple classification of the various subtypes of UI is seen in Table 14.12. The basic pathophysiology of incontinence and various related definitions are discussed earlier in this chapter.

There are situations in which urethral incontinence cannot be considered merely as an isolated abnormality of either bladder contractility or sphincter resistance. These situations, listed in Table 14.13, are more complicated to deal with because they are more difficult to diagnose and because one entity may adversely affect or compromise treatment of the other. The most common of these is DO with outlet obstruction. This occurs almost exclusively in the male. The incidence of DO in series of

TABLE 14.12 Classification of Urinary Incontinence

1. Extraurethral
    a. Fistula (vesicovaginal, ureterovaginal, urethrovaginal)
    b. Ectopic ureter
2. Urethral
    a. Functional
        1) Because of physical disability
        2) Because of lack of awareness or concern
    b. Bladder abnormalities
        1) Overactivity
            i. Involuntary contractions
            ii. Decreased compliance
            iii. Hypersensitivity with incontinence
    c. Outlet abnormalities
        1) Stress urinary incontinence (SUI)
        2) Intrinsic sphincter deficiency
        3) Urethral instability
        4) Postvoid dribbling
            i. Urethral diverticulum
            ii. Vaginal pooling of urine
    d. Overflow incontinence

TABLE 14.13 Combined Problems Associated with Incontinence

Detrusor overactivity (DO) with outlet obstruction
DO with impaired bladder contractility
Sphincteric incontinence with impaired bladder contractility
Sphincteric incontinence with DO

patients with outlet obstruction secondary to prostatic enlargement ranges from 50% to 80%. Treating only the DO in these patients may result in worsening symptoms. On the other hand, when the outlet obstruction is relieved in such patients, there is a high reversal rate of the bladder status, although this reversion generally takes between 1 and 6 months and may take as long as 12 months. Neil Resnick and Subbarao Yalla described the phenomenon of DHIC (detrusor hyperreflexia during filling/storage with impaired contractility during emptying) as occurring especially in frail, elderly, incontinent patients. These patients may have significant trabeculation, but their detrusor contracts poorly during voluntary micturition. Because bladder contractility is impaired, a vigorous pharmacologic approach usually used for involuntary bladder contractions may not be appropriate for this entity. Sphincter incontinence in an individual with impaired bladder contractility should alert the clinician to the possibility of the requirement of permanent CIC following surgical repair. Depending on the patient's ability and willingness to carry out intermittent catheterization, this may drastically alter an individual's usual treatment program for sphincter incontinence if the simpler, noninvasive therapeutic measures have failed. Sphincter incontinence can coexist with DO in a number of circumstances and with varying effects. Such bladder overactivity has been cited as one of the most common causes of "failure" of an operation for stress incontinence. Whether these urodynamic findings really do indicate that such an operation is likely to fail is an important question because an affirmative answer would mandate a very careful urodynamic evaluation in all such patients and would doubtless decrease the enthusiasm for corrective surgery in such patients who have coexistent SUI. If an individual has mixed incontinence (MUI) (both SUI and DO) and the SUI component is clearly predominant, correction will result in improvement or cure of the DO related incontinence in 50%–70%. However, de novo DO can occur after such surgery. Patients with SUI who also have decreased compliance do not seem to fare well after surgery to correct just the SUI. The decreased compliance generally does not change, and if it was refractory to nonsurgical therapy before, it will remain that way, at least in our experience.

A variant and more complicated form of such a combination may occur following radical pelvic surgery. Such patients may have a combination of decreased compliance with impaired bladder contractility (from the standpoint of emptying potential) with an open and nonfunctional smooth sphincter area and obstruction by residual striated sphincter tone that is not subject to voluntary induced relaxation. These patients often leak across the distal sphincter area and are unable to empty their bladders because, although they have an increased detrusor pressure, they have nothing that approximates a true coordinated and sustained bladder contraction. They often present with UI, which is characteristically most manifest with increases in IAP. This is usually most obvious in women because the prostatic bulk often masks a deficit in men in urethral closure function.

One additional fact with respect to definition bears mention. The traditional perspective on UI fails to account for instances in which symptoms of urinary frequency and urgency are present without the involuntary loss of urine. Overactive bladder (OAB) is the ICS term that describes the symptoms of urgency, with or without urgency incontinence, usually with frequency and nocturia. This can further be categorized as OAB wet (with urinary urge incontinence [UUI]) or dry (without UUI). The prevalence of OAB is approximately the same in men and women, but as a percent of overall prevalence, OAB wet is more common in women. The management (evaluation and treatment) of OAB is basically the same as that of DO.

Prevalence rates for the most inclusive definitions of UI in women 15 years and older range from 5% to 69%, with daily rates ranging from 4% to 14%. In older women, mixed and urgency incontinence predominate, whereas in younger and middle-aged women, stress (effort-related) incontinence predominates. Established and suggested risk factors for UI in women include age, pregnancy, parity, obstetric factors, hormonal status, LUT symptoms, neurologic disease, hysterectomy, obesity, functional impairment, constipation, chronic respiratory disease, cognitive impairment, and smoking. Genetic factors, some related to connective tissue disorders, may also play a role. In men the prevalence of UI (inclusive definition) has been reported to range from 3% to 39%, with general agreement that the prevalence is less than half that in women. Urgency incontinence predominates (40%–80%), followed by mixed UI (10%–30%), and SUI (less than 10%). Risk factors include age, LUT symptoms and infections, functional and cognitive impairment, neurologic disorder, and prostatectomy. In general, the prevalence of some UI in nursing home residents of both sexes is estimated at higher than 50%. UI imposes a significant psychosocial impact on individuals, their families, and caregivers. Quality of life, as measured by both generic and LUT-specific indices, is adversely affected by UI to a significant degree. The primary spheres affected are (1) self-esteem, (2) ability to maintain an independent lifestyle, (3) social interactions with friends and family, (4) activities of daily life, and

(5) sexual activity. A brief description of the more common types of UI is as follows:

Outlet-related incontinence in women: Classically, sphincteric incontinence in the female patient had been categorized into (1) SUI and (2) what was originally described by McGuire and Woodside as type III stress incontinence, now referred to as *intrinsic sphincter deficiency (ISD)*. Classical SUI is associated with hypermobility of the vesicourethral junction due to poor pelvic support and an outlet that is competent at rest but loses its competence only during increases in IAP. Classical ISD describes a bladder neck and proximal urethra which is nonfunctional or very poorly functional at rest. The division between these two situations, however, is not absolute, and virtually all "experts" agree that every case of sphincteric incontinence in the female involves varying proportions of SUI and ISD. The original implication of classical ISD was that a surgical procedure designed to correct only urethral hypermobility would have a relatively high failure rate as opposed to one designed to provide urethral compression and/or coaptation. SUI is a condition that arises from damage to muscles and/or nerves and/or connective tissue within the pelvic floor. Urethral support is important—the urethra normally being supported by the action of the levator ani muscles through their connection to the endopelvic fascia of the anterior vaginal wall. Damage to the connection between this fascia and muscle, damage to the nerve supply, or direct muscle damage can therefore influence continence. Bladder neck function is similarly important, and loss of normal bladder neck closure can result in incontinence despite normal urethral support. In older writings, the urethra was sometimes ignored as a factor contributing to continence in the female, and the site of continence was thought to be exclusively the bladder neck. However, in some continent women, urine enters the urethra during increases in abdominal pressure. The continence point in these women is at the midurethra, where urine is stopped before it can escape from the urethral meatus. With urethral hypermobility, there is weakness of the pelvic floor. During increases in IAP, there is descent of the bladder neck and proximal urethra. If the outlet opens concomitantly, SUI ensues. In the classic form of urethral hypermobility, there is rotational descent of the bladder neck and urethra. However, the urethra may also descend without rotation (it shortens and widens), or the posterior wall of the urethra may be pulled open while the anterior wall remains fixed. It should be noted, however, that urethral hypermobility is often present in women who are not incontinent, and thus, the mere presence of urethral hypermobility is not sufficient to make a diagnosis of a sphincter abnormality unless UI is also demonstrated.

The "hammock hypothesis" of John Delancey proposes that for stress incontinence to occur with hypermobility, there must be a lack of stability of the suburethral supportive layer. This theory proposes that the effect of abdominal pressure increases on the normal bladder outlet, if the suburethral supportive layer is firm, is to compress the urethra rapidly and effectively. If the supportive suburethral layer is lax and/or movable, compression is not as effective. ISD denotes an intrinsic malfunction of the outlet sphincter mechanisms. In its most overt form, it is characterized by a bladder neck that is open at rest and a low VLPP and maximum urethral closure pressure and is usually the result of prior surgery, trauma with scarring, or a neurologic lesion. Urethral instability refers to the rare phenomenon of episodic decreases in outlet pressure unrelated to increases in bladder or abdominal pressure.

Outlet-related incontinence in men: In theory at least, categories of outlet-related incontinence in men are similar to those in the female. In reality, there is little if any information regarding the topic of urethral instability in the male. Sphincteric incontinence in the male is not associated with hypermobility of the bladder neck and proximal urethra but is rather more similar to what is termed *ISD* in the female. It is generally due to prostatectomy, pelvic trauma, or neurologic diseases.

Bladder-related incontinence in women: Bladder-related abnormalities causing UI consist of either DO or low bladder compliance. Neurologically, involuntary bladder contractions can be due to any lesion occurring above the sacral spinal cord. The cause(s) of idiopathic DO in women is (are) obscure. In addition to the etiologies noted previously (neurogenic voiding dysfunction), one subject that should be mentioned is the simultaneous occurrence of DO with SUI. The fact that minor or moderate components of DO, and sometimes major ones, often disappear after successful surgery for stress incontinence suggests that these two phenomena are causally related in many patients in an as yet unknown fashion.

Bladder-related incontinence in men: The pathophysiology of bladder-related incontinence in men is similar to that in women except that there is no known association between DO and stress incontinence in the male. There is, however, a unique association of DO with BOO in the men. The incidence of DO in men with outlet obstruction secondary to prostatic enlargement is approximately 50%. When the outlet obstruction is relieved in such patients, there is a high reversion rate of the bladder overactivity status (approximately 70%), although this reversion may take as long as 12 months.

Overflow incontinence: This is a descriptive term that denotes leakage of urine associated with urinary retention. This is more common in the male than female. The primary pathophysiology is actually a failure of emptying, leading to urinary retention with "overflow" incontinence, resulting from either continuous or episodic elevation of intravesical pressure over urethral pressure. This generally results from outlet obstruction or detrusor inactivity, either neurologic or pharmacologic in origin, or may be secondary to inadvertent overdistention of the bladder.

Management of urinary incontinence – General principles: Management of incontinence includes the processes of evaluation and treatment. Various algorithms are available for each, ranging from the simplest to the most complicated.

What is appropriate for one patient may not be appropriate for another. The level of complexity of the evaluation and management depends, as it does for all types of voiding dysfunction, on the following:

1. The clinical problem at hand
2. The prior treatment experience(s)
3. The patient's desire for treatment
4. The patient's goals of therapy
5. The patient's desire to avoid invasive procedures and/or complications
6. The patient's ability and desire to follow instructions or carry out specific tasks
7. The expected level of improvement under optimal circumstances
8. The health care provider's level of expertise

9. Environmental considerations
10. Economic considerations

Treatment of Lower Urinary Tract Dysfunction

GENERAL PRINCIPLES

There are only a discrete number of therapies available, and these are easily categorized on a functional "menu" basis according to whether they are used primarily to facilitate urine storage or emptying and whether their primary effect is on the bladder or the outlet (see Tables 14.7 and 14.8). The algorithms for the management of UI in various populations endorsed by the Sixth International Consultation on Incontinence (ICI) (2016) are reproduced in Tables 14.e1, 14.e2, 14.e3, 14.e4, 14.e5, 14.e6, and 14.e7. The letter grades in the tables refer to the various committee assessments using the Oxford Guidelines (Table 14.e8) adopted by the ICI. For any especially interested in this area, the most recent two-volume text is highly recommended (Abrams et al. 2017). A new edition will be published in 2021–2022. Brief comments will be made about selected, more commonly used categories, as well as for therapies that may be sex-specific. Specific therapy for BPH is considered in Chapter 15.

Note that inclusion in the lists does not necessarily imply majority agreement on efficacy. Treatment should always begin with the simplest most reversible form(s) of therapy, proceeding gradually up the ladder of complexity, with the knowledge that it is only the patient (and/or family) who is (are) empowered to say when "enough is enough." A perfect result need not be achieved. Satisfaction and avoidance of adverse outcomes are the goals. At every step, the patient and/or family must understand the potential benefits, practicalities, and risks of further therapy.

THERAPY TO FACILITATE BLADDER FILLING/ URINE STORAGE

1. Inhibiting bladder contractility, decreasing sensory input, and increasing bladder capacity (see Table 14.7)
   a. **Behavioral therapy, behavioral modification, and bladder training:** These terms are sometimes used interchangeably in describing nonmedical, nonsurgical methods to treat various types of LUT dysfunction. The term *behavioral therapy*

in our center includes (1) patient education about LUT function; (2) information about lifestyle changes or dietary modification (e.g., fluid restriction, avoidance of irritants); (3) so-called *bladder training* or *retraining*, which includes instituting intervals of timed voiding and gradually increasing these intervals; (4) pelvic floor physiotherapy with or without biofeedback, both to strengthen the pelvic floor musculature and to aid in the individual's ability to shut off an unwanted bladder contraction; and (5) for physically or mentally challenged individuals, scheduled toileting and/or prompted voiding. In patients with OAB, the pelvic floor physiotherapy is used primarily as an aid to patients in suppressing urgency and DO. They are taught to do "quick flicks" of the pelvic floor musculature in an effort to accomplish this. Putting all these things together involves establishing a regimen for the patient and combining all of these modalities, such that the patient voids according to a timed schedule that they can initially maintain. A bladder diary is an important part of this regimen and is useful in following the patient's progress. Periodically, the patient is asked to increase the intervals between micturition until an acceptable interval is reached without the symptoms of urgency or urgent incontinence interfering. Biofeedback is a technique that provides visual and/or auditory signals to an individual with respect to their performance of a physiologic process, in this case pelvic floor muscle contraction. Electromyography or vaginal pressure measurements are generally used. Despite the logic of biofeedback, some comprehensive reviews have failed to demonstrate the superiority of pelvic floor muscle-exercise instruction with biofeedback over pelvic floor exercise instruction alone. It is clear, however, that, whether considering stress, urge, or mixed UI, and using the number of incontinence episodes or the amount of urine lost as primary outcome indicators, behavioral therapy is capable of causing a significant reduction. Quoted figures range from 40% to 80%. We think of behavioral therapy as an overall program that can be used for the treatment of UI or bladder overactivity without UI. With sphincteric-related incontinence, obviously the patient should concentrate more on pelvic floor physiotherapy for the purpose of strengthening the pelvic floor musculature.

With OAB, with or without urge incontinence, the patient should concentrate more on the behavioral modification, using pelvic floor physiotherapy more as a tool to abort involuntary bladder contractions. Biofeedback is optional in either case. Weight loss in the overweight population can improve both SUI and UUI and should be a part of behavioral therapy where applicable. The success of behavioral therapy (modification) is proportional to the skill and experience of the therapist and the "hands-on" time the therapist spends with the patient.

b. **Pharmacologic therapy**: In general, drug therapy for LUT dysfunction is hindered by a concept that can be expressed in one word: *uroselectivity*, a term originated by Karl-Erik Andersson. For instance, the clinical utility of available antimuscarinic agents is limited by their lack of selectivity, responsible for the classic peripheral antimuscarinic side effects of dry mouth, constipation, blurred vision, tachycardia, and/or effects on cognitive function. Calcium channel blockers, potassium channel openers, and sensory antagonists would be ideal for the treatment of OAB if a receptor or channel could be found that was bladder specific. At the Sixth International Consultation on Urinary Incontinence, the committee on pharmacology "graded" the various drugs used for the treatment of UI according to the Oxford system (Table 14.14).

   1) **Antimuscarinic agents**: The physiologic basis for the use of anticholinergic agents is that the major portion of the neurohumoral stimulus for physiologic and presumably involuntary bladder contraction is acetylcholine-induced stimulation of postganglionic parasympathetic cholinergic receptor sites on bladder smooth muscle. In patients with OAB, the effects have been described as follows: (1) increase in the volume to the first involuntary bladder contraction, (2) decrease in the amplitude of involuntary bladder contractions, (3) increase in total bladder capacity, and (4) decrease in urgency and urgency incontinence episodes. The common view previously was that in overactive bladder-related detrusor overactivity (OAB-DO), these drugs act by blocking the muscarinic receptors on the detrusor muscle that are stimulated by acetylcholine,

TABLE 14.14 **Drugs Used in the Treatment of LUTS, OAB, and DO** ***Assessments According to the Oxford System (Modified)***

	Level of Evidence	Grade of Recommendation
Antimuscarinic Drugs		
Atropine, hyoscyamine	3	C
Darifenacin	1	A
Fesoterodine	1	A
Imidafenacin	1	A
Propantheline	2	B
Solifenacin	1	A
Tolterodine	1	A
Trospium	1	A
Drugs with Mixed Actions		
Oxybutynin	1	A
Propiverine	1	A
Flavoxate	2	D
Drugs Acting on Membrane Channels		
Calcium antagonists	2	D
K-channel openers	2	D
Antidepressants		
Imipramine	3	C
Duloxetine	2	C
Alpha-AR Antagonists		
Alfuzosin	3	C
Doxazosin	3	C
Prazosin	3	C
Terazosin	3	C
Tamsulosin	3	C
Silodosin	3	C
Naftopidil	3	C
Beta-AR Antagonists		
Terbutaline (beta 2)	3	C
Salbutamol (beta 2)	3	C
Mirabegron (beta 3)	1	A
Vibegron (beta 3)	1	A
PDE-5 Inhibitors[a]		
(Sildenafil, tadalafil, vardenafil)	1	B

Continued

TABLE 14.14 Drugs Used in the Treatment of LUTS, OAB, and DO—cont'd

	Level of Evidence	Grade of Recommendation
COX-inhibitors		
Indomethacin	2	C
Flurbiprofen	2	C
Toxins		
Botulinum toxin (neurogenic)[d]	1	A
Botulinum toxin (idiopathic)[d]	1	A
Capsaicin (neurogenic)[c]	2	C
Resiniferatoxin (neurogenic)[c]	2	C
Other Drugs		
Baclofen[b]	3	C
Hormones		
Estrogen	2	C
Desmopressin[e]	1	A

DO, Detrusor overactivity; *LUTS*, lower urinary tract symptoms; *OAB*, overactive bladder.

[a]Male LUTS/OAB

[b]Intrathecal

[c]Intravesical

[d]Bladder wall

[e]Nocturia (nocturnal polyuria), caution hyponatremia, especially in the elderly

(From Abrams P, Cardozo L, Wagg A, Wein A, eds. INCONTINENCE 2017, International Continence Society and International Consultation on Urological Diseases.)

released from activated cholinergic (parasympathetic) nerves. Thereby they decrease the ability of the bladder to contract. However, antimuscarinic drugs act mainly during the storage phase, decreasing urgency and increasing bladder capacity; during this phase, there is normally no parasympathetic input to the LUT. Antimuscarinic drugs increase and anticholinesterase inhibitors decrease bladder capacity. Antimuscarinic drugs seem primarily to affect the sensation of urgency during filling. This suggests an ongoing acetylcholine-mediated stimulation of detrusor tone in such individuals. If this is correct, agents inhibiting acetylcholine release or activity would be expected to contribute to maintenance of low bladder tone and sensation during filling with a consequent decrease in filling and storage symptoms unrelated to the occurrence of an involuntary contraction. Outlet resistance, at least as reflected by urethral pressure measurements, does not seem to be clinically affected. High doses of antimuscarinics can produce urinary retention in humans, but in the dose range needed for beneficial effects in OAB-DO, there is little evidence for a significant reduction of the voiding contraction in normal individuals. The only instance in which inhibition of efferent-induced bladder contraction is a positive consideration is in the patient with neurogenic DO who wets between intermittent catheterizations. In our experience it usually takes a higher-than-recommended dose of antimuscarinics to "quiet" the bladder and achieve continence in such individuals between catheterizations. The pure antimuscarinics (and drugs with combined actions—see next section) and their "ratings" by the ICI are seen in Table 14.14. There are many claims regarding superiority of one agent over another in terms of efficacy, tolerability, and safety. One must be careful to separate theoretical "edges" (marketing) from real ones. Because most antimuscarinics penetrate the blood brain barrier (quarternary ammonium compounds should be an exception), there are now documented concerns of a negative effect on cognitive function with prolonged usage, especially in individuals with an already high total anticholinergic load because of other medications. This has prompted many authorities to advocate for beta adrenergic agonist therapy (see below) as a first choice for drug treatment for OAB, especially in the elderly, and in those with evidence of some cognitive impairment.

2) **Agents with combined action:** A number of agents, grouped under the somewhat exotic term *musculotropic relaxant* or *antispasmodic*, are promoted as having more than an antimuscarinic action. These additional actions include smooth muscle inhibition in the laboratory at a site metabolically distal to the cholinergic receptor mechanism and what are referred to as *local anesthetic properties*. The former action may relate to some calcium channel blocking activity. It should be noted that these

latter two activities can be demonstrated in vitro, but it is extremely doubtful that, when administered orally, either of these activities contributes to the clinical efficacy of such agents; the efficacy is most likely due simply to the fact that the 1-A drugs in this category (see Table 14.14) are good antimuscarinic agents.

3) **Beta-adrenergic (β-AR) agonists:** Three cloned subtypes of β-ARs (β_1, β_2, β_3) have been identified in the detrusor of most species, including humans. Studies have revealed a predominant expression of β_3-AR in human detrusor muscle. The generally accepted mechanism by which β-ARs induce detrusor relaxation in most species is activation of adenylyl cyclase with subsequent formation of cyclic adenosine monophosphate (cAMP). However, there is evidence suggesting that in the bladder, K + channels, particularly BK_{Ca} channels, may be more important in β-AR mediated relaxation than cAMP. However, there is also evidence of inhibition of filling-inducing activity in both mechanosensitive A- and C-fiber primary bladder afferents, at least with mirabegron.

The in vivo effects of β_3-AR agonists on bladder function have been studied in several animal models. It has been shown that compared with other agents (including antimuscarinics), β_3-AR agonists increase bladder capacity with no change in micturition pressure and the residual volume.

The selective β_3-AR agonists mirabegron and vibegron ARE approved for treatment of OAB. Others are in various stages of development. In the OAB patients, these consistently improves mean number of micturitions and reduces the number of urgency incontinence episodes. They also have been shown also to increase mean voided volume per micturition. There have been no adverse effects on flow rate or detrusor contractibility during voluntary emptying. At this point there has been no increase over placebo reported for dry mouth or constipation. Hypertension is mentioned as a possible issue with mirabegron, along with potentially significant drug-drug interactions. There are certain clinical scenarios in which a

β_3 agonist may be preferable as first-line treatment for OAB, especially in an individual with outlet obstruction or DU. An antimuscarinic may be combined with a β3 agonist. We and others have found that adding a β3 agonist to the low dose of a titratable antimuscarinic produces about the same efficacy as escalating to the higher dose of antimuscarinics without a corresponding increase in side effects.

4) **Phosphodiesterase (PDE) inhibitors**: Drugs stimulating the generation of cAMP and cyclic guanosine monophosphate (cGMP) are known to relax smooth muscles, including the detrusor. Use of PDE inhibitors to enhance the presumed cAMP- and cGMP-mediated relaxation of LUT smooth muscle should then be a logical approach. Several well-designed and -conducted randomized controlled trials have confirmed that PDE inhibitors used for the treatment of ED also improve urinary symptom scores, especially in men with BPH. The exact mechanism(s) behind the clinical effect and the site(s) of action are as yet unknown. Although tadalafil is approved by the Food and Drug Administration (FDA) for the treatment of LUTs due to benign prostatic obstruction, more extensive and long-term experience with PDE inhibitors in the treatment of OAB symptoms is lacking.
5) **Tricyclic antidepressants**: The tricyclic antidepressants have been found by some to be useful agents for facilitating urine storage by both decreasing bladder contractility and increasing outlet resistance. There is disagreement about the latter function but general agreement about their utility in decreasing bladder contractility. All of these agents possess varying degrees of three major pharmacologic actions: (1) they block the active transport system responsible for the reuptake of released amine neurotransmitters serotonin and norepinephrine; (2) they have central and peripheral anticholinergic effects at some but not all sites; and (3) they are sedatives, an action that occurs, presumably, on a central basis but is perhaps related to antihistaminic properties. At histamine receptors, however, they also are antagonistic to some extent. Imipramine has prominent systemic anticholinergic effects but

only a weak antimuscarinic effect on bladder smooth muscle. This action could be mediated centrally because an increase in serotonin concentration in the spinal cord could cause a decrease in bladder contractility, or it could be related to a direct inhibitory effect on bladder smooth muscle itself. In any case, the effects of imipramine on bladder smooth muscle do not appear to be mediated by an antimuscarinic effect. There may be a rationale for combining the use of such agents with an antimuscarinic drug before abandoning pharmaceutical treatment in cases where antimuscarinics or agents with combined actions have not produced the desired effect. If imipramine or any of these agents is to be utilized, one must pay careful attention to the adverse event profile, *especially* the potential for serious cardiac effects. The current use of such agents for treatment of OAB is infrequent.

6) **Intravesical therapy to decrease bladder contractility:** One way of achieving a more bladder-selective response is to administer a drug intravesically. This has been easily done in the laboratory with multiple agents and has been done clinically with oxybutynin.

   Most series are small but report definite beneficial effects with seemingly fewer side effects. Although the drug is absorbed into the circulation and effective serum levels can be measured, the first-pass metabolism through the liver is less. It is thought that the primary liver metabolite of oxybutynin is responsible in large part for the side effects, and thus, these would be less using this mode of administration. This is obviously cumbersome and requires catheterization to carry out. It may be, however, that with this mode of administration, those drugs with a theoretical combined action would be able to exert some direct effect on smooth muscle because of the high local concentration, whereas with oral administration, they would not.

7) **Botulinum toxin:** Botulinum A toxin (BoNT) is an inhibitor of the release of acetylcholine and probably other neurotransmitters at the neuromuscular junctions of autonomic nerves in smooth muscle and of somatic nerves in striated muscle. It does this by interacting with

the protein complex necessary for docking vesicles. This results in decreased muscle contractility and muscle atrophy at the injection site. A sensory blockade also seems to occur. The chemical denervation is reversible, and regeneration takes place over 3 to 9 months. There are seven subtypes of BoNT; subtype A has the longest duration of action. Its use is approved in the United States as the proprietary Botox. The intradetrusor injection of BTX-A has been reported by a number of investigators to be efficacious and safe in the treatment of both neurogenic and idiopathic DO. Dosage schedules and sites of injection vary, and a careful read of the source articles is recommended (e.g., Andersson and Wein, Chapter 120, *Campbell-Walsh-Wein Urology,* 12th edition). The botulinum toxin molecule cannot cross the blood-brain barrier. A potential side effect is spread to nearby muscles, particularly when high volumes are used. Distant effects can also occur, but distant or generalized weakness due to intravascular spread is very rare. Caution is recommended in those with disturbed neuromuscular transmission or on treatment with aminoglycosides.

8) **Desmopressin:** This is a synthetic vasopressin analogue that lacks significant vasoconstrictor action. It does exert a pronounced antidiuretic effect. It is widely used as a treatment for primary nocturnal enuresis and can be useful in adults with significant and bothersome nocturia, specifically those with nocturnal polyuria. Attention should be paid to its adverse event profile, particularly the possibility of hyponatremia, especially in the elderly. A large literature exists with respect to the pros and cons of using this for nocturia, especially in the elderly (see Chapter 119, Marshall and Weiss, *Campbell-Walsh-Wein Urology 12*[th] *edition*).
9) **Drugs affecting sensory input:** One attractive modality of therapy for OAB and bladder hypersensitivity, especially in an individual who retains the ability to voluntarily initiate a detrusor contraction, is to depress sensory neurotransmission. Capsaicin is the active ingredient of red peppers and, in sufficiently high concentrations, causes desensitization of C-fiber sensory afferents by

initially releasing and emptying the stores of neuropeptides, which serve as sensory neurotransmitters and then by blocking further release. C-fiber afferents act as the primary sensory pathway in patients with voiding dysfunction secondary to SCI, some other neurologic diseases, and in response to other noxious stimuli. Because of the initial release of neuropeptides after intravesical administration of the drug, capsaicin causes intense local symptomatology and often requires anesthesia for administration. In addition, although beneficial effects have been reported, these effects are not universal, although positive effects, when they result, have been reported to last for 2 to 7 months. Resiniferatoxin (RTX) is a compound with effects similar to those of capsaicin and is approximately 1000 times more potent than capsaicin in producing desensitization, but only 100 to 300 times more potent in producing inflammation. Available information suggests intravesical therapy may be effective in both neurogenic and idiopathic DO. At present, apparent formulation and supply problems seem to have hindered further investigations. Botulinum toxin injection into the detrusor has been discussed previously. The ideal drug for filling/storage abnormalities would be an agent which any noxious allows normal sensation and which allows voluntary micturition.

10) **Estrogens:** There are a number of theoretical reasons that estrogens may be useful in the treatment of postmenopausal women with both bladder- and outlet-related incontinence and in the treatment of the symptoms of OAB without incontinence. Estrogens have been used for years in this manner; however, few controlled trials have been performed to confirm that estrogen is of benefit. Estrogen has an important physiologic effect on the female LUT, and its deficiency may be an etiologic factor in the pathogenesis of a number of conditions. However, the use of estrogens alone to treat UI has given disappointing results. In fact, postmenopausal systemic hormone therapy increases the risk for UI. Both estrogen plus progestin and estrogen

alone decrease risks for fractures but increase risks for stroke, thromboembolic events, gallbladder disease, and UI. Estrogen plus progestin also increases the risk for breast cancer and probable dementia, whereas estrogen alone decreases the risk for breast cancer. The differences, though significant, are numerically small. Whether local administration (vaginal) can produce beneficial LUT change is a question still waiting to be answered in a double-blind controlled manner. If a positive response results for stress or urge incontinence or for symptoms of OAB without incontinence, the proper dosing schedule and preparation need to be established along with proof that local therapy does not carry any of the risks of systemic administration. Most agree that topical estrogen therapy produces positive results for atrophic vaginitis, some symptoms of which are confusable with those of OAB.

c. **Electrical stimulation:** ES has been utilized in three areas of treatment for LUTS: (1) to inhibit bladder contractibility and urgency; (2) to increase sphincter resistance; and (3) to facilitate bladder contraction in certain cases of nonobstructive urinary retention. A complete discussion of all types of ES can be found in Chapter 122 (Heesakkers et al, *Campbell-Walsh-Wein Urology. 12th edition)*.

   1) **Neuromodulation – sacral neuromodulation:** This refers to the use of mild electrical impulses to stimulate the sacral nerve roots associated with voiding function (primarily S-2, S-3) with resultant modulation of voiding and continence reflex pathways. The exact mechanism of action is unknown; for suppression of DO, the locus of modulation and "readjustment" is thought to be the CNS after activation of afferent pathways. The initial use of SNM involved a two-stage procedure: placement of a temporary or permanent lead for external stimulation with a test period, followed, if successful results occurred by implantation of a subcutaneous pulse generator capable of being activated by a programmable external unit. The original device was FDA approved as the InterStim system in 1997 for refractory UUI and subsequently for urgency-frequency syndrome and

nonobstructive urinary retention. A one-stage procedure can be used at present. Depending on the definitions utilized, initial success rates have ranged from 40% to 80% in this difficult group of patients with refractory storage conditions. Adverse events do occur, and potential patients must be made aware of these.

2) **Posterior tibial nerve stimulation (PTNS):** This is another type of ES utilized for DO and OAB symptomatology. The posterior tibial nerve contains fibers that originate from the same sacral roots that innervate the bladder. Activation of these is achieved by a percutaneous needle activated by a low-voltage stimulator. Treatment includes weekly sessions of 30 minutes for 8 to 12 weeks followed, in some centers if effective, by maintenance sessions every 4 to 6 weeks. Reasonable success, albeit with relatively short-term follow-up, has been achieved. Obviously, a transcutaneous stimulator would be a great step forward.

3) **Other forms of ES:** The success of SNM and PTNS for storage disorders has prompted the investigation of ES on other nerves, stimulation of which has been shown to favorably affect LUT function in patients with OAB (e.g., pudendal and dorsal genital). Acupuncture has been utilized as well, and the principle may be the same.

d. **Interruption of innervation**

1) **Subarachnoid block:** This is no longer used for urologic indications. Historically, this was used to convert a state of severe somatic spasticity to flaccidity and to abolish AH. As a by-product, DO was acutely converted to areflexia. The obvious disadvantage of this type of procedure was a lack of neurologic selectivity. Additionally, the conceptually simple result of an areflexic bladder with normal compliance very often was not maintained, as decreased compliance occurred.

2) **Sacral rhizotomy and selective sacral rhizotomy:** Selective sacral rhizotomy was originally introduced as a treatment to increase bladder capacity by trying to abolish only the motor supply responsible for involuntary bladder contractions. Nonselective sacral rhizotomy often affected sphincter, sexual, and lower extremity function. There

was still a problem in obtaining a truly selective result, and, therefore, this procedure has fallen out of favor. Deafferentation using a dorsal or posterior rhizotomy is generally used as a part of an overall plan to simultaneously rehabilitate storage and emptying problems in patients with significant SCI or disease. ES may be used in these patients to produce bladder emptying. Dorsal root ganglionectomy has also been mentioned in this regard. Surgical treatment of bladder overactivity by *peripheral bladder denervation* was popularized in the early 1980s. A variety of techniques were proposed to partially or totally denervate (or more correctly neurologically decentralize) the bladder. These have been largely abandoned because, although some of these techniques had a high initial success rate in controlling bladder overactivity and related incontinence, the relapse rate was quite high. In addition, the long-term response to the neurologic procedure was sometimes associated with a type of neural plasticity, resulting in decreased bladder compliance.

e. **Augmentation cystoplasty**: Creation of a low-pressure, high-capacity bladder reservoir by incorporation of a detubularized bowel segment is an important modality of treatment in LUT reconstruction and in the treatment of refractory filling/storage problems. Adequate reservoir function can generally be achieved. Complications can arise including inadequate emptying or urinary retention, mucus accumulation and stones, electrolyte imbalance, recurrent infection, and the possibility of rare malignant change. Contraindications to augmentation enterocystoplasty include (1) urethral disease precluding intermittent catheterization, (2) unwillingness or inability to perform intermittent catheterization, (3) renal failure, (4) significant bowel disease, and (5) poor medical status precluding surgery. Autoaugmentation or detrusor myomectomy refers to a procedure whose purpose is to increase bladder capacity by, in essence, creating a large bladder diverticulum by removal of a section of the outer layer of the bladder wall down to the mucosa. This has the obvious advantage of not requiring bowel resection and anastomosis, but opinion is divided as to the efficacy of this procedure in increasing reservoir function in adults.

2. **Increasing outlet resistance**
   a. **Pelvic floor muscle training (PFMT):** Although behavioral therapy without pelvic floor physiotherapy has been shown to significantly reduce the incidence and amount of stress incontinence in females, the portion of a behavioral therapy program that has received most attention for sphincteric incontinence is PFMT. The literature is remarkably consistent in describing a significant improvement rate in 50% to 65% of patients treated with PFMT, sometimes known as *Kegel exercises* (after Arnold Kegel, a gynecologist). For hypermobility-related stress incontinence in the female and for stress incontinence in the male, it is certainly worthwhile to try pelvic floor exercise along with the rest of the behavioral therapy program as an initial or adjunctive form of treatment. For women with a significant element of ISD, and for men with gross urinary leakage, it is conceptually doubtful whether significant improvement would occur in even a minority of such patients. However, it is also certain that such therapy would not hurt either, and such exercises may in fact allow the individual to be able to exert greater control over the detrusor reflex as well. As mentioned previously, it has never been objectively shown whether biofeedback, using either EMG or pressure displays, adds to careful and periodic personal instruction and supervision.
   b. **Electrical stimulation:** Intravaginal and anal ES have been reported to treat storage failure by increasing outlet resistance and decreasing bladder contractility. In this case, the mechanism is said to involve stimulation of the striated pelvic floor musculature through branches of the pudendal nerve. Most reviews have come to the conclusion that no consistent objective evidence supports the value of pelvic floor physiotherapy plus ES over pelvic floor physiotherapy alone in the general population of patients with sphincteric incontinence. It may be that some subgroups might benefit (i.e., those who are unable to isolate their pelvic floor muscles and who therefore cannot correctly perform PFMT).
   c. **Pharmacologic therapy**
      1) **Alpha-adrenoreceptor agonists:** The theoretical basis for pharmacologic therapy of sphincteric incontinence is

the preponderance of α-adrenergic receptor sites in the smooth muscle of the bladder neck and proximal urethra. When stimulated, these should produce smooth muscle contraction. Such stimulation can alter the urethral pressure profile by increasing maximum urethral profile and maximum urethral closure pressure. Historically, α-adrenergic agonists (such as ephedrine and phenylpropanolamine) lack selectivity for urethra alpha-receptors and may increase BP and cause sleep disturbances, headache, tremor, and palpitations. Although there are reports in the literature of efficacy with these agents, the Committee on Pharmacology of the Sixth International Consultation on Incontinence did not recommend any of these agents for the treatment of stress incontinence (Table 14.15).

2) **Estrogen:** As previously described, systemic menopausal estrogen therapy is not recommended for use to treat UI of any type (see Table 14.15). Topical vaginal estrogen can improve symptoms associated with the genitourinary syndrome of menopause (GUSM) including urgency and irritative voiding.
3) **Antidepressants**
   i. **Imipramine**, among several other pharmacologic effects (see earlier discussion), inhibits the reuptake of

TABLE 14.15 Drugs Used in the Treatment of Stress Incontinence *Assessments According to the Oxford System (Modified)*

Drug	Level of Evidence	Grade of Recommendation
Clenbuterol	3	C
Duloxetine	1	B
Ephedrine	3	D
Estrogen	2	D
Imipramine	3	D
Methoxamine	2	D
Midodrine	2	C
Norephedrine (phenylpropanolamine)	3	D

(From Abrams P, Cardozo L, Wagg A, Wein A, eds. INCONTINENCE 2017, International Continence Society and International Consultation on Urological Diseases.)

norepinephrine and 5-hydroxytryptamine (5-HT) in adrenergic nerve endings. In the urethra, this can be expected to enhance the contractile effects of endogenous norepinephrine on urethral smooth muscle. Theoretically, such an action may also influence the striated muscles in the urethra and pelvic floor by effects on the spinal cord level (Onuf nucleus). Imipramine can cause a wide range of potentially dangerous side effects, especially regarding the cardiovascular system, and should be used with caution. No randomized controlled trials on the effects of imipramine in SUI seem to be available. The Sixth ICI recommends against such usage.

ii. **Duloxetine hydrochloride:** This is a combined norepinephrine and serotonin reuptake inhibitor, which has been shown to significantly increase urethral sphincter muscle activity during the filling/storage phase of micturition in a cat model. Bladder capacity was also increased in this model, both effects mediated centrally through motor efferent and sensory afferent modulation. There are several randomized controlled trials documenting the efficacy of duloxetine in the treatment of stress incontinence. "Cure" and improvement rates exceed those of placebo, but so do adverse events and to a higher degree. Persistence has been a problem with moderate-to-severe incontinence (more than 15 episodes per week). Duloxetine is licensed in Europe for treatment of SUI in women. It was withdrawn from the FDA consideration process in the United States, although it is available at a lower dose for treatment of major depressive disorder, diabetic peripheral neuropathic pain, generalized anxiety disorder, fibromyalgia, and chronic musculoskeletal pain.

d. **Vaginal and supportive and perineal occlusive devices and urethral plugs:** Support of the bladder neck in the female resulting in improved continence is possible with intravaginal devices that have not been reported to cause significant LUT obstruction or morbidity. Bladder supports (Impressa®), tampons, continence pessaries, and intravaginal devices specifically designed for bladder neck support have been used. Ideally, support devices would reduce any degree of urethrovaginal prolapse and/or urethral hypermobility by supporting the anterior vaginal wall and therefore the urethrovesical junction and bladder neck to control stress incontinence. Although comparative studies are limited, information about vaginal support devices should be included in the treatment options when counseling women with SUI. It is generally agreed that such devices work best in individuals with minimal to moderate leakage. Despite the compressive effect of these devices on the urethra and bladder neck, difficulty voiding is uncommon. Regular examination of women wearing continence pessaries is important to recognize vaginal ulceration or mucosal irritation secondary to prolonged compression.

Occlusive devices: These can be broadly divided into external and internal devices, referring to whether the device itself occludes the urethra or bladder neck from the outside or has to be inserted per urethra. There have been many patterns of external occlusive devices available for use in the male, but all seem to take the form of a clamp that is applied across the penile urethra. The Baumrucker and Cunningham clamps are basically double-sided foam cushions that squeeze the penile urethra between the two arms. The Baumrucker clamp uses a Velcro-type system. Another type of compression device that is size adjustable encircles the penis and stops the flow of urine when it is inflated with air. Soft tissue damage by excess compression can occur with these clamps, and thus, their use is extremely risky in patients with sensory impairment. Their prime use is in men with sphincteric incontinence, however if applied tightly enough, the patient can occlude the urethra under any circumstances—although with a distinct danger of retrograde pressure damage. Occlusive devices for female sphincteric incontinence have been mentioned (and mostly discarded) since the late 1700s. Multiple intravaginal occlusive devices have been described, all of which historically consisted of rather bizarre-looking configurations of silicone and plastic with a dual purpose: to stay in the vagina and to compress the urethra. None of these seem to have stood the test of time. Another interesting concept that proved to be poorly functional was an inflatable pad held firmly against the perineum by straps attached to a waistband, fitted to the individual patient. Inflation of the pad with a cuff resulted in an elevation and compression of the perineum. The simplest of the more recently introduced devices is a continence control pad or external urethral occlusion device. A hydrogen-coated foam pad is placed over the external urethral meatus. Another type of device is a meatal suction or occlusion device. The concept is to create by suction a measured amount of negative pressure, causing coaptation of the urethral wall. Neither has achieved popularity.

Intraurethral Devices, or Urethral Plugs. These are inserted into the urethra to block urinary leakage. Similarities among these devices include (1) a means to prevent intravesical migration (a meatal plate or tab at the meatus), (2) a mechanism to maintain the device in its proper place in the urethra (spheres, inflatable balloons, or flanges on the proximal end), and (3) a device or mechanism to permit removal for voiding (a string or pump). Most patients utilizing external meatal occlusive devices or intraurethral devices have reported dryness or improvement in the laboratory and on continence diaries. Long-term results, however, are limited, and complaints of discomfort and UTI are common. These devices have not gained popularity and currently do not have a place in the usual algorithm of conservative management of female sphincteric incontinence.

The characteristics of an ideal occlusive or supportive device would include (1) efficacy; (2) comfort; (3) ease of application, insertion, and removal; (4) lack of interference with adequate voiding; (5) lack of tissue damage; (6) lack of infection; (7) no compromise of subsequent therapy; (8) cosmetic acceptance (unobtrusive); and (9) lack of interference with sexual activity. An ideal device does not exist and limitations of currently available options include (1) the patient's reluctance to "put anything inside me or on me"; (2) inconvenience (frequent removal and self-insertion for voiding, with a requirement for periodic replacement [sometimes very difficult] by the health care provider); (3) fear of discomfort; (4) fear of infection and/or bleeding; (5) cost (poor coverage for these devices); and (6) perceived lack of long-term success.

e. **Nonsurgical periurethral compression (bulking)**: Urethral bulking is a minimally invasive treatment option for SUI that can be effective in well-selected patients. It is believed to work by promoting mucosal coaptation due to the injection of material to "bulk" or thicken the submucosal layer of the urethra. The procedure was first described in 1938, but it was not until the introduction of collagen as an injectable implant material that it became highly utilized. Traditionally, urethral bulking was reserved for patients with ISD in the absence of urethral hypermobility. Generally, this was proven urodynamically with low ALPPs of less than 60–65 cm H_2O. Because of the minimally invasive nature of the procedure and the low complication rate, use was extended to patients with all types of SUI. In the current era, however, the higher efficacy of the synthetic midurethral sling, combined with its minimal morbidity compared with the prior surgical options, has lessened the interest and enthusiasm for bulking therapy. Nonetheless, bulking may be an appropriate treatment option for some patients. These include poor surgical candidates such as the frail elderly, patients with poor detrusor contractility putting them at high risk for postoperative retention, patients who are unable to discontinue anticoagulation therapy, those requesting local anesthetic, young women desiring future vaginal delivery, those patients who are unable to restrict physical activity for a formal postoperative recovery, those who have mild, persistent SUI after a previous antiincontinence surgery, and those with very mild symptoms.

Administration of the bulking agent is generally performed with a needle passed transurethrally through cystoscope into the submucosa of the proximal urethra and bladder neck. Different locations are selected for implantation (e.g., 2, 6, and 10 o'clock or 12, 4, and 8 o'clock) to allow concentric coaptation of the urethra. Periurethral techniques have also been described in which the needles are passed lateral to the urethral meatus and urethroscopy assists in localizing the injection to the proximal urethra or bladder neck. Many patients can tolerate administration of a bulking agent using local anesthesia with 2% viscous lidocaine jelly injected into the urethral lumen. Several agents have come in and out of use over the years primarily because the ideal bulking agent does not yet exist. This ideal agent would be nonimmunogenic, permanent, nonmigratory, nonerosive, noninflammatory, easily stored, easily injected, and have a high safety profile and no long-term side effects. Currently available agents include Macroplastique (nonbiodegradable silicone hydrogel), Durasphere (carbon-coated zirconium beads), Coaptite (calcium hydroxyapatite gel), and Bulkamid (polyacrylamide hydrogel). Collagen is no longer available for use.

Most clinical studies report short-term efficacy of up to 75% in women with a substantial decrement after 1 year. Complications of bulking include dysuria, hematuria, periurethral abscess, urinary retention, product migration, extrusion, and urethral prolapse. The results of off-label use in men have not been optimal, especially in cases of post prostatectomy incontinence.

f. **Retropubic suspension in women with or without prolapse repair:** The exact pathophysiology of SUI is unknown; however, loss of normal anatomic support of the urethra and bladder neck and ISD are both believed to be factors.

Retropubic suspension procedures restore the position of the bladder neck and proximal urethra to the retropubic space and are generally recommended in the setting of urethral hypermobility with the descent of the bladder neck and urethra out of the retropubic space and into the vagina with increases in IAP. Repositioning and securing the bladder neck and proximal urethra was thought to allow equal pressure transmission to the bladder and urethra during increases in IAP promoting continence. In addition, it is felt that the contraction of pelvic floor muscles to create urethral compression is more effective in the setting of a well-supported and suspended bladder neck and urethra.

The Burch colposuspension is the most common of the retropubic procedures and involves elevation of the anterior vaginal wall and paravesical tissue toward the iliopectineal line (Cooper's ligament) of the pelvis. The Tanagho modification describes sutures on each side of the midurethra and bladder neck to loosely approximate the vagina to Cooper's ligament. Excellent short-term continence is achieved with this procedure and at 5 years, "dry rates" are about 70%. A Marshall-Marchetti-Krantz (MMK) procedure, rarely performed today due to risk of osteitis pubis, suspends the bladder neck to the periosteum of the symphysis pubis. A vagino-obturator shelf (VOS) anchors the vagina to the internal obturator fascia and is essentially a combination of the Burch procedure and a paravaginal defect repair, a procedure aimed at restoration of pelvic fascial attachments of the vagina to the lateral pelvic sidewall. A minimally invasive laparoscopic approach to retropubic suspension has produced similar short-term success as the open repair, but long-term data are lacking. The introduction of the minimally invasive mesh sling essentially ousted the Burch colposuspension from practice; however, as controversy over the use of synthetic mesh continues and patients request mesh free alternatives rise, we may see a resurgence of this operation.

g. **Sling procedures**: Ed McGuire deserves credit for popularizing the urethral sling procedure and, more importantly, concepts that relate to its utilization. McGuire was among the first to conceptualize, in logical fashion, the fact that there was a category of women who leaked with effort, who were not well repaired by standard suspension procedures. These were patients who had poor intrinsic sphincter function, irrespective of mobility, and whose urethral function at that time could be semiquantitated only with the urethral pressure profile. He later developed the concept of ALPP to better quantitate sphincteric resistance in patients with stress incontinence. The noncircumferential compression afforded by the sling provides treatment for patients with poor urethral closure function and poor urethral smooth muscle function. Although originally described through a retropubic approach, these are done most commonly through a vaginal approach today. Initially, the use of the sling procedure was restricted to patients who satisfied the definition of intrinsic sphincter dysfunction and who did not have stress incontinence associated with urethral hypermobility. However, as individuals have come to believe that stress incontinence due to hypermobility and intrinsic sphincter dysfunction were but two ends of the spectrum and that the great majority of individuals had some combination of the two, the sling procedure became, for some, a logical choice for the correction of stress incontinence of all types. The sling provides an adequate suburethral supporting layer (see prior description of the hammock hypothesis) and thus corrects hypermobility-related incontinence and ISD. The sling itself can be made of autologous fascia (rectus or fascia lata), and recently a variety of other materials (cadaveric fascia, dura, synthetic materials) have been used, some with success and some with problems.

h. **Synthetic midurethral slings**: Midurethral synthetic slings, otherwise known as *tension-free vaginal tape procedures*, were born from the integral theory proposed by Petros and Ulmsten. This theory postulates that damage to the pubourethral ligaments, damage to the suburethral vaginal hammock, and weakening of the pubococcygeus muscle impair midurethral function and anterior urethral wall support, thus resulting in UI. Damage and weakening can be the result of pelvic surgery, parturition, aging, or hormonal manipulation. This minimally invasive approach to stress incontinence surgery utilizes synthetic monofilament, polypropylene mesh with optimum porosity to allow fibrous ingrowth and inflammatory cell migration to support the midurethra. The procedure can be performed on an outpatient basis under local, regional, or general anesthesia. Several "kits" are available utilizing slightly different insertion needles or trocars to facilitate passage of the mesh from the vaginal space to either the retropubic or obturator space or vice versa from the retropubic or obturator space into the vaginal space. The mesh is placed at the level of the midurethra using a midline vaginal incision. Tension-free placement is insured by placing a surgical instrument between the urethra and mesh prior to securing the mesh in place. Careful cystoscopy is required in all sling-placement procedures to rule out inadvertent injury to the bladder or urethra. Success rates range widely depending on the definition of success used but are generally felt to be 81% to 90% at greater than 3 years follow-up. Complication rates are generally low, and these range from bladder injury to mesh erosion to de novo urgency symptoms. Mesh complications have attracted broad interest from patient advocacy groups, the media, and legal authorities. Meta-analyses have calculated composite mesh erosion rates for midurethral slings to be between 2% and 4%; however, the use of mesh for pelvic organ prolapse and abdominal hernia repair has led to confusion over the specific attributable risk of sling mesh for those who do not fully understand the surgical procedures being performed, the mesh products being used, and the size and location of the mesh implanted. Without a doubt, the public perception of mesh is negative, and many women request mesh free alternatives.

A little digression about the use of mesh in pelvic prolapse and SUI surgery. The FDA approved vaginal mesh kits for surgical treatment of prolapse in 2001. By 2005, there were multiple mesh kits on the market, as transvaginal mesh prolapse repairs became popular. In 2008, after learning of complications associated with this procedure, FDA released a public health notification with recommendations to decrease risk, manage complications, and educate patients. In 2011, FDA released a communication regarding 2874 related complications with transvaginal mesh and stating that this was not associated with improved symptomatic outcomes or quality of life as compared to native tissue prolapse repair and was associated with unique risks. In April 2019, FDA stopped manufacturers from producing mesh devices for pelvic prolapse repairs and from selling and distributing these products. In multiple countries as of the time of this writing, there is a total ban on the use of vaginal mesh for any purpose. In the United States, no action has been taken regarding mesh for correction of SUI with a midurethral sling, and the Society of Urodynamics, Female Pelvic Medicine and Urogenital Reconstruction (SUFU) and the American Urogynecologic Society (AUGS) have issued a combined position statement that the polypropylene mesh midurethral sling is the recognized worldwide standard for the surgical treatment of SUI. The statement goes on to say that the procedure is safe, effective, and has improved the quality of life for millions of women.

The advantage of autologous tissue is complete biocompatibility with extremely rare urethral erosion or vaginal extrusion. The disadvantage is the increased operative time to harvest the tissue, increased postoperative pain, and the rare but potential seromas or hematomas at the harvest site.

Rectus fascia is harvested through a Pfannenstiel incision which allows easy attainment of an approximately 1.5 cm by 8 cm piece of rectus fascia. Fascia lata is also a suitable material for a pubovaginal sling and can be harvested through a skin incision over the iliotibial tract. Sutures are placed on each end of the harvested sling. The sling is placed through a vaginal incision in the location of the proximal urethra or bladder neck. The retropubic space is entered bluntly to allow finger guidance of a ligature carrier from the suprapubic space to the vaginal incision. The ligature carrier allows passage of the sutures on the end of the sling through the retropubic space. Variable degrees of sling tension are possible with this approach ranging from no tension to compression. Applying the correct amount of tension is the "art" of this surgery and requires an individualized approach to each patient and surgeon experience. Cystoscopy is required after placement of the sling to ensure inadvertent entry into the urinary tract did not occur. Cure rates from this surgery range from 67% to 97% with high patient satisfaction rates.

i. **Bladder outlet reconstruction:** This is primarily a historical treatment in adults. Reconstruction of the bladder outlet is one possible method of restoring sphincteric incontinence in patients with ISD. This technique was introduced by Young in 1907, and was subsequently modified by Dees, Leadbetter, and Tanagho. Procedures utilizing the Young-Dees principle involve construction of a neourethra from the posterior surface of the bladder wall and trigone. In the male, the prostatic urethra affords additional substance for closure and increase in outlet resistance. The Leadbetter modification involves proximal reimplantation of the ureters to allow more extensive tubularization of the trigone. Tanagho described a procedure based on a similar concept but using the anterior bladder neck to create a functioning neourethral sphincter. "Success rates" of between 60% and 70% were reported, but it is difficult to know what success means and what the real long-term success rates are.

j. **Artificial urinary sphincter (AUS):** Control of sphincteric UI with implantable prosthetics has evolved rapidly over the last 30 years. Clearly, the most significant contribution was the introduction, by F. Brantley Scott and coworkers, of a totally implantable artificial sphincter mechanism that could be used in adults and children of both sexes but is most commonly used in men following prostate surgery. This was originally introduced in the early 1970s. The end result of the biomechanical evolution of this device currently is most frequently utilized for postprostatectomy incontinence, but use of the device has been championed by various clinicians for refractory sphincteric incontinence of virtually every etiology, assuming bladder storage is or can be converted to normal. The sphincter consists of an inflatable cuff that fits around the urethra (generally) or the bladder neck, a reservoir that generally is placed under the rectus muscle, and an inflate/deflate pump or bulb that transfers fluid from the cuff to the reservoir, allowing refilling of the cuff from the reservoir over a 3- to 4-minute period. The pump is placed in the scrotum or the labia. High success rates have been achieved by experienced surgeons. The incidence of mechanical malfunction and infection, although it was initially high, is quite low in contemporary series with the latest iteration. Techniques such as trancorporal placement have been developed to allow replacement of a sphincter in men who experience urethral atrophy at the cuff site.

k. **Perineal sling in men:** For the treatment of male SUI, most often after radical prostatectomy, the male perineal sling has emerged as a viable patient option. The male perineal sling is a minimally invasive surgical technique that involves the placement of a compressive sling at the level of the bulbar urethra. Traditionally, this was generally anchored to the descending pubic rami, most often with bone screws; however, new techniques utilize trocar passage much like the female sling. With this technique, unlike the AUS, there is nothing for the patient to manipulate. Because of the minimal dissection that is needed, one theoretical benefit is less chance for any urethral complications. It also appears to be safe in those who have a previous artificial urinary sphincter or radiation therapy. Success rates have varied widely depending on the definition of continence used and surgeon experience. Few complications have been noted, including perineal/scrotal numbness (usually self-limited), infection, and bone screw dislodgment. A review of the literature on male perineal slings suggests that this is another effective option in the treatment of male SUI; however, it may be best reserved for those men with only mild-to-moderate incontinence.

l. **Closure of the bladder outlet:** This is generally an end-stage procedure suitable for an individual whose outlet is totally incompetent and uncorrectable by medical or conventional surgical means. This can result from chronic indwelling urethral catheters in women, multiple failed antiincontinence procedures, or extensive tissue loss from extirpative mesh procedures. It is also sometimes used in individuals who can be put into retention but who cannot catheterize themselves per urethra. In this latter condition and in the circumstance of an incompetent urethra in an individual with adequate hand control who desires to be dry, a continent catheterizable abdominal stoma can be created. Augmentation cystoplasty can be carried out at the same time. For individuals lacking adequate hand control or the cognitive facilities necessary for intermittent catheterization or who simply do not want to carry out catheterization, a chimney-type conduit of bowel is created emanating from the bladder with an abdominal stoma that drains into an appliance.

3. **Circumventing the problem**
   a. **Antidiuretic hormone–like agents:** These have been mentioned under the category of pharmacologic therapy for nocturia and for short-term usage in OAB or neurogenic patients. Another "trick" utilized in an individual with significant nocturia is to try to adjust diuretic dosage, utilizing a short-acting diuretic sometime in the afternoon, the object being to reduce the amount of fluid mobilized after the individual goes to bed.
   b. **Intermittent catheterization:** Popularization of intermittent catheterization as a treatment modality has made possible many of the other therapeutic options for the treatment of voiding dysfunction that are now commonplace. Originally introduced by Guttman in the treatment of SCI patients as a method of reducing UTI, credit needs to go to Jack Lapides for advocating and popularizing the use of clean CIC for all types of voiding dysfunction in which such circumvention of storage or emptying failure is necessary. The details (types of catheters, intervals, cleansing and sterilization regimens, and prophylaxis or not) are specific to practitioner and institution.
   c. **Indwelling urethral or suprapubic catheters:** These are generally used for short-term bladder drainage. The use of a small-bore catheter for a short time, does not, with proper care, seem to adversely affect the ultimate outcome. Occasionally, more often in female patients, an indwelling catheter is a last resort type of therapy for long-term bladder drainage. A contracted fibrotic bladder may be the ultimate result; bladder calculi may form on the catheter; urethral complications in the female may include urethral dilation because of the temptation to replace each catheter with a larger diameter one to prevent leakage around the catheter consequent to bladder spasm. A suprapubic catheter does not obviate urethral leakage and does not provide better drainage in patients with sphincteric incontinence. It may be easier to wear, but it is more difficult to replace. There is still some controversy as to whether long-term indwelling

catheterization, especially in the female, in the neurologically challenged population, is associated with a poorer outcome with respect to either significant upper and lower tract complications or quality of life. It must be kept in mind that development of carcinoma of the bladder in patients with long-term indwelling catheter drainage is possible, and so adequate monitoring of such patients is necessary.

d. **External collecting devices:** These are useful only in the male. A suitable external collecting device has not yet been devised for the female. Care must be taken in individuals with sensory impairment to avoid necrosis of the penis because of an inappropriately tightly fitting device.

e. **Absorbent products, diapers, pads:** It is difficult to know whether to label pads and absorbent products as a treatment for refractory incontinence or as a convenient "bail-out." They are used for both. Huge amounts are currently spent in the United States yearly for pads and absorbent products. Absorbent products that collect and contain urine due to failure to store are commonly utilized as a first-line defense and daily management option for individuals experiencing incontinence. Unlike feminine hygiene products that are designed to absorb menstrual blood, these products are specifically designed to absorb and contain urine. Current technology of absorbent incontinence products mitigate the potential clinical complications from incontinence, such as incontinence-associated dermatitis and tissue injury in the perineal area.

These products are sex-specific and particularly useful in supporting persons who are not candidates for treatments or interventions and, therefore, remain incontinent. To meet the varied needs of individuals and their lifestyles, these products include a variety of designs, absorbency levels, and options for use.

Over the past decade, as acuity levels and comorbidities have increased with the aging population, there is rising demand for even more products, making absorbent products one of the fastest-growing household products. The adult absorbent product market was valued at 4.9 billion US dollars in 2019.

f. **Urinary diversion:** This is a last resort for these patients and is in a category known as "desperate measures." The diversion can utilize the patient's own bladder for storage if the outlet is competent or closure can be accomplished, or a continent catheterizable reservoir can be constructed totally of bowel. Sometimes, the tried-and-true intestinal conduit (Bricker or bilateral ureteroileostomy) will represent, all things considered, the best choice for an individual patient. The usually listed standard indications for supravesical urinary diversion include (1) progressive hydronephrosis or intractable upper tract dilation (which may be due to obstruction at the ureterovesical junction or to VUR that does not respond to conservative measures), (2) recurrent episodes of sepsis, and (3) intractable filling and storage or emptying failure when CIC is impossible.

THERAPY TO FACILITATE BLADDER EMPTYING AND VOIDING

1. **Bladder related (increasing intravesical pressure or facilitating bladder contractility)**

   DU continues to be a major problem without a satisfactory solution.

   a. **External compression, Valsalva:** Such voiding is unphysiologic and is resisted by the same forces that normally resist stress incontinence. Adaptive changes (funneling) of the bladder outlet generally do not occur with external compression maneuvers of any kind. Increases in outlet resistance may actually occur. The greatest likelihood of success with this mode of therapy (although some would say it should never be used) is in the patient with an areflexic and hypotonic or atonic bladder and some defunctionalization of the outlet (smooth or striated sphincter or both). Such a patient not uncommonly has stress incontinence as well. The continued use of external compression or Valsalva maneuver implies that the intravesical pressure between attempted voidings is consistently below that associated with upper tract deterioration. This may be an erroneous assumption, and close follow-up and periodic evaluation are necessary to avoid this complication.

b. **Promotion or initiation of reflex contractions:** In most types of SCI characterized by DO, manual stimulation of certain areas within sacral and lumbar dermatomes may provoke a reflex bladder contraction. The most effective classic method of doing so is rhythmic suprapubic manual pressure. If the pressure characteristics of such induced voiding are favorable, and induced emptying can be carried out frequently enough so as to keep bladder volume and pressure below the level dangerous for upper tract deterioration, the incontinence can be "controlled," and, conceptually, this amounts to a form of timed voiding in these neurologically impaired patients. Some clinicians still believe that the establishment of a rhythmic pattern of bladder filling and emptying by maintaining a copious fluid intake and by periodically clamping and unclamping an indwelling catheter or by intermittent catheterization can "condition" or "train" the micturition reflex. This concept, in our opinion, has yet to be proven, and it may be that the prime value of such programs is to focus attention on the urinary tract and ensure an adequate fluid intake.

c. **Pharmacologic therapy**

1) **Parasympathomimetic agents:** Many acetylcholine-like drugs exist. However, only bethanechol chloride exhibits a relatively selective action on the urinary bladder and gut with little or no action at therapeutic dosages on ganglia or the cardiovascular system. It is cholinesterase resistant and causes a contraction in vitro of smooth muscle from all areas of the bladder. Although anecdotal success in rare patients with voiding dysfunction seems to occur, attempts to facilitate bladder emptying in a series of patients where bethanechol chloride was the only variable have been disappointing. In adequate doses, bethanechol chloride is capable of eliciting an increase in tension in bladder smooth muscle, as would be expected from in vitro studies, but its ability to stimulate or facilitate a physiologic bladder contraction in patients with voiding dysfunction has been unimpressive. It is difficult to find reproducible urodynamic data that support a general recommendation for the use of bethanechol chloride in any specific category of patients.

2) **Other pharmacologic treatments:** One could construct a "wish list" of other potential pharmacologic avenues for facilitating bladder contractility or the micturition reflex. In the cat at least (see previous discussion) there is a sympathetic reflex elicited during filling that promotes urine storage partially by exerting an α-adrenergic inhibitory effect on pelvic parasympathetic ganglionic transmission. Alpha-adrenergic blockade, theoretically, then could facilitate transmission through these ganglia and thereby enhance bladder contractility, or, simply by decreasing outlet resistance. Alpha-adrenergic blockers are sometimes given for the "treatment" of urinary retention, using these rationales, but whether relief of retention occurs because of the use of these agents or simply simultaneously is unknown. Because endogenous opioids have been hypothesized to exert a tonic inhibitory effect on the micturition reflex at various levels, narcotic antagonists offer possibilities for stimulating reflex bladder activity. This concept has never been translated into successful clinical use. Prostaglandins contribute to the maintenance of bladder tone and bladder contractile activity. Some subtypes cause an in vitro and in vivo bladder contractile response and some cause a decrease in urethral smooth muscle tone. Intravesical prostaglandin use has been reported to facilitate voiding in postsurgical patients. A number of conflicting positive and negative reports exist, and double-blind placebo studies are obviously necessary to settle this controversy.

d. **Electrical stimulation**

Stimulation directly to the bladder or spinal cord originated in the 1940s but met with failure. Fibrosis related to the electrodes, bladder erosion, electrode malfunction, or other equipment malfunction was common. The spread of current to other pelvic structures with stimulus thresholds lower than that of the bladder resulted in undesirable stimulation of a number of bodily processes.

Stimulation to the nerve roots has been pursued for the last 40 years, initially by Brindley, Tanagho, and Schmidt for the treatment of voiding dysfunction. Anterior sacral root stimulation, in combination with dorsal rhizotomy or dorsal root ganglionectomy, has become a practicality and a reality, especially in patients with SCI. Prerequisites for such usage are (1) intact neural pathways between the sacral cord nuclei of the pelvic nerve and the bladder and (2) a bladder that is capable of contracting. The champions of these techniques deserve much credit for pursuing and developing their ideas over the years, in the face of much negative opinion as to the possibility of their ultimate success. Although these techniques are still in a phase of evolution, they are currently practical and hold much promise for the future.

Intravesical electrostimulation is an old technique that has been resurrected with some very interesting and promising results. The mechanism of action is totally unknown, and it is similar to neuromodulation in two respects: the vague way in which it is defined and the definition of its mechanism of action. Patients with incomplete central or peripheral nerve lesions and with at least some neural pathways between the bladder and cerebral centers are candidates for this technique. One conceptualization of the mechanism of efficacy invokes the involvement of an artificial activation of the micturition reflex, with repeated activation producing an "upgrade" of the micturition reflex.

e. **Reduction cystoplasty**: The problem of myogenic decompensation has suggested surgical reduction to some investigators because the chronic overstretching affects mainly the upper free part of the bladder, and the nerve and vessel supply enter primarily from below. Thus resection of the dome (or doubling this over) does not influence the function of the spared bladder base and lower bladder body. This technique would seem to be most effective when the detrusor was underactive rather than acontractile and greatly distended, and measures to decrease outlet resistance might be required in addition to achieve adequate emptying. Anecdotal success stories aside, the risk-benefit ratio of this procedure has not been established.

2. **Outlet Related (Decreasing Outlet Resistance)**
   a. **At a site of anatomic obstruction:** These measures are all discussed in the chapters on BPH (Chapter 15) and urethral stricture disease (Chapter 11).

b. **At the level of the smooth sphincter:**

1) **Pharmacologic therapy:** Bob Krane and Carl Olsson promoted the concept of a physiologic internal sphincter partially controlled by tonic sympathetic stimulation of contractile α-adrenergic receptors in the smooth musculature of the bladder neck and proximal urethra. Further, they hypothesized that some obstructions at this level are a result of inadequate opening of the bladder neck and/or inadequate decrease in resistance in the area of the proximal urethra. They also theorized and presented evidence that α-adrenergic blockade could be useful in promoting bladder emptying in such a patient with an adequate detrusor contraction but without anatomic obstruction or detrusor-striated sphincter dyssynergia. Although most would agree that α-adrenergic blocking agents exert at least some of their favorable effects on LUT dysfunction by affecting the smooth muscle of the bladder neck and proximal urethra, some other information in the literature suggests that they may affect striated sphincter tone as well. These agents are also used to treat obstruction due to BPH by lowering prostatic smooth muscle "tone" and may have some secondary effects on bladder contractility in these patients as well, probably mediated through different receptor subtypes or at the level of the CNS.

Phenoxybenzamine was the α-AR antagonist originally used for the treatment of voiding dysfunction. Side effects affect approximately 30% of patients and include orthostatic hypotension, reflex tachycardia, nasal congestion, diarrhea, miosis, sedation, nausea, and vomiting (secondary to local irritation). Prazosin was the first potent selective α-AR antagonist used to lower outlet resistance. The potential side effects of prazosin are consequent to its α-AR blockade. Occasionally, there occurs a "first-dose phenomenon," a symptom complex of faintness, dizziness, palpitation, and, infrequently, syncope, thought to be caused by acute postural hypotension. Terazosin and doxazosin are two highly selective postsynaptic α_1-AR antagonists. They are readily absorbed with high bioavailability and a long plasma half-life, enabling their activity to be maintained over 24 hours after a single oral dose. Both of these agents have been evaluated with respect to their efficacy in patients with LUT symptoms and decreased flow rates presumed secondary to BPH. Their efficacy in decreasing symptoms and raising flow rates has been shown to be superior to placebo. Their safety profiles have been well documented as a result of their widespread use over several years for the treatment of hypertension. Side effects are related to peripheral vasodilatation (postural hypotension), and both drugs have to be started at a low dose and titrated to obtain an optimal balance between efficacy and tolerability. Dizziness and weakness are sometimes observed, and these are presumed secondary to CNS actions. These drugs are sometimes useful for the treatment of individuals with both outlet obstruction and hypertension.

Alfuzosin, tamsulosin, and silodosin, all highly selective α_1-AR blockers, were developed solely for the treatment of BPH. Reports suggest preferential action on prostatic rather than vascular smooth muscle. Marketing claims aside, whether there is any clinically relevant difference in the efficacy and side effect profiles of these individual agents and between them and the nonuroselective alpha-blockers remains a topic of controversy. These are discussed in more detail in Chapter 15.

2) **Transurethral resection or incision of the bladder neck/smooth sphincter:** The prime indication for transurethral resection or incision of the bladder neck is the demonstration of true obstruction at the bladder neck by combining urodynamic studies with either fluoroscopic demonstration of failure of opening of the smooth sphincter area or a micturitional profile showing that the pressure falls off sharply at some point between the bladder neck and the area of the striated sphincter. Bladder neck or smooth sphincter dyssynergia has been previously discussed, and it is this entity (occurring almost exclusively in males) that is the most common

indication for the current performance of transurethral incision or resection of the bladder neck. The preferred technique at this time in the male is incision of the bladder neck at the 4-5 o'clock and/or 7-8 o'clock position, with a single full-thickness incision extending from the bladder base down to the level of the verumontanum. Most clinicians would place the incidence of retrograde or diminished ejaculation somewhere between the reported incidences of 10% and 80%.

3) **Y-V Plasty of the Bladder Neck.** This is recommended or suggested only when a bladder neck resection or incision is desired and an open surgical procedure is simultaneously required to correct a concomitant disorder. This is rarely carried out.

c. **At the level of the striated sphincter**

1) **Behavioral therapy with or without biofeedback**: Behavioral therapy in this case is used to facilitate emptying in an individual with occult voiding dysfunction (characteristics of striated sphincter dyssynergia, but neurologically normal). A urodynamic display of striated sphincter activity can facilitate clinical improvement in a strongly motivated patient capable of understanding the instructions of biofeedback-assisted therapy, in this case pelvic floor relaxation.

2) **Pharmacologic therapy**: There is, unfortunately, no class of pharmacologic agents that selectively relaxes the striated musculature of the pelvic floor. Three different types of drugs have been used to treat voiding dysfunction secondary to outlet obstruction at the level of the striated sphincter: (1) benzodiazepines, (2) baclofen, and (3) dantrolene, all of which have been characterized under the general heading of antispasticity drugs. Baclofen and the benzodiazepines exert their actions predominantly within the CNS, whereas dantrolene acts directly on skeletal muscle. Unfortunately, there is no completely satisfactory oral form of therapy for alleviation of skeletal muscle spasticity. Although these drugs are capable of providing variable relief of spasticity in some circumstances, their efficacy is far from complete, and this, along with troublesome muscle weakness,

adverse effects on gait, and a variety of other side effects, minimizes their overall usefulness. Alpha-adrenergic blocking agents have also been hypothesized to exert an inhibitory effect on the striated sphincter, and this may be especially pronounced in those cases in which neuroplasticity with altered innervation of this area has occurred. Finally, botulinum toxin has been injected directly into the striated sphincter to reduce its tone, and the results have been impressive (see prior section on BTX).

3) **Surgical sphincterotomy**: The primary indication for this procedure is detrusor-striated sphincter dyssynergia in a male patient when other types of management have been unsuccessful or are not possible. A substantial improvement in bladder emptying occurs in 70% to 90% of cases. Upper tract deterioration is rare following successful sphincterotomy; vesicoureteral reflex, if present preoperatively, often disappears because of decreased bladder pressures and a reduced incidence of infection in a catheter-free patient with a low residual urine volume. An external collecting device is generally worn postoperatively, although total dripping incontinence or severe stress incontinence is unusual unless the proximal sphincter mechanism (the bladder neck and proximal urethra) has been compromised—by prior surgical therapy, the neurologic lesion itself, or as a secondary effect of the striated sphincter dyssynergia (presumably a hydraulic effect on the bladder neck itself). The 12 o'clock sphincterotomy remains the procedure of choice for a number of reasons. The anatomy of the striated sphincter is such that its main bulk is anteromedial. The blood supply is primarily lateral, and thus there is less chance of significant hemorrhage with a 12 o'clock incision. There is some disagreement about the rate of postoperative ED in those individuals who preoperatively have erections. Estimates utilizing the 3 o'clock and 9 o'clock technique vary from 5% to 30%, but whatever the true figure is, it is clear that most would agree that this complication is far less common (approximately 5%) with incision in the anteromedial position. Other complications may include significant hemorrhage and urinary

extravasation. Failure to attain satisfactory bladder emptying following external sphincterotomy may be due to inadequate or poorly sustained bladder contractility, a poorly done sphincterotomy, or persistent obstruction at the level of the bladder neck from unrecognized coexistent smooth sphincter dyssynergia. In these latter patients, bladder neck incisions, as described previously, may facilitate bladder emptying. Botulinum toxin A injection into the sphincter can achieve a similar benefit with fewer complications.

4) **Urethral overdilation:** Overdilation to 40 to 50 French in female patients can achieve the same objective as external sphincterotomy but is rarely used. If incontinence results, there is no suitable external collection device for women. It is sometimes used in young boys, when sphincterotomy is contemplated, and a similar stretching of the posterior urethra can be accomplished through a perineal urethrostomy. Observations indicate that, in myelomeningocele patients treated by this method, compliance can be improved by decreasing the outlet resistance.
5) **Urethral stent:** Permanent urethral stents to bypass the sphincter area have been utilized. There is little question that a significant decrease in detrusor leak pressure and residual urine volume occurs. The questions are long-term efficacy, ease of removal, and replacement when required, and the true incidence of the development of BOO afterwards.
6) **Pudendal nerve interruption:** This procedure, first described in the late 1890s, is seldom if ever used today because of the potential of undesirable effects consequent to even a unilateral nerve section (impotence, and fecal and stress incontinence).

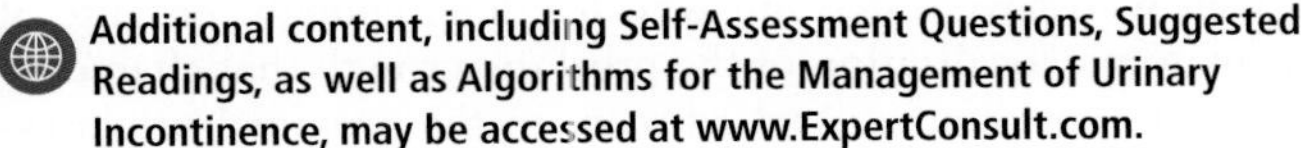
Additional content, including Self-Assessment Questions, Suggested Readings, as well as Algorithms for the Management of Urinary Incontinence, may be accessed at www.ExpertConsult.com.

Benign Prostatic Hyperplasia and Related Entities

Harcharan Gill, MD, FRCS, Stephen Mock, MD,
and Roger R. Dmochowski, MD, MMHC

General Considerations

The evaluation and management of symptoms related to bladder outlet and urethral obstruction are responsible for a large portion of any given urology practice. An etiologic categorization is seen in Table 15.1. Although some of these entities may be associated with abnormalities of the urinary sediment or a characteristic finding on physical examination, most present only with lower urinary tract symptoms (LUTS). The symptoms are remarkably nonspecific and are associated more so with some entities rather than others strictly because of their prevalence.

This chapter considers the most common of these, benign prostatic hyperplasia (BPH), and its related entities: benign prostatic enlargement (BPE) and benign prostatic obstruction (BPO). Bladder neck and smooth sphincter dyssynergia or dysfunction and striated sphincter dyssynergia have been previously considered in Chapter 14, and urethral stricture disease in Chapter 11.

Definitions and Epidemiology

BPH refers to a regional nodular growth of varying combinations of glandular and stromal proliferation that occurs in almost all men who have testes and who live long enough. Because of the anatomic localization of the prostatic growth that characterizes BPH—surrounding and adjacent to the proximal urethra—clinical problems can result. BPH can be defined in a number of ways, depending on the orientation of the user of the term.

Microscopic BPH refers to the histologic evidence of cellular proliferation. *Macroscopic BPH* refers to organ enlargement due to the cellular changes. BPH histopathologically is characterized by an increased number of epithelial and stromal cells in the periurethral area of the prostate, the molecular etiology of which is uncertain. The incidence of histologic or microscopic BPH is far greater than that of clinical or macroscopic BPH. BPH has also been referred to as *hyperplasia, benign prostatic hypertrophy, adenomatous hypertrophy, glandular hyperplasia,* and *stromal hyperplasia.*

Historically, the term *prostatism* was applied to almost all symptoms that reflected a micturition disorder in the older man. The term unfortunately implied that the cause of the problem was the prostate, which, in later years was found clearly not to be the case in many instances. The World Health Organization (WHO) sponsored consultations on BPH and has recommended changes to the terminology related to urinary symptoms and the prostate in elderly men. The term *LUTS (lower urinary tract symptoms)* was introduced by Paul Abrams and has been adopted as the proper terminology to apply to any patient, regardless of age or sex, with urinary symptoms but without implying the underlying problem. **LUTS were initially divided into "irritative" and "obstructive" symptoms, but it became obvious that there was a poor correlation between so-called obstructive symptoms and a urodynamic diagnosis of bladder outlet obstruction (BOO) and also between so-called irritative symptoms and a urodynamic diagnosis that related to definable abnormalities seen during filling and storage.** Additionally, the term *irritative* implied to some people an infectious or inflammatory process. Thus **the division of LUTS into "filling/storage symptoms and emptying/voiding symptoms" evolved** (see Chapter 14).

The terminology with respect to prostate characteristics has also changed. Paul Abrams was the first to suggest a reconsideration of the use of the term *BPH* and a redefinition of the terminology. He pointed out that BPH was a histologic diagnosis that had been shown to occur in 88% of men older than 80 years. He added that, in some patients, the prostate gland enlarged, and this condition should be distinguished from BPH and referred to as *BPE.* In approximately half of these patients with BPE, he stated that true BOO resulted, a condition that should be termed *BPO.* BPH was previously an all-encompassing term that included prostate size, benign prostate histology, and all filling/storage or voiding/emptying symptoms thought to be related to the prostate pathophysiologically in the adult male. The current terminology recognizes the imprecise and misleading implications of the initial usage of this phrase. The terminology related to the prostate is currently expressed as follows:

1. *BPH*—benign prostatic hyperplasia: This term is used and reserved for the typical histopathologic pattern that defines the condition.
2. *BPE*—benign prostatic enlargement: This refers to the size of the prostate, specifically the prostatic enlargement due to a benign cause, generally histologic BPH. If there is no prostatic histologic examination available, the term *prostatic enlargement* should be used.
3. *BPO*—benign prostatic obstruction: This is a form of BOO. This term may be applied when the cause of the outlet obstruction is known to be BPE due to a benign cause, generally histologic BPH. *BOO* is a functional term for any cause of subvesical obstruction. The WHO-sponsored consultation on BPH recommended the generic phrase *LUTS suggestive of BPO* to describe elderly men with filling/storage or voiding/emptying problems likely to be caused by an obstructing prostate. It should be noted that there are other causes of BOO than prostatic enlargement (see Table 15.1).

Autopsy data indicate that anatomic (microscopic) evidence of BPH is seen in about 25% of men aged 40 to 50, 50% of men aged 50 to 60, 65% of men aged 60 to 70, 80% of men aged 70 to 80, and 90% of men aged 80 to 90.

Estimates of the prevalence of clinical BPH vary widely, probably because of the varying thresholds used to define the presence of BPH on the basis of symptoms and/or urodynamics (no uniform definition) or on the basis of the rate of prostatic surgery. It has been classically stated that 25%–50% of individuals with microscopic and macroscopic evidence of BPH will progress to clinical BPH. Depending on which definition is used, the prevalence of clinical BPH in an individual community in men aged 55 to 74 years may vary from less than 5% to more than 30%. Only 40% of this group, however, complain of LUTS, and only about 20% seek medical advice because of them. The number of individuals who receive treatment for clinical BPH varies according to the threshold for providing such treatment, a threshold that can vary widely in different parts of the world and in different parts of the

TABLE 15.1 Bladder Outlet and Urethral Obstruction: Etiology

Prostate
Benign prostatic enlargement
Cancer
Other infiltrative processes
Bladder Neck and Proximal Urethra
Contracture, fibrosis, stricture, stenosis
Dyssynergia/dysfunction
Smooth sphincter
Striated sphincter
Secondary hypertrophy of bladder neck
Compression
Distended vagina and uterus
Extrinsic tumor
Calculus, mucus, foreign body
Ectopic ureterocele
Polyp
Posterior urethral valve
Distal Urethra
Contracture, fibrosis, stricture, stenosis, calculus, foreign body
Anterior urethral valve

United States. As treatments become less invasive, this number can be expected to rise.

Only age and the presence of testes are positively correlated with the development of BPH. Obesity may be positively correlated with prostate volume. Most agree that cirrhosis is inversely correlated, probably because of decreased plasma testosterone (T) levels. **A positive association between LUTS secondary to BPO and erectile dysfunction (ED) seems to be real, but whether this is simply age related or not is less certain.** There are no consistent correlations for dietary factors, vasectomy, prior sexual history, smoking, or other disease states. **BPH does appear to have an inheritable genetic component,** although the specifics are yet to be elucidated.

Prostatic Size and Morphology Pertinent to Benign Prostatic Hyperplasia

Although some prostatic growth occurs throughout life, the prostate changes relatively little in size until puberty, when it undergoes rapid growth. Autopsy studies indicate that the normal adult prostate plateaus at a volume of approximately 25 mL at age 30. This remains relatively stable until approximately age 50, after which increasing volume is observed, such that the average prostate volume is approximately 35 to 45 mL at age 80.

Throughout developmental life the prostate maintains its ability to respond to endocrine signals, undergoes rapid growth at puberty, and maintains its size and tissue androgen receptor levels. In some individuals, abnormal growth subsequently occurs, which may be either benign or malignant. The mechanisms of normal and abnormal growth have yet to be resolved but are thought to involve multiple growth promoting and inhibiting factors ultimately controlling cell replication, cell cycle control, cell aging, cell senescence, and cell death, both necrosis and apoptosis. A full discussion of the factors relating to prostate physiology and growth can be found in Chapter 90 of *Campbell-Walsh Urology*, 10th edition ("Development, Molecular Biology, and Physiology of the Prostate").

The size of the prostate is not linearly correlated to either urodynamic evidence of BOO or the severity of symptoms.

The adult prostate is a truncated cone with its base at the urethrovesical junction and its apex at the urogenital diaphragm. The prostate is pierced by the urethra, which angles forward at the verumontanum, and by the paired ejaculatory ducts, which join the urethra at its point of angulation. A lobular configuration of the prostate was originally described by Lowsley, based on studies of the human fetal prostate. A posterior, two lateral, an anterior, and a middle lobe were described. Although this description was used by urologists for years because it seemed to bear some relationship to endoscopic and gross surgical anatomy, **distinct lobes do not exist in the prepubertal and normal adult prostate**. The concept of a lobular structure has been replaced by one based on concentric zones that have morphologic, functional, and pathologic significance. McNeal and associates from Stanford have done the most to expand our understanding of adult prostate morphology, describing the zonal anatomy based on examination of the gland in different planes of section (Fig. 15.1). The urethra represents the primary reference point, dividing the prostate into an anterior fibromuscular and a posterior glandular portion. The anterior fibromuscular stroma comprises up to one third of the total bulk of the prostate. It contains no glandular element. This fibromuscular stroma has

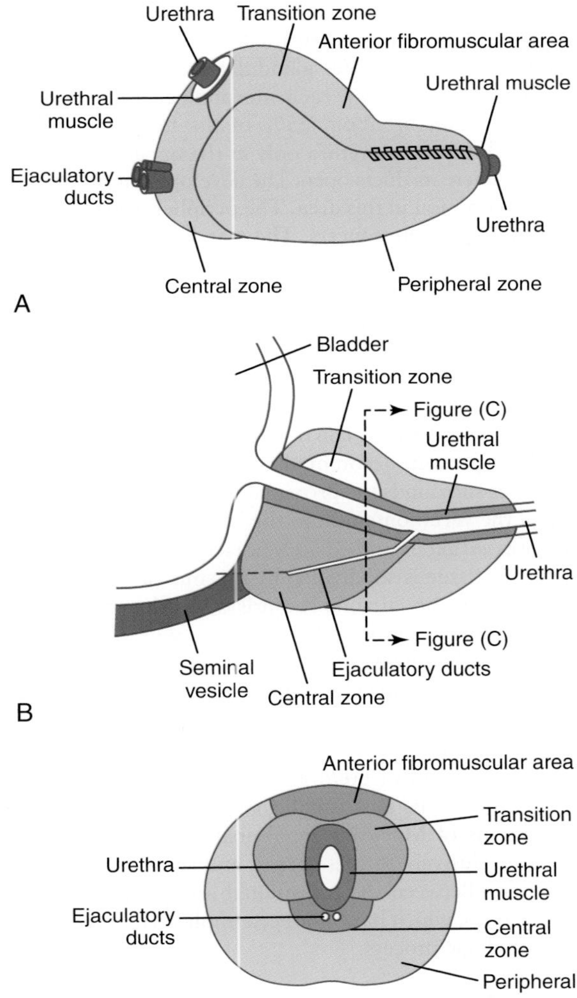

FIGURE 15.1 Prostatic zonal anatomy after McNeal. Schematic (A), sagittal cross-section (B), and transverse cross-section (C). (From Hanno P, Malkowicz SB, Wein A, eds. *Benign Prostatic Hyperplasia, Clinical Manual of Urology.* New York: McGraw Hill; 2001, F15-1, 441.)

not been linked to a specific pathologic process. The two principal regions of the glandular prostate are defined as the peripheral zone (approximately 75% of total glandular volume) and the central zone (approximately 25%), each morphometrically distinct. The central zone makes up about 25% of the functioning glandular prostate. It contains the urethra only at the upper end of the verumontanum, where its ducts open. The development of carcinoma is relatively uncommon in this area. **The peripheral zone is the site of origin of most prostate cancers. The glandular tissue that participates in the BPH nodule formation is derived exclusively from the branches of a few small ducts, representing approximately 5% to 10% of the glandular prostate, that join the urethra at or proximal to its point of angulation.** Urethral angulation at the most proximal extent of the verumontanum displaces the proximal urethral segment from the secretory gland mass anteriorly and into the anterior fibromuscular stroma. The resulting space between the urethra and glandular prostate accommodates a cylindrical smooth muscle sphincter that surrounds the proximal segment of the urethra from the base of the verumontanum to the bladder neck. All nodules of BPH develop within or immediately adjacent to this smooth muscle layer, and this tissue is subdivided by this muscle into two discrete regions. The transitional zone comprises less than 5% to 10% of the total glandular volume and consists of two separate lobules of tissue immediately outside of the smooth muscle layer, located laterally and extending somewhat ventrally. A tiny periurethral region (less than 1% of the total glandular prostate) contains glands that are entirely contained within the smooth muscle layer from just proximal to the point of urethral angulation to the bladder neck. This periurethral zone is so small that it is not pictured in many other renditions of McNeal's zonal anatomy. The origin of BPH is confined exclusively to these areas, and some cancers may also originate here. Between the transitional and peripheral zones are the central zones, which have not been implicated in the origin of a specific pathologic process.

Etiologic Theories of Benign Prostatic Hyperplasia: Pathophysiology

Clinically detectable BPH nodules arise from a variety of adenomas in the transitional and periurethral zones. As these grow, they may outwardly compress the anterior fibromuscular stroma and areas in the peripheral and central zones. A so-called *surgical capsule* develops between the hyperplastic nodules and the compressed glandular tissue and serves as a plane of cleavage. This serves as a useful landmark in open or transurethral surgical treatment. The etiologic factors responsible for BPH nodule induction and further development are unclear. However, a number of factors are obviously involved, although the magnitude of their importance and their interactions remains to be fully elucidated. What follows is the briefest of descriptions of the major factors mentioned, gleaned mostly from the work of Walsh, Coffey, and their group at Johns Hopkins; Grayhack, Lee, and the group at Northwestern; and Cunha and others. A complete discussion of prostate physiology and the pathophysiology of BPH can be found in Chapters 90 and 91 of *Campbell-Walsh Urology*, 10th edition ("Development, Molecular Biology, and Physiology of the Prostate" and "Benign Prostatic Hyperplasia: Etiology, Pathophysiology, Epidemiology, and Natural History").

HORMONES

There is no question that a functioning testis is a prerequisite for the normal development of the prostate in animals and humans. Males castrated before puberty do not develop BPH. BPH is rare in males castrated before the age of 40. Androgen deprivation in older men reduces prostate size. Patients with diseases that result in impaired androgenic production or metabolism have reduced or minimal prostatic growth. Although other endocrine factors are no doubt involved, the androgenic influence on prostatic growth and function is obviously central, although endocrine evaluation of the aging male has uncovered no recognizable surge in androgen secretion. The prostate develops from the urogenital sinus during the third fetal month under the influence of dihydrotestosterone (DHT) produced from fetal T via 5-alpha reductase. During development, there is a close but incompletely understood interaction between the stromal and epithelial components. DHT is produced from T in the stroma cell and has an autocrine effect there and a paracrine effect in the epithelial cell. These effects are thought to include induction of multiple growth factors and alteration in the extracellular matrix. Prostate growth and maintenance of size and secretory function are stimulated by serum T, converted within the prostate to DHT, a compound whose relative androgenicity is higher. Free plasma T enters prostatic cells by diffusion and is rapidly metabolized to other steroids. More than 90% is irreversibly converted to the main prostatic androgen, DHT, by the enzyme 5-alpha reductase. DHT or T is bound to specific androgen receptors in the nucleus, when activation of the steroid receptor occurs.

Originally, an abnormal accumulation of DHT in the prostate was hypothesized as a primary cause of BPH development. However, Coffey and Walsh showed that human BPH occurs in the presence of normal prostatic levels of DHT. Estrogen-androgen synergism has been postulated as necessary for prostatic growth, as have other steroid hormones and growth factors. Although much remains to be elucidated regarding the hormonal interactions and necessities for the induction and maintenance of BPH, it is clear that clinically a reduction in prostate size of approximately 20% to 30% can be induced by either interfering with androgen receptor binding or metabolism.

STROMAL-EPITHELIAL INTERACTION THEORY

This theory, first introduced by Cunha and associates, postulates that a delicate stromal-epithelial balance exists in the prostate, and that stroma may mediate the effects of androgen on the epithelial component, perhaps by the production of various growth factors and/or autocrine and paracrine messengers.

STEM CELL THEORY

This is attributed to Issacs and associates and hypothesizes that BPH may result from abnormal maturation and regulation of the cell renewal process. In simple terms, this postulates that abnormal size in an aged prostate is maintained not by the increase in the rate of cell replication but rather by a decrease in the rate of cell death. Hormonal factors, growth factors, and oncogenes all influence this balance of replication and cell death. The exact interaction of these and possibly other factors and what determines the setting points for the level of cells in the prostate and their rates of growth, replication, and death are of major importance in understanding both BPH and prostate cancer.

STATIC AND DYNAMIC COMPONENTS OF PROSTATIC OBSTRUCTION

It is extremely important to understand the concepts of the two prostatic components contributing to BOO caused by BPO. The *static component* is due to bulk and includes elements of the stromal and epithelial cells and extracellular matrix. Androgen ablation, at least in short-term studies, affects primarily the epithelial cell population volume. Long-term effects on stromal and matrix volume and effects on aspects of stroma and matrix other than volume have not been excluded, however. Therapeutic modalities that reduce the size of the prostate, or "make a hole," or enlarge one are directed primarily toward this bulk component.

The *dynamic component* of obstruction refers to the contribution of prostatic smooth muscle. The tension of prostatic smooth muscle is mediated by alpha-1 adrenergic receptors, most of which are in the prostatic stroma. Alpha-1 receptors also exist in the smooth muscle of the bladder neck and the prostatic capsule. Activation of these contractile receptors can occur either through circulating catecholamine levels or through adrenergic innervation. Prostatic intraurethral pressure can be reduced experimentally by as much as 40% after systemic administration of an alpha-receptor antagonist. This dynamic component may be responsible for the well-recognized variation in symptoms over time experienced by many patients and may account for exacerbation of symptoms experienced by some individuals in response to certain foods, beverages, change in temperature, and levels of stress.

This two-component idea was first popularized by Marco Caine and later developed by Herb Lepor and Ellen Shapiro, resulting in the successful application of selective alpha-adrenergic blocking agents for the treatment of BPH symptoms. **The ratio of stroma to epithelium in the normal prostate is approximately 2:1, and in BPH approximately 5:1.** These data for BPH are derived primarily from small resected prostates; the ratio for larger glands with epithelial nodules may be lower. Although the smooth muscle content of stroma has not been precisely determined, a significant proportion of the stroma is in fact smooth muscle.

Lower Urinary Tract Symptoms

LUTS is a rubric, introduced by Abrams, to replace the term *prostatism*, which implied that the prostate was responsible for most (or all) symptomatic voiding complaints in men. LUTS with its subdivisions, filling/storage symptoms and voiding/emptying symptoms, have replaced the terminology of *irritative* and *obstructive* symptoms, both rather imprecise terms that imply an etiology that may be incorrect. **Voiding/emptying symptoms include impairment in the size and force of the urinary stream, hesitancy and/or straining to void, intermittent or interrupted flow, a sensation of incomplete emptying, and terminal dribbling, although the last by itself seems to have little clinical significance. Filling/storage symptoms include nocturia, daytime frequency, urgency, and urgency incontinence. Emptying/voiding symptoms are the most prevalent, but filling/storage symptoms are the most bothersome to the patient** and interfere to the greatest extent with daily life activities.

LUTS associated with BPE and BPO are, however, not simply solely due to BOO. Such symptoms are due, in varying proportions in different individuals, to obstruction, obstruction-related changes in detrusor structure and function, age-related changes in detrusor structure and function, and changes in neural circuitry that may occur secondary to these factors.

Signs of Benign Prostatic Hyperplasia

1. Detectable anatomic **enlargement of the prostate** on physical examination or imaging is generally, but not always, the correlate of symptom-producing BPH. However, **no clear relationship exists between the degree of anatomic enlargement and the severity of urodynamic changes.**
2. *Bladder changes* secondary to obstruction can occur. These consist of *bladder wall thickening*, *trabeculations* (which are also associated with involuntary bladder contractions), and *bladder diverticula* (which could also be congenital). Bladder *calculi* can develop. Bladder *decompensation* can occur, and gross bladder *distention* can result. Chronically increased residual urine volumes may result and may contribute to frequency and urgency and persistent urinary infection. Acute urinary retention may supervene. Azotemia may result from

upper tract changes. There is an increased incidence of lower urinary tract infections (UTIs) in obstructed patients.

3. *Upper tract changes* of ureterectasis, hydroureter, and/or hydronephrosis can result. These can result either from secondary vesicoureteral reflux, sustained high-pressure bladder storage without reflux, and sustained high-pressure attempts at emptying. Ureteral obstruction could also occur secondary to muscular hypertrophy or angulation at the ureterovesical junction. Hematuria may arise from dilated veins coursing over the surface of the enlarged adenomatous prostate.

Urodynamics of Bladder Outlet Obstruction

The urodynamics of BOO are described in Chapter 14. Patients with BPO characteristically exhibit decreased mean and peak flow rates, an abnormal flow pattern characterized by a long, low plateau, and elevated detrusor pressures (P_{DET}) at the initiation of and during flow. They may or may not have residual urine. Approximately 50% of such patients are found to have detrusor overactivity during filling. Pressure flow urodynamics testing (UDS) can demonstrate detrusor underactivity. In this circumstance, it usually cannot be determined whether obstruction exists or existed prior, accounting for the detrusor dysfunction—a major issue. Specialized variations of UDS, either with or without video, are often helpful to separate BPO from other forms of outlet obstruction (see Chapter 14).

RESIDUAL URINE VOLUME

If the residual urine volume is significant, its reduction is important in the evaluation of results of treatment of BPO. For many with a significant residual volume, it is impossible to differentiate deficient bladder contractility from outlet obstruction as the primary cause, without a pressure flow study. Most agree that a large residual urine volume reflects a degree of bladder dysfunction, but it is difficult to correlate residual urine with either specific symptomatology or other urodynamic abnormalities. The most popular noninvasive method of measurement is ultrasonography. The error for ultrasound has been estimated at 10% to 25% for bladder volumes greater than 100 mL and somewhat worse for smaller volumes. Residual urine volumes in an individual patient at different times can vary widely. Reflux and large diverticula may complicate the accuracy of measurement. Paul Abrams and colleagues, after a thorough review of the subject, concluded that elevated residual urine has a relation to prostatic obstruction, although not a strong one, as supported by the following observations.

1. Elevated residual urine is common in the elderly of both sexes.
2. The absence of residual urine does not rule out severe obstruction.
3. Elevated residual urine does not have a significant prognostic factor for a good operative outcome. Volume of more than 300 mL may correlate with unfavorable outcome.

What constitutes an abnormal residual urine? The International Consultation on BPH concluded that a range of 50 to 100 mL represents the lower threshold to define abnormal. There is discussion ongoing as to the concept that it may be more clinically meaningful to describe residual urine volume as a percent of bladder capacity rather than as an absolute number.

UROFLOWMETRY

Significant disagreement exists regarding what constitutes an adequate urodynamic evaluation of LUTS in the male and whether a urodynamically quantifiable definition of obstruction is necessary or desirable before beginning treatment. Of all these urodynamic studies, uroflowmetry seems to excite the least controversy. **Although diminished flow may be caused by either outlet obstruction or impairment of detrusor contractility, and outlet obstruction may certainly exist in the presence of a normal flow, it is acknowledged that most men with BOO do have a diminished flow rate and altered flow pattern.**

What is a normal flow rate? Paul Abrams and Derek Griffiths originally proposed that, empirically, peak flow rates of less than 10 mL/sec were associated with obstruction; peak flow rates greater than 15 mL/sec were not associated with obstructed voiding; and peak flow rates between 10 and 15 mL/sec were equivocal. Although this proposal has been widely used, it is generally acknowledged that flow rates at any level may be associated with either obstruction or lack of obstruction. Studies are cited showing that 7% to 25% of patients referred with LUTS had high flow BOO.

Potential problems related to uroflow include the following:

1. Many patients do not or will not void in a volume sufficient for accurate measurement.
2. Others void with an interrupted stream or with postvoid dribbling, which makes interpretation of the endpoint of micturition difficult, casting some element of subjectivity into the calculation of average flow rate.
3. Some patients are unable to relax sufficiently to void in the same manner in which they would in the privacy of their own bathroom.
4. A considerable discrepancy may exist between the first and subsequent measures of mean and peak flow.
5. The flow parameter measured noninvasively and in the course of pressure flow studies in the same individual may vary considerably.

Flow data changes can be expressed in terms of absolute change, percent change, or as cumulative frequency distribution. Clearly important is the initial flow number, the value of which may make the absolute or percent change look better or worse. In other words, raw data must be expressed along with the other frills that may be added to embellish flow data. It should be noted also that **it is unknown what change in flow is necessary to give the impression of mild, moderate, or marked improvement.**

Because voiding events may be different from point to point in an individual's life, a variety of flow nomograms have been constructed to facilitate comparison of them. It should be noted that many nomograms and tables of "acceptable flow rates" are available for various age groups. Many believe that the Siroky nomogram, commonly used in the United States, overestimates peak and average flow rates for older men and therefore underestimates the number of older men with BOO. Other nomograms include the Drach peak flow nomogram and the Liverpool and Bristol nomograms. It is doubtful that consistency will be achieved among flow nomogram makers. However, one of the systems supported by at least a portion of urodynamicists should be utilized for comparison following treatment of BPO.

CYSTOMETRY AND PRESSURE FLOW STUDIES

Filling cystometry provides information on sensation, compliance, and the presence of and threshold for involuntary bladder contractions and urodynamic bladder capacity. Compliance is generally not affected in patients with BPO, but as mentioned previously, approximately 50% of such patients will have involuntary bladder contractions.

On a logical basis, BOO would seem to be defined by the relationship between flow rate and detrusor contractility. **Outlet obstruction is best characterized by a poor flow rate in the presence of a detrusor contraction of adequate force, duration, and speed. With obstruction, P_{DET} during attempted voiding generally rises, flow rates generally fall, and the shape of the flow curve becomes more like a plateau than a parabola.** However, marked disagreement exists about the utility of pressure flow urodynamic measurements in the prediction of success of a given treatment and in the assessment of treatment results. Authorities who make an excellent case for the use of various types of pressure flow studies in evaluating patients with LUTS and favorably affecting outcomes include Abrams and associates; Blaivas, Coolsaet, and Blok; Jensen, Neal, and colleagues; Schafer and coworkers; and Rollema and Van Mastrigt. Some add other mathematical means to augment the relationships observed on a simple plot of P_{DET} versus flow. Equally forceful arguments against the utility of such measurements are made by Andersen, Bruskewitz, and colleagues; Graverson and coworkers; and McConnell. Jensen did an exhaustive review of the subject of urodynamic efficacy in the evaluation of elderly men with prostatism. One conclusion was that, in this group, interpretation of pressure flow data using the nomogram of Abrams and Griffiths (see Chapter 14) revealed a significantly better subjective outcome for surgery in patients classified as *obstructed* than in those classified as *unobstructed* (93.1% versus 77.8%, $P < .02$). Others have also demonstrated better outcomes for surgery in urodynamically obstructed men than in those with no obstruction.

Successful treatment of BPO by prostatectomy is generally correlated with a reduction in the P_{DET}. The corresponding detrusor pressure at maximum flow (P_{DET} at Q_{MAX}) and the peak flow rate (Q_{MAX}) are the most common and most important pressure flow variables reported. Consideration of the entire pressure flow plot or other complex mathematical manipulations and graphic representation may, in fact, prove to be more accurate and informative ways of looking at this relationship and may narrow further the diagnostic gray zone between BOO and decreased detrusor function. The problem is that there is not just one such program, but a number of them, with intense competition among their creators in the literature.

SYMPTOMATIC VERSUS URODYNAMIC IMPROVEMENT

The data from pressure flow studies can be reported either as raw changes in individual parameters (e.g., Q_{MAX}, P_{DET}, P_{DET} at Q_{MAX}), as a change in category or number designating the grade or severity of obstruction, or by a visual demonstration of change on the nomogram itself. Aside from the utility (or nonutility) of these measurements in assessing the outcome of BPH treatment, a **global question referable to these studies seems to be whether the evaluation of the average older man with LUTS is more likely to lead to a better treatment outcome if urodynamic studies are performed.** In other words, can urodynamic studies predict the outcome of various treatments for LUTS, including watchful waiting? The critical question, when considering a given analysis of pressure-flow data, is: Are patients with LUTS in whom treatment in the form of outlet ablation fails the same as those whose detrusor contractility is judged ineffective by the criteria under consideration? If the answer to this question is no, then the relevance of the analysis is in question, unless it can predict which patients will worsen or which patients will have undesirable sequelae, or it can predict which modalities are apt to be more successful in treatment than others. In our opinion, we who perform urodynamics have done a remarkably poor job of looking into this aspect of outcome analysis.

One final consideration should be mentioned—a seeming dissociation that may occur between symptomatic and urodynamic improvement. This has been most noticeable in data concerning pharmacologic agents. The fact that symptomatic improvement occurs that is seemingly out of proportion to the amount of urodynamic improvement may, in fact, indicate that a given treatment is not equal to the current gold standard of prostatectomy or that the results will be of shorter duration. **However, one important possibility to consider is that the actual symptoms which we will attribute to BPO have much less to do with urodynamically defined obstruction than is thought, and their relief with**

these other types of treatment has to do more with the correction of some ill-defined mechanism within the prostate and/or prostatic urethra that is not directly related to the amount of mechanical obstruction. Alternatively, it may not be necessary to reduce outlet obstruction by the amount achievable by prostatectomy to significantly improve symptomatology and prevent bladder or upper tract deterioration.

The Natural History of Benign Prostatic Hyperplasia and its Alteration

Although LUTS due to BPO may be progressive over time, spontaneous improvement can occur in an untreated patient, and thus, the course may be highly variable. Combining data from a number of reports of the natural history of untreated LUTS/BPO, one can conclude that over a 1- to 5-year period, approximately 15% to 30% of patients with clinical BPH will experience subjective improvement; 15% to 55% will have no change; and 15% to 50% will experience some worsening in their symptomatology. Data suggest that over 3 to 5 years, 15% to 25% of patients will show an increase in flow rates; 15% will have no change; and 60% to 70% will have some worsening. Placebo responses of 20% to 40% have consistently been reported over the years for drug therapy.

Although BPH is rarely life threatening, it is generally considered to be a slowly progressive disease. Although many patients may do perfectly well with watchful waiting over long periods of time, the natural history of the disease can include undesirable outcomes. More recently, attention has been focused not only on evaluating the acute positive effects of treatment but on stabilizing symptoms, reversing the natural progression of BPH, and avoiding acute or undesirable events. The outcome measures recorded generally include (1) progression of symptoms, or signs, or both; (2) the occurrence of acute urinary retention; and (3) the need for surgical intervention. Progression can be measured in terms of any of the parameters used to assess outcome acutely or subacutely. A matched control group is obviously valuable in this regard because the use of historical control subjects is less than ideal. Acute urinary retention is probably the event most feared by men with BPH. Reported occurrences range from 0.004

to 0.13 episodes per person-year, with a 10-year cumulative incidence rate ranging from 4% to 73%. Others report the incidence of retention in 3 years to be 2.9% and cite incidences in the literature as low as 2% in 5 years and as high as 35% in 3 years. Progression to the point of requiring surgical intervention is an obvious undesirable outcome, but little data are available regarding the incidence of this outcome, especially because the definitions of surgery and the indications and triggers for different types of "make a hole" therapy other than prostatectomy are continually changing.

Evaluation of Lower Urinary Tract Symptoms Suspected to Be Due to Benign Prostatic Hyperplasia

The essentials of our initial evaluation include history, digital rectal and focused physical examinations, urinalysis, urine cytology in those with significant irritative symptoms, serum creatinine, renal ultrasound if creatinine is abnormal, and a standardized symptom assessment, such as the American Urological Association Symptom Score (AUASS) or International Prostate Symptom Score (IPSS) (Fig. 15.2). **Currently no absolute consensus exists as to routine prostate-specific antigen (PSA) measurement in men with LUTS. PSA can be useful for two reasons: prostate cancer screening and as a parameter for prognostic value for BPH progression and response to treatment.** Prostate cancer screening is addressed in Chapter 16. **PSA is a surrogate for prostate volume in the absence of cancer and a predictor of the risk of acute urinary retention and the ultimate need for surgery in men with LUTS secondary to BPO.** In any case the benefits and risks of PSA measurement, including the issues of false negative and positive results, should be discussed with the patient. The US Preventive Services Task Force issued a recommendation against PSA-based screening for prostate cancer, whereas the American Urological Association (AUA) guideline recommended shared decision-making for men aged 55 to 69 years who are considering PSA screening, and proceeding based on a man's values and preferences.

Men who do not have absolute or near-absolute indications for treatment (see the following discussion), and have an AUASS

AUA Symptom Index (range from 0 to 35 points).

	NOT AT ALL	LESS THAN 1 TIME IN 5	LESS THAN HALF THE TIME	ABOUT HALF THE TIME	MORE THAN HALF THE TIME	ALMOST ALWAYS
1. Over the last month how often have you had a sensation of not emptying your bladder completely after you finished urinating?	0	1	2	3	4	5
2. Over the last month, how often have you had to urinate again less than 2 hours after you finished urinating?	0	1	2	3	4	5
3. Over the last month, how often have you found you stopped and started again several times while urinating?	0	1	2	3	4	5
4. Over the last month, how often have you found it difficult to postpone urinating?	0	1	2	3	4	5
5. Over the last month, how often have you had a weak stream while urinating?	0	1	2	3	4	5
6. Over the last month, how often have you had to push or strain to begin urinating?	0	1	2	3	4	5

A

7. Over the last month, how many times did you most typically get up to urinate from the time you went to bed until the time you got up in the morning?	0, none	1 time	2 times	3 times	4 times	5 or more times

AUA symptom index score: 0–7 mild; 8–18 moderate; 19–35 severe symptoms.

TOTAL [ ]

QUALITY OF LIFE DUE TO URINARY SYSTOMS

	DELIGHTED	PLEASED	MOSTLY SATISFIED	MIXED ABOUT EQUALLY SATISFIED AND DISSATISFIED	MOSTLY DISSATISFIED	UNHAPPY	TERRIBLE
1. If you were to spend the rest of your life with your urinary condition just the way it is now, how would you feel about that?	0	1	2	3	4	5	6

QUALITY OF LIFE ASSESSMENT INDEX (QOL) =

B. Quality of life assessment recommended by the World Health Organization.

B

FIGURE 15.2 **American Urological Association *(AUA)* Symptom Index for benign prostatic hyperplasia.** (From Hanno P, Malkowicz SB, Wein A, eds. *Benign Prostatic Hyperplasia, Clinical Manual of Urology*. New York: McGraw Hill; 2001, T15-2, 389-390.)

of less than or equal to 7 (mild symptoms), do not need further evaluation or active treatment but should be followed on a watchful waiting program. In patients with more severe symptoms or who are being considered for active treatment, urodynamics may be desirable. The simplest of these, flowmetry and residual urine volume, are now considered optional in primary management by the AUA Practice Guidelines Committee and the 6th International Consultation on BPH. We consider endoscopic examination of the lower urinary tract to be reasonable if other lower urinary tract pathology is suspected or prior to invasive treatment when the choice of treatment or chances of success or failure depend on the anatomic configuration and/or intraurethral size of the prostate. Algorithms from the AUA Guidelines Committee and the 6th International Consultation on New Developments in Prostate Cancer and Prostate Diseases are seen in Figs. 15.3 and 15.4.

SYMPTOMS AND SYMPTOM SCORES

Symptoms have classically formed the initial database on which to formulate evaluation of potential outlet obstruction, indications for active treatment, and evaluation of the results of treatment. Symptom quantitation is difficult, and meaningful comparison of symptoms before and after treatment is even harder. The concept of a symptom score or severity table for BPH was first developed by an ad hoc group formed by the Food and Drug Administration (FDA) in 1975; the initial recommendations were published in 1977. Investigators have evaluated every factor imaginable with such scoring tables, eliminating some symptoms and adding others, changing the weights and definitions of the severity of various symptoms, considering some symptoms separately, or dividing the symptoms into storage and voiding groups. **There is generally no provision in a symptom score for considering what actually changed most recently to bring the patient to the physician, what is in fact most annoying to the patient, and what he wants corrected most, or what effect the overall symptom complex, or any one symptom, has on his quality of life (QoL), general activities of daily living, or any activity in particular (such as sexual activity).**

Through its original Measurement Committee, the AUA formulated indices that address many of the issues relevant to symptom scores and produced a symptom index that has become

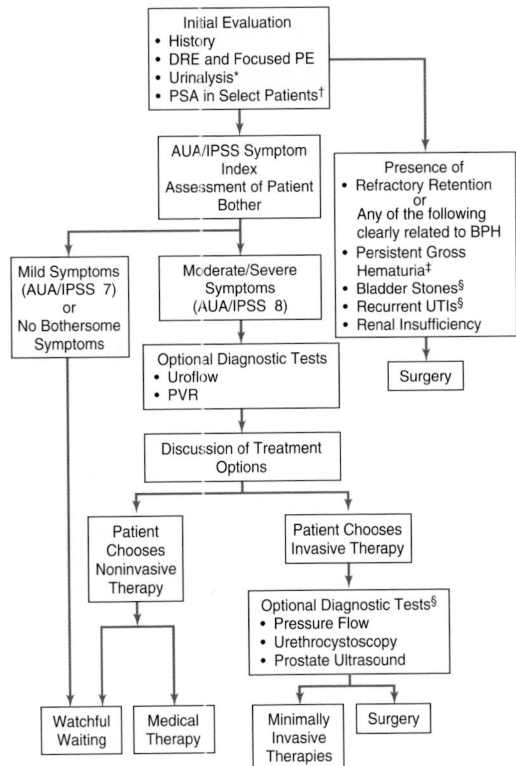

*In patients with clinically significant prostatic bleeding, a course of a 5α-reductase inhibitor may be used. If bleeding persists, tissue ablative surgery is indicated.
†Patients with at least a 10-year life expectancy for whom knowledge of the presence of prostate cancer would change management or patients for whom the PSA measurement may change the management of voiding symptoms.
‡After exhausting other therapeutic options as discussed in detail in the text.
§Some diagnostic tests are used in predicting response to therapy. Pressure-flow studies are most useful in men prior to surgery.

AUA, American Urological Association; DRE, digital rectal exam; IPSS, International Prostate Symptom Score; PE, physical exam; PSA, prostate-specific antigen; PVR, post-void residual urine; UTI, urinary tract infection.

FIGURE 15.3 AUA Practice Guidelines Committee algorithm for benign prostatic hyperplasia *(BPH)* diagnosis and treatment. (Data from McVary KT, Roehrborn CG, Avins AL, et al. Update on AUA guidelines for the management of benign prostatic hyperplasia. *J Urol.* 2011;185:1793–1803.)

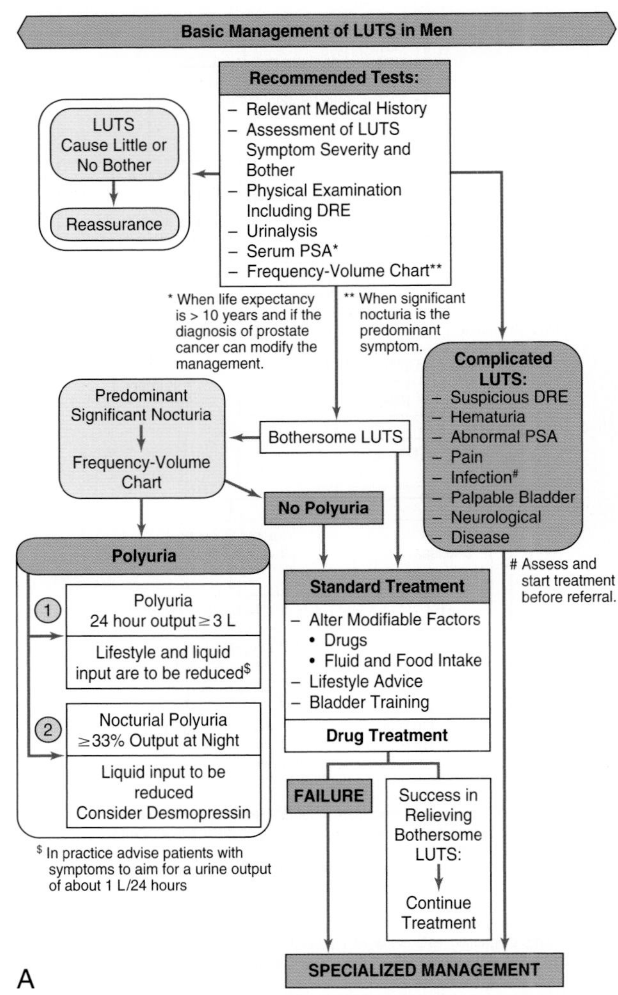

FIGURE 15.4 Algorithms for basic (A) and specialization

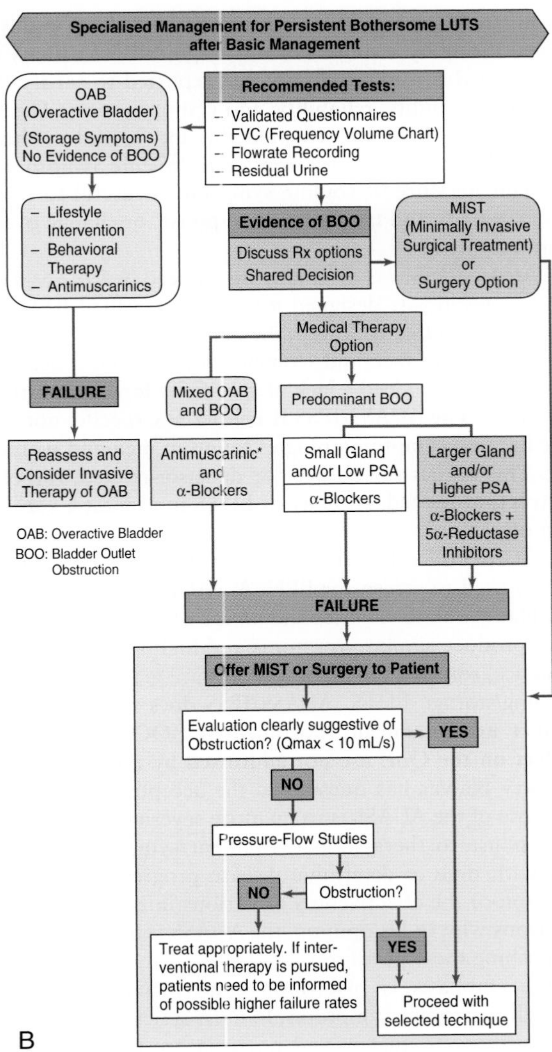

FIGURE 15.4, cont'd (B) management of lower urinary tract symptoms *(LUTS)* in men. *DRE*, Digital rectal examination; *PSA*, prostate-specific antigen. (From Abrams P, Chapple C, Khoury S, Roehrborn C, de la Rosette J. Evaluation and treatment of lower urinary tract symptoms in older men. *J Urol.* 2013;189(1 Suppl):S93-S101.)

widely utilized (see Fig. 15.2). **This index correlates highly with the global rating by a subject of the magnitude of urinary problems attributed to BPH and has been reported to satisfy the requirements of validity, reliability, and responsiveness.** The WHO Consultation on BPH has adopted this index, and in this context, it is referred to as the *International Prostate Symptom Score (IPSS)*. **This measure of voiding symptoms is useful to ascertain symptom severity and treatment of response, or change over time without treatment.**

The AUASS/IPSS was originally introduced in 1992 as a symptom index specifically designed for what was called *BPH* at that time. In the years that followed, the questionnaires were administered to samples of men and women, however, and it became obvious that there is **indeed a lack of specificity for LUTS attributed to BPO/BPE. The AUASS/IPSS is neither sex specific nor disease specific because symptomatologies found in men and women are similar.** This argues for an age- or detrusor-related, rather than an obstruction-related, etiology of LUTS in at least a substantial portion of patients.

The AUASS/IPSS does not make the diagnosis of BPH, and it cannot be used to screen for BPH. A variety of primary and secondary bladder abnormalities and nonprostatic causes of obstruction can produce similar symptoms and high symptom scores. In our practice, some of the highest scores are generated by women with filling/storage LUTS. **AUASS/IPSS does not correlate with or predict urodynamically documented BOO. Bothersomeness and effect on the QoL are not addressed by the AUA questionnaire.** Jerry Blaivas has questioned the accepted statements that the purpose of the AUASS is to quantify severity of disease, document response to therapy, assess patient symptoms, follow the patient with time to determine disease progression, and follow comparison of the effectiveness of various interventions. He lists four reasons why, in his opinion, the AUASS is not a good tool for accomplishing these purposes:

1. Undue emphasis is placed on emptying/voiding compared with filling/storage symptoms. In most series on LUTS in older men, urinary frequency and nocturia are the most common symptoms, and coupled with urge and urge incontinence, they seem to be the most troublesome. Only three of the seven questions relate to these symptoms. Urgency incontinence,

which most would consider the most bothersome symptom, is not mentioned.

2. No means exists for quantitating how badly the symptoms bother the patient. An example cited is that a man who voids every half hour during the day, has urgency and urge incontinence half of the time, and gets up three times a night to void scores only 11 of 35 points, yet has severe symptoms. A man who voids three times daily, hesitates, stops and starts, and has a weak stream and sensation of incomplete emptying but no nocturia, urgency, or incontinence scores 20 of 35 points, even if he empties completely, yet has mild-to-moderate symptoms.
3. The symptom score does not consider the possibility that urinary frequency and nocturia may not reflect any dysfunction or may not be related to the lower urinary tract because many persons void frequently by habit or by choice and do not consider daytime frequency or nocturia to be a symptom.
4. Changes in the symptom score are not necessarily a good measure of therapeutic efficacy because treatment of the most bothersome symptoms may be diluted by the response of symptoms that cause relatively no bother. An example cited is that in many of the original studies on drug treatment of BPH, there was no effect whatever of drug versus placebo on the two most troublesome symptoms (nocturia and frequency) and yet there was a statistically significant effect on the overall symptom score.

Change in symptom score is currently the most featured data in any clinical trial but what constitutes a significant change may be viewed differently by patient, investigator, gatekeeper or specialty physician, statistician, manufacturer, and the FDA. In the original publication about the AUASS, the index was noted to decrease from a preoperative mean of 17.6 to 7.1 in 4 weeks after prostatectomy and to 5 at 3 months. (Results of symptom scores can be reported in terms of absolute change or percent change from the pretreatment value.) The higher the pretreatment symptom score, the lower the percent change of a given absolute change. To compare symptom score changes, either absolute numbers or percentages, between groups, the pretreatment symptom scores clearly must be about the same.

QUALITY-OF-LIFE INDICES

Perhaps the softest, but maybe the most important, outcome measure to gauge the overall effect of clinical BPH on an individual and the efficacy of treatment for BPH is quality of life. **Most men seek treatment for BPH because of the bothersome nature of their symptoms that affect the quality of their lives.** Symptom severity does not necessarily correlate with bothersomeness or QoL indices. No consensus has been reached as to the optimal tool to record and compare disease-specific QoL measures in patients with LUTS.

One question on the QoL issue has been included by the International Consensus Committee to assess the impact of symptoms on QoL in clinical practice (see Fig. 15.2). This has been a consistent recommendation since the first WHO Consultation on BPH in 1991. Although the Committee recognized that this single question could not capture the global impact of LUTS on QoL, it was believed that this might serve as a valuable starting point for a physician-patient conversation concerning this issue.

Indications for Treatment

Indications for *surgery* have varied widely over time, and the current climate is much more conservative than existed 10 to 20 years ago. **Certain absolute or near-absolute indications exist;** they are refractory or repeated urinary retention, related azotemia, significant recurrent gross hematuria, related recurrent or residual infection, bladder calculi, and large related bladder diverticula. All of these assume that the bladder is indeed contractile. In our opinion, a large residual urine volume that is increasing can also be considered an indication.

Without an absolute or near-absolute indication, or combinations of these, the bothersome nature of the symptomatology is generally what prompts the patient to request, or the physician to suggest, treatment. Pathologic urodynamic findings may certainly be influential as well. Once the option of treatment is chosen, the risks and benefits of all applicable modalities must be discussed with the patient, and the patient must ultimately decide among these. General medical status and comorbid conditions may significantly influence this decision. **In general, the more definitive the expectation of a positive outcome is, the more**

invasive the procedure and the greater the risk. The term *watchful waiting* has replaced *no treatment*. Ideally each patient would be presented with a chart or other informational medium that describes each possible accepted treatment in terms of the expected likelihood of improvement, the magnitude of improvement, the likelihood of side effects (incontinence, impotence, retrograde ejaculation, and others), and the incidence of reoperation (if a procedure).

Treatment of Benign Prostatic Hyperplasia and Related Entities

The treatment options are summarized in Table 15.2. The natural history determines the results that can be expected from watchful

TABLE 15.2 Treatment Options for Clinical Benign Prostatic Hyperplasia

Watchful Waiting (Observation)
Pharmacologic
Reducing prostate smooth muscle tone (the dynamic component)
Alpha-1 adrenergic antagonists
Reducing prostate bulk (the static component primarily)
Estrogen
LHRH agonists/antagonists
5-alpha-reductase inhibitors
Antiandrogens
Aromatase inhibitors
Growth factor inhibitors (theoretical)
Unknown Mechanisms
Phytotherapy
Other
Mechanical and Surgical
Prostatic urethral stents
TUMT
Transurethral water-induced thermotherapy
Interstitial Therapy
TUNA
Laser energy
High-intensity focused ultrasound

Continued

TABLE 15.2 Treatment Options for Clinical Benign Prostatic Hyperplasia—cont'd

Ethanol Injection
Transurethral resection and incision by:
Laser (laser TURP, TUIBN-P)
Electrosurgery (TURP, TUIBN-P)
Electrovaporization (TUVP)
Ultrasound Aspiration
Open prostatectomy

LHRH, Luteinizing hormone releasing hormone; *TUMT*, transurethral microwave thermotherapy; *TUNA*, transurethral needle ablution; *TURP*, transurethral prostatectomy; *TUIBN-P*, transurethral incision bladder neck-prostate; *TUVP*, transurethral vaporization of prostate.

waiting. It is clear that symptoms do tend to wax and wane and that a substantial number of men will have at least short-term stability or improvement of symptoms. The literature would suggest that, at least over a 5-year period, more than 50% of patients either have improved or exhibited no change on the basis of subjective criteria. However, clinical progression, which can include worsening of symptom score, acute urinary retention, need for invasive surgical treatment, renal insufficiency, and recurrent UTI, does develop and varies based on certain factors, including age, severity of symptom score, PSA, and prostate size. Development of urodynamic parameters to predict those patients who will worsen is clearly of paramount importance. The most commonly used, but not all, therapies are discussed.

ASSESSING THE RESULTS OF TREATMENT

The outcome measures utilized to assess the results of treatment are seen in Table 15.3. Symptom scores and urodynamic parameters are most commonly used. QoL improvement and alteration of natural history are currently rarely utilized, an unfortunate state of affairs. It must be recognized, however, that different segments of the population will have different priorities and orientations and may draw different conclusions regarding relative value or efficacy from the same set of outcomes (Table 15.4).

TABLE 15.3 Outcome Measures to Assess the Results of Treatment for Benign Prostatic Hyperplasia and Related Entities

Symptoms and symptom scores
Quality-of-life indices
Correction of undesirable sequelae (e.g., azotemia)
Urodynamic indices
Size (for bulk-reducing therapy)
Alteration of natural history
Adverse effects
Cost and cost-effectiveness

TABLE 15.4 Populations with Different Viewpoints on Evaluation of Outcomes Following Any Type of Treatment

Patient
Family
Treater
Referrer
Friend
Manufacturer
Competitor
Person in the street
Agency for Health Care Policy and Research
Food and Drug Administration (FDA)

WATCHFUL WAITING

The AUA guideline on BPH issued a standard recommendation that states patients with mild symptoms of LUTS secondary to BPH (AUASS score less than 8) and patients with moderate or severe symptoms (AUASS 8 or greater) who are not bothered by their LUTS should be managed using a strategy of watchful waiting. This is a management strategy in which a patient is monitored by his physician but receives no active treatment for BPH. **The rationale for this lies in the fact that the progression of symptoms or deterioration of QoL occurs in only a portion of men, and treatment intervention is still effective, even when delayed.** The natural history of BPH and the impact of watchful waiting can be seen in the Veterans Administration Cooperative Study that randomized men with moderate symptoms to transurethral resection of the prostate (TURP) versus watchful waiting. During 3 years of follow-up, 17% of the watchful waiting group had treatment failure (defined as acute urinary retention, high postvoid residual [PVR] urine, or high symptom score) versus 8.2% in the TURP group. The Medical Therapy of Prostate Symptoms (MTOPS) trial demonstrated a similar failure rate in the placebo arm and of which, age (> 62 years), larger prostate (> 31 g), and higher baseline PSA values (> 1.6 mg/dL) correlated with progression. While helpful to predict risk, these factors should not be used as sole determinants of the need for active therapy.

ALPHA-ADRENERGIC ANTAGONISTS

Pharmacologic studies and receptor cloning have identified at least three alpha-1 adrenergic receptor subtypes in the lower urinary tract: alpha-1_a, alpha-1_b, and alpha-1_d. In the prostate, alpha-1_a receptors are found predominantly in the stroma, alpha-1_b in the glandular epithelium, and the alpha-1_d in stroma and blood vessels. The alpha-1_a subtype is the predominant one (about 70%) in stromal tissue. The alpha receptors are found also in the smooth muscle of the bladder base and proximal urethra and in the spinal cord and ganglia as well. The extraprostatic sites of alpha receptors and the lack of absolute receptor or organ selectivity account for their side effects when used for the treatment of LUTS. **The beneficial effects of alpha-blockers in the treatment of BPH are assumed primarily to result from a direct antagonism of alpha-adrenergic–induced tone in the stromal smooth muscle, resulting in a decrease in outlet resistance.**

Some of the history of the development of the use of alpha-blockers for the male LUTS patient can be found in Chapter 14. Commonly used preparations now include alfuzosin, doxazosin, terazosin (once daily), and tamsulosin (once daily). **The percentage of improvement in the total symptom score with these agents ranges from 30% to 45%, with a placebo effect of 10% to 30%. The improvement in maximum flow varies from 15% to 30%, with placebo showing 5% to 15%. It should be noted that numerically these translate into relatively small increments. Potential side effects include dizziness, asthenia, orthostatic hypotension, nasal congestion, and abnormal ejaculation.** Sexual function is complex and is frequently reduced in patients with LUTS/BPH. Alpha-blockers lack major effects on sexual desire and data are inconsistent on effects on erectile function. An effect is demonstrated in the domain of ejaculatory dysfunction, with rates as high as 28% in the case of tamsulosin. However, claims abound as to superiority of individual products. The AUA guidelines committee concluded that the alpha-blockers mentioned previously are appropriate treatment options for patients with LUTS secondary to BPH and that all four agents had equal clinical effectiveness with slight differences in the adverse event profiles. Also despite the in vitro specificity of the available drugs, it does not imply an advantage for the improvement of LUTS or the minimization of side effects. Acceptable head-to-head trials are scarce.

5-ALPHA REDUCTASE INHIBITORS

The rationale for the use of 5-alpha-reductase inhibitors (5αRI) is that the embryonic development of the prostate is dependent on DHT, to which T is converted by the enzyme 5αR. Both T and DHT bind to the androgen receptor, although DHT does so with greater affinity and is considered the more potent of the two. The ligand-receptor complex initiates transcription and translation, thus promoting cellular growth and contributing to the condition of BPH. **Two isoenzymes exist. Type 2 is found mainly in the prostate, and type 1 in extraprostatic tissues. Finasteride is a competitive type 2 inhibitor; dutasteride inhibits both types 1 and 2 5αR.** Finasteride reduces serum DHT by about 70% and prostate DHT by 80% to 90%, and dutasteride reduces serum DHT by more than 90%. Finasteride does not reduce DHT levels to castrate levels because circulating T is converted to DHT by type 1 isoenzymes that exist extraprostatically. This reduction results in an increase in apoptosis and atrophy and generally shrinkage of the gland ranging from 15% to 25% at 6 months. This atrophy is most pronounced in the glandular epithelial component of the prostate, which is the source of the production and release of PSA and, as a result, is responsible for the approximately **50% decrease in serum PSA.** Although the number of clinical trials with finasteride is much greater, most agree that clinical efficacy seems comparable at this point: volume reduction of 18% to 26% (placebo—2 to + 14), IPSS reduction of 3.3 to 4.5 (placebo—1.3 to 2.3), and peak flow increase of 1.9 to 2.2 (placebo—0.2 to 0.6). **Both are reported to decrease the long-term risk of acute urinary retention**

and the need for surgery by up to 50% to 60% in patients with enlarged prostates (baseline numbers were, however, small). These benefits are seen primarily in men with enlarged prostates (over 30–40 cc). Side effects include decreased libido, ejaculatory disorders, and ED, all with a reported incidence of 5% to 6% and reversible on discontinuation of therapy (data primarily from finasteride studies). The two agents have not been directly compared specifically with respect to efficacy and tolerability.

COMBINED THERAPY

Is combination therapy (alpha-blocker plus 5αRI) more effective than either alone? A Veterans Administration Cooperative Study by Lepor et al. compared placebo, finasteride, terazosin, and finasteride plus terazosin. The mean group differences for all patients between finasteride and placebo were not statistically significant for the AUA symptom index, symptom problem index, BPH impact index, and peak flow rate. The changes for terazosin were significant versus placebo and versus finasteride. The group mean differences between combination therapy and terazosin for all measures other than prostate volume were significantly in favor of terazosin. The volume decrease was 20% in their finasteride and combination groups. The AUASS improvement was 2.6 units for placebo, 3.2 for finasteride, 6.6 for terazosin, and 6.2 for the combination; peak flow rate change was 1.4, 1.6, 2.7, and 3.2 mL/sec, respectively. Finasteride supporters argue that the apparent lack of efficacy in this study was due to a relatively small mean prostate volume in the population studied. For the men with volumes larger than 50 mL, there was a mean increase in Q_{MAX} of 2.5 mL/sec and a mean decrease in AUASS of 2.9, both significantly different from those of comparable men in the placebo group.

The **Medical Therapy of Prostate Symptoms** study looked at the question of whether long-term therapy of BPH with placebo, doxazosin, finasteride, or doxazosin plus finasteride would prevent or delay disease progression, which was defined as a four-point rise in AUASS, 50% increase in baseline creatinine, acute urinary retention (AUR), two or more UTIs within 1 year, urosepsis due to BOO, or socially unacceptable incontinence. **Based partly on the result of this study, the AUA guideline committee issued an option statement that combination therapy is an appropriate**

and effective treatment for patients with LUTS associated with demonstrable prostatic enlargement based on volume measurement, PSA level as a proxy for volume, and/or enlargement on digital rectal examination (DRE). Combination therapy appeared more effective than alpha-blocker monotherapy in relieving and preventing the progression of symptoms. **The overall risk of progression was reduced** by 39% for doxazosin (D), 34% for finasteride (F), and 67% for a combination. The risk of retention was reduced by 31% for D, 67% for F, and 79% for D + F. **The risk of surgery was reduced by 64% for F and 67% for F + D. Doxazosin alone did not reduce the risk of surgery over placebo. AUASS and Q_{MAX} improved significantly more in the combination therapy group compared with the monotherapy groups, whereas adverse events were similar across treatment groups to previously reported studies. Patients more likely to benefit are those with larger prostates and higher non–cancer-related PSA values,** although absolute thresholds are yet uncertain.

The CombAT (Combination of Avodart and Tamsulosin) trial randomized approximately 5,000 men to receive tamsulosin 0.4 mg versus dutasteride 0.5 mg versus combination therapy with both. Inclusion criteria required patients to have an IPSS score greater than 12, a PSA between 1.5 and 10 ng/mL, and a prostate volume by transrectal ultrasound (TRUS) greater than 30 g. The recently published 4-year follow-up data demonstrated, irrespective of baseline subgroup, the incidence of AUR or BPH-related surgery was higher among patients treated with tamsulosin compared with dutasteride and combined therapy and generally the lowest for patients on combined therapy. Across treatment groups, incidence was higher for those with baseline IPSS scores greater than 20, PSA value greater than 3 ng/mL, and prostate volume greater than 40 mL. Clinical progression followed a similar trend, with higher rates among men receiving tamsulosin than dutasteride or combined therapy.

ANTICHOLINERGIC AGENTS

In the human bladder, the muscarinic receptor subtypes M2 and M3 are primarily responsible for bladder contraction. Blockage of this interaction by anticholinergic agents results in reduction in smooth muscle tone and improved symptomatology of overactive bladder (OAB). An overlap exists between the LUTS secondary to BPH and those of OAB such that the AUA guideline issued its use as an option and stated it is an appropriate and effective alternative for the management of LUTS secondary to BPH in men without an elevated PVR and when LUTS are predominately irritative. In a meta-analysis that assessed the safety and efficacy of anticholinergic agents either as monotherapy or in combination with an alpha-blocker in men with LUTS related to BPH, minimal changes were reported in Q_{MAX} and IPSS scores, a minimal increase in PVR, and no convincing increase in AUR rates.

COMPLIMENTARY AND ALTERNATIVE MEDICINE

Complimentary and alternative medicine (CAM) for the treatment of LUTS generally consists of phytotherapeutic preparations in the form of dietary supplements that include extracts of saw palmetto plant (*Serenoa repens*) and stinging nettle (*Urtica dioica*), among others. The mechanism of action is unknown but may be related to modulation on prostaglandin synthesis or alterations in growth factor–induced proliferation. Most of these preparations involve various components extracted by various techniques, yielding different concentrations and complicating their comparison among different manufacturers. Additionally, these manufacturers are exempted from prospective oversight from the FDA, and thus, the quality and purity of these supplements are not rigorously monitored. However, they have great appeal to patients because they are assumed to be “natural” products and are available over the counter. Use varies according to the severity of the symptoms, with CAM being given to patients with the lowest IPSS and combination therapy with alpha-blocker and 5αRI for those with the highest IPSS. The recent AUA guidelines issued a consensus statement that no dietary supplement or other nonconventional therapy is recommended for the management of LUTS secondary to BPH, either due to lack of proven effect or insufficient evidence to offer clear clinical guidance.

NONMEDICAL MANAGEMENT

This category has rapidly expanded in the last three decades. A number of new technologies and techniques have emerged, although some have been phased out or replaced. These can be broadly grouped into *minimally invasive and surgical*.

Minimally invasive: Transurethral microwave thermotherapy (TUMT), transurethral needle ablation (TUNA), water vapor thermal therapy, prostatic urethral lift (PUL), transurethral electrosurgical incision of the prostate (TUIP), transurethral electrovaporization of the prostate (TUVP), photoselective vaporization of the prostate (PVP).

Surgical: Simple prostatectomy (open or robotic) TURP, holmium laser enucleation of the prostate (HoLEP), thulium laser enucleation of the prostate (ThuLEP), Aquablation.

An alternative classification is **hospital based vs office based.** The former does not always imply inpatient care. A number of these techniques are done in surgery centers as outpatient procedures.

Hospital based: Simple prostatectomy (open or robotic) TURP, PVP, HoLEP, ThuLEP, Aquablation, TUIP, TUVP.

Office based: TUMT, PUL, water vapor thermal therapy.

Balloon dilatation was tried and approved in the late 1980s. However, lack of any durable response and early complications resulted in rapid abandonment of this technology.

Prostatic stents were approved for use in BPH, but due to urothelial overgrowth, encrustation, and difficulty in removing, they are no longer available in the market. However, a number of new stent-like devices are undergoing trials and may be available in the near future.

MINIMALLY INVASIVE THERAPIES: THERMAL THERAPIES

Radiofrequency, lasers, or steam can be used as a source of thermal energy. These were first introduced in the 1990s and included coagulative lasers, microwave, and radiofrequency energy. At temperatures lower than 45°C, coagulation necrosis of normal tissue does not occur. Irreversible cellular damage begins to occur above 45°C. Coagulation can take up to an hour to occur at temperatures minimally above this level. At 60 to 100°C, coagulation is rapid, and at 100°C, it is virtually instantaneous. At temperatures higher than 100°C, tissue vaporization is produced. The tissue effects of laser energy are produced by the virtually instantaneous attainment of temperatures higher than 60°C to create coagulation necrosis and above 100°C to create vaporization. The types of laser commonly utilized for clinical BPH treatment include potassium-titanyl-phosphate laser (KTP), a free beam treatment with high energy density to create vaporization without concurrent deep coagulation, and pulsed holmium: yttrium-aluminum-garnet (Ho:YAG), which causes thermomechanical vaporization and can be used as a cutting tool. The Neodymium-doped yttrium-aluminum-garnet (Nd:YAG) laser is infrequently used, given that its poor absorption by water and body pigments allows for relatively deep tissue penetration. This poor absorption in a fluid medium causes thermal coagulation of the surface tissue and of areas just under the surface.

Thermal therapies include TUMT, TUNA, water vapor thermotherapy, PVP, holmium laser ablation of the prostate (HoLAP), and TUVP.

TRANSURETHRAL MICROWAVE THERMOTHERAPY

This was the most commonly utilized method of energy ablation in the *office setting*. A large body of literature supports both the efficacy and the very low rate of significant side effects of these therapies. These systems are based on urethral catheters that house a microwave transducer just proximal to the anchoring balloon and thus dwell within the prostate during treatment. Newer systems have evolved to include higher energy levels and concomitant urethral cooling systems to offset these higher energy effects on adjacent tissue. After placement of this catheter and a rectal temperature sensor, **the microwave is activated to heat the prostate adenoma to a target temperature of at least 45°C for an extended period of time (30–45 minutes).** This causes coagulation necrosis and subsequent reduction in the size of the adenoma allowing for improved peak flow and reduction of symptom score that is durable in one report up to 11 years. **Results are encouraging but still do not match those of TURP.** Systemic review of randomized controlled trials (RCTs) with 540 patients revealed a pool mean Q_{MAX} increase from 7.9 to 13.5 mL/sec after TUMT versus 8.6 to 18.7 mL/sec after TURP. Representative results from studies with follow-up greater than 5 years include an increase in Q_{MAX} from 6.7 to 11.4 mL/sec and 6.5 to 8.9 mL/sec, and a decrease in IPSS from 21 to 7.4 and 22.5 to 11.9. However, conflicting results abound as a result of a heterogenous mix of studies that differ in size, follow-up, outcome measure, and model of TUMT system. Generally, the newer systems appear to have improved efficacy and longer durability but study dropouts can be significant and may suffer from selection bias. Thus results may be misleading if analysis is performed only on these best "responders." These procedures are performed in the office setting with only local anesthesia via lidocaine jelly. However, many patients initially require an indwelling urethral catheter for a few days post procedure due to problems with urinary retention caused initially by edema, though this is decreasing in the newer systems with a post-TUMT catheterization rate less than 20% in some studies. Additionally, urinary symptoms require 6 to 12 weeks to improve posttreatment. Side effects and complication profiles are generally very low with this form of therapy but the durability is less than desired. There is a significantly higher risk of requiring additional BPH treatment compared with TURP.

TRANSURETHRAL NEEDLE ABLATION OF THE PROSTATE

TUNA of the prostate is also an **office-based procedure in which radiofrequency energy is used to ablate prostatic adenoma.** The system is based on a cystoscopy-like device that allows the surgeon to visualize the prostatic urethra and then deploy electrodes into the parenchyma of the prostate that deliver radiofrequency to heat the prostate to 80 to 100°C. Each cycle, lasting about 5 minutes, creates an area of necrosis that is rather small and thus requires multiple lesions to be created in a systematic fashion to debulk the prostate. However, the reduction in prostatic volume is less than initially anticipated because the BPH histology is likely replaced with a scar, leaving a modest volume reduction. Total treatment times range from 30 to 60 minutes. **Randomized trials have shown effectiveness both subjectively and objectively.** More than 500 patients have been observed for 12 months and had an average Q_{MAX} improvement of 77% and a symptom score improvement of 58%. Durable results were seen at the 5-year follow-up that included a Q_{MAX} change from 8.8 to 13.5 mL/sec and a AUASS change from 20 to 11.7, though these results have to be carefully interpreted because only 28% of the initial study group was available. **The AUA guideline panel concluded, based on these trials, that the symptom improvement is significant and sustained for both TUNA and TURP, but with somewhat greater improvement in the symptom score for TURP.** Side effects are also mild and generally self-limited; post treatment urinary retention occurs at a rate between 13.3% and 41.6%, and irritative voiding symptoms occur in about 40% of patients but generally resolve and last between 1 and 7 days. Sexual dysfunction and stricture are rare, but, as for TUMT, retreatment rates are higher from TUNA than TURP, with 14% of patients who underwent TUNA requiring a reoperation within 2 years. The lack of long-term durability of response has resulted in abandonment of this procedure.

WATER VAPOR THERMAL THERAPY

Unlike TUMT and TUNA that utilize conductive heat transfer, the mechanism of action for the water vapor system is convective heat transfer due to the thermodynamic properties of water. Water vapor is delivered through a retractable vapor needle via emitter holes in the transurethral device. This is done in 9-second bursts to the transition zone of the prostate, where, via convection, it diffuses evenly throughout the target tissue. The depth of the needle penetrating is approximately 10 mm.

In an RCT, currently with a 3-year follow-up, there was a mean improvement of IPSS of 11 points, a mean Q_{MAX} improvement from 9.7 mL/s to 13.2 mL/s, and a mean PVR improvement from 81.5 mL to 55.1 mL ($P < .001$). Side effects reported include a decrease in ejaculatory volume, which was reported by 2% of participants. At 36 months, no de novo ED was reported, but dysuria was reported by 1% of participants. At 48 months, there was a significant change in IIEF-EF scores compared to baseline ($P = .03$), but there was not a significant change at the other follow-up intervals.

This procedure is commonly done in the office under prostate block or conscious sedation. Patients require a catheter for 3 to 7 days post procedure.

PHOTOSELECTIVE VAPORIZATION OF THE PROSTATE

The KTP laser (wavelength 532 nm) is utilized during this procedure. **This wavelength is highly absorbed by oxyhemoglobin, thus allowing efficient tissue vaporization with excellent hemostasis.** A specialized side-firing laser fiber is utilized cystoscopically to focus the energy into the prostate causing vaporization of all vascularized tissue. Representative results from one of the few randomized trials comparing PVP and TURP at 1 year show a similar improvement in Q_{MAX} (approximately 115%), 61% versus 53% decrease in IPSS, catheterization time of 13.3 versus 44.7 hours ($P < .001$), and a significant decrease in length of hospital stay (1.09 versus 3.6 days, $P < .001$). Additionally, costs were reported to be 22% less in the PVP group. Advantages include excellent hemostasis allowing use on anticoagulated patients, no risk of TUR syndrome, and a quick learning curve. Side effects are minimal. Drawbacks include difficulty of resection of very large glands (> 80 g).

HOLMIUM LASER ABLATION OF THE PROSTATE

The HoLAP procedure is a modification of the HoLEP that also requires a continuous flow resectoscope, high-powered holmium laser, and, instead of an end-firing laser fiber, a side-firing laser fiber. During this procedure, the laser fiber is employed to vaporize the surface tissue of the adenoma via continuous delivery of laser energy. With the minimal depth of penetration of the holmium energy, this approach can be time consuming; however, it does provide bloodless, immediate debulking of adenoma. Single group cohort studies involving HoLAP and TURP indicate that the Q_{MAX} improved in both groups, with improvements sustained at up to 24 months follow-up and similar in both groups. Drawbacks include difficulty in treatment of prostates greater than 80 g in size.

TRANSURETHRAL ELECTROVAPORIZATION OF THE PROSTATE

This technique that is very similar to TURP involves substitution of the resection loop of the resectoscope with a broad-based, rolling electrode that can be swept over the surface of the prostate while the electrical current is activated. The high-power density that is transmitted literally vaporizes the underlying tissue. This technique requires more time than resection, and thus, in most studies, prostate size was less than 60 g. TUVP decreases risks of hemorrhage and TUR syndrome because vessels are sealed during vaporization. The desiccated base, however, is less susceptible to further vaporization. No tissue is recovered during the procedure. In the published trials comparing TURP to TUVP, improvements in symptom score and peak flow rates have been demonstrated but generally with no difference between the two treatment groups for up to 1 year of follow-up. Sexual side effects, incontinence rates, stricture, and bladder neck contracture rates are similar to those following TURP but postoperative duration of catheterization, hospital stay, hematuria, transfusion rate, and retrograde ejaculation were lower for the TUVP group.

MINIMALLY INVASIVE NONTHERMAL THERAPIES: NONTHERMAL PROSTATIC URETHRAL LIFT

This procedure involves altering the prostate urethral anatomy without ablating tissue. It is an office-based procedure that requires urethral analgesia, but some centers use mild sedation as well. PUL utilizes transprostatic suture implants delivered by a hand-held device through a specially designed cystoscope. The implants are composed of two T-shaped bars, with one on each side of a length of suture. They are deployed with one bar located outside the prostate capsule and the other within the prostatic urethral lumen. The tension between the two bars pulls the lumen of the prostatic urethra toward the capsule, compresses the prostate parenchyma, widens the prostatic urethral lumen, and improves symptoms. The urethral side of the implant epithelializes within 12 months and thus encrustation is not a problem. In an early RCT—the L.I.F.T study—comparing PUL to sham, the mean change from baseline IPSS (MD: −5.2; CI: −7.45, −2.95) and improvements in IPSS-QoL (MD: 1.2; CI: 1.7, −0.7) favored PUL.

Q_{MAX} at 3 months was higher for those who underwent PUL (4.3 mL/s) compared to sham (2.0 mL/s; $P = .005$). Of the participants randomized to PUL, 5-year follow-up data demonstrated slight decreases in mean IPSS and QoL scores. Early side effects included dysuria, hematuria, pelvic pain/discomfort, urgency, bladder spasm, UTI, and urinary retention.

In a later randomized study comparing PUL to TURP, a lower proportion of individuals in the PUL group responded to treatment at 12 months follow-up compared to TURP, as measured by the IPSS reduction goal of ≥ 30% (73% versus 91%; $P = .05$).30. At 24 months follow-up, the mean difference between PUL and TURP was 6.1 points (CI: 2.2, 10.0) favoring TURP; however, changes in IPSS-QoL were similar between groups at all follow-up intervals. Additionally, Q_{MAX} was significantly lower in participants allocated to PUL at all follow-up intervals. Both these studies excluded patients with prostates ≥ 80 g or obstructive middle lobe.

TRANSURETHRAL ELECTROSURGICAL INCISION OF THE BLADDER NECK AND PROSTATE

For patients with smaller prostates (less than 30 g) this procedure involves simply incising through the bladder neck from a point distal to the ureteral orifices to the lateral edge of the verumontanum. The incision(s) can be performed with either electrocautery or holmium laser energy at the 5 or 7 o'clock position or on one side of the midline only. Ideal candidates are those with little lateral lobe hypertrophy, no median lobe hypertrophy, and a high posterior lip of the bladder neck. In suitable candidates, improvement in peak flow rates is approximately the same, global improvement rates slightly less (80%–95% versus 85%–100%), retrograde ejaculation much less but can vary based on the number of incisions (0%–37%), and bladder neck contracture much less (1%). Impotence has been rarely reported, and incontinence is seen in 0% to 1% of patients. This is certainly an underutilized procedure; based on historical statistics, nearly 80% of patients undergoing TURP in the United States have less than 30 g of tissue resected. A single RCT is available that compared TUIP to TURP in subjects whose prostate was less than 30 g. With 2 years of follow-up, both groups improved significantly in symptom score and peak flow rate, but no difference in outcome was noted between the two groups.

SURGICAL PROCEDURES

Surgery represents the most invasive option for the management of LUTS. It is typically performed in the operating room setting, requiring either general or regional anesthesia, and is associated with the greatest risks for morbidity and higher costs. Surgery is appropriate for moderate-to-severe LUTS, AUR, or other BPH-related complications and is generally reserved for those who have failed medical therapy. Surgical management has evolved from extirpative surgery toward less invasive, endoscopic procedures utilizing laser energy that represent efficacious alternatives with lower perioperative morbidity. This includes a generally shorter postoperative duration of catheterization and length of hospital stay.

TRANSURETHRAL RESECTION OF THE PROSTATE

This remains the gold standard of treatment for symptoms of BPH. This technique uses a resection loop and electrosurgical generator capable of delivering cutting and coagulating current. The lower-voltage, continuous-cutting waveform instantaneously vaporizes a path through the tissue and does not result in significant coagulation. The coagulation current consists of short segments of higher-voltage, lower-current energy, resulting in deeper penetrative heating and hemostasis. A literature reviews showed that **resection via electrocautery loop by a transurethral route has a 75% to 96% chance of improvement of symptoms, with the degree of improvement 4 on a scale of 4. Modern series reporting risks of TURP have shown significant improvement.** The Veterans Affairs Cooperative Study on TURP remains the most definitive study on the efficacy and safety of TURP. In this RCT comparing TURP with watchful waiting, improvements at the 3-year follow-up were noted for symptom score, Q_{MAX}, and multiple QoL measures in favor of TURP. Relative risk of treatment failure was 0.48 favoring TURP. The rate of urinary incontinence was 1% (which was similar to the watchful waiting group) and an overall decline in sexual function that was identical to the watchful waiting group. Hemorrhage requiring transfusion occurred in 1%. The incidence of bladder neck contracture and urethral stricture was 3.2%. Retrograde ejaculation is common and occurs in 50% to 95%. No mention was made of patients suffering from TUR syndrome, **a potentially devastating complication that is caused by intravascular absorption of irrigating fluids. Dilutional hyponatremia and fluid overload can occur leading to bradycardia, neuromuscular dysfunction, seizures, coma, and death. If suspected, immediate treatment with intravenous saline, IV mannitol, and loop diuretics should be instituted.** Additionally, patients can expect to stay in the hospital for 1 to 3 days postsurgery with an indwelling catheter during that time. Newer procedures are being refined to help decrease these risks and morbidity. Bipolar resection of the prostate utilizes a specialized resectoscope loop that incorporates both the active and return electrodes. This design limits the dispersal of current flow and allows for the use of 0.9% sodium chloride as the irrigation fluid. Meta-analysis of RCT that compared the two techniques noted overall poor trial quality, and while long-term efficacy evaluation of bipolar TURP was not possible, the occurrence of TUR syndrome and postoperative clot retention was significantly less than for monopolar TURP.

HOLMIUM LASER ENUCLEATION OF THE PROSTATE

The addition of high-powered holmium lasers (80–100 W) has enabled urologists to perform prostate resection. Holmium energy (wavelength 2120 nm) allows actual resection and debulking of adenoma in a similar fashion to standard TURP. Holmium energy has a minimal depth of penetration (0.4 mm) but divides tissue in a nearly bloodless fashion. **The HoLEP procedure utilizes a continuous flow resectoscope with an end-firing 550-micron fiber that enables enucleation of the prostate in a fashion similar to open suprapubic prostatectomy. The laser fiber is used to incise the prostate adenoma down to capsule, and then entire lobes of the prostate are enucleated and pushed into the bladder. Once the entire adenoma is resected, a tissue morcellator is used cystoscopically to remove the prostate piecemeal. Significant advantages include excellent hemostasis, results equivalent to standard TURP, no risk of TUR syndrome (saline irrigation), and a shortened hospital stay.** Patients who are fully anticoagulated can be treated using this approach. Generally, the results compare favorably to open prostatectomy in an experienced group; the 5-year follow-up results of a RCT comparing the two for patients with prostates greater than 100 g had similar findings with a mean AUASS of 3 and a mean Q_{MAX} of approximately 24 mL/sec. Late complications and reoperative rates were similar as well. At 7 years of follow-up comparing HoLEP versus TURP in those with a mean TRUS of approximately 70 mL, mean AUASS (8 versus 10.3) and Q_{MAX} (22 versus 17.8 mL/sec) were similar. While operative time for HoLEP was longer (62.1 versus 33.1 min, $P < .001$), the amount of resected tissue (40.4 versus 24.7 g, $P < .05$), duration of catheterization (17.7 versus 44.9 h, $P < .01$), and length of hospital stay (27.6 versus 49.9 h, $P < .001$) favored the HoLEP group. **Drawbacks are a significant learning curve and a need for a high-power laser and morcellation.**

HOLMIUM LASER RESECTION OF THE PROSTATE

The holmium laser resection of the prostate (HoLRP) procedure involves resection of the prostatic adenoma using a holmium laser fiber and a specially adapted resectoscope. Two-year follow-up in an RCT comparing HoLRP with TURP yielded no difference between the two groups in AUASS or Q_{MAX}. No recent studies have been published for HoLRP, suggesting it has been displaced by HoLEP. The AUA guideline groups these four aforementioned laser therapies together and grades them as an option and as appropriate and effective treatment alternatives to TURP and open prostatectomy in men with moderate-to-severe LUTS. The guideline says the choice of approach should be based on the patient's presentation anatomy, the surgeon's level of training and experience, and discussion of potential benefits and risks for complications.

AQUABLATION

Aquablation surgery utilizes a robotic handpiece with a waterjet, console, and conformal planning unit (CPU). Using a biplanar TRUS, mapping of the area of resection is planned out. A high-pressure jet of saline is then released at right angle to the handpiece. The CPU then adjusts the flow rate to alter the depth of penetration based on the mapped area of ablation. After hydroresection hemostasis is achieved with elecrocautery. The technique is not in the minimally invasive surgical treatment (MIST) category, as patients must undergo general anesthesia and the risk of bleeding remains significant. There is a lower risk of retrograde ejaculation compared to TURP. This may be due to decreased tissue removal at the verumontanum or possibly from protecting the bladder neck. In RCTs comparing aquablation to TURP with 6-month, 1-year, and 2-year outcomes, aquablation significantly improved IPSS, IPSS-quality of life (IPSS-QoL), maximum urinary flow rate (Q_{MAX}) and PVR from baseline to last follow-up in all prospective studies. At 2-year follow-up, aquablation showed non-inferior symptom relief compared to TURP, with a lower risk of anejaculation favoring aquablation and no significant differences regarding other complications including blood transfusion rates.

OPEN PROSTATECTOMY

This increasingly infrequently utilized option for BPH is clearly the most invasive but may still be the treatment of choice for prostates larger than 100 g. This operation, first described by Fuller in 1894, is performed through a lower midline incision and allows complete, intact removal either through the bladder or through the anterior capsule of the prostate. However, the morbidity of the procedure stemming from complications, including retrograde ejaculation, impotence, UTI, transfusion, stricture, incontinence, bladder neck contracture, ureteral obstruction, and persistent urine leak, makes this operation generally less attractive and thus less often performed. When compared with TURP, open prostatectomy is associated with lower retreatment rates and more complete removal of prostatic adenoma. Recent publications report the viability of laparoscopic and robotic-assisted transvesical prostatectomy. However, this experience is still limited to small case series, but it appears symptom improvement is comparable to the open approach while with significantly less total blood loss, duration of catheterization, and length of hospitalization but at the expense of longer operative time.

OTHER THERAPIES

Prostate Stents

A number of new temporary or permanent devices are currently being developed and tested in Europe and the United States. These are likely to get approved in the next few years as either temporary or permanent treatments for BPH. *iTind* is a temporarily implanted nitinol device deployed for 5 to 7days. It is deployed via a flexible cystoscopy without sedation or general anesthesia and works by remodeling the prostatic urethra. It has been approved by the FDA. Other devices that are in clinical trial include Butterfly, Prodeon and Zenflow.

Prostate Artery Embolization

Although this is a minimally invasive procedure, it requires a highly skilled interventional radiologist and can be a lengthy procedure. It also has a steep learning curve and very limited long-term data. Apart from some urologic complications the patient may get large amounts of radiation during the procedure. The AUA guidelines do not recommend prostate artery embolization (PAE) for the treatment of LUTS secondary to BPH, as it is not supported by current data and trial designs, and benefit over risk remains unclear. Therefore, PAE is not recommended outside the context of clinical trials.

CONCLUSION

It is clear that the age of significant morbidity for treatment for BPH has ended. A number of new techniques and technologies have been introduced into the nonmedical armamentarium of the urologist. The primary change has not only been to reduce the morbidity but to shift treatment to office-based procedures under local anesthesia or sedation only. In addition, there has been an increased involvement of the patients in decision-making with the great number of choices that are now available. Although long durability and low morbidity of the procedure have been the major goals of the urologists, patients often choose a procedure with less sexual effects and office based over durability. In addition all treatments are geared to improving patients' symptoms and QoL (IPSS), and emphasis on improving flow rates to above "normal" is considered less important. In the future, patients will likely be presented with a checklist of the advantages and disadvantages of each type of management. The number of surgical and mechanical therapies dictates, however, that no one practitioner will have expertise with all of these, but rather each will have their "favorites," based on sound reasoning and results.

Additional content, including Self-Assessment Questions and Suggested Readings, may be accessed at www.ExpertConsult.com.

Adult Genitourinary Cancer: Prostate and Bladder

Ruchika Talwar, MD, David J. Vaughn, MD, Alan J. Wein, MD, PhD (Hon), FACS, and Thomas J. Guzzo, MD, MPH

Prostate Cancer

GENERAL CONSIDERATIONS

Prostate cancer is the most common cancer in men and the second greatest cause of cancer mortality in men. One in nine men will be diagnosed with prostate cancer; however, only 1 in 41 will die from prostate cancer. Prostate-specific antigen (PSA) screening has led to a dramatic stage shift over the last few decades, with most men currently presenting with low-risk, organ-confined disease. PSA screening led to an increase in the detection of indolent prostate cancer as evidenced by the discrepancy between lifetime risk of prostate cancer diagnosis compared to that of prostate cancer mortality. Early detection likely improves outcomes in a subset of men; however, overtreatment of indolent cancer is now recognized as a potential drawback of screening. For those with localized disease, definitive therapy provides excellent oncologic outcomes. For those patients with intermediate or high-risk cancer for whom the risk of disease recurrence after local therapy is significant, combined modality therapy may be beneficial. The nature of biochemical recurrence after local treatment is being better defined, allowing for the stratification of these patients. Treatment of advanced disease has classically been provided through some form of androgen ablation and cytoreductive chemotherapy; however, recent advances in the treatment of locally advanced and metastatic prostate cancer have redefined our treatment paradigms in this patient population, and will likely continue to do so.

INCIDENCE

In 2019 there were an estimated 174,650 new cases of prostate cancer and approximately 31,620 cancer-related deaths in the United States. Experts anticipate that by 2030, there will be 1.7 million new cases and nearly 500,000 deaths worldwide. After the rapid increase in detected cases after the introduction of PSA testing, the number of incident cases has decreased to its present level. The death rate from prostate cancer has decreased by approximately 25% in the past decade, likely secondary to a combination of early detection, stage migration, adoption and effectiveness of curative therapy, as well as increased death rates from alternative causes.

PROSTATE-SPECIFIC ANTIGEN SCREENING

PSA screening has been in widespread use in the United States for two decades. While we have definitely noted a stage migration toward that of lower risk, clinically localized disease, the benefit of screening remains controversial. Recently the results of two large randomized PSA screening studies have been reported with conflicting results. The Prostate, Lung, Colorectal, and Ovarian (PLCO) screening trial randomized 76,693 men in the United States to receive annual prostate cancer screening versus usual care. **After 7 to 10 years of follow-up, there was no difference in prostate cancer mortality between the screened and unscreened groups.** However, the methodology of this study has been heavily criticized. Notably, there was a significant contamination rate in the control group, with up to 90% of men in the control arm undergoing at least one PSA test prior to randomization on subsequent analyses. Furthermore, the biopsy rate was only approximately 40% in men who were positively screened. The European Randomized Study of Screening for Prostate Cancer (ERSPC) randomized 162,387 men from 7 European countries to receive PSA screening versus no screening. **With a mean follow-up of 8.8 years, a 20% relative risk reduction from prostate cancer mortality was reported in the PSA-screened group.** The number needed to screen to prevent one prostate cancer death was 1410, and the number needed to treat was 48. However, these numbers have proven to be lower with greater follow-up, with a number needed to invite to screening of 570, and a number needed to diagnose of 18.

The negative findings in the PLCO study, the high number needed to treat in the original ERSPC analysis, and the potential morbidity associated with prostate biopsy and definitive treatment led the US Preventive Services Task Force (USPSTF) to recommend against population-based PSA screening for prostate cancer in 2012. Given the aforementioned flaws in the original trials, follow-up analyses, and advocacy of the urologic community, the USPSTF has since upgraded their recommendation to a Grade C. As of 2018, they recommend a shared decision-making approach to screening in men 55 to 69 years of age. In men above the age of 70, they maintained their recommendation against screening. The American Urological Association (AUA) has also recently updated their clinical guidelines on prostate cancer screening, making the following recommendations:

1. PSA screening in men under the age of 40 is not recommended.
2. Routine screening in men between the ages of 40 and 54 years at average risk is not recommended.
3. For men 55 to 69 years old, the decision to undergo PSA screening involves weighing the benefits of reducing the rate of metastatic prostate cancer and prevention of prostate cancer death against the known potential harms associated with screening and treatment. For this reason, shared decision-making is recommended for men aged 55 to 69 years who are considering PSA screening, and proceeding based on a man's values and preferences. The greatest benefit exists in the 55 to 69 year age group, and urinary biomarkers, imaging, and risk calculators are available to identify men at risk for more aggressive cancers.
4. To reduce the harms of screening, a routine screening interval of 2 years or more may be preferred over annual screening in those men who have participated in shared decision-making and decided on screening. As compared to annual screening, it is expected that screening intervals of 2 years preserve the majority of benefits and reduce overdiagnosis and false positives.
5. Routine PSA screening is not recommended in any man over age 70 or any man with less than a 10- to 15-year life expectancy.

EPIDEMIOLOGY

Prostate cancer is distributed in a very uneven manner with regard to race. **Black Americans have the highest mortality rate from**

this disease, which is also highly prevalent in the Caribbean and Africa. There is a significant contrast to native Asian men who have the lowest disease incidence and death rate from this condition. Although lower than in other ethnic groups, prostate cancer incidence and disease mortality demonstrate an upward trend in Asian countries. White men in the United States and Europe have an intermediate rate of disease expression, with the highest incidence rate and disease mortality found in northern Europeans.

1. Age: The autopsy incidence of prostate cancer can be significant by the fourth decade of life and is at least 30% in men older than the age of 50 years and more than 70% by the eighth decade of life. Clinical detection occurs at earlier ages because of increased awareness and more intense disease screening. More significant disease may be found in Black Americans at an earlier age.
2. Family history: **A twofold greater risk for developing prostate cancer exists in those individuals with a first-degree relative with prostate cancer.** This climbs to almost ninefold if three first-degree relatives are affected. Risk also exists if second-degree relatives have a diagnosis of prostate cancer. Alterations in specific genes or genetic loci may contribute to the development of disease. Hereditary prostate cancer is usually defined as multiple affected family members and a distribution along several generations. Approximately 5% to 10% of prostate cancer cases are attributable to high-risk inherited genetic factors.
3. **Geography**: Data suggest an inverse relationship between latitude and the incidence of prostate cancer. Northern populations have a greater level of disease, and it is hypothesized that it is related to the lower vitamin D levels secondary to less exposure to ultraviolet radiation. This may also be due to dietary changes or other factors. Native Black populations in Zaire have lower levels of prostate cancer compared to ethnic Zairians living in Belgium.

ETIOLOGY

1. The genetic factors responsible for prostate cancer are being actively investigated. At this time a few candidate prostate cancer genes have been identified, yet the majority of data suggest that subtle changes in several different genes involved in

such vital areas as steroid metabolism or detoxification may have an aggregate effect on prostate cancer disposition.

a. BRCA-2 familial mutations have been linked with more aggressive localized disease and faster progression to metastatic disease with poor outcomes. In addition, germline mutations in ATM, PALB2, and CHEK2 have also been associated with an increased risk of prostate cancer.
b. Mutations in the HOXB13 gene (17q21–22) have been shown to be significantly more common in men with familial forms of the disease. The lifetime risk of developing prostate cancer in carriers of this mutation ranges between 30% and 60%.
c. HPC1/RNASEL (1q24–25) and PG1/MSR1 (8p22–23) are potential prostate cancer-specific susceptibility genes, which functionally deal with inflammatory and infectious processes. Their exact roles in cancer etiology are under intense scrutiny. HP1C, which is an autosomal dominant gene, has been reported to have a fairly high penetrance in genetic carriers.
d. Chromosomal rearrangements similar to those seen in certain sarcomas have been identified in prostate tumors. Gene fusions resulting in androgen-driven oncogenic gene products suggest a new method of tumor pathogenesis. This is exemplified in the fusion/rearrangement of TMPRSS2 with ETS transcription factor genes. TMPRSS2-ETS fusion has been identified in up to 50% of PSA-detected tumors. The utility of TMPRSS2-ETS fusions as a prognostic marker is yet to be elucidated but is under investigation.
e. Androgen receptor CAG repeat length, alterations in SRD5A2 (5-alpha reductase-2), and cytochrome p450 genes associated with steroid metabolism (Cyp 3A4, Cyp 19A1, Cyp 17A1) have some relative impact on prostate cancer susceptibility alone or in concert.
f. Data suggest that the GSTM1-null phenotype may increase prostate cancer risk in smokers.

2. Androgens: In normal situations, these heavily influence the development of the prostate and have a role in the maintenance of normal function. Studies on androgen levels have been conflicting but have suggested higher testosterone levels or dihydrotestosterone/testosterone ratios in Black American

men. Exposure to androgens at certain developmental time periods is likely critical in prostate cancer carcinogenesis. Mutations or alterations in the androgen receptor (CAG repeats) may also be unequally distributed among individuals in populations, affecting response to testosterone. Meta-analyses suggest that shorter CAG repeats lead to higher risk of disease, with an OR of 1.21.

3. Diet: High intake of animal fat is associated with increased prostate cancer risk. Conversely the intake of soy products (isoflavonoids, phytoestrogens, Bowman-Birk inhibitor) may affect the development and progression of prostate cancer. Migration studies of Asians moving west demonstrate an increase in prostate cancer incidence compared to that of White populations in the same area. Studies in other tumor systems on vitamin E and selenium showed a one-third to two-third decrease in prostate cancer incidence, respectively. However, studies specifically designed to evaluate the effect of vitamin E and selenium in prostate cancer have not demonstrated a preventative association.
4. Insulin-like growth factor (IGF) system: These are peptides similar in structure to proinsulin that modulate proliferation, apoptosis, and tissue repair. IGF-1 and IGF-2 combine with one of six binding proteins (usually IGFBP3). Several studies have demonstrated that elevated serum levels of IGF-1 are associated with a higher risk of prostate cancer. The relative impact of the IGF axis on prostate cancer development or detection is currently unclear.
5. Inflammation: A growing body of investigation suggests that chronic inflammatory processes may play a role in the pathogenesis of prostate cancer. A pathway from normal tissue to proliferative inflammatory atrophy (PIA), to prostatic intraepithelial neoplasia (PIN), with resultant invasive prostate cancer has been proposed.

PATHOLOGY

The proposed pathway from inflammatory atrophy to invasive disease is a working hypothesis under investigation. Evidence for high-grade PIN as a precursor of invasive disease has grown stronger with further genetic and biochemical research. PIN is the proliferation of the acinar epithelium, and high-grade PIN is associated with the subsequent diagnosis of prostate cancer in approximately 20% of patients. Although the natural history of this condition is incompletely defined, patients should be counseled regarding the association between high-grade PIN and prostate cancer, and repeat prostate biopsy should be considered within 1 to 3 years after an initial diagnosis of multifocal (not focal) high-grade PIN.

1. Adenocarcinoma: The majority of prostate tumors are adenocarcinoma, which develops from the acinar glands. The majority of these arise from the peripheral zone of the prostate gland, yet up to 25% may originate in the central gland from the central and transitional zones.
2. Mucinous variant: If more than 25% of the representative tissue has mucin-containing glands, this designation may be given. It is purported to have an equal or worse outcome than classic adenocarcinoma.
3. Signet cell carcinoma: This is another adenovariant with rapid progression and poor prognosis.
4. Endometrioid or ductal carcinoma: A variant that usually presents at advanced stage with papillary-like growth; ductal carcinoma generally has a poor prognosis.
5. Small cell carcinoma: A neuroendocrine variant of prostate carcinoma, this often presents with normal PSA values. Although the general prognosis is poor, it may respond to platinum-based therapy.
6. Urothelial carcinoma: This may arise from the distal prostatic ducts. It usually manifests as an extension of primary bladder cancer. Stromal invasion carries a poorer prognosis than ductal infiltration.
7. Prostate sarcoma: This is a very rare tumor, generally designated as leiomyosarcoma. Recent data demonstrate c-kit positive staining in several cases suggesting potential therapy with Gleevec.
8. Hematologic malignancies: Leukemia and lymphoma variants are rare.
9. Metastases: Malignant melanoma, colorectal carcinoma, and pulmonary metastases have been documented.

GRADING AND STAGING SYSTEM

1. **The Gleason grading system, originally the gold standard grading system for prostate adenocarcinoma, has gone through**

several recent changes. When tumors were diagnosed as incidental findings after transurethral resection of prostate (TURP), lower grade designations were commonly assigned. However, needle biopsy specimens and surgical specimens are usually assigned a grade from 3 to 5. The two most common patterns are added together to provide a Gleason score with the grade of the most predominant tumor listed first. This provides stratification of score 7 lesions as 3 + 4 or 4 + 3, which can have some prognostic implications, but led to confusion among clinician and patients alike, especially in the context of active surveillance. Recently, the Gleason grade group system has become the endorsed scale by the International Society of Urologic Pathologists (ISUP) and World Health Organization (WHO).

Grade Group System	Gleason Grade System
Grade Group 1	Gleason 3 + 3
Grade Group 2	Gleason 3 + 4
Grade Group 3	Gleason 4 + 3
Grade Group 4	Gleason 8 (4 + 4, 3 + 5, or 5 + 3)
Grade Group 5	Gleason 9–10 (4 + 5, 5 + 4, 5 + 5)

2. Staging is generally designated by the TNM system (Tables 16.1 and 16.2). This provides a general description of tumor extent, yet may not fully represent the degree of tumor volume or the significance or insignificance of microscopic tumor extension beyond the prostatic capsule. Often the designation of organ confinement, extracapsular extension, and the degree of margin positivity, with some sense of the overall tumor volume, better describes lesions that are similar yet might be categorized more divergently.

SIGNS AND SYMPTOMS

Screen-detected prostate cancers are typically asymptomatic. In more advanced stages, they may be associated with urinary obstructive symptoms or hematuria. Bone pain is common in those patients with metastatic disease. A nodule on the prostate or induration of the gland is a hallmark sign on physical examination. It is not always specific for a carcinoma and can underestimate the extent of disease when it does represent a carcinoma.

TABLE 16.1 TNM Classification

TNM 2002	Histologic Description
Tis	Carcinoma in situ
Ta	Epithelial confined, usually papillary
T1	Invading lamina propria
T2a, b	Invasion of the muscularis propria: 2a: superficial invasion 2b: deep invasion
T3a, b	Perivesical fat invasion: 3a: microscopically 3b: macroscopically
T4a, b	Invasion of contiguous organs: 4a: prostate, vagina, uterus 4b: pelvic sidewall, abdominal wall
NO	No lymph node involvement
N1	Single ≤ 2 cm
N2	Single > 2 cm, ≤ 5 cm Multiple ≤ 5 cm
N3	Single or multiple > 5 cm
M0	No distant metastases
M1	Distant metastases

TABLE 16.2 TNM Definitions

TNM 2002	Definitions
T1	Tumor an incidental histologic finding
T1a	< Gleason score 7 < 5% of tissue resected Tumor an incidental histologic finding
T1b	> Gleason score 7 > 5% of tissue resected
T1c	Tumor identified by needle biopsy (e.g., for elevated serum PSA)
T2	Tumor confined within the prostate
T2a	Tumor involves one lobe or less
T2b	Tumor involves more than one lobe
T3	Tumor extends through and beyond the prostate capsule
T3a	Unilateral extracapsular extension
T3b	Bilateral extracapsular extension
T3c	Tumor invades seminal vesicle(s)
T4	Tumor is fixed or invades adjacent structures other than seminal vesicles

PSA, Prostate-specific antigen.

NATURAL HISTORY

1. Until recently the natural history of prostate cancer, especially for earlier stage disease, has been difficult to discern. Several longitudinal studies and clinical trials have provided greater information in that regard. Information regarding high-grade PIN continues to accrue and suggests that there is a progression rate from this entity to clinical cancer in a reasonable number of patients.
2. The data from the Connecticut tumor registry provide reasonable information for natural history and depict significantly worse outcomes in those individuals with higher Gleason scores.
3. Follow-up from Scandinavian, non-PSA screen-detected patient cohorts have reported a 33% rate of metastatic progression and a 21% rate of prostate cancer mortality at 15 years for patients undergoing watchful waiting. An updated analysis at 23 years suggested a 43.3% rate of metastatic progression and a 31.3% rate of prostate cancer mortality in the WW group.
4. In patients with classic metastatic bone disease, the median survival is 27 to 33 months. Mortality is 75% at 5 years and 90% at 10 years. Recent data suggest that androgen-independent prostate cancer in the presence of metastatic disease has a median survival of 16 months.

DIAGNOSIS AND STAGING/PROSTATE-SPECIFIC ANTIGEN SCREENING

1. Digital rectal examination (DRE): This is a classic component of the physical examination that, by itself, is not sensitive or specific for prostate cancer. A palpable nodule can have an approximately 50% chance of being a carcinoma. Conversely, a normal DRE does not exclude the possibility of prostate cancer.
2. Transrectal ultrasound (TRUS): Multiple studies have demonstrated that TRUS is sensitive yet not specific for the detection of prostate cancer. The classic finding is a hypoechoic lesion that in general has a 30% chance of being positive for carcinoma. Prostate cancer can also present as an isoechoic or hyperechoic lesion. The most important use of TRUS is in aiding transrectal guided needle biopsies of the prostate gland.
3. Serum markers: The classic marker for prostate cancer was acid phosphatase. The enzymatic test was elevated in 70% of

patients with extracapsular and metastatic prostate cancer. The more sensitive radioimmunoassay of this enzyme is not as useful for detecting extracapsular disease and has no value as a screening test for prostate cancer. PSA is the most useful marker in the detection and monitoring of prostate cancer and is discussed in detail separately.

4. Prostate needle biopsy: Prostate biopsy is most commonly performed via a transrectal ultrasound-guided approach, although MRI-guided prostate biopsies are being increasingly adopted (discussed later). The sampling of a minimum of 12 cores of tissue is considered the standard of care. The procedure is generally well tolerated; however, biopsy-associated complications include hematuria, hematospermia, hematochezia, urinary retention, and, rarely, sepsis. **Postbiopsy sepsis is becoming more common with the emergence of fluoroquinolone-resistant bacteria.** The percentage of positive cores, line length, or line percentage of cancer per core can provide further predictive information with regard to staging and outcomes.
5. Bone scan: Before a lesion can be seen on a conventional radiograph, it must have replaced bone mass by 30% to 50% and be 10 to 15 mm in diameter. Plain film correlates of suspicious areas are often obtained. In some cases dedicated magnetic resonance imaging (MRI) or computed tomography (CT) imaging can resolve equivocal cases. Patients with a PSA value less than 10 ng/mL rarely demonstrate metastases.
6. CT and MRI: CT scans of the pelvis may be used for assessing metastatic disease in higher risk prostate cancer. Endorectal MRI was shown to provide additional staging information in those patients with intermediate PSAs and greater than 50% positive needle-core biopsies. However, significant advancements in MRI technique, specifically with 3 Tesla magnets, have obviated the need for endorectal coil use. Dynamic contrast enhancement and diffusion-weighted imaging have improved the detection of suspicious areas in the gland. The development of Prostate Imaging Reporting and Data System (PI-RADS) has standardized the reporting of such lesions, with scores ranging from 1 (least suspicious) to 5 (most suspicious).
   a. Given the utility of MRI in the detection of prostate cancer, imaging guided biopsies have been integrated into clinical practice. The use of fusion technology allows real-time

ultrasound guidance, superimposing the MRI image, so that a three-dimensional reconstruction can be formed and the suspicious lesion can be effectively targeted. In addition, an experienced operator can also perform targeting of the lesion without any specialized equipment, using a technique termed cognitive fusion.

b. The advantage of MRI-guided prostate biopsy lies not just within the increased detection of prostate cancer overall. Specifically, effective MRI use results in increased detection of clinically significant disease and avoidance of clinically insignificant diagnoses. The PROMIS trial from the United Kingdom, published in 2017, found that MRI-guided biopsies had a higher sensitivity than TRUS biopsies, 93% vs 48% and negative predictive value, 89% vs 74%. The multicenter European and North American PRECISION trial demonstrated a higher rate of clinically significant cancer detection, and lower insignificant cancer detection with the use of MRI versus TRUS biopsy.

7. Prostate-specific antigen
   a. Biochemical characteristics: PSA is a 240 amino acid single-chain glycoprotein that has a molecular weight of 34 kD. It is coded on chromosome 19 (6 Kb: 4 introns, 5 exons) and is homologous to members of the kallikrein gene superfamily and is designated human kallikrein 3 (hK3). It is a serine protease.
   b. Physiology: PSA liquefies the seminal coagulum that is formed after ejaculation. A substrate produced in the seminal vesicles has been identified. PSA has activity like chymotrypsin and trypsin. The half-life of PSA is 2.2 to 3.2 days.
   c. Marker properties: There is no PSA level that indicates zero risk of having prostate cancer. Initially a PSA value of 4.0 ng/mL was used as a cutoff point for biopsy. A value above 2.6 ng/mL in younger men has also been used as a trigger for biopsy. Serum values are not generally altered by DRE but can be affected by recumbency, urologic instrumentation, ejaculation, and prostate biopsy. Nonmalignant conditions that affect PSA levels include prostatitis, prostate infarction, and benign prostatic hypertrophy (BPH).
   d. General clinical use: The principle use of PSA is in disease detection. The most specific use for PSA is the monitoring

of patients after radical prostatectomy. Postoperative baseline values should be in the undetectable range. Residual disease is suggested by any detectable postoperative levels, and values greater than 0.2 ng/mL suggest biochemical failure of therapy. It is also used to monitor the response to radiation therapy.

8. Biomarkers: The lack of disease specificity associated with serum PSA testing has led to investigation of more specific markers for prostate cancer.
   a. Blood-based biomarkers: Since PSA released from malignant cells has been shown to have higher rates of coupling with serum proteases, the proportion of free and bound PSA has been used as a screening biomarker. In a multi-institutional, prospective study, a free PSA cutoff of 25% in PSA values ranging from 4 to 10 ng/mL identified 95% of malignancies while avoiding 20% of unnecessary biopsies. Human kallikrein peptidase (hK2) has also been used as a prostate cancer blood-based marker. Its function is to activate PSA through protein cleavage. Due to its similar amino acid structure, it shares a similar affinity for prostatic tissue, and has increased expression in malignant tissue. Combining free/total PSA and a multi-kallikrein panel, the 4K score, has shown to have an increased cancer detection rate.
   b. Circulating tumor cells/DNA: Antibody staining for cluster differentiation proteins and cytokeratins has been shown to be a poor prognostic indicator in prostate cancer. Detection of androgen-reception splice variants correlate with resistance to systemic therapy in metastatic prostate cancer, and may have treatment implications.
   c. Urine-based biomarkers: PCA3, a prostate-specific microRNA detectable in the urine after a DRE, had a higher specificity for malignancy than PSA. A challenge in its interpretability, however, is that it is reported as a continuous score. Therefore, it is most useful as a two-threshold test, with emphasis placed on its negative predictive value in scores < 20 and its positive predictive value in scores > 60.

CANCER PREVENTION

1. General considerations: Because prostate cancer is relatively common, chemoprevention strategies for this disease are

reasonable. However, because such therapies are delivered to large groups of cancer-free subjects, toxicity must be extremely low or nonexistent. Estimates for the number of patients requiring treatment to prevent one case of cancer demonstrate the broad range of such therapies. Given the incidence of prostate cancer in the United States, 500 men would have to be treated with an agent that could reduce cancer of the prostate by 50% to avoid one cancer. Chemoprevention strategies may therefore require additional considerations such as a focus toward higher risk populations.

2. 5-Alpha-reductase inhibition: A major phase III chemoprevention trial, the Prostate Cancer Prevention Trial (PCPT), demonstrated a 24.8% reduction in period prevalence of prostate cancer in patients using 5 mg of finasteride (type II) daily compared to placebo. However, the prevalence of higher grade prostate cancer was 25% higher (6.4% versus 5.1%), dampening this overall positive result. The reasons for this increase in higher grade disease remain to be fully explained but have hindered widespread adoption of 5-alpha-reductase inhibition as chemoprevention. The REDUCE trial using dutasteride, a type I and type II 5-alpha-reductase, also demonstrated a reduction in prostate cancer detection (23% compared to placebo).
3. Toremifene: This agent is a synthetic estrogen receptor modulator (SERM) that in phase IIb/III trials demonstrated the ability to reduce the progression of those patients with high-grade PIN to prostate cancer by 22%. A more recent phase III trial including men with a history of high-grade PIN did show a 10.2% relative risk reduction for prostate cancer compared to placebo; however, it was not statistically significant.
4. Selenium and vitamin E: In large phase III chemoprevention trials targeting other primary tumors, a secondary end-point analysis demonstrated that selenium reduced the incidence of prostate cancer by 63% in a study targeting skin cancer, and vitamin E reduced prostate cancer by 32% in a lung cancer study. This provided the basis of the SELECT trial. This trial was discontinued early, as it clearly demonstrated no risk reduction with either selenium or vitamin E supplementation.
5. Lycopene: This agent is a water-soluble antioxidant. There are several lines of evidence but no conclusive proof that it may have an impact on prostate cancer chemoprevention.

6. Antiinflammatory agents: General nonsteroidal antiinflammatory drugs (NSAIDs) and cyclooxygenase (COX)-2 inhibitors demonstrate antiprostate cancer activity in the laboratory but are not under current consideration for study as chemopreventive agents because of their additional side effects.
7. Soy and other isoflavones: The components of soy may have anticancer properties, and epidemiologic studies support the potential for risk reduction by the inclusion of these substances in the diet.

OUTCOME PROGNOSIS AND STRATIFICATION

Several statistical approaches to the stratification of patients with regard to outcomes based on clinical data have been developed. Approaches using multiple regression analysis, nomograms (Fig. 16.1), and neural networks have been employed for several different scenarios for prostate cancer. Hybrids of these methods have also been tested. In general the correlation of these models to individual outcomes is in the 0.7 to 0.75 range. Nomogram strategies may provide more individualized information. All of these methods may be useful in better directing patient choices and the use of additional therapies in the future.

TREATMENT OF LOCALIZED DISEASE

1. General considerations: In discussing treatment for prostate cancer it is important to consider patient factors such as age and general performance status as well as tumor factors such as Gleason score, initial serum PSA, and estimated clinical volumes and stage of the tumor. If a patient has less than a 50% chance for surviving 10 years due to other comorbidities, it is difficult to measure the positive effect of treatment. Patient tolerance for the side effects of different therapies also has to be considered. It is best when patients come to a treatment decision based on consultation and input from both surgical and radiation oncology services. The stage shift in tumors due to PSA detection strategies has resulted in 5-year disease-free survival for active therapies of nearly 100%.
2. Watchful waiting: This approach has generally been reserved for men with significant comorbidities that limit their overall survival and those unwilling to consider other forms of treatment. With 15-year follow-up, the SPCG-4 trial of surgery

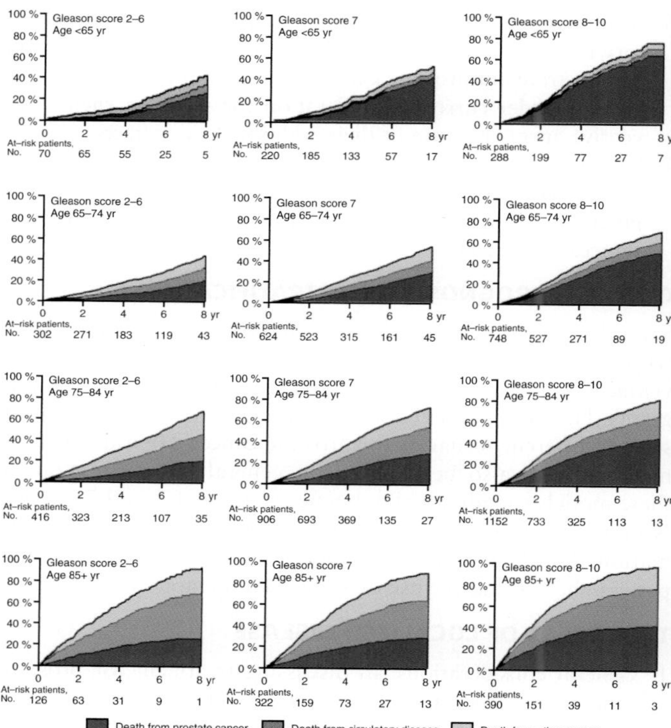

FIGURE 16.1 Cumulative mortality from prostate cancer and other causes after diagnosis of locally advanced prostate cancer, stratified by age and Gleason score. (From Akre O, Garmo H, Adolfsson J, et al. Mortality among men with locally advanced prostate cancer managed with noncurative intent: a nationwide study in PCBaSe Sweden. *Eur Urol*. 2011;60:554-563.)

versus watchful waiting demonstrated improved outcomes for those undergoing radical prostatectomy including metastasis rate (11.7% risk reduction), disease-specific survival (6.1% reduction), and overall survival at 10 years (6.6% reduction). These findings were more pronounced in patients younger than the age of 65 years. With 23-year follow-up, these results were further corroborated with even wider improvements in outcomes.

3. Active surveillance: With the significant stage shift in prostate cancer, the prevalence of low-grade, low-volume cancer has increased significantly. It has been postulated that the majority of very low-risk prostate cancers pose little threat to an individual's mortality. In light of this, active surveillance has become an increasingly popular option for men with low-risk disease in an attempt to minimize the morbidity of treatment in those who are unlikely to die from prostate cancer. Active surveillance differs from that of watchful waiting in that there is strict surveillance by periodic DRE and PSA and repeat prostate biopsy, with the intent for curative intervention with progression to more aggressive disease characteristics. While active surveillance criteria vary from center to center, generally men considered appropriate candidates have: Grade Group 1 and low-volume Grade Group 2 disease; less than or equal to two positive biopsy cores; less than or equal to 50% of any core involved with cancer; a PSA of less than or equal to 10; and a PSA density of less than or equal to 0.15. Classic triggers for intervention are volume or grade progression on subsequent biopsy. PSA doubling time has also been used by some as an indication for intervention. Approximately 30% of men in the Johns Hopkins active surveillance cohort ultimately underwent therapeutic intervention (roughly three-quarters based on biopsy reclassification). With intermediate term follow-up, active surveillance has been reported to be a safe option for highly selected men with low-risk and/or low-volume disease.
4. Radical prostatectomy: This is an appropriate treatment choice for younger patients and for older patients who are very fit and desire this form of treatment. Generally, a chronologic age of 70 is used as a relative cutoff point, but decisions need to be individualized with respect to health status and anticipated life span. Surgical mortality is less than 0.2%, but 1% to 2% of patients may experience a pulmonary embolus or deep vein thrombosis. Surgical approaches include retropubic, perineal, robotic, and laparoscopic. With the widespread integration of robotic surgical platforms into both academic and community health systems across the country, the robotic approach has become the most widely utilized in the United States. Urinary incontinence may occur in up to 10% of patients. The potential for erectile dysfunction (ED) can be

decreased with surgical approaches that spare the cavernosal nerves; however, age and preoperative erectile function are also significant predictors of ED following surgery. A bladder neck contracture can occur in 2% to 3% of patients. Disease-specific survival is in the 95% range over 10 years.

5. Radiation therapy
   a. External beam radiation therapy (EBRT): This is an option for localized prostate cancer and is the treatment of choice for T3 disease and patients unfit for surgery. Significant technical advances, such as conformal radiation and intensity modulated radiation therapy (IMRT), have allowed for the increase in dose intensity yet a decrease in overall side effects. In general, it is administered in divided doses ranging from 70 to 80 Gy and is well tolerated. Approximately 3% to 5% of patients will experience persistent rectal or bladder symptomatology; greater than 60% of patients will develop ED within 2 years. Hematuria or hemorrhagic cystitis is a late development in a small percentage of patients.
   b. Interstitial brachytherapy: Ultrasound-guided transperineal brachytherapy has become an accepted modality for the treatment of localized prostate cancer. It is difficult to treat large prostate glands (greater than 50 cm^3) with this technique. Intermediate term results (10 years) suggest similar outcomes to surgery or EBRT in selected patients. The usual radiation sources are ^{125}I and ^{103}Pd. The principle urologic side effect is voiding dysfunction, which is usually short term but may be persistent. Those individuals with high International Prostate Symptom Score (IPSS) scores should not be considered for this technique.
6. Cryosurgical ablation of the prostate: This technique has undergone multiple modifications and is currently performed with small-caliber needles using freeze-thaw cycles employing argon and helium gas. More recent series show less morbidity and a decrease in chronic pelvic pain noted in early reports. While cryotherapy is of controversial utility in the primary setting, it has shown value in salvage cases for local recurrence after radiation therapy.
7. High-intensity focused ultrasound (HIFU): HIFU is currently under investigation for treatment of focal and localized disease. Early data demonstrate feasibility, yet data on intermediate- and

long-term outcomes and side effects are pending. HIFU is not currently Food and Drug Administration (FDA) approved in the United States for primary treatment.

8. Post treatment follow-up: Serum PSA is the single most important follow-up parameter in evaluating post treatment patients with either surgery or radiation.
   a. In surgery patients, the serum PSA should drop to an undetectable level. Occasionally very low persistent PSA findings that do not progress are noted. In most cases, if the serum PSA becomes detectable and rises above 0.2 ng/mL, the patient continues to show disease progression. Biochemical failure can predate clinical failure by 6 to 8 years. Newer data suggest that biochemical failure is a surrogate marker for ultimate clinical failure and survival. However, not all patients with biochemical failure will ultimately die of prostate cancer. Outcomes are heterogenic. Patients with high-grade disease who fail early and display a short doubling time may have a survival as short as 7 years, whereas patients who are late failures with lower moderate-grade disease who are progressing slowly may live as long as 19 years. Further follow-up is necessary to clearly define the true impact of biochemical failure.
   b. In general, response to radiation therapy is predicated on the pretreatment PSA and can be predicted by the post-treatment PSA. The closer to an undetectable value post treatment the better the overall outcome.
   c. There is a role for radiation therapy after postsurgical biochemical failures. Success is best when therapy is instituted before the PSA is greater than 1.0 ng/mL, and studies have also demonstrated improved therapeutic responses at even lower PSAs. Percentage for cure ranges between 30% and 50% in different series. Salvage surgery can be employed in radiation therapy failures.

TREATMENT OF BIOCHEMICAL AND CLINICAL FAILURE

1. In general, 25% of patients will experience a PSA recurrence in 10 years after local therapy. The exact definition of recurrence and the clinical significance of these outcomes have become somewhat clearer in the past several years. The yearly incidence of such patients in the United States is 50,000.

2. PSA failure in surgery: This definition ranges from any detectable PSA to 0.4 ng/mL. Low, stable detection of PSA may occur in postoperative patients and is often attributed to persistent benign tissue. Once the PSA value rises above 0.2 ng/mL, it rarely recedes. This value is therefore considered an absolute threshold for biochemical failure.
3. PSA failure in radiation patients: A strong definition for these patients has been more difficult to define due to the persistence of PSA detection after therapy and the kinetics involved in defining true progression from variations about a mean value. Nadir value plus two consecutive rises is the current operational definition, yet other definitions may be employed in the future.
4. Significance of biochemical failure: A rough guide to PSA failure in surgery patients suggests that there are approximately 8 years from biochemical failure to clinical failure, and 5 years from that point to cancer-related death. This could be stratified by time to failure from surgery, initial PSA and Gleason score of the tumor, and PSA doubling time. The range of values was from 7 to 19 years. Recent analysis places significant import on PSA doubling times, with a doubling time of 3 months as a surrogate marker for cancer-related death. This was noted in approximately 12% of surgery patients and 20% of radiation patients. A more recent analysis based on the stratification of time to failure (greater or less than 3 years), less or greater than Gleason score 8 cancer, and a PSA doubling time ranging from 3 to 15 months could separate out patients with a 2% to 99% chance of experiencing a prostate cancer-related death.
5. Treatment for biochemical failure
   a. Watchful waiting for late recurrence, slow velocity, long doubling-time tumors
   b. Salvage radiation therapy for surgery patients
   c. Androgen blockade for radiation patients with persistently rising PSA.

TREATMENT OF ADVANCED DISEASE

The gold standard for the initial treatment of metastatic prostate cancer is androgen ablation therapy. This can be accomplished with gonadotropin-releasing hormone (GnRH) agonists, bilateral orchiectomy, and more recently GnRH antagonists.

Diethylstilbestrol (DES) is no longer used because of increased cardiovascular risk associated with this agent. Toxicities of androgen ablation therapy include hot flashes, loss of libido, impotency, muscular atrophy, osteopenia, and osteoporosis. **Recently, first- and second-generation antiandrogens, inhibitors of androgen synthesis, and systemic chemotherapy have been demonstrated to improve outcomes in metastatic hormone-sensitive prostate cancer (mHSPC), shifting treatment paradigms considerably.**

1. Antiandrogens block the intracytoplasmic androgen receptor (AR). Nonsteroidal antiandrogens are traditionally utilized. First-generation agents such as flutamide, nilutamide, and bicalutamide are used for combination androgen blockage with luteinizing hormone-releasing hormone (LHRH) agonists, as they block the testosterone surge that is associated with such agents. Second-generation agents also block the AR, but additionally inhibit DNA binding and androgen-mediated gene transcription. These agents include enzalutamide and apalutamide. **Enzalutamide has been approved across the spectrum hormone-sensitive prostate cancer, both M0 and M1 states.** The PROSPER trial demonstrated an improvement in metastasis-free survival in men with non-metastatic hormone-resistent prostate cancer (nmHRPC). As such, apalutamide has recently been approved in M0 hormone-resistant disease.
2. Inhibitors of androgen synthesis inhibit enzymes along the cytochrome P450 steroid synthesis pathway. Ketoconazole, a nonselective P450-dependent pathway inhibitor, effectively decreases testosterone levels with continuous usage. However, after about 5 months of treatment, testosterone levels generally start to rise. Abiraterone, a more selective cytochrome P17 inhibitor, exerts its effect on 17 α-hydroxylase and C17,20-lyase, targeting cortisol and androgen production. **A landmark trial, LATITUDE, established the efficacy of abiraterone plus prednisone in men with newly diagnosed high-risk metastatic hormone-sensitive prostate cancer (MHSPC).** The agent was superior to androgen deprivation therapy (ADT) alone, extending median progression-free survival by approximately 18 months. The STAMPEDE trial also corroborated these results, leading to the inclusion of abiraterone into the guidelines for first-line therapy in this disease state.
3. Docetaxel, a taxane-based chemotherapeutic agent, was first approved for metastatic, hormone-resistant disease, which

will be discussed below. The CHAARTED randomized trial was the first to establish docetaxel's role in upfront therapy for MHSPC. In men randomized to docetaxel plus ADT versus ADT alone, the combination arm experienced a 10-month overall survival benefit. This survival advantage was most pronounced in the subset of men with high-volume disease. **The STAMPEDE trial again corroborated these results, with a 1.8-year survival benefit demonstrated, in comparison to a 1.1-year survival benefit in CHAARTED. This led to the inclusion of docetaxel as an upfront treatment for high-volume metastatic hormone-sensitive prostate cancer.**

In summary, according to the National Comprehensive Cancer Network (NCCN) guidelines, systemic options for metastatic hormone-sensitive prostate cancer include the following:

1. **LHRH agonist alone ± docetaxel**
2. **LHRH agonist plus first-generation anti-androgen ± docetaxel**
3. **LHRH antagonist ± docetaxel**
4. **LHRH agonist plus abiraterone**
5. **LHRH antagonist plus abiraterone**

Metastatic disease that progresses despite castration has been classically labeled as *hormone-refractory disease* (also called *androgen-independent* or *castrate metastatic*). As referenced earlier, in the last decade, cytotoxic chemotherapy in the form of docetaxel has been the standard of care in this setting. **The use of docetaxel in the metastatic, hormone-refractory setting is based on randomized trials demonstrating a modest (3-month) survival benefit.** Second- and third-generation chemotherapeutic agents, including cabazitaxel and satraplatin, have also been recently approved. For patients with or without visceral metastases, both abiraterone and enzalutamide can also be considered.

Immunotherapy has also emerged as a treatment option for advanced prostate cancer. Sipuleucel-T is the first cancer vaccine to gain FDA approval for metastatic, hormone-refractory prostate cancer. Phase III studies have demonstrated an approximately 4-month survival benefit in this therapy. Furthermore, in patients with microsatellite instability positive cancers, pembrolizumab may be utilized after a patient has progressed through another line of systemic therapy. While challenges remain on the immunotherapeutic front, including cost and a cumbersome delivery method, targeting prostate cancer with immunotherapy may hold promise in the advanced setting.

HRPC patients with bone metastases are at increased risk of skeletal complications including pathologic fracture and bone pain. A randomized trial demonstrated that administration of the bisphosphonate zoledronic acid decreases the risk of skeletal complications in men with progressive HRPC and bone metastases compared to placebo. More recently, the monoclonal antibody denosumab has been reported to reduce skeletal-related events in men on androgen-deprivation therapy. Advantages of denosumab, compared to bisphosphonates, are that it is administered subcutaneous and can also be given to patients with renal insufficiency. Important morbidity associated with bisphosphonate and denosumab therapy is osteonecrosis of the jaw (Table 16.3).

TABLE 16.3 The 2013 American Urological Association guidelines for PSA screening

The 2013 American Urological Association guidelines for PSA screening include:

1. PSA screening in men under the age of 40 is not recommended.
2. Routine screening in men between ages 40 and 54 years at average risk is not recommended.
3. For men 55–69 years old, the decision to undergo PSA screening involves weighing the benefits of preventing prostate cancer mortality in 1 man for every 1000 and screened over a decade against the known potential harms associated with screening and treatment. For this reason, shared decision-making is recommended for men 55–69 years old who are considering PSA screening, and proceeding based on the patient's values and preferences.
4. To reduce the harms of screening, a routine screening interval of 2 years or more may be preferred over annual screening in those men who have participated in shared decision-making and decided on screening. As compared to annual screening, it is expected that screening intervals of 2 years preserve the majority of benefits and reduce overdiagnosis and false positives.
5. Routine PSA screening is not recommended in men over age 70 or any man with less than a 10–15-year life expectancy.
    - Postbiopsy sepsis is becoming more common with the emergence of fluoroquinolone-resistant bacteria.
    - Generally, men considered appropriate candidates have Gleason score $\leq$ 6 disease, $\leq$ 2 positive biopsy cores, $\leq$ 50% of any core involved with cancer, a PSA of $\leq$ 10, and a PSA density of $\leq$ 0.15.

Carcinoma of the Bladder

GENERAL CONSIDERATIONS

Bladder cancer is the second most common urologic malignancy. The majority of cases are urothelial carcinoma, and 65% to 75% of new cases are Ta (mucosal only), T1 (lamina propria invasion), or carcinoma in situ (CIS) (flat, noninvasive). These lesions were previously grouped as "superficial" tumors, but their distinct biology warrants the stratification of these lesions. The remainder is muscle-invasive tumors. Transurethral resection (TUR) of these lesions is the principal form of diagnosis and therapy for bladder cancer. Nonmuscle invasive lesions are often further treated with intravesical therapy to reduce the risk of disease recurrence and progression. A single perioperative intravesical treatment with mitomycin C reduces the risk of tumor recurrence. Recurrent Ta, initial T1, and CIS lesions may be treated with bacille Calmette-Guérin (BCG) intravesical immunotherapy, which can decrease tumor recurrence and reduce tumor progression. Muscle-invasive disease and treatment-resistant T1 and CIS lesions are best treated with radical cystectomy and some form of urinary diversion. Combined chemotherapy and radiation approaches are useful in select patients and those who cannot tolerate surgery. Advanced disease responds to platinum and paclitaxel-based chemotherapy regimens, but sustained complete responses are rare.

EPIDEMIOLOGY

In 2018, the United States had 81,190 new cases of bladder cancer yearly with approximately 17,240 cancer deaths. Bladder cancer is the 10th most frequent cancer worldwide with a yearly incidence of 549,393 new cases.

Three percent of men will develop bladder cancer over their lifetime, and just under 1% will die from their disease. In women, these rates are estimated to be 1.1% and less than 0.5%, respectively. Although more common in men, women have been shown to present with more advanced disease. They also have worse outcomes, stage for stage, than their male counterparts. Racial and ethnic disparities are also evident; although bladder cancer is most common in White Americans (1.5× that of Black Americans; 2× that of Hispanic Americans), Black patients are more likely to present with invasive disease.

ETIOLOGY

1. Tobacco exposure: **Tobacco use confers a two- to threefold increased risk of developing bladder cancer.** The polycyclic aromatic hydrocarbon, 4-aminobiphenyl, has been suggested as the most significant carcinogen in tobacco. Latency is approximately 20 years, and risk reduction occurs with smoking cessation.
2. Industrial exposure: The first link of industrial exposure and cancer was made between bladder cancer and aniline dyes. Textile printing and rubber manufacturing have also been established with this tumor. Major carcinogens found in such environments are 2-naphthylamine, 4-aminobiphenyl, and 4-nitrobiphenyl.
3. Age: The median age at diagnosis is 70 years. Bladder cancer is rare in persons younger than 40 years of age and tends to be less aggressive in younger age groups.
4. Chemotherapy: Cyclophosphamide and ifosfamide have been associated with the development of bladder cancer. The presence or absence of hemorrhagic cystitis is not associated with the likelihood of developing cancer. The use of reducing agents (mesna), hydration, and catheter drainage during therapy have probably decreased the development of cancer with these agents.
5. *Schistosoma haematobium:* Infection is common in many areas of North Africa, and the deposition of ova in the bladder leads to inflammation and the development of carcinoma. Inflammation in the presence of nitrites from bacterial activity is also implicated. Additionally, heavy tobacco use and exposure to nitrate-containing fertilizers are endemic in these areas. The majority of these tumors are squamous carcinoma.
6. Chronic irritation and infection: Chronic infection carries a slightly increased risk of developing bladder cancer, and those patients with a chronic indwelling Foley catheter have a 10- to 20-fold increase in developing bladder cancer (primarily squamous). Premalignant changes can be noted after a few years, and yearly cystoscopic evaluations are recommended.
7. Genetic predisposition: Differences in metabolism of toxins rather than germline mutations play a role. N acetyltransferase 2 (slow acetylators), glutathione S-transferase M1 homozygous deletions, and CYP2A1 expression all add to risk.

8. Pelvic irradiation: This is associated with an approximate 10% increased risk of developing bladder cancer. Newer methods of conformal radiation may lessen the risk to nontarget organs.
9. Additional risks: Arsenic in the water supply, the ingestion of the Chinese herb *Aristolochia fangchi*, and ingestion of ochratoxin A (in bracken fern) may also contribute to the development of bladder tumors. Ingestion of phenacetin is associated with the development of upper urinary tract transitional cell carcinoma (TCC).

PATHOLOGY

1. Normal urothelium demonstrates basal, intermediate, and superficial cells. There are usually seven cell layers.
2. Hyperplasia is generally described as thickened mucosa without cellular atypia.
3. Urothelial dysplasia: Preneoplastic changes in the basal and intermediate layers with the presence of cell cohesion, yet some architectural disruption; progresses to frank neoplasia in 15% to 20% of cases.
4. Carcinoma in situ (CIS): This is a cytologically malignant flat lesion with prominent disorganization of cells, loss of cell cohesion, loss of cellular polarity, and coarse chromatin. Pagetoid, small cell, and large cell variants have been described. CIS is a noninvasive lesion, but if it is left untreated, 20% to 83% of patients will progress to invasive carcinoma.
5. Urothelial papilloma: This is a benign exophytic neoplasia with normal-appearing urothelium on a fibrovascular core. It usually appears as solitary lesions. An inverted papilloma growth variant also exists.
6. Papillary urothelial neoplasm of low malignant potential (PUNLMP): This is similar to papilloma but with increased cellularity; it is associated with an occasional propensity for recurrence progression and rare mortality.
7. Papillary urothelial neoplasm low grade: Papillary morphology with variable architecture and mitoses at all levels; altered CK20 expression FGFR3 mutations in 80% of cases.
8. Papillary urothelial neoplasm high grade: Marked architectural disorder with papillary fusion and variable cell number thickness; demonstrates significantly more molecular alterations.

9. Stromal invasion (T1): Tumor invades the lamina propria but not the muscularis propria. Attempts at subdivision have been made with regard to depth of lesion, vascular invasion, and muscularis mucosa involvement.
10. Invasive urothelial carcinoma: Tumor invasion into true muscularis propria; almost exclusively high grade; tumor front may be "pushing" or tentacular.
11. Squamous carcinoma: This uncommon cancer (3%–7%) is distinct from squamous metaplasia. It is associated with chronic irritation or schistosomiasis and has a greater tendency for local recurrence when treated.
12. Adenocarcinoma: This is a rare tumor (1%–2%) associated with urachal carcinoma at the bladder dome. It is necessary to rule out gastrointestinal (GI) tract or breast metastases before designating it as a primary tumor.
13. Small cell carcinoma: This has a neuroendocrine origin. It is highly aggressive with presentation at high pathologic stage and responds poorly to any therapy.
14. Micropapillary carcinoma: This is an aggressive variant of bladder cancer that resembles papillary serous carcinoma of the ovary. Noninvasive and invasive presentations have been reported.

GRADING AND STAGING SYSTEM

1. The WHO 2015 grading system is the most widely accepted grading system. It categorizes tumors into low or high grade, allowing for ease of interpretation.
2. Staging is best achieved with the TNM classification, which subdivides the different levels of muscle invasion and extravesical extension.
3. **Grade, followed by stage, is the most significant predictor of recurrence and progression.**

NATURAL HISTORY

The natural history of bladder tumors with regard to recurrence and progression is closely related to the stage and grade of the lesion. The distinct classifications of noninvasive tumors as opposed to lumping them as superficial lesions demonstrate these differences.

1. Low-grade Ta lesions
   a. Noninvasive low-grade lesions account for 25% to 50% of bladder tumors. Those lesions defined as PUNLMP demonstrate a recurrence rate of 30% to 50%, but with

5- to 10-year follow-up, with minimal episodes of progression noted. In low-grade lesions, tumor multiplicity, recurrence at 3-month cystoscopy, and tumor size greater than 3 cm are factors favoring recurrence.

b. Low-grade Ta lesions carry a 50% to 70% risk of recurrence and a 1% to 5% risk of progression after 5 years.

2. High-grade Ta lesions
   a. These lesions account for 3% to 18% of most series with an average incidence of 6%. This is a difficult tumor to distinguish pathologically, and on comparative review, many of these lesions (up to three-fourths) are restaged as T1 lesions.
   b. These lesions demonstrate an 80% risk of recurrence and 50% risk of tumor stage progression.
3. CIS
   a. These lesions account for 5% to 10% of all superficial bladder cancer, and by definition are noninvasive, high-grade tumors.
   b. A suggestion of clinical subtypes has been made: primary disease, secondary CIS (detected after prior papillary disease), and concurrent CIS (CIS in the presence of papillary tumors). Primary disease accounts for 30% of cases, secondary 42%, and concurrent 28%. The distinction of primary asymptomatic unifocal CIS and symptomatic multifocal primary CIS has also been advanced.
   c. **Overall, 54% of patients with CIS progress to muscle-invasive disease.** If left untreated, the rate of progression rises to 80%.
   d. Asymptomatic patients account for 25% of patients, whereas 40% to 75% of patients will have irritative bladder symptoms.
4. T1 bladder tumors
   a. T1 lesions comprise 25% to 30% of superficial bladder tumors. **They will recur in up to 80% of cases and demonstrate tumor progression in 30% to 50% of cases.** Those with deep invasion to the layer of the muscularis mucosa have a more aggressive history with a progression rate of 40% and 5-year survival of 50%.
   b. Rebiopsy of T1 lesions can result in upstaging of the initial lesion in 30% to 60% of cases. This is especially true when no muscle is noted on the initial biopsy. Persistent tumor on

repeat biopsy can also be a poor prognostic indicator for response to therapy.

5. Muscle-invasive disease

Patients with muscle-invasive disease demonstrate stage progression and tumor metastases to lymph nodes, lung, liver, and bone. The majority of untreated patients (80%–90%) will demonstrate a cancer-related death in 2 to 3 years.

SIGNS AND SYMPTOMS

1. The most common symptom of bladder cancer is microscopic or gross hematuria followed by irritative bladder symptoms. Bladder masses can also be found as incidental findings on imaging examinations or as incidental findings during a cystoscopic examination.
2. **Hematuria in some form is noted in 85% of cases of bladder cancer.** Bladder masses on imaging can represent stones or polypoid cystitis. Additionally, the absence of a mass on imaging does not rule out the presence of a bladder tumor, which may not be detected because of tumor size or incomplete filling of the bladder.

DIAGNOSIS OF BLADDER CANCER

1. The evaluation of a suspected bladder mass should consist of an imaging exam, visual inspection of the urothelium, and cytologic evaluation of the urine. The role of additional urine-based tumor markers, both for the diagnosis and surveillance of bladder cancer, continues to evolve.
2. Historically, the imaging modality for the urinary tract has been the intravenous urogram (pyelogram). With improvements in technology, the CT urogram and MR urogram have become very popular; the AUA Guidelines for hematuria evaluation recommends CT urogram to clear the upper tracts. Ultrasound resolution is too low to discern small upper tract lesions or many bladder lesions and does not evaluate the ureters. In the case of renal insufficiency, an ultrasound can evaluate the renal parenchyma, and the urinary tract can be evaluated with retrograde pyelograms and cystoscopy. Recent studies have demonstrated that ultrasound can safely replace CT urogram in some low-risk patients with microscopic hematuria.

3. Urinary cytology: This cellular evaluation has poor overall sensitivity but is very specific for high-grade disease and CIS. Although the performance characteristics are rather poor for low-grade, low-stage lesions, high-grade tumors, and CIS, which may not be easily seen on cystoscopy, can be detected with a sensitivity in the 80% range and a specificity of 90% to 95%.
4. Cystoscopy: Endoscopic evaluation of the urothelium can be carried out by rigid or flexible optical scopes that allow one to examine the urethra, prostatic fossa, and bladder lining. It is the "gold standard" for the evaluation of the urinary tract lining; however, it is not 100% accurate. Small tumors and areas of CIS may be missed on exam.
    a. To improve the detection of smaller papillary tumors and CIS, enhanced cystoscopic techniques have been developed. Blue light cystoscopy uses hexaminolevulinate (HAL), a fluorescent porphyrin that accumulates in neoplastic tissue. Although more Ta tumors were detected with this technique, the greatest benefit was seen in the detection of CIS.
    b. Narrow band imaging (NBI) filters light into both blue (415 nm) and green (540 nm) wavelengths, which are absorbed by hemoglobin. This allows selective penetration of superficial tissue structures, highlighting the interface between mucosal surface and microvasculature. NBI has also shown a mild benefit over traditional white light cystoscopy.

DISEASE SCREENING AND TUMOR MARKERS

1. Hematuria screening: No prospective studies demonstrate a decrease in bladder cancer-related deaths as a function of screening. Comparisons of screened and unscreened populations suggest a shift in the detection from T2 to high-grade noninvasive disease with serial dipstick hematuria screening. This suggests that high-risk populations such as male smokers or those with high-risk occupational exposures and older than 50 years may benefit from this activity.
2. Tumor markers: Several protein-based and genomic-based markers have been evaluated for their role in the detection and surveillance of bladder cancer. A few have FDA approval for the monitoring of bladder cancer. In general, the protein markers have high sensitivity but lack specificity as tumor markers. They are more sensitive than urine cytology for the detection

of lower grade tumors and often less sensitive than cytology for high-grade disease or CIS. The performance of the protein-based markers can be degraded by inflammation and hematuria. False-positive tests create test anxiety but in some cases may detect disease before it is clinically evident. False-negative tests result in missed diagnosis and tumor progression. In general, these markers have the potential to make detection and monitoring of bladder cancer more precise, but no marker has been definitively established in this role.

a. Protein-based markers
   1) NMP22: This is a nuclear mitotic protein that is released in urine. It has been available as a laboratory test and now a point-of-contact test. A general cutoff value has been 10 U/mL, but different values have been used. The specificity ranges between 60% and 80%, and the sensitivity ranges between 18% and 100%. It is approved as an aid in the diagnosis of patients at risk for bladder cancer and for disease monitoring.
   2) BTA: This test detects a complement factor H-related protein and complement factor H. It exists as a point-of-contact test and a standard enzyme-linked immunosorbent assay (ELISA). Sensitivity ranges from 10% to 90%, and sensitivity is near 90% in healthy patients. This, however, is degraded by inflammation and hematuria to the 50% range. It is not useful for the detection of disease and is approved as an aid in managing bladder cancer.
   3) Hyaluronic acid-hyaluronidase (HA-HAase): This test measures HA and HAase ELISA assays. It has an 83% sensitivity and 90% specificity in detecting bladder cancer. It appears to be less affected by inflammation or hematuria, and false-positive studies have a 10-fold risk of tumor recurrence within 5 months. It has yet to undergo multicenter trials.
   4) ImmunoCyt: An immunocytologic evaluation of exfoliated cells with three antibodies. This test in conjunction with cytology has a combined sensitivity of 90% and specificity of 79%. This falls off, however, in patients with hematuria, cystitis, or BPH.
   5) CxBladder: A urine assay measuring microRNA fragments HOXA12, CDC2, MDK, CXCR2, and

IGFBP5. This test has a sensitivity and specificity of about 85%.

b. Genomic-based markers
   1) UroVysion test, fluorescent in situ hybridization (FISH): This is a multitarget FISH assay that evaluates alterations in ploidy with three chromosome enumeration probes 3, 7, and 17 and one locus-specific identifier 9p21 (p16 locus). Sensitivity is between 60% and 100% for low- to high-grade tumors, and specificity is approximately 95%. It is approved for the detection and monitoring of bladder cancer.
   2) Microsatellite analysis: This assay evaluates loss of heterozygosity at several loci in the genome. Sensitivity ranges between 72% and 97%. Specificity is high in healthy populations but may be altered in cystitis and BPH. No standardized set of markers is in use and prospective studies are in progress.

CLINICAL STAGING AND IMAGING

1. TUR: TUR by the method of electrocautery is the classic method for initial treatment and staging of bladder tumors. A blended current of cutting and cautery is employed, and an effort to resect the entire tumor with deep muscle biopsy is made. The potential for bladder perforation exists and generally may be treated by prolonged catheterization when extraperitoneal. Intraperitoneal perforation may require an open repair. Patients can demonstrate hematuria and irritative symptoms for several weeks after the procedure.
2. Random biopsies: The routine use of random biopsies has not been established, yet they can be useful in determining the extent of disease such as CIS and the presence of disease in sites such as the prostatic urethra. They have a greater role in higher grade and stage noninvasive lesions. It is less common to detect disease from normal-appearing areas of the bladder when low-grade Ta lesions are present.
3. Fluorescence cystoscopy: Compared to standard white light cystoscopy, this method requires the use of a blue light and the photosensitizer hexaminolevulinate. As discussed earlier, this approach allows for better visualization of CIS and small tumors which can be missed with white light cystoscopy. Some studies have shown a

decrease in tumor recurrence using this technique. Fluorescence cystoscopy may also be useful in patients with a persistently positive cytology and a negative white light cystoscopy.

4. CT scanning and MRI scanning do not provide precise information regarding clinical stage (invasive). Sensitivity is in the 70% to 90% range with specificity in the similar range. Accuracy is in the 55% to 85% range. Operational characteristics for defining lymph node status are somewhat higher. These modalities are also useful for demonstrating the absence or presence of hydronephrosis.
5. Bimanual examination under anesthesia: This maneuver is still valuable in assessing the status of patients with muscle-invasive tumors and provides information with regard to tumor extent and pelvic or abdominal wall involvement.

THERAPY IN GENERAL

1. TUR
2. Surgical excision alone may be adequate in the treatment of low-grade Ta disease. Fulguration about the perimeter of resection and care in avoiding gross perforation enhance the effectiveness of this technique.
3. Laser ablation of bladder tumors
   a. This is an effective method of treating bladder lesions, but a major drawback is the lack of pathologic specimen. It has advantages for patients on anticoagulation therapy and causes less pain and no obturator reflex. Neodymium-doped yttrium aluminum garnet (Nd:YAG) laser is popular for this purpose.
4. Intravesical chemotherapy instillation
   a. General considerations: Cytotoxic chemotherapy agents have been administered within the bladder with the objective of eradicating existing tumors, preventing the recurrence of treated tumors, and possibly preventing or delaying tumor progression. The ideal agent would be nontoxic, effective in a single dose, and inexpensive. No such ideal agent exists, but several agents demonstrate activity against noninvasive lesions.
   b. The summary analysis of multiple studies looking at the efficacy of chemotherapy demonstrates that in the short term these agents reduce recurrence by 14% to 17%. Over 3 to 5 years, this effect is reduced to approximately 7%.

Several large series of intravesical chemotherapy with a median survival follow-up of nearly 8 years demonstrate that there is no advantage to inhibiting tumor progression with this form of therapy. Most of these data are compiled from six-course administrations. Data evaluating combined or sequential chemotherapy generally demonstrate no therapeutic advantage but an increase in side effects. Some work on sequential mitomycin and gemcitabine suggests some potential synergy. Combined chemotherapy and immunotherapy have likewise shown additive value.

c. Immediate instillation of single-dose therapy. **A meta-analysis of seven clinical trials demonstrated that immediate instillation of a single dose of intravesical chemotherapy (most commonly mitomycin C) can decrease Ta and T1 tumor recurrence by approximately 39%.** This was most effective in patients with a single tumor, but it had some effect on patients with multiple lesions. The principal impact on recurrence occurred over the first 2 years. The mechanism is probably through an inhibition of tumor reimplantation after TUR. This form of therapy is contraindicated if a bladder perforation is noted during tumor resection. BCG cannot be used in this approach because of the possibility of intravascular inoculation and possible sepsis. However, perioperative gemcitabine use was recently shown to result in a 34% recurrence reduction with a more favorable risk profile.

5. Optimization of therapy
   a. Attempts to optimize therapy include dehydration prior to instillation, alkalinization of urine, administration of small volumes of intravesical fluid, and maximum dwell times. Studies with mitomycin C suggest that this can improve time to recurrence and recurrence-free survival. Additionally, research is progressing with drug delivery enhanced by electromotive administration and thermotherapy.
6. Common intravesical chemotherapy agents
   a. Mitomycin C: An alkylating agent that inhibits DNA synthesis by cross-linking, mitomycin C is cell cycle nonspecific. The molecular weight is 334 kD; therefore there is negligible systemic absorption. The most frequent side effects are chemical cystitis in up to 40% of patients and

palmar rash or other cutaneous symptoms in up to 10% of patients. It is usually administered as 40 mg in 40 mL of solution.

b. Doxorubicin: This is an anthracycline antibiotic that binds DNA base pairs and inhibits topoisomerase II and protein synthesis. It has a high molecular weight of 580 kD, and 25% to 50% of patients can develop chemical cystitis. The usual dose is 50 mg in 30 mL of solution with ranges reported from 30 to 100 mg.
c. Thiotepa: One of the first intravesical agents, thiotepa is an alkylating agent and is not cell cycle specific. At a molecular weight of 189 kD, it can be absorbed systemically causing thrombocytopenia in 3% to 13% of patients and leukopenia in 55% of patients. The usual dose is 30 mg in 15 mL of sterile water.
d. Valrubicin: This is a lipophilic, semisynthetic analogue of doxorubicin that demonstrates a 21% response in BCG refractory patients. This agent is FDA approved in this specific population.
e. Newer agents, such as gemcitabine and taxanes: Gemcitabine, a deoxycytidine analogue (2′,2′-difluoro-2′ deoxycytidine), has shown single agent activity in advanced bladder cancer. In BCG refractory patients, a SWOG trial has demonstrated a 2-year disease-free survival rate around 20%. Intravesical taxanes have also demonstrated similar results in this heavily pre-treated population.

7. BCG therapy

BCG is an attenuated strain of *Mycobacterium bovis* developed in 1921 and used as a tuberculosis vaccine. In 1976, BCG's efficacy against non–muscle-invasive bladder cancer (NMIBC) was demonstrated by Dr. Alvaro Morales. **Collective series demonstrate a 60% to 80% response rate against CIS, a 45% to 60% chance of eradicating residual papillary disease, and a 40% improvement over TUR alone for disease prophylaxis.**

The exact mechanism of BCG action is incompletely understood. Direct cell contact is necessary, and it appears that a TH1 immune pathway is predominant. Some activation of TH2 pathways is also seen, as is nitric oxide synthetase (NOS) activity. Recruitment of polymorphonucleocytes to the area of inflammation may provide further cytotoxic agents for tumor cell killing.

No data demonstrate the optimal schedule for BCG therapy. The most commonly accepted program has been designated the *6 + 3* program consisting of 6-week induction therapy followed by three booster treatments at 3- to 6-month intervals anywhere from 2 to 3 years. Irritative side effects can be significant and limit the long-term application of this strategy.

BCG appears to be the only intravesical agent that can decrease tumor progression. This has been demonstrated in meta-analysis and is powered by those clinical series in which maintenance BCG in some form was administered. The persistence of this effect over the long term (10–15 years) is questionable. The effect of BCG on overall patient survival so far demonstrates no advantage.

BCG produces irritative bladder symptoms in 90% of patients. Other symptoms include hematuria, low-grade fever, malaise, and nausea. Treatment with isoniazid and fluoroquinolones may be required. Patients with high fever (greater than 103°F or 39.4°C) require hospitalization and treatment with isoniazid 300 mg and rifampin 600 mg. A fluoroquinolone may also be used. BCG sepsis is rare, occurring in early series in 0.4% of patients. Patients with sepsis are treated with isoniazid, rifampin, and ethambutol 1200 mg daily plus a fluoroquinolone. Steroid therapy may be added. Additionally, one should consider and cover for gram-negative sepsis. Severe side effects may be reduced when direct intravascular absorption can be avoided such as traumatic catheterization, administration of BCG in the presence of an active urinary tract infection (UTI), or administration early after TUR.

Anatomically protected sites include the prostatic urethra and the distal ureters. Limited series suggest that a TUR of the bladder neck and prostatic fossa can provide better access for BCG, allowing a response in 50% to 80% of patients with superficial or ductal involvement.

8. Systemic therapy

Checkpoint inhibitors, which also have an emerging role in the management of systemic disease, have been under investigation for the use of NMIBC. By disrupting the interactions between the PD-L1/PD-1 receptor-ligand pathways, these agents stimulate cytotoxic T-cell function against tumor cells. In the KEYNOTE 057 trial, 75% of patients with CIS who failed intravesical immunotherapy with BCG had a complete response lasting over 6 months. Pembrolizumab was recently FDA approved for certain patients with BCG refractory bladder cancer and CIS.

TREATMENT OF LOW-GRADE TA DISEASE

1. The contemporary data suggest that such patients should be treated with a single perioperative intravesical instillation of a chemotherapeutic agent as described previously, unless there is evidence of a bladder perforation.
2. If the tumor is visually completely resected, immediate reresection is not warranted.
3. Little evidence supports the use of BCG in these patients. Patients with recurrent disease, especially multiple recurrences and/or associated CIS, may benefit from BCG therapy.
4. Small low-grade recurrences may be treated by office fulguration.
5. Cystoscopy disease status at 3 months and tumor size greater than 3 cm predict recurrence and possible progression.

TREATMENT OF HIGH-GRADE TA DISEASE AND CARCINOMA IN SITU

1. Evidence-based data are sparse for the treatment of high-grade Ta lesions because of the small percentage of overall tumors.
2. Immediate intravesical instillation is warranted with second-look cystoscopy and transurethral resection of bladder tumor (TURBT) with possible bladder mapping and BCG therapy with maintenance for persistent or recurrent high-grade Ta disease.
3. Consider cystectomy for original high-grade Ta if there is progression to T1 disease or CIS after BCG.
4. Maintain long-term, close (6-month) follow-up.
5. BCG demonstrates a 72% to 90% complete response in patients with only CIS. Initial response does not predict durability because up to 50% of patients may recur or progress.
6. Intravesical chemotherapy demonstrates a 35% to 53% response rate with wide variance about that interval given the studies evaluated.

7. TUR alone demonstrates a 0% durable response at 3 years.
8. In trials comparing BCG to chemotherapy, 68% of BCG and 49% of chemotherapy patients demonstrate a complete response. The BCG response is durable in 68% of patients compared to 47% of chemotherapy patients. Overall, disease-free rates at nearly 4 years are 51% for BCG and 27% for chemotherapy.
9. Maintenance therapy with BCG results in an improvement in complete response from 55% to 84%. Maintenance consists of a 3-week course of therapy every 6 months for 2 to 3 years. Patients may experience complications of bladder dysfunction. Decreased dose therapy (1/3, 1/10, 1/30, 1/100 of normal dose) may allow completion of therapy.
10. Disease progression in CIS is reduced by at least 35% with BCG. This effect is more prominent early. Long-term effects are less clear.
11. Treatment of BCG failures includes further therapy with valrubicin, additional therapy with intravesical interferon and BCG, or cystectomy. Valrubicin responses are in the 20% range. Forty percent to 50% of BCG failures may respond to combined BCG and interferon. Photodynamic therapy is a historical option. As discussed previously, systemic therapy with pembrolizumab has demonstrated durable complete responses lasting greater than 6 months in those with BCG-unresponsive CIS with or without papillary tumors.

TREATMENT OF T1 DISEASE

1. Repeat TURBT for staging is mandatory. Intravesical immediate instillation of chemotherapy should be performed even with suspected T1 lesions.
2. Immediate cystectomy versus BCG
   a. Argument for cystectomy is 30% upstaging in multiple series. Chemotherapy is associated with 33% progression and is not a good option unless patient cannot tolerate a cystectomy.
   b. BCG treated T1 disease associated with an average of only 12% recurrence (0%–35%). Overall treatment failure, including any recurrence, is 40% to 50%.
   c. Immediate cystectomy carries the morbidity and mortality of cystectomy. Surgery does not provide 100% 5-year survival (85%–90%).

d. Some stratification of high-grade T1 may be useful. Those with accessible, unifocal tumors, no CIS, and less than T1 disease on reTURBT may benefit from initial therapy. Those with multifocal disease, concomitant CIS, residual T1 on reTURBT, and tumors in difficult locations may benefit from cystectomy.

3. BCG therapy
   a. BCG failure may require stratification.
      1) Refractory disease: Worsening or nonimproved disease at 3 months or persistent disease at 6 months
      2) Resistant disease: Recurrent or persistent at 3 months but of lesser intensity; cleared at 6 months
      3) Relapsing: Recurrent after disease-free status achieved at 6 months
      4) Intolerant: Persistent or recurrent disease after less than adequate treatment because of patient tolerance
   b. Overall a second course of BCG may be useful in high-grade T1 patients, but therapy should not persist beyond two courses due to a significant risk of progression.

CYSTOSCOPIC SCHEDULE AND UPPER URINARY TRACT FOLLOW-UP

1. Cystoscopic schedules have been developed on the basis of authority opinion. Usually patients undergo cystoscopy every 3 months for the first 1 to 2 years, every 6 months for the next year, and either yearly exams thereafter or an exam every 6 months for 5 years in high-risk patients. A recurrence calls for a return to evaluations every 3 months.
2. Data on low-grade Ta disease suggest that evaluations can be of lesser intensity, often once at 3 months and at 12 months, followed by yearly visual exams. Although irritating, patients are willing to forego regular cystoscopy on the basis of the results of a tumor marker only if that marker would be 95% accurate. Cystoscopy findings at 3 months also influence patterns of recurrences.
3. Upper tract disease is uncommon in low-grade Ta disease yet can occur in more than 20% of patients with high-grade disease or CIS. Actuarial recurrence of upper v disease has been reported as high as 40% over 15 years in high-risk patients. Upper tract imaging yearly or every other year is indicated for the intermediate time frame for such patients.

TREATMENT OF T2 AND GREATER DISEASE

1. Radical cystectomy
   a. This is the standard of care in treating muscle-invasive bladder cancer. A radical cystectomy entails en bloc removal of the bladder, prostate, seminal vesicles, and proximal urethra. If the prostatic urethra is involved with tumor, a total urethrectomy is also carried out. This can also be performed as a subsequent separate procedure. An intact urethra is monitored by routine urethral cytology and/or urethroscopy in the postoperative period.
   b. Organ removal surgery has been associated with significant perioperative and postoperative morbidity. When analyzing data from Medicare claims, studies have demonstrated that radical cystectomy has the second highest 30-day readmission rate of all surgical procedures. Therefore, ongoing studies regarding the role of preoperative optimization, termed "prehabilitation," are gaining significant interest.
   c. In females, an anterior exenteration is performed that includes removal of the bladder, entire urethra, and anterior vaginal wall, a total abdominal hysterectomy and bilateral salpingo-oophorectomy. Recently, some surgeons have adopted gynecologic-sparing approaches in women with lower risk disease; however, studies regarding long-term safety and efficacy of this approach are ongoing. An en bloc pelvic lymph node dissection starting at the aortic bifurcation or common iliac vessels is performed in both sexes. The risk of recurrence for patients with radical cystectomy alone is shown in Fig. 16.2.
   d. Urinary diversion is an integral component of the procedure and accounts for most of the long-term postoperative morbidity. The major forms of diversion include a standard ileal conduit, colon conduit, or continent urinary diversion, which may be cutaneous or orthotopic. Operative mortality for radical cystectomy and urinary diversion is roughly 1% to 3%. Early and late postoperative complications range from 10% to 50%.
2. Neoadjuvant chemotherapy
   a. Recurrence rates in patients who undergo radical cystectomy alone for muscle-invasive disease approach 50%. Therefore, organ removal alone is not sufficient to prevent

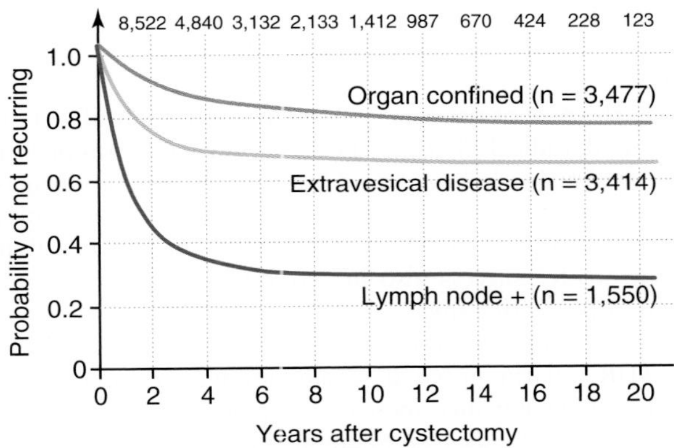

FIGURE 16.2 Kaplan-Meier (KM) curve. (From Bochner BH, et al. Postoperative nomogram predicting risk of recurrence after radical cystectomy for bladder cancer. *J Clin Oncol*. 2006;24:3967-3972.)

recurrence and progression in a large subset of patients. Cisplatin-based neoadjuvant chemotherapy has demonstrated a 6% overall survival benefit and a complete response rate of approximately 30%. Administration of neoadjuvant, as opposed to adjuvant, chemotherapy has several advantages. These will be discussed in a subsequent section.

3. Partial cystectomy
   a. This technique may be employed on a very selective basis for circumscribed lesions usually in the dome of the bladder where a 1- to 2-cm free margin may be obtained without requiring a further procedure such as ureteral reimplantation. This procedure can be overextended in the hope of preserving a normal lower urinary tract. This should not be the case in the present era of continent urinary diversion.
4. Radiation therapy
   a. Definitive radiation therapy has been employed in invasive bladder cancer. Overall, durable complete responses are 40% and are much poorer stage for stage than those obtained with surgery. Interstitial radiation therapy (iridium

needles) has been employed primarily in Europe. Careful patient selection is necessary to obtain success.

5. TUR
   a. In the case of patients who are severely medically compromised, radical TUR may be an appropriate form of therapy for invasive lesions. In addition, laser irradiation may be employed in this situation. A complete response may be obtained in as many as 20% to 30% of patients. Reports of greater success also incorporate salvage cystectomy as part of the therapy.
6. Combined modality therapy
   a. TUR, platinum-based combination chemotherapy, and EBRT have gained increased popularity over the past several years. Studies have demonstrated survival rates equivalent to that of cystectomy in highly selected populations. Patients ideally suited for this approach typically classically have unifocal tumors, no CIS, a complete TUR, and no hydronephrosis. Furthermore, this approach may also be preferred in frail, elderly patients with comorbidities that would complicate organ removal surgery.

URINARY DIVERSION

1. General considerations

   Urinary diversion is an integral part of urinary reconstruction and urologic oncology. Such surgery can be technically advanced and is associated with potential long-term and short-term complications. Additionally, careful consideration must be given to the physiologic costs of diverting the urinary tract and the appropriate selection of patients for a particular procedure. Urinary diversion can consist of simple diversion of the ureters to the skin, diversion of urine into the alimentary tract, or diversion of urine into an isolated segment of bowel serving as a conduit or reservoir for urine. There is no one preferred method of performing urinary diversion; therefore fundamental principles of reconstruction must be understood to appropriately apply these techniques in a given situation.
2. History

   During the mid and late 19th century many efforts were made to divert urine into the alimentary tract in an attempt to treat congenital malformations such as bladder exstrophy or conditions such as bladder cancer. Multiple complications occurred due to technical limitations in the preantibiotic era. The ureterosigmoidostomy of Robert Coffey provided one of the first reasonable methods of diverting the urinary system. Metabolic complications and the development of adenocarcinoma at the ureter-bowel junction discouraged further widespread use of this technique. The ileal loop urinary conduit described by Eugene Bricker in 1950 became the standard form of urinary diversion over the next several decades. Different techniques of continent urinary diversion have since been developed and modified by multiple individuals. The application of continent diversion has been further aided by the acceptance of clean intermittent catheterization as an appropriate form of urinary drainage.

3. General physiologic considerations
   a. Renal function

      Approximately 30% of patients will experience long-term (5–15 years) renal deterioration after urinary diversion. It must be remembered, however, that not all renal units associated with a diversion are normal preoperatively. This deterioration can be hastened by high static pressures within the reconstructed urinary tract, reflux, or chronic infection. Many of the metabolic abnormalities described below first became manifest or are exacerbated by patients displaying a serum creatinine greater than 2 ng/dL. Care must therefore be taken when considering such patients for urinary diversion.
   b. Infection

      The majority of patients with a urinary diversion will display urine colonized with bacteria. In general there is no concomitant symptomatic infection, and this situation is best left untreated. Repeated therapy for asymptomatic colonization can lead to infection with stone formation or severely resistant strains of bacteria. This may necessitate the use of parenteral antibiotics. Classically 4% to 6% of patients with urinary diversions may eventually die of urosepsis.

c. Urolithiasis

This may occur in 2% to 10% of patients with urinary diversions. The presence of foreign bodies, especially staples, provides a nidus for stone formation. Stones also have a greater tendency to form in patients with *Proteus* UTIs and in patients with hyperchloremic metabolic acidosis.

4. Metabolic considerations

a. Electrolyte abnormalities

These occur secondary to the interaction of urine with a particular bowel epithelium. The altered transport of different ions gives rise to particular metabolic abnormalities.

1) Colon: The classic abnormality seen in ureterosigmoidostomy is hyperchloremic metabolic acidosis. It was first recognized by Ferris and Odel in 1950. The condition can be seen in as many as 80% of patients and is exacerbated by the large surface area of the colon exposed to urine. Essentially, a significant amount of bicarbonate equivalents is lost into the colonic urine with the absorption of chloride from the urine. This condition can lead to a severe acidosis that is exacerbated by compromised baseline renal function. Another less recognized complication can be total body potassium depletion and hypokalemia. Furthermore, elevated ammonia levels may develop in patients secondary to bacterial overgrowth. This is best treated by adequate urinary drainage and/or treatment with neomycin or lactulose.

2) Ileum: Hyperchloremic metabolic acidosis is also seen in patients with ileal conduits. Although the findings are less severe, they can be present in as many as 70% of patients with ileal conduits. Again, patients with impaired baseline renal function will display a greater propensity toward metabolic derangement.

i. Monitoring: McDougal and Koch emphasize the potential implications of long-term subtle metabolic abnormalities such as growth retardation and osteomalacia. The exact timing for intervention in subtle acidosis is not clear, especially in elderly adults treated for cancer, yet these issues are of great concern in the pediatric and young adult population.

ii. Treatment: Hyperchloremic acidosis is treated by alkalizing agents such as oral sodium bicarbonate, Polycitra, or Shohl solution. If a sodium cannot be tolerated, cyclic adenosine monophosphate (cAMP) inhibitors such as nicotinic acid and chlorpromazine may be employed. Although sodium overload is avoided with such therapies, potential side effects such as peptic ulcer disease and tardive dyskinesia can occur.

3) Jejunum: Use of this bowel segment is associated with a hyponatremic, hypochloremic, hyperkalemic, metabolic acidosis. This is due to a loss of salt and an increase in potassium and hydrogen ions. A feed-forward mechanism is established by the initial loss of salt and water, followed by a renin-aldosterone response to the hypovolemia. The permeable jejunal epithelium is presented with a low-sodium, high-potassium urine, which facilitates further body loss of sodium into the conduit and reabsorption of potassium. Initial management requires fluid resuscitation followed by long-term sodium chloride supplementation.

4) Stomach: This bowel segment has been employed in urinary diversion or bladder augmentation in several different configurations. It has been employed predominantly in the pediatric population. The advantages of using stomach include compensation for preexisting metabolic acidosis, conversation of GI absorptive area, and decreased mucus production. The most common metabolic side effect is a hypokalemic, hypochloremic, metabolic alkalosis such as that seen with prolonged nasogastric suction. It is best managed with good oral fluid intake.

5. Other considerations

a. Neoplasia

Reports of adenocarcinoma in patients with ureterosigmoidostomies were first made in 1929. This event will occur in approximately 10% of such patients with a latency period of 10 to 20 years. Because serial screening was not performed, original reports displayed generally advanced disease with up to a 36% mortality rate. Although the lesion is usually at the ureter-colon junction, it is difficult to discern the issue of origin. The etiology of these carcinomas is poorly understood. Cases of carcinoma have been reported in ileal conduits and cystoplasties. The long-term implications for continent diversion are unknown.

b. Drug absorption

A large bowel segment provides a significant reabsorptive area for many chemicals. This is important because many patients undergoing chemotherapy for bladder cancer may be at risk for intoxication. Methotrexate, which is used with vinblastine, Adriamycin, and cisplatin in the MVAC regimen, has been reported to cause toxicity. Anticonvulsant agents may also be reabsorbed by the bowel of a urinary diversion.

c. Vitamin B_{12} metabolism

Vitamin B_{12} is absorbed primarily in the terminal ileum, which is often isolated from the alimentary tract when constructing a continent reservoir. Because usual body reserves are adequate for approximately 5 years, this is not an immediate postoperative concern, but it must be addressed with regard to replacement therapy in patients over the long term. The 15- to 20-cm segment employed in a standard ileal conduit usually does not deplete the absorptive distal ileum still in continuity with the alimentary tract.

d. Hematuria-dysuria syndrome

This is a complex of symptoms in patients with a diversion or bladder augment from a gastric segment, which includes bladder spasm, urethral pain, gross hematuria, and skin irritation. The etiology is incompletely understood yet is probably related to the secretion of gastric acid. The activation of pepsinogen to pepsin at a low pH has been proposed as the urothelial irritant. It is best treated by oral hydration and histamine blockade. This syndrome is partially related to hypergastrinemia, which can be demonstrated in gastric segment diversions. Ulceration is another possible problem with these segments.

6. Mechanical considerations
   a. Neuromuscular activity
      Bowel segments have an intrinsic coordinated contractile activity that must be taken into consideration when constructing conduits. It is a physiologic property that is disadvantageous for the active storage of urine. For continent reconstruction, the splitting of bowel on its antimesenteric border and its reconfiguration are meant to cause a zero net resultant pressure vector, thus preventing directional flow of urine. Additionally, a general discoordination of contraction activity occurs and thus lowers intraluminal pressure. This discoordination is the primary mechanical effect of reconfiguration, but its long-term efficacy is questionable because several studies suggest the return of coordinated activity fronts over time.
   b. Geometric aspects
      Much of the effectiveness in creating high-volume, low-pressure reservoirs by bowel reconfiguration may be accomplished by the fact that detubularization essentially approximates a sphere. This is the maximized volume for a given surface area, and the sphere has a larger radius than the tube of the bowel. The law of Laplace states that for a given wall tension, a larger radius will result in lower intraluminal pressure, which is the goal of a continent pouch with regard to continence and the prevention of upper tract deterioration.
7. Forms of urinary diversion (noncontinent)
   a. Ileal conduit
      Since its introduction in 1950, the ileal conduit has become the reference standard for urinary diversion. Approximately 15 to 20 cm of terminal ileum is isolated from bowel continuity, allowing this bowel segment to serve as a conduit or passageway to the skin. General complications are listed in the following.
      1) Cutaneous considerations: The loop may be matured at the skin as a Brooke ostomy or as a Turnbull loop. The latter is useful in patients with a thick abdominal wall. One of the several ostomy appliances is attached

to this site. Appropriate preoperative marking on the abdominal wall and care in constructing the stoma bud are important to avoid difficulties with patient comfort and skin care. Stomal stenosis is the most common long-term complication of cutaneous urinary diversion.

2) Ureteral considerations: The ureteral/enteral anastomosis is a potential site for complications. A direct anastomosis between the bowel and ureter with mucosa-to-mucosa apposition is the preferred method of construction. Early ureteral leakage was a significant and morbid complication of this procedure that has been reduced by greater attention to technique and the use of ureteral diversion stents in the perioperative period. Ureteral stenosis is not uncommon and may require balloon dilation or re-anastomosis.

b. Colon conduit

A portion of colon may be employed as a urinary conduit. The potential for hyperchloremic acidosis exists but is reduced if short segments of colon are used. When employed in conjunction with a full pelvic exenteration, a bowel anastomosis may be avoided. A transverse colon conduit is a very useful alternative in patients with heavily irradiated bowel. This segment is usually away from most radiation fields and provides a healthy alternative to possibly damaged ileum. Nonrefluxing ureteral anastomoses may be constructed with the use of tinea coli, but the potential for ureteral obstruction exists.

c. Jejunal conduit

The jejunum has been employed as an alternative segment in cases of radiated bowel. Due to its permeability characteristics, it is prone to severe metabolic complications previously described and is not generally employed in urinary diversion.

d. Cutaneous ureteral diversion

This is a direct form of urinary diversion generally complicated by stenosis at the level of the skin and by potential difficulties with collection appliances.

8. Continent urinary diversion
   a. General goals
      1) Adequate capacity reservoir
      2) Low-pressure reservoir
      3) Urinary continence during normal activities
      4) Volitional emptying
   b. General construction
      1) Cutaneous urinary diversion
      2) Orthotopic urinary diversion
   c. Continence mechanisms
      1) Intussuscepted nipple valve
      2) Fixed resistance
      3) Flap valve—Mitrofanoff principle
      4) Pelvic floor external sphincter (orthotopic)
   d. Ureterosigmoidostomy
   e. This is one of the original forms of urinary diversion and can be considered continent urinary diversion in the broad sense. It is rarely applied in developed countries because of the metabolic and neoplastic complications previously described. Recent modifications of this procedure have included J-pouch alteration of the sigmoid colon or the use of detubularized ileal patches to increase local capacity and decrease tenesmus.
   f. Cutaneous continent diversion
   g. In this form of diversion, a reservoir or ileum, a colon, or a combination of both is constructed from detubularized bowel and brought to the skin as a discrete, flush, catheterizable stoma. The site may be paraumbilical or just above the pubic hairline. In the case of a thick or distorted abdominal wall, the umbilicus is the preferred site. The site must be catheterized every 4 to 6 hours to avoid over distention. In addition to the standard complications of urinary diversion, patients may develop eccentricity of the catheterization pathway or incontinence requiring revision of the site. Initial series reported revision rates of 25% to 30% but these have decreased to a 5% to 15% range.
      1) Indiana pouch: A detubularized segment of cecum and colon acts as a storage reservoir whose continence is maintained by fixed resistance established at the ileocecal valve and distal ileum. The tapered distal ileum

serves as the catheterizable limb. Ease of construction and a low complication profile make this a popular form of diversion. Capacity is lower than that seen with ileal pouches, and a potential for chronic diarrhea exists (5%) because of the removal of the ileocecal valve and colonic tissue.

2) Penn pouch: In this form of diversion, the appendix is used in a tunneled method and acts as a flap valve (Mitrofanoff principle) to provide urinary continence. This recapitulates the natural course and mechanism of the ureter as it enters the bladder. Issues of pouch capacity and diarrhea are similar to those seen in the Indiana pouch. The appendix may not be a suitable catheterizable limb in all adults.

3) Monti procedure: The use of a transversely tubularized bowel segment (TTBS) increases the range and flexibility for the construction of a catheterizable limb in a cutaneous continent urinary reconstruction. A 2.5-cm segment of small bowel can be detubularized and transversely retubularized to create long, relatively narrow bowel segments, which can be implanted in a urinary reservoir and brought to the skin. When necessary, two segments can be attached in series to gain additional length. This is an extension of the Mitrofanoff principle, which uses a small-diameter tube implanted in a flap valve fashion to provide continence.

4) Pouch hygiene: As previously stated, forms of urinary diversion are subject to bacterial colonization. In continent reservoirs, this may proceed to frank pouchitis and pyelonephritis if emptying is inefficient or incomplete. Furthermore, most bowel segments continue to produce mucus for at least 1 year, which can be a source of obstruction leading to dysfunction and infection. The potential for such difficulties can be reduced by simple maneuvers such as daily pouch irrigation with saline solution by the patient after a routine catheterization.

h. Orthotopic continent diversion

i. This is a form of continent reconstruction based on the striated external sphincter as the primary continence mechanism. A high-capacity, low-pressure system is essential for an optimal result. Potential complications include enuresis in 5% to 10% of patients (because of relaxation of the pelvic floor during deep stages of sleep) and tumor recurrence at the urethral margin necessitating major surgical revision. Pouches may be constructed of pure ileum (hemi-Kock pouch, ileal neobladder) or mixed segments of large and small bowel (Mainz pouch).

1) Urodynamics: Functional studies reveal excellent capacity, storage, and efficient emptying with a combination of pelvic floor relaxation and abdominal straining. The potentially large capacity of these pouches can make a patient inattentive to the need for voiding. If the reservoir is chronically overdistended, the ability to empty is compromised and may necessitate the need for intermittent catheterization. Upper tract deterioration is primarily avoided by having low static pressures in the pouch and avoiding pouch-ureter reflux. Reflux may be further prevented by an intussuscepted nipple.
2) Female orthotopic diversion: The technique of orthotopic diversion has recently been extended to female patients. Careful pathologic studies have suggested that the absence of CIS or lack of tumor involvement in the trigone or bladder neck is associated with a lack of tumor in the female urethra. Although a concern for urinary incontinence was an initial issue, it has been noticed that many of these patients will develop partial or complete urinary retention. Patients tend to be equally divided: one-third void normally with or without occasional catheterization, one-third experience complete urinary retention, and one-third have stress urinary incontinence. No significant problems with urethral recurrence have been reported.

TREATMENT OF ADVANCED DISEASE

1. Chemotherapy for metastatic disease

Urothelial cancer is a moderately chemotherapy-sensitive malignancy. Prognostic risk factors (sometimes called the Bajorin risk factors) for patients with metastatic disease include visceral metastases (bone, lung, liver) and Karnofsky performance status less than 80% (greater than ECOG 2). Patients are classified as having zero, one, or two risk factors. Patients with zero risk factors treated with cisplatin-based chemotherapy have a median survival of 33 months, and some derive long-term benefit from chemotherapy. Patients with two risk factors have a median survival of 9 months and are unlikely to derive long-term benefit from chemotherapy. An important point is that results of chemotherapy trials including response rate and survival are clearly influenced by patient selection; randomized trials should stratify for these risk factors.

MVAC is the historic standard of care. MVAC is associated with significant toxicity. The combination of gemcitabine and cisplatin has been demonstrated to result in a similar survival but with less toxicity than MVAC. A regimen of dose-intense MVAC has not demonstrated improved overall survival over standard-dose MVAC, although higher complete response rates were noted.

Because cisplatin is nephrotoxic, this agent should not be used in patients with significant renal impairment. Approximately one-quarter of patients with advanced urothelial cancer are not candidates for cisplatin because of renal insufficiency. The combination of paclitaxel plus carboplatin can be used in these patients but has less therapeutic efficacy.

There is no standard effective second-line chemotherapy option for patients with advanced urothelial cancer. Therefore, researchers began assessing the role of immune checkpoint inhibitors in advanced urothelial carcinoma.

Under normal circumstances, T cells exhibit CTLA-4, an immune checkpoint molecule that binds to receptors on antigen presenting cells (APCs), preventing T-cell proliferation. In order to modulate this response, programmed cell death 1 (PD-1) receptors are expressed on T cells. It is thought that tumor cells have high levels of PD-L1; upon binding with PD-1 on host T cells, they inactivate these cells. By interrupting either the CTLA-4/APC or PD-1/PD-L1 interaction, immune checkpoint inhibitors upregulate cytotoxic T cells that results in immune driven tumor death.

Promising results in clinical trials led to the FDA approval of first-line atezolizumab, a PD-L1 inhibitor, and pembrolizumab, a PD-1 inhibitor, for platinum ineligible patients with metastatic disease. Additional agents, including CTLA-4 inhibitors, have been approved for second-line therapy in advanced disease. These agents are also currently being evaluated in the postcystectomy population as an adjuvant treatment for patients with high-risk features.

2. Neoadjuvant and adjuvant chemotherapy

   Patients with muscle-invasive bladder cancer are at risk of developing metastatic disease, even after cystectomy. Postcystectomy pathology demonstrating extravesical disease or lymph node metastases is associated with an increased risk of recurrence and distant metastases. Systemic chemotherapy has been studied to determine if it can eradicate micrometastatic disease in the earlier disease setting.

   Neoadjuvant chemotherapy refers to chemotherapy given before cystectomy. A meta-analysis of multiple randomized trials demonstrated that neoadjuvant chemotherapy is associated with an absolute survival advantage of about 6% at 5 years. Neoadjuvant therapy can also be given to downstage locally advanced tumors.

   Adjuvant chemotherapy refers to systemic chemotherapy administered after cystectomy. Small trials suggest benefit, but a sufficiently powered randomized trial of surgery alone versus surgery plus adjuvant chemotherapy has not been performed.

   Finally, a small trial from MD Anderson Cancer Center compared neoadjuvant MVAC with adjuvant MVAC and determined that survival was similar with both approaches.

CLINICAL PEARLS

Bladder Cancer

- Tobacco use confers a two- to threefold increased risk of developing bladder cancer.
- Stage and grade are both significant predictors of recurrence and progression in bladder cancer.
- Hematuria in some form is noted in 85% of cases of bladder cancer.
- Intravesical BCG therapy has an initial clinical response rate of 60% to 80% for CIS.
- Neoadjuvant chemotherapy is associated with a 5% absolute survival advantage for patients with muscle-invasive bladder cancer.

DIFFERENTIAL DIAGNOSIS

Elevated PSA

- BPH
- Prostate cancer
- Prostatitis
- Recent urologic instrumentation
- Recent ejaculation
- Urinary tract infection

Additional content, including Self-Assessment Questions and Suggested Readings, may be accessed at www.ExpertConsult.com.

Adult Genitourinary Cancer: Renal and Testicular

Ruchika Talwar, MD, David J. Vaughn, MD, Alan J. Wein, MD, PhD (Hon), FACS, and Thomas J. Guzzo, MD, MPH

Neoplasms of the Kidney

GENERAL CONSIDERATIONS

The paradigm in diagnosis, evaluation, and management of renal cell carcinoma (RCC) has evolved significantly over the last several decades. Whereas 30 years ago the diagnosis of RCC was predicated on clinical signs and symptoms, the **majority of renal tumors are now diagnosed incidentally on imaging performed for other reasons.** The identification of iatrogenic renal insufficiency associated with radical nephrectomy has rendered nephron-sparing techniques the preferred treatment for small renal masses. Active surveillance of small renal masses has also emerged as an option for select patients. Although RCC remains the prototype for tumors resistant to radiation and chemotherapy, an expanding number of molecular- and immune-targeted therapies are now available.

INCIDENCE AND EPIDEMIOLOGY

There were approximately 73,750 new cases of RCC in 2020 and 14,830 deaths attributable to the disease. **The incidence of RCC has increased over the last several decades with a stage migration toward lower-stage, smaller tumors.** Despite this downward stage migration, there has yet to be a demonstrable decrease in kidney cancer–related mortality rates.

RCC represents 2% to 3% of all malignancies, with a male-to-female ratio of 2:1 and a peak incidence in the fifth to seventh decade of life. Most RCC cases are sporadic, but a number of hereditary conditions are associated with various renal tumors (Table 17.1). In general, RCC in hereditary syndromes has an

TABLE 17.1 Hereditary Syndromes Associated With RCC

Syndrome Name	Gene Involved	Renal Tumors	Other Manifestations
Von Hippel-Lindau (VHL) disease	VHL gene (3p25-26)	Clear cell RCC in 50% of patients (also type 1 papillary RCC)	Cysts of the epididymis and pancreas, cerebellar hemangioblastomas, retinal angiomas, and pheochromocytoma
Hereditary papillary RCC	c-MET proto-oncogene (7q31)	Type 1 papillary RCC	None described
Hereditary leiomyomatosis and RCC	Fumarate hydratase (1q42)	Type 2 papillary RCC	Cutaneous and uterine leiomyomas
Birt-Hogg-Dubé (BHD) syndrome	BHD1 gene/folliculin (17p12q11)	Chromophobe RCC, oncocytoma, hybrid oncocytic cells (also clear cell RCC seen)	Cutaneous fibrofolliculomas, lung cysts with spontaneous pneumothorax
Tuberous sclerosis complex (TSC)	TSC1/TSC2 tuberin	Angiomyolipomas (AMLs; 60%–80% of patients), renal cysts (20%–30% of patients), RCC (< 1%)	Facial angiofibroma, subependymal nodules epilepsy, mental retardation

RCC, Renal cell carcinoma.

autosomal-dominant inheritance pattern with variable penetrance. RCCs associated with hereditary syndromes generally present at an earlier age and are more likely to be bilateral and multifocal. Although these hereditary conditions are uncommon (4% to 6% of all patients with RCC), they have been essential in improving RCC tumor biology.

ETIOLOGY

Tobacco use is the strongest known risk factor for RCC, with users having an approximately twofold increased risk. Hypertension and obesity have also been associated with RCC in large epidemiologic studies. Furthermore, the association of increased incidence of RCC with acquired renal cystic disease secondary to end-stage renal disease (ESRD)/dialysis has been debated; many practitioners advocate performing periodic imaging in dialysis patients.

PATHOLOGY: RENAL TUMORS

1. RCC
   a. RCC represents nearly 80% of solid renal tumors. Several distinct histologic patterns have been observed. The most common histopathologic entities are clear cell (conventional) RCC followed by papillary RCC. Both are thought to arise from the proximal convoluted tubular epithelium. Less commonly observed are chromophobe RCC and collecting duct carcinoma, which arise from components of the distal nephron. Other rare subtypes are also recognized. Sarcomatoid differentiation occurs in up to 5% of RCC, may be present with any subtype, and carries significant negative prognostic value.

      Grossly, RCC is usually round and contained within a fibrous pseudocapsule. Most sporadic tumors are solitary and unilateral, but up to 5% of patients will develop bilateral tumors. RCC has a unique predilection for venous involvement, with up to 10% harboring tumor thrombus at presentation.

   b. Clear cell (conventional) RCC: **This is the most common histology accounting for 70% to 80% of all RCC. It is associated with an allelic loss of the Von Hippel-Lindau (VHL) gene.** Grossly, tumors appear yellow or gray-tan in color with variable areas of hemorrhage, necrosis, or cystic changes. Microscopically, they are composed predominantly of cells with clear eosinophilic or granular cytoplasm, containing glycogen, cholesterol, and phospholipids. In general, clear cell RCC has a worse prognosis than papillary and chromophobe RCC after adjustment for grade and stage.

c. Papillary RCC: This comprises 10% to 15% of newly diagnosed RCC, but accounts for a higher percentage in patients with end-stage and acquired renal cystic disease. Papillary RCC is more likely to be multifocal or bilateral than other histologies. Two distinct subtypes are recognized: type 1 and type 2 papillary RCC. They are associated with two different familial RCC syndromes (see Table 17.1). Papillary type 1 tumors are associated with activation of the *MET* proto-oncogene (chromosome 17), whereas papillary type 2 tumors are associated with mutations in the fumarate hydratase gene. Type 2 papillary RCC tends to be the more aggressive variant.

d. Chromophobe RCC: This represents 3% to 5% of RCC and is associated with multiple chromosome losses. Histologically, a defining feature is its perinuclear "halo." Chromophobe RCC histology may be confused with oncocytoma, a benign renal lesion. Chromophobe RCC tends to have a better prognosis than clear cell and papillary subtypes.

e. Collecting duct carcinoma: This is a rare but very aggressive RCC subtype, representing less than 1%. It tends to occur in younger patients, and up to half have metastasis at presentation.

f. Renal medullary carcinoma: This is a highly aggressive tumor seen in young Black Americans with sickle cell trait. It may represent a variant of collecting duct carcinoma and carries a very poor prognosis.

2. Oncocytoma

a. Accounting for approximately 5% of all renal tumors, oncocytomas are well-circumscribed parenchymal masses composed of densely acidophilic cells that show mitochondrial hyperplasia on electron microscopy. They may be bilateral in up to 5% of cases. In contrast to RCC, the principal genetic alteration appears to involve changes in mitochondrial DNA and translocation of chromosome 14. Grossly, they are mahogany brown in color, encapsulated, and may contain a dense central scar extending in a stellate pattern, which may be identified in cross-sectional imaging. Oncocytomas are benign and can be managed conservatively; however, their preoperative clinical diagnosis is often unreliable, and a definitive diagnosis may be made on frozen section or percutaneous biopsy due to histologic similarities to chromophobe RCC.

3. Angiomyolipoma (AML)
   a. These benign lesions composed of fat, muscle, and blood vessels can generally **be identified by the presence of macroscopic fat on computed tomography (CT) scan.** Although lesions are generally identified as incidental radiographic findings, patients may present with acute flank pain or hemorrhagic shock due to spontaneous renal or retroperitoneal hemorrhage. Treatment is based on tumor size and patient symptoms. **Asymptomatic tumors smaller than 4 cm may be managed expectantly. However, symptomatic tumors or those greater than 4 cm should undergo selective embolization, percutaneous ablation, or nephron-sparing surgery (NSS).** Some large central tumors not amenable to nephron-sparing strategies may require radical nephrectomy.
   b. Tuberous sclerosis, an autosomal-dominant mutation in either 9p34 or 16p13, is the most common genetic cause of hereditary AML. Patients often have multiple and bilateral renal AMLs, making NSS of paramount importance. Everolimus, a mammalian target of rapamycin (mTOR) inhibitors, has been shown to decrease the size of AML and is Food and Drug Administration (FDA) approved for the treatment of AML in patients with tuberous sclerosis.
4. Sarcoma
   a. Sarcomas constitute 2% to 3% of malignant renal parenchymal tumors. They are more common in women. Differentiation from RCC is difficult. The predominant subcategory is leiomyosarcoma. The preferred treatment remains radical nephrectomy with wide negative margins.
5. Lymphoma
   a. B-cell non-Hodgkin lymphoma will occasionally present as an infiltrative renal mass. It is uncommon for leukemia to present as a primary renal lesion.

6. Metastasis
   a. The most common metastases to the kidneys are primary carcinomas of the lung, breast, and uterus, and melanoma. Metastatic lesions appear poorly vascularized and display irregular borders on imaging studies. A percutaneous biopsy of the renal mass may be warranted in patients with signs of progression from their other malignancy or in masses that do not demonstrate contrast enhancement on imaging studies.

GRADING AND STAGING

The Fuhrman grading system is commonly used to classify nuclear features of RCC. It ranges from grades I (well differentiated) to IV (poorly differentiated) and is contingent on nuclear size, nuclear outline, and presence of nucleoli. The most common staging system for RCC remains the American Joint Committee on Cancer (AJCC) TNM system (Table 17.2). Major changes occurred in the 10th edition, including subdivision of T2 tumors and reclassification of tumors with lymphatic involvement, tumor thrombus, and adrenal metastasis. **Pathologic stage remains the single most important prognostic factor**. Other important considerations are tumor size, grade, subtype, presenting symptoms, and patient factors. Whereas 5-year survival for patients with T1a disease is between 90% and 100%, survival drops to 50% to 70% in patients with T3a disease, and to 20% or less in patients with nodal or distant metastatic disease.

CLINICAL PRESENTATION

Greater than 50% of all RCCs are found as asymptomatic incidental masses on imaging studies obtained for another purpose. The classic triad of hematuria, flank pain, and a palpable mass was historically seen in approximately 10% of patients but is now a very rare presentation. Systemic symptoms of unintentional weight loss, fever, anemia, and night sweats suggest the presence of metastasis. Tumor thrombus can obstruct drainage of the testicular vein, producing a right-sided or noncollapsible varicocele. Paraneoplastic syndromes may occur in advanced disease, including hypercalcemia from parathyroid-like hormone production, hypertension, polycythemia, and Stauffer syndrome, or nonmetastatic hepatic dysfunction.

TABLE 17.2 AJCC Eighth Edition Staging System for Renal Cell Carcinoma

Primary Tumor (T)

TX—Primary tumor cannot be assessed

T0—No evidence of primary tumor

T1—Tumor 7 cm or less in greatest dimension, limited to the kidney

T1a—Tumor 4 cm or less in greatest dimension, limited to the kidney

T1b—Tumor > 4 cm but not > 7 cm in greatest dimension, limited to the kidney

T2—Tumor > 7 cm in greatest dimension, limited to the kidney

T2a—Tumor > 7 cm but 10 cm or less in greatest dimension, limited to the kidney

T2b—Tumor > 10 cm, limited to the kidney

T3—Tumor extends into major veins or perinephric tissues but not into the ipsilateral adrenal gland and not beyond Gerota fascia

T3a—Tumor grossly extends into renal vein or segmental (muscle-containing) branches, or tumor invades perirenal and/or renal sinus fat but not beyond Gerota fascia

T3b—Tumor grossly extends into the vena cava below the diaphragm

T3c—Tumor grossly extends into the vena cava above the diaphragm or invades into the wall of the vena cava

T4—Tumor invades beyond the Gerota fascia (including contiguous extension into the ipsilateral adrenal gland)

Regional Lymph Nodes (N)

NX—Regional lymph nodes cannot be assessed

N0—No regional lymph node metastasis

N1—Metastasis in regional lymph node

Distant Metastasis (M)

M0—No distant metastasis

M1—Distant metastasis

AJCC, American Joint Committee on Cancer.

(From Rini BI, McKiernan JM, Chang SS, et al. Kidney. In: Amin MB, ed. *AJCC Cancer Staging Manual*. 8th ed. New York: Springer; 2017:739.)

IMAGING EVALUATION

The most common renal mass is a benign cyst, identified in approximately 50% of patients over 50 years of age. A mass not meeting ultrasound criteria for a simple cyst should be evaluated with a dedicated renal CT scan or magnetic resonance imaging (MRI) with thin cuts. Renal cysts are classified by the Bosniak system (Table 17.3).

1. Diagnostic studies
   a. CT: Precontrast and postcontrast thin-slice CT images should be obtained. Contrast-enhanced imaging takes advantage of the neovascularity of most renal neoplasms. **Enhancement of greater than 15 Hounsfield units is worrisome, and the presence of enhancement must prompt immediate consideration of RCC.** The presence of macroscopic fat, defined as regions of attenuation of less than −20 Hounsfield units, indicates the presence of AML. In addition to characterizing the primary renal tumor, CT provides information on lymph node involvement, perinephric extension, and venous involvement. High-speed spiral CT technology permits three-dimensional (3D) renal reconstruction and CT angiography, which may

TABLE 17.3 Bosniak Classification of Cystic Masses

Category	Description	Risk of Malignancy
Bosniak I	Simple cyst; measuring water density; does not enhance; contains no calcifications	< 2%
Bosniak II	Minimally complex cyst; thin wall (< 1 mm); no enhancement, although may contain several hairline septa; hyperdense cyst	< 5%
Bosniak IIF	Indeterminate; complex cyst with thicker septa	~ 25%
Bosniak III	Suspicious indeterminate; thicker, regular, nodular walls with thicker, regular calcifications and septations	~ 50%
Bosniak IV	Malignant; nodular or solid component	> 90%

be very useful in preparation for either NSS or laparoscopic renal surgery.

b. Renal ultrasound: Ultrasound is an inexpensive and noninvasive modality used to distinguish cystic from solid renal masses. A simple cyst will be smooth with a definite border of imperceptible thickness, be absent of internal echogenicity, and should display acoustic enhancements beyond the posterior wall.
c. MRI: This is an alternative to CT for evaluation of renal masses and is particularly useful for those with iodinated contrast allergies. Enhancement seen after gadolinium contrast on T1-weighted images is characteristic of RCC. MRI is also effective in demonstrating the presence and extent of renal vein or vena caval tumor thrombi. Whereas contrast-enhanced MRI was historically performed in patients with renal insufficiency, it is now avoided because of the risk of nephrogenic systemic fibrosis with gadolinium administration in patients with chronic kidney disease (CKD).
d. Angiography: Classic angiography has been largely replaced by magnetic resonance angiography or 3D CT angiography in the evaluation of the renal vessels. However, renal angioembolization may be useful before radical nephrectomy for very large central tumors or in the presence of bulky hilar adenopathy.
e. Radionuclide imaging: This may be useful in determining the presence of a pseudotumor. Renal pseudotumors can results from multiple causes, but the most common is hypertrophied column of Bertin. Pseudotumors appear with a uniform distribution of radioisotope uptake on radionuclide imaging, whereas benign cysts and true renal tumors will appear as photon-deficient areas of uptake.
f. Percutaneous biopsy: Historically, biopsy was performed only if a renal mass was suspected to be lymphoma, metastasis, or abscess. In recent years, percutaneous biopsy has been revisited. Nearly one-third of small renal masses are benign, and the majority of the remaining two-thirds are frequently low-grade tumors. Most contemporary series show greater than 90% accuracy with biopsy, with complication rates less than 2%. Biopsy provides valuable information on grade and histologic subtype, both of which can

be used for treatment planning, especially in the setting of active surveillance and cryoablation.

2. Clinical staging
   a. The initial workup and clinical staging, according to the National Comprehensive Cancer Network (NCCN) guidelines, consists of a history, physical exam, complete blood count, comprehensive metabolic panel, urinalysis, chest imaging, and a contrast-enhanced cross-sectional imaging of the abdomen and pelvis. A bone scan may be obtained in symptomatic patients or those with elevated alkaline phosphatase. If neurologic symptoms or extensive metastatic disease is present, a brain MRI should be considered. For renal masses that are suspicious for urothelial origin, dedicated urothelial imaging (including urogram or pyelograms), urinary cytology, and ureteroscopy should be considered.

TREATMENT

1. Small renal masses and localized disease (T1-T2)
   a. Surgical management
      1) A dramatic change in the treatment of clinical T1 renal masses has occurred over the last several years. At one time NSS was reserved only for those with absolute indications, including preexisting renal insufficiency or solitary kidney. With improvements in our understanding of the risk of CKD following radical nephrectomy, **NSS has emerged as the preferred treatment for small renal masses.** Most studies demonstrate similar oncologic outcomes with greater preservation of renal function with partial nephrectomy compared to radical nephrectomy. Local recurrence rates are less than 5%. Furthermore, several series have shown that tumor enucleation can maximize parenchymal sparing and still provide adequate oncologic outcomes. The operative morbidity of partial nephrectomy is similar to radical nephrectomy, but with the potential for slightly greater blood loss and urinary leak. Renal ischemia remains a concern during partial nephrectomy. Ischemia can be avoided in select cases by not clamping or selectively clamping segmental arteries. Renal cooling can be used

to convert warm ischemia to cold ischemia, thereby decreasing the metabolic rate of the kidney with the goal of avoiding acute tubular necrosis (ATN). Although ischemic time is important, **the amount of renal parenchyma that is preserved is the most important factor that the surgeon can modify for long-term renal function preservation.**

2) **Radical nephrectomy is now generally reserved for large tumors or tumors not amenable to partial nephrectomy.** Components of radical nephrectomy include early vascular ligation and en bloc removal of the kidney, surrounding Gerota fascia, and proximal ureter. Recent data suggest that ipsilateral adrenalectomy is unnecessary in the presence of a normal-appearing adrenal gland that does not appear to be involved radiographically or intraoperatively.

3) The role of lymphadenectomy at the time of renal surgery remains poorly characterized. It may provide a small benefit in controlling micrometastatic disease in select patients, but a well-performed randomized trial (EORTC 30881) failed to show any survival benefit attributable to the routine application of lymphadenectomy. The surgical approach to a renal mass depends on tumor and patient characteristics but also upon surgeon experience. Laparoscopic partial and radical nephrectomy can be performed using a transperitoneal or retroperitoneal approach with pure laparoscopy, hand-assistance, or robotic assistance.

b. Tumor ablation techniques

1) Percutaneous or laparoscopic ablation using cryosurgery or radiofrequency offers reduced morbidity and more rapid recovery when compared to surgical excision. These benefits, however, are balanced with somewhat higher rates of local recurrence. Between-series comparisons are difficult because reliable histologic and pathologic staging is not performed with ablative techniques. Tumor size is also an important predictor of success; therefore ablative therapy is generally reserved for renal masses less than 4 cm. Ablation was typically reserved for patients of advanced age and significant

comorbidity; however, the 2017 American Urological Association (AUA) guidelines state that thermal ablative techniques are an acceptable treatment option for renal masses smaller than 3 cm, even in healthy patients.

c. Active surveillance
   1) With the increasing number of incidentally identified renal masses, particularly in comorbid elderly patients, active surveillance for small renal masses has emerged as a reasonable management strategy. The median growth rate for most small renal masses is less than 0.3 cm/year, and for biopsy-proven RCC, it is only approximately 0.4 cm/year. Tumors less than 3 cm may be monitored with serial imaging every 6 to 12 months. Increased growth kinetics and surpassing a size threshold are typical indications for intervention. Early series demonstrate a low risk of metastatic dissemination in small renal masses under active surveillance. The 2017 AUA guidelines include active surveillance as an option for small, solid Bosniak 3 and 4 cysts, as well as in renal masses smaller than 2 cm in young, healthy patients. Renal mass biopsy may play an important role in the shared decision-making process.

2. Locally advanced RCC
   a. Inferior vena caval tumor thrombus: Inferior vena cava extension occurs in 4% to 10% of patients with newly diagnosed RCC, more commonly in patients harboring clear cell RCC. In the absence of vascular wall invasion or metastasis, an aggressive surgical approach with nephrectomy and tumor thrombectomy is advocated. Advanced surgical techniques can be successful, usually with thoracoabdominal, chevron, or midline approaches to permit complete vascular control. Cardiopulmonary bypass with or without hypothermic cardiac arrest can be used for bulky intrahepatic or suprahepatic lesions. MRI, multiplanar CT scan, or transesophageal echocardiography (TEE) should be performed as close to surgery as possible to evaluate the extent of the thrombus because progression can affect the surgical approach. Operative mortality ranges from 1.4% to 14%, with 30% to 40% postoperative complications such as sepsis, retroperitoneal hemorrhage, or hepatic dysfunction.

b. Adjuvant systemic therapy: There have been many studies exploring adjuvant-targeted therapy after nephrectomy for high-risk patients; only sunitinib, a vascular endothelial growth factor (VEGF) inhibitor, has been shown to demonstrate a disease-free survival advantage without any overall survival benefit. Current ongoing trials exploring the use of immunotherapy in the adjuvant setting will likely provide further guidance on the role of postsurgical systemic therapy in high-risk patients.

3. Metastatic RCC
   a. Motzer criteria: Patients with metastatic disease can be categorized into low, intermediate, and poor risk based upon published criteria. Such criteria include metastasis-free interval from nephrectomy, performance status, number and location of metastases, and select laboratory values. Often referred to as the Motzer criteria, this risk-stratification scheme was initially described in patients receiving immunotherapy but has recently been validated in patients receiving VEGF-targeted therapy.
   b. Cytoreductive nephrectomy: The role for radical nephrectomy in patients with metastatic RCC in the current era of targeted systemic therapy remains unclear. Historically, cytoreductive nephrectomy was performed in individuals with an excellent performance status undergoing immunotherapy. Two randomized controlled trials conducted by SWOG and EORTC have demonstrated a benefit of nephrectomy and interferon compared to interferon alone; however, the CARMENA study, randomizing patients to surgery followed by targeted therapy versus targeted therapy alone, suggests that poor prognosis patients may not benefit from cytoreductive nephrectomy. Given that sunitinib is no longer the preferred initial therapy in metastatic disease, the clinical implications of the CARMENA trial are inconsistent. Recent paradigm shifts suggest that upfront systemic therapy, followed by cytoreductive nephrectomy, may be of benefit.
   c. Metastasectomy: Approximately 1% to 4% of patients with metastatic disease will have a solitary metastasis or oligometastasis, for which surgical resection provides a 5-year survival between 30% and 50%.

d. Systemic therapy: The chemorefractory nature of RCC likely arises from the expression of multidrug resistance efflux pump proteins. RCC is, however, an immunogenic tumor, and the use of immunotherapy was the cornerstone of systemic therapy for many years. Interferon-alpha provides a 15% partial response rate, but complete response is very rare; therefore it is no longer commonly used. High-dose interleukin-2 is associated with durable, complete response with long-term survival in select patients. A response rate in the 10% to 20% range has been demonstrated, but treatment is associated with major toxicities, including adult respiratory distress syndrome (ARDS) as a result of the capillary leak syndrome. Some centers still offer high-dose interleukin-2 to young patients with good performance status who have metastatic clear cell RCC. Inpatient admission, frequently to ICU-level settings, is required during administration to monitor for toxicity and provide supportive care.
e. Efforts have also focused on leveraging knowledge of the molecular mechanisms by which RCC develops, leading to the usage of molecular-targeted therapies that inhibit angiogenesis and cell cycle regulation. Tyrosine kinase inhibitors (TKIs) that target VEGF-mediated pathways, such as sunitinib, sorafenib, and pazopanib have been used for metastatic and high-risk localized disease. Everolimus is an mTOR inhibitor that was reserved as a second-line therapy for patients refractory to TKIs. Temsirolimus, another mTOR inhibitor, is approved for poor-risk metastatic RCC. Using RECIST criteria, multiple studies have revealed fairly consistent response rates to various TKIs, on the order of 30% to 40%. However, the use of immune checkpoint inhibitors has revolutionized our approach to the treatment of both metastatic and high-risk localized disease. These agents modulate molecular interactions to upregulate the body's innate immune response. Nivolumab coupled with ipilimumab, a combined PD-L1/CTLA-4 blockade, demonstrated superiority to sunitinib and is currently a first-line treatment option for patients with metastatic clear cell RCC. In the CheckMate 214 trial, patients who received combination therapy versus sunitinib were shown to have

an objective response rate of 42%, and a complete response rate of 9%. The KEYNOTE-426 trial demonstrated the role of axitinib plus pembrolizumab, a VEGF inhibitor with a PD-1 inhibitor, appeared to be better tolerated with a complete response rate of 5.8%. Ongoing trials will continue refine our understanding of the role of these agents in the front-line setting.

FOLLOW-UP AFTER TREATMENT

Practice patterns for RCC follow-up vary dramatically between centers. Because cross-sectional imaging is usually required, cost and radiation exposure can vary widely between surveillance protocols. The NCCN recommends a history, physical, and comprehensive metabolic panel every 6 months for 2 years, then annually for 5 years. According to the NCCN, imaging of the chest, abdominal, and pelvis should be obtained 2 to 6 months from treatment and then only as indicated. The authors advocate for an individualized approach based on patient and tumor characteristics.

Urothelial Tumors of the Renal Pelvis and Ureter

GENERAL CONSIDERATIONS

The urinary tract is lined by urothelial cell epithelium from the most proximal calyces to the proximal urethra. In this section, attention is given to the tumors of the renal collecting system and the ureter. It is essential that urothelial tumors of the renal pelvis and ureter be understood in the broad context of urothelial cell carcinoma (UCC), which is discussed in greater detail in the section on bladder cancer (see Chapter 16). Although UCC of the upper tract shares similarities to urothelial carcinoma of the bladder (UCB), several distinct differences merit consideration.

INCIDENCE

Upper tract UCC (UTUCC) accounts for 5% to 7% of all renal tumors and 5% to 10% of all urothelial cancers. The exact incidence of UTUCC is largely unknown because renal pelvis tumors are generally included in data on all renal tumors. Although the incidence of UTUCC is **thought to be increasing over the last several decades, it remains a rare tumor type. Patients with a history of UCB have a 2% to 4% chance of developing upper tract tumors (synchronous or metachronous); however, this increases up to 25% in patients with carcinoma in situ (CIS) of the bladder or in patients with high-grade tumors adjacent to the ureteral orifices. Following radical cystectomy, an approximately 7% chance of developing UTUCC exists, with the preponderance of this risk being in the first 3 to 4 years after cystectomy.** Patients with high-grade non–muscle-invasive bladder cancer should undergo routine upper tract surveillance, given the increased risk of developing upper tract disease. Nonetheless, the optimal intensity of upper tract surveillance remains largely unknown. It is the authors' practice to perform upper tract surveillance every 1 to 2 years in high-risk patients. Conversely, patients with a history of an incident upper tract tumor have a 20% to 50% chance of eventually developing UCB. For this reason, routine surveillance cystoscopy is necessary in all patients with UTUCC. Metachronous bilateral UTUCC occurs in 2% to 4% of patients with UTUCC.

ETIOLOGY AND NATURAL HISTORY

As in UCB, chemical carcinogenesis is the most important factor in the development of UTUCC. Because of the relatively short transit time of urine through the upper tracts, lesions of the upper tract occur much less often than bladder lesions. Similarly, distal ureteral tumors are more common than proximal. Ureteral UCC occurs in the distal, mid, or proximal ureter in 70%, 20%, and 5% of cases, respectively.

Similar to UCB, the most common risk factor is smoking. Tobacco use is associated with at least a twofold increase in the relative risk for the disease, but this risk may be up to sevenfold higher in long-term, heavy smokers. An uncommon but notable risk factor for the development of UTUCC is Balkan nephropathy, an inflammatory lesion of the renal interstitium endemic to the Balkan region. Balkan nephropathy is characterized by multiple, often bilateral, low-grade upper tract urothelial tumors that may be associated with aristolochic acid intake. Abuse of phenacetin, an analgesic medication withdrawn by the FDA, is considered a historical risk factor for the disease. A few hereditary conditions are associated with UTUCC, including Lynch syndrome II, which is characterized by the early development of nonpolyposis colonic tumors and additional extracolonic neoplasms.

Depth of invasion is the single most important prognostic factor in UTUCC 5-year survival ranges from 100% for noninvasive tumors (Ta) to 40.5% for tumors invading beyond the muscularis (T3). Because of the relative paucity of muscle wall thickness compared to the bladder, UTUCC is considered more likely to be of advanced stage at presentation. Interestingly, the renal parenchyma is thought to prevent spread of T3 tumors in the renal pelvis compared to UTUCC in the ureter.

CLINICAL PRESENTATION

Between 60 to 98% of patients present with either microscopic or gross hematuria. Flank pain can occur in up to 30% of patients, which may be due to obstruction secondary to tumor, blood clot, or a combination of both. Only 15% of UTUCC is identified incidentally; however, these tumors are likely to manifest clinically because UTUCC is rarely discovered at autopsy.

PATHOLOGY AND STAGING

UTUCC and UCB share common pathologic subtypes. The TNM staging systems for UTUCC is analogous to that of UCB (Table 17.4). However, clinical staging in UTUCC is extremely difficult given the technical challenges associated with endoscopic sampling.

DIAGNOSIS

1. Radiographic studies: UTUCC will appear as a radiolucent filling defect in 50% to 75% of cases. CT urography (CTU) has become the most commonly used imaging modality to identify upper tract urothelial tumors. CT urogram can help to differentiate a renal parenchymal mass from a renal pelvic mass, and a ureteral tumor from a radiolucent calculus. Nonetheless, **the distinction between a UTUCC and a central renal parenchymal mass is frequently challenging and commonly requires endoscopic evaluation.** MR urography (MRU) can be used as a substitute for CTU in patients unable to receive iodinated contrast. CT and MR urograms provide useful staging information, including the presence of lymphadenopathy, and

TABLE 17.4 AJCC Eighth Edition Staging System for Upper Tract Urothelial Carcinoma

Primary Tumor (T)
TX—Primary tumor cannot be assessed
T0—No evidence of primary tumor
Ta—Papillary noninvasive carcinoma
Tis—Carcinoma in situ
T1—Tumor invades subepithelial connective tissue
T2—Tumor invades the muscularis
T3—Renal pelvis tumor invades beyond muscularis into peripelvic fat or the renal parenchyma
T3—Ureter tumor invades beyond muscularis into periureteric fat
T4—Tumor invades adjacent organs or through the kidney into perinephric fat

Regional Lymph Nodes (N)[a]
NX—Regional lymph nodes cannot be assessed
N0—No regional lymph node metastasis
N1—Metastasis in a single lymph node 2 cm or less in greatest dimension
N2—Metastasis in single lymph nodes > 2 cm but not > 5 cm in greatest dimension; or multiple lymph nodes, none > 5 cm in greatest dimension
N3—Metastasis in a lymph node > 5 cm in greatest dimension

Distant Metastasis (M)
M0—No distant metastasis
M1—Distant metastasis

[a]Note: Laterality does not affect the N classification.
AJCC, American Joint Committee on Cancer.
(From McKiernan JM, Hansel DE, Bochner BH, et al. Renal pelvis and ureter. In: Amin MB, ed. *AJCC Cancer Staging Manual*. 8th ed. New York: Springer; 2017:749.)

extent of invasion. Despite this, CTU has been shown to mis-stage nearly 40% of patients.

Prior to the widespread adoption of CTU, intravenous excretory urography (IVU) was commonly used. Additionally, retrograde pyelography can be used to evaluate the upper urinary tracts in patients unable to receive intravenous contrast because of CKD, although MRU is also an option. Retrograde pyelograms are also indicated to evaluate pyelocalyceal and ureteral segments not adequately visualized on excretory urography, given the greater sensitivity for the identification of small filling defects.

DIFFERENTIAL DIAGNOSIS

Differential diagnosis of upper urinary tract filling defects includes:

Air
Papilloma
Malakoplakia
Sloughed papilla
Secondary metastasis
Uric acid or matrix calculi
Extrinsic compression (vessels, adenopathy, retroperitoneal fibrosis)
Urinary tuberculosis
Ureteritis or pyelitis cystica
Inverted papilloma
Sarcoma

2. Ureteroscopy: Endoscopic evaluation permits direct visualization and biopsy of the upper tract urothelium. Tumor morphology has some correlation to tumor stage and grade; papillary tumors are more likely to be low grade and noninvasive, whereas sessile tumors are more likely to be high grade and invasive. Urinary cytology is collected prior to biopsy. Given the difficulties in endoscopic sampling, clinical staging remains a challenge. However, **tumor grade on biopsy has been shown to correlate with risk for invasion and may serve as a surrogate. Low-grade tumors are far less likely to be invasive.** These findings have implications for therapy because small, low-grade lesions are frequently amenable to endoscopic laser ablation.
3. Brush biopsy and cytology: This is usually performed during pyeloureterography and may be done by an urologist or radiologist. Although the combination of an upper tract filling defect and a positive renal wash cytology in the same side is sufficient evidence for definitive surgical treatment, ureteroscopy may identify multifocal tumors. A positive renal cytology in the absence of urothelial filling defects mandates further evaluation with ureteroscopy.

TREATMENT OF UTUCC

Multiple treatment options exist for patients with UTUCC, and treatment choice should be individualized based upon disease characteristics, baseline renal function, and functional status.

1. Radical nephroureterectomy with excision of a bladder cuff: Nephroureterectomy remains the preferred treatment for tumors of the renal pelvis and proximal ureter that are large, high grade, and invasive. Furthermore, nephroureterectomy should be considered for tumors that are not amenable to endoscopic ablation. During radical nephroureterectomy, the entire distal ureter, including the intramural portion, should be removed en bloc given the unacceptably high risk of recurrence within a remnant ureteral stump (30% to 60%). Concomitant adrenalectomy may be deferred if preoperative imaging and intraoperative examination reveal the adrenal gland to be normal. The open procedure may be performed via a single thoracoabdominal incision or a two-incision approach (flank and infraumbilical midline).
2. Laparoscopic, hand-assisted laparoscopic, and robotic-assisted laparoscopic nephroureterectomy: These minimally invasive techniques have been popularized and are the preferred approach at many academic and community centers. Although the minimally invasive approach to the kidney is of clear benefit, the laparoscopic management of the bladder cuff remains controversial. Some have advocated that the safest approach includes bladder cuff excision using an open approach via the kidney extraction incision. This may be performed extravesically or through a transvesical approach. Other approaches to the bladder cuff include complete transurethral resection of the intramural ureter and cauterization with endoscopic stapling. These techniques may reduce operative time and avoid an additional incision; however, there are few high-quality data upon which to evaluate the comparative effectiveness and harms of various techniques. Regardless of technique, it is essential to remove the specimen en bloc within a "closed" system because UCC can implant on nonurothelial surfaces. There have been case reports of trocar site and peritoneal seeding after laparoscopic nephroureterectomy when oncologic principles were violated.
3. Endoscopic management: For low-volume, low-grade tumors, a retrograde ureteroscopic approach is preferred. A percutaneous antegrade approach may be considered for larger tumors

in the renal pelvis and proximal ureter, although this is associated with greater morbidity. Regardless of the approach, cytology should be collected and the tumor should be biopsied prior to laser ablation or fulguration. Multiple biopsies are usually required considering the small yield of endoscopic forceps. Although stage cannot be assessed with ureteroscopic biopsies, tumor grade has been found to correlate well with tumor stage. Specifically, approximately 90% of low-grade tumors are found to be noninvasive compared to 30% of high-grade (grade 3) tumors. Greater than 50% of patients suffer recurrence within the ipsilateral collecting system, and, as such, strict surveillance is essential. Over 30% of patients initially managed endoscopically progress to radical nephroureterectomy. These patients do not appear to be at increased risk for metastatic disease compared to those undergoing upfront nephroureterectomy.

4. Ureterectomy: This may be indicated for patients who are not candidates for endoscopic management but who have a compelling indication for NSS. Ureterectomy can be performed open or with various laparoscopic techniques. Segmental ureterectomy with ureteroureterostomy may be considered for proximal or midureteral tumors; however, the ureter distal to the anastomosis remains at high risk for recurrence. For distal tumors, a complete distal ureterectomy can be performed with a direct ureteroneocystostomy. If the length of excised ureter is longer, then a psoas hitch with or without Boari flap can be employed. A downward nephropexy has also been used to reduce the distance of the ureteral defect. Less common approaches include subtotal ureterectomy with ileal interposition or renal autotransplantation.
5. Lymphadenectomy: Regional lymph nodes may be removed at the time of radical nephroureterectomy with little additional operative time and minimal morbidity. However, unlike UCB where an adequate lymphadenectomy provides a clear survival benefit at time of radical cystectomy, the therapeutic benefits of lymphadenectomy for UTUCC have not yet been demonstrated in prospective, randomized trials. This may be because the lymphatic drainage for the renal pelvis and ureter is less well defined and dissection boundaries are variable. Lymphadenectomy does provide valuable prognostic information in

UTUCC, particularly when considering adjuvant chemotherapy. Furthermore, multiple recent studies have demonstrated that lymph node yield may be a consistent predictor of survival. Node-positive patients almost invariably develop early distant metastasis.

6. Chemotherapy
   a. Intrarenal and intraureteral therapy: Instillation of immunotherapeutic and chemotherapeutic agents has been used in an effort to decrease the risk of ipsilateral recurrence after endoscopic management. The same agents used for UCB are used for UTUCC (bacille Calmette-Guérin [BCG] and mitomycin). However, unlike UCB where improvements in recurrence have been clearly demonstrated, data on the use of intrarenal topical therapy remain sparse. The lack of benefit in UTUCC may be the result of insufficient patients in trials or from inadequate delivery systems to the upper tracts. Agents can be instilled through a nephrostomy tube (often after percutaneous management) or retrograde via ureteral reflux by way of stenting.
   b. Systemic chemotherapy: Similar to UCB, urothelial tumors of the upper tract are chemosensitive, and the chemotherapy regimens are modeled after those used in UCB. The historical standard for the management of metastatic UCC is MVAC (methotrexate, vincristine, Adriamycin [doxorubicin], cisplatin) chemotherapy, but combination chemotherapy with cisplatin and gemcitabine has proven to be equivalent with respect to efficacy and results in considerably less morbidity. Unfortunately, many patients with UCC are "unfit" to tolerate cisplatin, largely secondary to baseline renal insufficiency. Radical nephroureterectomy, even more so than radical cystectomy, is likely to reduce renal function, precluding many patients from receiving cisplatin in the adjuvant setting. This has led to increased interest on neoadjuvant cisplatin-based regimens. Prospective trials are ongoing to evaluate the long-term efficacy of adjuvant and neoadjuvant chemotherapy in patients with UTUCC.
7. Follow-up

Patients should be examined every 3 months for at least a year with a history, physical examination, cystoscopy, urinalysis, and cytology. If NSS is undertaken, close endoscopic surveillance is required because up to 75% of early recurrences can be missed with imaging alone. Because synchronous or metachronous bilateral disease can be seen in up to 4% of patients, regular urothelial imaging (CTU, MRU, or retrograde pyelogram) is required at least yearly. Depending on stage, grade, and presence of recurrence, follow-up intervals for UTUCC can be increased in a similar fashion to UCB surveillance to every 6 months for years 2 and 3, then yearly after. Chest radiographs and abdominopelvic cross-sectional imaging are initially obtained every 6 months and then yearly.

Testicular Tumors

GENERAL COMMENTS

Approximately 95% of testis tumors are derived from germ cells, whereas the rest arise from stromal cells. Germ cell tumors (GCTs) of the testis are broadly classified as seminoma or as nonseminoma because of differences in tumor biology and treatment paradigms. **Seminomas are exquisitely sensitive to radiation therapy, whereas both seminoma and nonseminomatous germ cell tumors (NSGCT) respond well to platinum-based combination chemotherapy**. Retroperitoneal lymphadenectomy continues to play an important role in the treatment of NSGCT in both the pre- and postchemotherapy settings and for seminoma in the postchemotherapy setting. Furthermore, the tumor markers beta-human chorionic gonadotropin (beta-HCG) and alpha-fetoprotein (AFP) play an essential role in diagnosis, staging, and treatment planning.

INCIDENCE

In 2013 there will be an estimated 7920 new cases of testis cancer with only 370 deaths attributed to the disease, largely owing to the effectiveness of multimodality therapy.

ETIOLOGY

No definitive cause of testis cancer has been identified, but several risk factors are well established. Cryptorchidism is associated with a four- to sixfold increased risk of developing the disease.

While the preponderance of risk is in the undescended testis, a slightly increased risk of testicular cancer is in the contralateral descended testis. It has been hypothesized that testicular dysgenesis might play a role in the development of testicular cancer, which may explain the link between male factor infertility and increased testicular cancer risk.

Men with a first-degree relative with testicular cancer also have increased risk for the disease. Furthermore, men with a personal history of testicular cancer are at an increased risk for tumor development in the contralateral testis. While the development of a metachronous testis is uncommon, close surveillance by monthly self-examinations is strongly advocated.

EPIDEMIOLOGY

Testicular cancer is most frequently observed in young men and is the most common solid tumor in men between the ages of 20 and 40. Smaller peak incidences exist for men older than 60 years. The incidence of testis cancer is five times higher in White Americans than Black Americans. Additionally, there exists considerable geographic variation in the incidence of testis cancer, with the highest rates observed in Scandinavian countries.

NATURAL HISTORY

GCTs typically arise from areas of intratubular germ cell neoplasia (ITGCN), the testis cancer equivalent of CIS. From these lesions, GCTs may invade beyond the basement membrane to eventually replace some or all of the testicular parenchyma. Epididymal and spermatic cord involvement rarely occurs because tumor growth is contained by the tunica albuginea. **Approximately 50% of patients with ITGCN will progress to an invasive GCT within 5 years, and between 5% and 9% of patients with GCT will have ITGCN in the contralateral testis. Contralateral testis biopsy is no longer advocated; however, the finding of contralateral ITGCN should merit aggressive surveillance or consideration of treatment.** The finding of microlithiasis on ultrasound may be associated with the presence of ITGCN; however, less than 2% with microlithiasis will develop testis cancer.

All GCTs identified in adults should be treated as malignant neoplasms. Metastatic dissemination most often occurs via the lymphatic route, typically first to the retroperitoneum. Several decades ago, the long-term survival rate for advanced testicular cancer was less than 10%, but now it is greater than 90% after the introduction of platinum-based combination chemotherapy. The majority of patients who die from testicular cancer do so within 3 years of diagnosis.

PATHOLOGY

1. Germ cell neoplasms
   a. Seminoma
      1) Classic seminoma: **Classic seminoma accounts for approximately 85% of identified seminomas and 30% of all testicular GCTs.** Mixed tumors that contain any NSGCT components should be classified as NSGCT regardless of the proportion of seminoma. **Approximately 15% will also contain syncytiotrophoblastic elements, which may produce HCG. Thus the finding of an elevated HCG does not preclude the diagnosis of pure seminoma.** Conversely, AFP should never be elevated in a pure seminoma, and therefore regardless of orchiectomy pathology, an elevated AFP should prompt the treating physician to consider the patient to have NSGCT. Peak incidence for seminoma is seen in the fourth and fifth decades of life, one decade later than NSGCT. Grossly, seminomas appear as well-defined, yellow-tan tumors.
      2) Spermatocytic seminoma: Typically seen in older patients (50% are older than 50 years), spermatocytic seminomas account for less than 1% of all testicular tumors. Although it was once considered as a subtype of seminoma, **however, it is now classified as a distinct classification.** These lesions are not thought to arise from ITGCN. These tumors carry a favorable prognosis with little to no propensity for metastatic dissemination.
      3) Anaplastic seminoma: This is also **no longer considered a distinct subtype of seminoma.** While these tumors typically present at a later stage than classic seminoma, when adjusted for stage this pathologic subtype does not carry any prognostic importance.
   b. Embryonal carcinoma
      1) This represents approximately 3% of pure GCTs but may be a component of up to 25% of mixed GCTs.

Embryonal carcinoma is the most undifferentiated NSGCT cell type and is considered an aggressive tumor type that is associated with a high rate of disease progression and metastasis. The proportion of embryonal carcinoma is generally considered to associate with a higher risk of occult metastatic disease in patients with clinical stage I NSGCT.

c. Teratoma
   1) These tumors may be composed of endodermal, mesodermal, or ectodermal elements. It is the second most common testis tumor in children after yolk sac tumor. Teratoma may be classified as mature or immature depending on the degree of differentiation. Teratoma is not responsive to either radiotherapy or chemotherapy, and therefore metastatic deposits can only be cured with surgery. Many arise from transformation of NSGCT after chemotherapy. Teratoma may undergo malignant transformation to develop into a teratocarcinoma or grow to result in deleterious local effects, the latter described as *growing teratoma syndrome*.

d. Choriocarcinoma
   1) This typically represents less than 1% of all NSGCT. It usually presents with metastatic disease and very high serum levels of HCG. **Choriocarcinoma has the propensity to metastasize hematogenously, and, as such, lung and brain metastases are common.** Because of tumor vascularity, brain metastasis is associated with a 4% to 10% risk of intracranial hemorrhage during chemotherapy.

e. Yolk sac tumor
   1) This is the most common NSGCT in children. It is a rare tumor type in its pure form but may be present in up to 25% of mixed GCTs. Nearly all yolk sac tumors produce AFP, but not HCG. Approximately 50% of yolk sac tumors have the pathognomonic finding of Schiller-Duval bodies on microscopy.

2. Nongerm cell neoplasms
   a. Specialized gonadal stromal tumors
      1) Leydig cell tumor: This constitutes 1% to 3% of all testis tumors; it may present with gynecomastia because of the aromatization of excess androgens produced by

the tumor. Approximately 10% of adult Leydig cell tumors are malignant; however, these tumors never are considered malignant in prepubertal patients. Histologic determination of malignancy is unreliable; therefore malignancy is often only identified by the presence of metastases.

2) Sertoli cell tumor: This is less than 1% of testis tumors, and 10% are malignant. As with Leydig cell tumors, histology is unreliable, and malignancy is identified by the presence of metastases.
3) Gonadoblastoma: This is associated with a dysgenetic gonads and patients suffering from disorders of sex development. Bilateral orchiectomy is indicated because 50% of such gonads will develop into malignant GCTs.

STAGING

Unique to testis cancer, the AJCC staging system includes a separate category for tumor marker status to aid in identifying patients with high risk for relapse (Table 17.5). Fortunately, the vast majority of men with newly diagnosed testis cancer enjoy favorable 5-year survival. Indeed, the 5-year survival rate for patients with clinically localized disease is 99%, for patients with nodal

TABLE 17.5 AJCC Eighth Edition Staging System for Testicular Cancer

Primary Tumor (T)[a]
The extent of primary tumor is usually classified after radical orchiectomy, and for this reason a pathologic stage is assigned.
pTX—Primary tumor cannot be assessed
pT0—No evidence of primary tumor (e.g., histologic scar in testis)
pTis—Intratubular germ cell neoplasia (CIS)
pT1—Tumor limited to the testis and epididymis without vascular or lymphatic invasion; tumor may invade the tunica albuginea but not the tunica vaginalis
pT2—Tumor limited to the testis and epididymis with vascular or lymphatic invasion; tumor extending through the tunica albuginea with involvement of the tunica vaginalis
pT3—Tumor invades the spermatic cord with or without vascular and lymphatic invasion
pT4—Tumor invading the scrotum with or without vascular and lymphatic invasion

Continued

TABLE 17.5 AJCC Eighth Edition Staging System for Testicular Cancer—cont'd

Regional Lymph Nodes (N)
Clinical
NX—Regional lymph nodes cannot be assessed
N0—No regional lymph node metastasis
N1—Metastasis with a lymph node mass 2 cm or less in greatest dimension; multiple lymph nodes, none > 2 cm in greatest dimension
N2—Metastasis with a lymph node mass > 2 cm but not > 5 cm in greatest dimension; or multiple lymph nodes, any one mass > 2 cm but not > 5 cm in greatest dimension
N3—Metastasis with a lymph node mass > 5 cm in greatest dimension

Distant Metastasis (M)
M0—No distant metastasis
M1—Distant metastasis
M1a—Nonregional nodal or pulmonary metastasis
M1b—Distant metastasis other than to nonregional lymph node and lungs

Serum Tumor Markers (S)
SX—Marker studies not available or not performed
S0—Markers within normal limits
S1—LDH < 1.5 × N[b] and HCG (mIU/mL)< 5000 and AFP < 1000 (ng/mL) < 1000
S2—LDH 1.5–10 × N or HCG (mIU/mL) 5000–50,000 or AFP (ng/mL) 1000–10,000
S3—LDH > 10 × N or HCG (mIU/mL) > 50,000 or AFP (ng/mL) > 10,000

[a]Note: Except for pTis and pT4, extent of primary tumor is classified by radical orchiectomy. TX may be used for other categories in the absence of radical orchiectomy.
[b]N indicates the upper limit of normal for the LDH assay.
AFP, Alpha-fetoprotein; *AJCC*, American Joint Committee on Cancer; *CIS*, carcinoma in situ; *HCG*, human chorionic gonadotropin; *LDH*, lactate dehydrogenase.
(From Brimo F, Srigley JR, Ryan CJ, et al. Testis. In: Amin MB, ed. *AJCC Cancer Staging Manual*. 8th ed. New York: Springer; 2017:727. [Corrected at 4th printing, 2018.])

metastases is 96%, and for patients with distant metastatic disease is 72%.

CLINICAL PRESENTATION

The most common presenting symptom is a painless testicular mass. A 4- to 6-month delay in presentation is not uncommon; however, treatment delay is associated with more advanced disease and worse outcomes. **Approximately 10% to 15% of patients will present with symptoms of metastatic disease, such as cough, abdominal or supraclavicular mass, back pain, and lymphadenopathy**. Certainly, any young male presenting with a retroperitoneal mass should undergo thorough evaluation of the scrotal contents. Gynecomastia may be present in up to 2% of men secondary to elevation of HCG or the effect of tumor estradiol synthesis with Leydig cell tumors.

DIAGNOSIS AND STAGING

1. Transscrotal ultrasound can confirm the presence of an intraparenchymal testicular mass, rule out benign processes such as a hydrocele or epididymitis, and effectively evaluate the contralateral gonad. The incidence of bilateral GCT is approximately 2% with the majority of bilateral tumors arising in a metachronous fashion. Pathologic discordance between primary tumors bilaterally can occur in 30% of such cases.
2. Radical inguinal orchiectomy: Treatment of the primary tumor requires early clamping of the spermatic cord near the internal ring and complete removal of the testis. **While partial orchiectomy may be considered in select cases, the standard of care remains radical inguinal orchiectomy**. Scrotal orchiectomy or percutaneous biopsy should never be performed because of the theoretical risk of alteration to the lymphatic drainage of the testis resulting in inguinal metastases.
3. **Staging imaging involves a posterior anterior (PA) and lateral chest x-ray (CXR) and CT scan of the abdomen and pelvis with contrast.** In the absence of lymphadenopathy on CT of the abdomen and pelvis, a CT scan of the chest is generally not preferred. Additionally, brain MRI and nuclear medicine bone scan should be considered if clinically indicated. Lastly, sperm banking should be discussed with patients before undergoing chemotherapy or radiation therapy.
4. Tumor markers
   a. Over all stages, 90% of patients with nonseminomatous tumors will have an elevation of HCG and/or AFP. After therapy, tumor markers should display a logarithmic pattern of decrease in accordance with their half-lives. Sustained elevation of markers or slow decreases after orchiectomy or retroperitoneal lymph node dissection (RPLND)

suggests residual disease; however, normalization of markers is not definite evidence of complete surgical cure.

b. HCG: This is a heterodimeric protein with immunologically distinct chains. Circulating levels are extremely low (1 ng/mL) in normal males. The syncytiotrophoblastic tissue of some GCTs produces HCG. It can therefore be detected in almost all choriocarcinomas, 40% to 60% of embryonal cell carcinomas, and 5% to 10% of pure seminomas. The half-life for HCG is roughly 24 hours. Because beta-HCG shares structural homology with luteinizing hormone (LH), spurious elevations may occur in patients with hypogonadism secondary to gonadal failure.

c. AFP: This is an oncofetal protein detected in testis and liver tumors. It is produced by yolk sac elements that may or may not be histologically recognized. This substance is *not* produced in pure choriocarcinoma or pure seminoma. The presence of elevated AFP in a patient with histologic seminoma precludes the diagnosis of pure seminoma. The half-life of AFP is 5 to 7 days.

d. Lactate dehydrogenase (LDH): This general cellular enzyme is not specific for testicular lesions but is thought to correlate with tumor burden. It may play some role in monitoring patients with advanced seminoma and in marker negative patients with NSGCT and persistent disease.

TREATMENT AFTER ORCHIECTOMY

1. Seminoma

   a. Clinical stage I: Approximately 80% of patients diagnosed with seminoma will have clinical stage I disease. Seminomas are sensitive to both radiation and platinum-based chemotherapy. **Accepted treatment options for clinical stage I include surveillance, primary radiotherapy, and primary chemotherapy with single-agent carboplatin.** Fortunately, the long-term cancer control is nearly 100% with any of these modalities. **The decision whether to pursue surveillance or active treatment rests in the presence or absence of risk factors for disease progression, the individual patient's preferences, and the morbidity associated with each therapeutic strategy.** Risk factors for disease progression in seminoma include tumor size greater than 4 cm and rete testis invasion. Patients with zero, one, or both risk factors have a 5-year relapse risk of 12%, 16%, and 32%, respectively.

1) Surveillance: This involves careful monitoring with initiation of treatment at the first sign of disease progression. Monitoring includes frequent tumor markers, chest radiographs, and abdominopelvic CT scans at prespecified intervals, which grow longer with increasing time since diagnosis. Given the fact that relapse-free survival for all patients with clinical stage I seminoma is approximately 80%, surveillance prevents overtreatment, and thus the morbidity of either chemotherapy or radiotherapy, in 8 out of 10 men. Additionally, cancer-specific survival after salvage therapy approaches 100%, lending further support to surveillance. Treatment at the time of relapse is dictated by the stage at relapse and requires chemotherapy, radiotherapy, or both. Surveillance for clinical stage I seminoma is limited by the need for long-term observation given that relapse after 5 years is not uncommon. There is some concern over the long-term consequences of multiple CT scans required for surveillance. Unlike NSGCTs, serum tumor markers have limited utility with detecting recurrence in seminoma.
2) Primary radiotherapy: This generally involves delivery of approximately 25 Gy in a "dog leg" pattern to the retroperitoneum and ipsilateral pelvis. Recurrence within the radiation field occurs in less than 1% of the cases, thereby obviating the need for frequent abdominopelvic CT scans after radiotherapy. Side effects include acute toxicity of treatment (nausea, vomiting, hematologic), oligospermia, and hematologic abnormalities. The incidence of secondary malignancy has been estimated to be as high as 18% within 25 years of radiation.
3) Primary chemotherapy: Primary chemotherapy involves one or two cycles of single-agent carboplatin as an alternative to radiation. This approach is associated with a 5-year relapse-free survival over 90% with less late toxicity compared to radiation. Because relapse usually occurs within the retroperitoneum, abdominopelvic CT

scan cannot be excluded in follow-up surveillance as it can be for primary radiation.

i. Clinical stage IIA and IIB: From 10% to 15% of patients with seminoma will have CSIIA-B. Standard treatment at most centers is "dog leg" radiation with 25 to 35 Gy.

ii. Clinical stage IIC and III: See later.

iii. Postchemotherapy residual mass: See later.

2. Nonseminomatous GCTs
   a. Clinical stage I: As in clinical stage I seminoma, numerous therapeutic options exist for men with clinical stage I NSGCT, including surveillance, primary RPLND, and primary chemotherapy. Again, long-term survival is nearly 100% for RPLND, primary chemotherapy, and surveillance, so treatment decision-making must be individualized to optimize patient satisfaction. For 70% to 80% of patients, orchiectomy alone will be curative. To avoid overtreatment, a risk-adapted approach is used at most centers. Risk factors for occult metastasis include the presence of lymphovascular invasion in the orchiectomy specimen and predominance of embryonal carcinoma (usually greater than 40% to 45%) in the orchiectomy specimen.
      1) Surveillance: Given the high cure rate with orchiectomy alone and excellent salvage rate in relapsed patients, surveillance is a reasonable option for most patients, particularly those without risk factors for occult metastasis. As in any disease requiring long-term observation, one disadvantage of surveillance is the need for long-term cross-sectional imaging, with the associated risk of secondary neoplasia. The use of MRI technology has reduced this risk, although multiple factors contribute to the ability to use serial MRI, including familiarity of the operating radiologist. High rates of noncompliance with surveillance protocols have been reported, and certainly the ability of each patient to commit to observation should be evaluated prior to undertaking surveillance.
      2) RPLND: This provides effective control of the most common site of metastasis, the retroperitoneum. The incidence of teratoma is 15% to 25% for those with occult metastasis. Only RPLND can treat teratoma because it is

resistant to both chemotherapy and radiation. Different RPLND templates have been proposed based on lymphatic drainage of the involved testis. Controversy exists over the use of unilateral templates. Only the full bilateral template is associated with a low enough retroperitoneal recurrence rate (less than 2%) that abdominopelvic CT scan can be eliminated in follow-up surveillance. Nerve-sparing techniques can reduce but not eliminate the risk of retrograde ejaculation. RPLND can be technically challenging and is best reserved for high-volume centers.

3) Primary chemotherapy: Two cycles of bleomycin, etoposide, and cisplatin (BEP) offer the greatest chance of relapse-free survival; however, long-term surveillance with abdominopelvic CT is still required to monitor for retroperitoneal recurrence. While the presence of teratoma on the orchiectomy specimen has been associated with its presence in the retroperitoneum, the absence of teratoma on the orchiectomy specimen does not rule out the presence of retroperitoneal teratoma. As previously mentioned, teratoma is resistant to chemotherapy and remains subject to surgical control. It is important to recognize the risk of late cardiovascular toxicity and secondary malignancy with chemotherapy; however, the incremental risk associated with two cycles of BEP remains largely unknown.

b. Clinical stage IS: The presence of elevated serum tumor markers after orchiectomy without clinical evidence of metastatic disease is treated as clinical stage IIC-III (see later).

c. Clinical stage IIA and IIB: Both RPLND and induction chemotherapy (Etoposide/cisplatin [EP] × 4, BEP × 3) offer excellent overall survival rates to patients with radiographically evident nodal disease. Induction chemotherapy is generally preferred in patients with elevated tumor markers or in the presence of bulky lymphadenopathy (greater than 3 cm), and RPLND is preferred as initial therapy for those at high risk of harboring teratoma but low risk for systemic disease. For patients who do not fall into either of these groups, the decision between RPLND and induction chemotherapy is controversial and in all cases should be tailored to individual patient preferences.

1) Benefits of primary RPLND include that it allows the 15% to 35% of patients with pathologically negative

lymph nodes to avoid unnecessary chemotherapy and it eliminates the need for future therapy in approximately 30% of patients with teratoma. The disadvantage of primary RPLND largely surrounds surgical morbidity, in particular, a considerable risk of ejaculatory dysfunction (10% to 20%).

2) Induction chemotherapy with BEP × 3 or EP × 4 results in a complete response for 60% to 80% of patients. Furthermore, chemotherapy regimens are relatively well established, and, compared with RPLND, have potentially less variation with regard to treatment quality. The disadvantage of induction chemotherapy remains the late toxicity associated with chemotherapy and, if relapse occurs, the possibility of establishing chemoresistance.

3. Postchemotherapy residual mass:
   a. Seminoma: **Residual masses are present on 60% to 80% of abdominopelvic CT scans in seminoma patients after first-line chemotherapy; however, the majority of these masses will spontaneously involute within 18 months.** The use of RPLND in the treatment of postchemotherapy residual disease remains controversial. There is a significant desmoplastic reaction within the retroperitoneum from chemotherapy rendering postchemotherapy RPLND for seminoma technically challenging. Furthermore, unlike NSGCT, there is less concern for teratoma and malignant transformation with seminoma. For masses smaller than 3 cm in size, the risk of viable tumor is less than 5%. Fluorodeoxyglucose positron emission tomography (FDG-PET) has demonstrated the ability to identify which seminoma patients with a residual mass have a viable tumor. Therefore observation can be safely employed for seminoma patients with residual masses less than 3 cm and for masses greater than 3 cm that are PET-negative.
   b. NSGCT: Management of the postchemotherapy mass in patients with NSGCT is considerably different than for patients with seminoma. Approximately 40% to 70% of patients have a residual mass greater than 1 cm after chemotherapy. **The distribution of histologies in residual NSGCT masses is as follows: 40% necrosis, 45% teratoma, and 15% viable malignancy.** Therefore at our institution, patients with a postchemotherapy mass greater than 1 cm

will undergo a postchemotherapy RPLND. Unlike in seminoma where the risk of teratoma is quite low, the significant risk of teratoma renders FDG-PET unreliable given the fact that teratoma is not PET-avid. Thus FDG-PET is not recommended for use in patients with NSGCT. **Complete resection of the residual mass is paramount, and bilateral RPLND should be performed with the use of nerve-sparing techniques wherever possible.**

4. Advanced testicular cancer
   a. Clinical stage IIC and III seminoma and NSGCT are treated similarly with induction chemotherapy, according to the International Germ Cell Consensus Classification of risk (Table 17.6). Chemotherapy regimens are platinum

TABLE 17.6 International Germ Cell Consensus Risk Classification for Metastatic Germ Cell Tumor

Prognosis	Seminoma	NSGCT
Good	Any primary; without nonpulmonary visceral metastasis; normal AFP, any HCG or LDH	Testis/retroperitoneal primary; without nonpulmonary visceral metastasis with good tumor markers: AFP < 1000 ng/mL, HCG < 5000 mIU/mL, LDH < 1.5× upper limit normal
Intermediate	Any primary; nonpulmonary visceral metastasis present; normal AFP, any HCG or LDH	Testis/retroperitoneal primary; without nonpulmonary visceral metastasis; with intermediate markers: AFP 1000–10,000 ng/mL, or HCG 5000–50,000 mIU/mL, or LDH 1.5×–10× upper limit normal
Poor	No patients with seminoma are classified as poor risk	Mediastinal primary; or nonpulmonary visceral metastasis present; or poor tumor markers: AFP > 10,000 ng/mL, or HCG > 50,000 mIU/mL, or LDH > 10× upper limit normal

AFP, Alpha-fetoprotein; *HCG*, human chorionic gonadotropin; *LDH*, lactate dehydrogenase.

based with cisplatin being superior to carboplatin in randomized trials for advanced testicular cancer. Attempts have been made to avoid bleomycin in low-risk patients because of the pulmonary toxicity.

1) Seminoma: Ninety percent of advanced seminoma is classified as good risk and can be treated with BEP × 3 or EP × 4 for a 5-year overall survival of 91%. The 10% of advanced seminoma with nonpulmonary metastasis is classified as intermediate risk and treated with BEP × 4 for a 5-year overall survival of 79%. Poor prognosis tumors do not exist for seminoma.
2) NSGCT: For good-risk patients, BEP × 3 or EP × 4 has a 5-year overall survival of greater than 90%. BEP × 4 is the standard for intermediate risk and poor risk with 5-year overall survival rates of 79% and 48%, respectively. Etoposide-ifosfamide-cisplatin (VIP) × 4 has been also been used for intermediate- and poor-risk NSGCT; however, it is limited by increased hematologic and genitourinary toxicity.

5. Patient surveillance
6. For detailed guidelines concerning various surveillance protocols, see the NCCN Clinical Practice Guidelines in Oncology (www.nccn.org).

Additional content, including Self-Assessment Questions and Suggested Readings, may be accessed at www.ExpertConsult.com.

Adult Genitourinary Cancer: Urethral and Penile

Zachary L. Smith, MD

Penile Cancer

GENERAL CONSIDERATIONS

Penile cancer remains an uncommon diagnosis in the United States, representing only 0.5% of all malignancies. Nonetheless, the disease accounts for up to 10% of all male cancers in the developing world. In the United States, there was an estimated 2200 cases of penile cancer in 2020 with approximately 440 deaths from the disease, a rate that has increased over the last decade. Penile cancer has been described in men of all ages, with a sharp increase in incidence in the fifth decade of life. Because of its rarity, little high-quality evidence exists upon which to base clinical practice.

1. **Benign lesions**
   a. **Bowenoid papulosis:** This is an uncommon form of penile intraepithelial neoplasia thought to be caused by human papillomavirus (HPV) type 16. It presents with raised, hyperpigmented papules usually on the penile shaft in younger men. **Although histology of this lesion resembles squamous cell carcinoma in situ (CIS), the course of Bowenoid papulosis is universally benign.** Unlike the similarly named Bowen disease, Bowenoid papulosis never progresses to an invasive carcinoma. Given the benign course of this disease, less morbid interventions such as simple excision, cryoablation, topical 5-fluorouracil, or laser photocoagulation are recommended.
2. **Premalignant lesions**
   a. **Condyloma acuminata (genital warts):** These lesions are caused by HPV infection and may involve the glans, prepuce, or shaft of the penis. They are generally considered

benign papillomatous growths; however, HPV virus types 16, 18, 31, 33, 35, 39, 45, 51, 52, 58, and 59 are associated with anogenital cancers. They are exophytic in nature and do not invade deeper tissues. Several topical treatment options are available for condyloma, including podophyllotoxin 0.5%, trichloroacetic acid, imiquimod 5% cream. Patients who desire immediate wart removal or those with lesions refractory to topical therapy are candidates for cryoablation with liquid nitrogen, local excision with electrofulguration, or CO_2 laser ablation. **It is important to note that treatment of condyloma has not been proven to diminish transmission between partners nor prevent progression to malignancy.** Prevention should be reinforced in all patients with condyloma due to the high risk of transmission through sexual contact and the etiologic association of HPV infection with cervical cancer in women. The HPV quadrivalent vaccine was found to be safe in males and females between the ages of 9 and 26 years. It is recommended for the prevention of condyloma acuminata in both genders. The incidence of cervical cancer is expected to decrease over time with the widespread utilization of the HPV vaccine. A decrease in the incidence of other HPV-associated anogenital cancers, including penile cancer, is also expected; however, further study will be required to document these epidemiologic phenomena.

b. **Buschke-Löwenstein tumor:** This lesion is also known as *giant condyloma acuminatum* or *verrucous carcinoma.* **Buschke-Löwenstein tumors differ from standard condyloma acuminatum in that they do invade deep structures. They harbor very low metastatic potential but often become locally destructive and require resection.** A penile-sparing approach should be undertaken, though due to the nature of the tumor may not be achievable. Due to the high rate of recurrence, patients should be surveilled regularly after resection.

c. **Leukoplakia:** This term describes a white cutaneous plaque that may be hypertrophic or atrophic. It typically results from chronic irritation. **Leukoplakia is considered a premalignant condition to the development of squamous cell carcinoma (SCC).** 10%–20% of lesions show evidence of dysplasia. Circumcision and surgical excision are the preferred treatments, but radiation therapy has also been used.

d. **Balanitis xerotica obliterans (BXO):** This subcategory of lichen sclerosus atrophicus involving the male genitalia is associated with destructive inflammation, phimosis, urethral stricture, meatal stenosis, and penile SCC. These hypopigmented, papular, or atrophic appearing lesions typically involve the glans penis, meatus, or fossa navicularis. **BXO most commonly presents in middle-aged uncircumcised men complaining of meatal stenosis, penile pain, painful erections, or dyspareunia. Initial management should include biopsy to exclude the presence of carcinoma, followed by topical steroids.** 2.3%–5.8% of BXO patients progress to SCC; therefore, long-term follow-up and self-examination are recommended, with low threshold for biopsy of any suspicious lesions.

e. **Pseudoepitheliomatous micaceous and keratotic balanitis:** This lesion is a variant of balanitis that appears as thick, adherent scales on the glans. While usually asymptomatic, the patient can experience disruption of the urinary stream and irritation of the skin. This condition is not associated with HPV and its etiology is currently unknown. The lesion should be biopsied for confirmation and can be treated with local excision, laser ablation, 5FU cream, steroids, or cryoablation depending on the stage, size of lesion, and patient preference. Even with a response to therapy, this lesion tends to recur and the patient should be surveilled with physical exam and repeat biopsies if necessary.

f. **Cutaneous horn:** This lesion is one that is usually found on the face and scalp but in rare cases can occur on the penis. It presents as a solid, protuberant, horn-like keratin outgrowth. **There is an association with HPV 16 infection and thus is also associated with SCC.** The lesion should be excised with a margin of tissue at the base to prevent recurrence and to assess for malignancy. Postoperatively, the patient should be surveilled for recurrence of the lesion at first with office follow-up, then by self-exam.

3. CIS

a. **Erythroplasia of Queyrat:** If involving the glans or prepuce, CIS is also known as Erythroplasia of Queyrat. These lesions appear as well-marginated, velvety red patches but may develop into painful ulcers. **There is a 10%–33% rate of progression to invasive carcinoma of the penis and this should be treated. However, progression to metastatic disease is rare.** If noninvasive on biopsy, consider local treatment with topical 5FU, 5% imiquimod cream, laser ablation, or local excision with a 5-mm margin. If invasive on biopsy, proceed to management of invasive penile carcinoma.

b. **Bowen disease:** If involving the penile shaft, CIS is known as Bowen disease. On exam, Bowen disease appears as scaly, erythematous, well-marginated plaques. Some lesions appear ulcerated or crusted. As with Erythroplasia of Queyrat, metastasis is rare but 5% of lesions progress to invasive carcinoma. **Lesions on the prepuce can be safely treated with circumcision.** Although the standard management of CIS remains local excision with a 5-mm margin, other alternatives include laser ablation, topical 5-fluorouracil, and imiquimod cream. These alternatives achieve acceptable local control with organ preservation. It is essential to perform a deep biopsy to rule out invasive carcinoma, as mentioned earlier.

4. Other

a. **Kaposi sarcoma of the penis: Kaposi sarcoma is associated with human herpesvirus 8 (HHV 8) and is highly associated with immunosuppression.** Lesions are painful, bluish in color, can bleed, and can even cause urethral obstruction. Kaposi sarcoma is sometimes the presenting symptom of HIV infection that has progressed to AIDS, but is associated with other types of immunosuppression as well. Lesions will often recede if the immunosuppression is reversed. Treatment includes excision and radiation, though if a large area is involved partial penectomy may be necessary.

b. **Melanoma of the penis:** Like all penile cancers, melanoma of the penis is rare. It presents as blue-black or reddish brown papules, plaques, or ulcers, typically on the glans penis. Due to the high risk of metastasis, a diagnosis of melanoma requires wide local excision with margins dependent on Breslow depth. This often may require partial or total penectomy. Additionally, these patients will typically require modified bilateral inguinal lymph node dissection or sentinel lymph node biopsy. Contrarily, if the melanoma is confined to the prepuce, circumcision followed by close surveillance may be a reasonable treatment plan, again dependent on invasiveness.

c. **Sarcoma of the penis:** Sarcoma of the penis is exceedingly rare, and with many sarcomas, presentation is varied. Wide excision with partial penectomy is recommended for superficial tumors, but if deeper structures are invaded, total penectomy must be pursued. Regional and distant metastases are rare in this disease.

d. **Paget disease of the penis:** Paget disease of the penis is a rare condition that is associated with other primary genitourinary (GU) malignancies. It presents with a well-demarcated erythematous plaque that can only be identified as Paget disease on histology. Treatment includes wide local excision with intraoperative frozen section, as well as thorough workup for possible occult GU malignancy. If the disease is invasive on initial biopsy, neoadjuvant chemotherapy may be considered.

e. **Basal cell carcinoma of the penis:** This entity is exceedingly rare with only 30 reported cases in the literature. However, outcomes are excellent, with simple resection being curative in all studied cases.

f. **Metastases to the penis:** The penis is a relatively rare site of metastasis for any malignancy and the primary anatomic location are the corporal bodies, given the hematogenous spread of many cancers. Due to tumor obstruction of vascular, priapism can be a presenting symptom, as can penile swelling and urinary obstruction. Metastasis involving the penis is usually an advanced finding with regard to the primary tumor, and the majority of patients presenting with penile metastasis are deceased within 1 year. Any surgical intervention in this setting is palliative.

5. **Invasive squamous cell carcinoma of the penis**

a. **Etiology:** The development of penile carcinoma has long been associated with poor hygiene and exposure to irritants, carcinogens, or possible viral pathogens. **Neonatal circumcision has been shown to be protective against the development of penile cancer; however, adult circumcision fails to provide the same risk reduction.** Infection with

HPV 16 or HPV 18 is also thought to be a risk factor for penile cancer and is associated with 30% to 60% of penile carcinomas. Lichen sclerosis, tobacco usage, and genital ultraviolet radiation are also associated with penile carcinoma development. Penile SCC has *not* been proven to be associated with marijuana use, alcohol use, or non-HPV STDs (Table 18.1).

b. **Natural history overview:** Carcinoma of the penis usually begins as a small lesion on the glans or prepuce, and diagnosis is often delayed, given inattention to personal hygiene or anxiety and shame related to the finding (Table 18.2). Invasion is usually direct and capable of destroying surrounding tissue. **Metastases from penile cancer travel via the lymphatics in an invariable pattern: first to superficial inguinal lymph nodes, then deep inguinal nodes, then pelvic nodes. The right and left lymphatic drainage systems are interconnected, so metastatic deposits may travel to the contralateral lymphatic landing zones at every level.** Distant metastases typically occur late in the disease after inguinal lymph nodes become clinically evident.

TABLE 18.1 Risk Factors for Invasive SCC of the Penis

Uncircumcised or circumcised after adolescence
Phimosis
Tobacco use (all forms)
Number of sexual partners
HPV positivity (types 16, 18, 31, 33)
Lichen sclerosis
UV light exposure

HPV, Human papillomavirus; *SCC*, squamous cell carcinoma; *UV*, ultraviolet light.

TABLE 18.2 Lesion Frequency by Location

Location	Percentage
Glans	48%
Prepuce	21%
Corona	6%
Shaft	< 2%

Typically the primary lesion must erode Buck fascia to achieve hematogenous spread. The most common sites of distant metastasis include the bone, liver, and lung. Metastases to solid organs or bones occur in less than 10% of cases. Death is usually secondary to involvement of regional nodes, which results in skin necrosis, chronic infection, sepsis, malnutrition, or hemorrhage secondary to erosion into the femoral vessels. **If untreated, most patients will die within 2 years of diagnosis.**

c. **Clinical features:** The primary penile lesion may assume the appearance of a nodule, wart-like exophytic growth, or ulceration. **Phimosis is present in as many as 50% of patients and may obscure the lesion, contributing to delays in detection.** Between 15% and 50% of patients with carcinoma of the penis have a delay in presentation of over 1 year from onset of symptoms. **Lymph nodes are palpably enlarged in nearly 50% of patients.**

Diagnosis depends on an adequate tissue biopsy or tumor excision. The tumor should be assessed for depth of invasion, lymphovascular invasion, perineural invasion, and histologic grade. Penile carcinoma is broadly classified into high grade and low grade by Broders' classification. These histologic features of the biopsy have important prognostic significance and help determine the need for subsequent inguinal lymph node management.

Histologic subtypes are varied and contribute to overall prognosis. Approximately **70–80% of tumors exhibit low-grade histology.** A high-grade tumor on histology correlates with a higher risk of nodal metastasis and is associated with a higher stage at diagnosis. Additional high-risk histologic features include lymphovascular and perineural invasion; these are associated with increased risk of nodal metastases (Table 18.3).

TABLE 18.3 Subtypes of Penile Cancer

Favorable	Intermediate	Unfavorable
Verruciform	Typical squamous	Basaloid Sarcomatous

d. **Diagnosis:** Preoperative staging of penile cancer can be challenging. Tumor size, location, fixation, and involvement of the corporal bodies should be assessed by physical examination. Laboratory studies should include chemistries, as **hypercalcemia of malignancy can be seen in penile cancer and must be treated.** Contrast-enhanced penile magnetic resonance imaging (MRI) is the most sensitive imaging modality for evaluating depth of invasion of the primary lesion and surgical planning. Careful bilateral palpation of the inguinal regions is of extreme importance and is highly sensitive for detection of nodal metastasis. **Computed tomography (CT) imaging of clinically negative groins has not been demonstrated to improve staging, except in patients whose body habitus precludes thorough physical exam.** If palpable inguinal adenopathy is present, CT chest/abdomen/pelvis is then helpful for surgical planning and identification of distant metastases. Fluorodeoxyglucose-positron emission tomography (FDG-PET) imaging and fine-needle aspiration (FNA) lymph node biopsy have not been proven to sufficiently aid decision-making prior to possible lymph node dissection.

e. **Staging:** Staging for penile carcinoma most commonly uses the unified Union Internationale Contre le Cancer (UICC) and American Joint Committee on Cancer (AJCC) staging system (Tables 18.4). Like many other malignancies, 5-year survival is largely contingent upon stage at presentation. Grading has been adapted from the grading system for skin cancer, where grades 1 and 2 represent low-grade cancers and grades 3 and 4 represent high grade. Patients with disease localized to the penis demonstrate 5-year survival rates of 80% to 90%, whereas patients with nodal disease

TABLE 18.4 Penile Cancer Survival

Stage at Presentation	5-Year Survival
Localized to penis	80%–90%
Nodal disease	50%–60%
Extranodal extension	5%–18%
Distant metastases	5%–15%

TABLE 18.5 AJCC Penile Cancer Staging

Primary Tumor	
Tx	Primary tumor cannot be assessed
T0	No evidence of primary tumor
Tis	Carcinoma in situ
Ta	Noninvasive verrucous carcinoma
T1a	Tumor invades subepithelial connective tissue without lymphovascular invasion and is not poorly differentiated (Grade 3–4)
T1b	Tumor invades subepithelial connective tissue with lymphovascular invasion or is poorly differentiated (Grade 3–4)
T2	Tumor invades corpus spongiosum
T3	Tumor invades corpus cavernosum
T4	Invasion of adjacent structures (scrotum, prostate, pubic bone)
Regional Lymph Nodes	**Clinical Stage**
cNx	Regional lymph nodes cannot be assessed
cN0	No palpable or visibly enlarged inguinal lymph nodes
cN1	Palpable, mobile, unilateral lymph node
cN2	Palpable, mobile, bilateral lymph nodes
cN3	Palpable fixed inguinal nodal mass or pelvic lymphadenopathy (unilateral or bilateral)
	Pathologic Stage
pNx	Regional lymph nodes cannot be assessed
pN0	No regional lymph node metastasis
pN1	Metastasis in single inguinal node
pN2	Metastasis in multiple or bilateral inguinal nodes
pN3	Extranodal extension of lymph node metastasis or pelvic lymph node metastasis (unilateral or bilateral)
Distant Metastasis	
M0	No distant metastasis
M1	Distant metastasis

Continued

TABLE 18.5 AJCC Penile Cancer Staging—cont'd

Stage	
0	Tis or Ta, N0, M0
1	T1a, N0, M0
2	T1b, T2, or T3, N0, M0
3	T1-3, N1, M0 or T1-3, N2, M0
4	T4 any N, M0 or any T, N3, M0, or any T, any N, M1

(From Amin MB, Edge S, Greene F, eds. *AJCC Cancer Staging Manual*. 8th ed. New York City, NY: Springer International Publishing: American Joint Commission on Cancer; 2017.)

and distant metastatic disease have 5-year survival rates of 50% to 60% and 5% to 15%, respectively. Greater lymph node density which is calculated as number of lymph nodes positive out of total nodes identified on pathology predicts worse survival (Tables 18.5).

f. **Treatment of primary lesion**

Suspicious penile lesions should undergo biopsy with a deep margin to ensure satisfactory staging. **An organ-sparing approach should only be considered in tumors with favorable features: Ta, Tis, or T1 with low-grade histology.** The goal for organ sparing is to maintain penile length, function, and aesthetics without compromising survival. Although acceptable oncologic outcomes can be achieved with this approach, these patients are at greater risk of local recurrence and must have close long-term follow-up. It is important to recognize that patient compliance and reliability with regard to long-term follow-up may limit the pursuit of penile-sparing techniques. Encouragingly, repeat organ-sparing techniques performed on recurrent tumors have been effective if implemented early.

1) **Limited surgical excision:** Although historically a 2-cm tumor margin was thought necessary, this has recently been challenged. **Several series have shown no detriment to oncologic outcomes with a margin as close as 5 mm, although a 1-cm margin is more commonly reported.** Intraoperative frozen sections should be performed to

ensure microscopically negative margins. Limited excision of glans or shaft lesions can be performed with or without the use of grafts or flaps for reconstruction depending on size of defect. Lesions confined to the prepuce may be treated by circumcision alone with satisfactory oncologic outcome. Recurrence rate in this population is between 4% and 9%.

2) **Glans resurfacing:** This minimally invasive procedure consists of subdermal dissection of skin and connective tissue from the corpus spongiosum. This procedure is primarily recommended for treatment of CIS. **Positive margins are common, but these are treatable with topical therapy.**
3) **Topical creams:** Both 5-fluorouracil cream and 5% imiquimod cream have been used to treat Tis or Ta penile cancer. 5% 5FU cream is applied BID (twice daily) for 2 to 6 weeks and 5% imiquimod cream is applied at night three times a week for 2 to 6 weeks. Close follow-up is necessary to confirm resolution of the lesion and monitor for recurrence.
4) **Laser ablation:** The four most widely used laser energy sources include the CO_2, argon, Nd:YAG, and potassium titanyl phosphate (KTP) lasers. The 0.1-mm depth of penetration of the CO_2 laser makes it suboptimal for treatment of penile carcinoma, with recurrence rates as high as 50%. Conversely, the Nd:YAG laser results in protein denaturation at a depth of up to 6 mm. Although overall recurrence rates after laser ablation have been reported around 8% for penile Tis and 10%–25% for T1 lesions, results from more contemporary series using the Nd:YAG laser with tumor base biopsies have been more encouraging, with recurrence rates below 7%. **Close surveillance and patient self-examination are paramount after laser ablation. Recurrences after laser treatment are best treated with wide local excision or partial penectomy.** Perioperatively, lesions can be treated with 3% acetic acid solution and will become acetowhite, allowing for precise targeting of the laser. Precautions should be taken to avoid exposure to aerosolized HPV given high co-occurrence rates. Further specifics of laser ablative treatment can be found in the National

Comprehensive Cancer Network (NCCN) Penile Cancer Guidelines.

5) **Mohs microsurgery:** This involves a layer-by-layer complete excision of the penile lesion in multiple sessions using a fixed tissue technique that theoretically offers improved precision and control of the negative margin while maximizing organ preservation. **Although results with Mohs microsurgery are comparable to limited excision with intraoperative frozen section, this is only recommended for Ta, Tis, and T1 disease less than 3 cm.** Consider for a patient with a small, superficial lesion on the proximal shaft who would otherwise require total penectomy given location but is otherwise relatively low risk.
6) **Radiation:** Both external beam radiation therapy (EBRT) and brachytherapy are therapeutic options for patients with localized penile carcinoma. **Rate of local control is significantly worse than with penectomy; however, there is a high rate of organ preservation and salvage resection after radiation is possible.** Often circumcision is necessary to provide exposure of the lesion and to prevent postradiation complications. EBRT is limited by the need for penile immobilization but has less operator dependence than brachytherapy. Interstitial radiation has been used successfully to treat penile carcinoma with a variety of radioisotopes, including radium-226, iridium-192, and cesium-137. Data from a number of centers show that penile conservation may be achieved in up to 83% of patients, with 5-year local recurrence rates varying between 24% and 57%. The pathologic variables associated with treatment failure in most studies are the presence of corporal invasion and tumor size greater than 4 cm. Although some series reported 5-year disease-free survival rates as high as 78%, delayed side effects have been reported in up to 53% of patients. **The most common complications of penile radiotherapy include urethral stricture disease (45%) and penile necrosis (23%).** Indications for treatment of groin lymphadenopathy are the same as for surgery; however, only tumor biopsy information is available rather than full pathologic stage from resection. Prophylactic radiation to the groins is not recommended; however, adjuvant radiation after

inguinal node dissection is reasonable. Radiation can also play a palliative role for symptomatic inguinal nodes or bone metastases.

6) **Partial or total penectomy: Penectomy should be considered for tumors 4 cm or larger, high-grade histology, or T2 invasion of the glans or corpora.** With both total and partial penectomy, ensuring at least a 1-cm tissue margin proximal to the tumor is critical. Local wedge resection has a 50% recurrence rate compared to 8% or less with partial penectomy. In bulky T3 and T4 tumors, or if the tumor location is such that amputation would leave a penile stump inadequate for voiding or sexual activity, a total penectomy with perineal urethrostomy is preferred.

g. **Nodal management**

For patients with invasive penile carcinoma, the most important prognostic factor is the presence and extent of inguinal lymph node metastases. For clinically positive groins, inguinal lymph node dissection alone can be curative without addition of adjuvant or neoadjuvant chemoradiotherapy. In certain clinical situations, prophylactic lymph node dissection is appropriate, but this procedure carries significant morbidity and should not be done in every case. **Complications from lymphadenectomy remain considerable and include skin necrosis, necrosis of reconstructive flap, thromboembolism, wound infection, and lymphedema.** As may be expected, bulky lymphadenopathy is associated with higher morbidity given the greater disruption of vascular supply and lymphatic drainage required for disease control. Advances in surgical techniques and postoperative management have reduced the complication rate, but it remains substantial. Surveillance of clinically negative groins, however, is associated with its own risks including significant rates of loss to follow-up, progression of disease to inoperable, and closure of the window to cure. **Unfortunately, salvage lymphadenectomy is rarely effective in the population that is status post resection and surveilled until palpable.**

1) **Palpable inguinal adenopathy:** Approximately 43% of patients with clinically positive groins will have evidence

of disease on surgical pathology, the remainder have reactive nodes. The timing of adenopathy can be helpful in determining treatment, as persistent or new palpable adenopathy after treatment of the primary lesion is likely to be metastatic in origin. Historically all patients were given a 4- to 6-week treatment course of antibiotics, and if adenopathy remained, they underwent lymphadenectomy. **Empiric antibiotic treatment is no longer recommended as it results in a delay of potentially curative intervention.** Therefore, current recommendations are to perform an FNA of enlarged lymph nodes at the time of or soon after the treatment of the primary tumor. The sensitivity and specificity of this technique are 93% and 91%, respectively. If FNA is negative but clinical suspicion remains high, consider repeat FNA, excisional node biopsy, or superficial node dissection with frozen section at the time of treatment of the primary lesion. Five-year survival is highly impacted by the nodal status (Table 18.6). For example, 5-year survival is 80% or better if fewer than two nodes are positive on surgical pathology, nodal involvement is unilateral, extranodal extension is not present, and there is no pelvic involvement. If palpable nodes are ≥ 4 cm in size and FNA or excisional biopsy is positive for metastasis, the NCCN recommends neoadjuvant chemotherapy with paclitaxel, ifosfamide, and cisplatin prior to lymphadenectomy.

2) **Nonpalpable lymph nodes:** As noted previously, inguinal lymph node dissection (ILND) is associated with an almost 80% 5-year overall survival rate for patients found to have minimal lymph node involvement on surgical pathology. However, ILND is associated with

TABLE 18.6 Penile Cancer Survival by Pathologic Nodal Stage

Nodal Burden	5-Year Survival
Negative on exam or histology	73%
< 2 nodes positive on pathology	72%–88%
2 nodes positive on pathology	10%–50%
Pelvic nodes on pathology	0%–15%

significant and potentially permanent morbidity. Thus, a risk-adapted approach should be undertaken to identify the 20% to 25% of patients harboring occult metastasis in clinically negative nodes, while avoiding overtreatment in the remaining 75% to 80% with truly negative nodes. **Patients are divided into low- and high-risk strata based on pathologic features of the primary penile tumor (Table 18.7).** Patients with Tis and Ta tumors have a low risk of metastasis (less than 16%) and can be managed expectantly (Fig. 18.1). Patients with corporal invasion (pT2) are at high risk for metastasis (greater than 64%). Patients with pT1 disease represent a heterogeneous cohort with heterogeneous outcomes and are thus at intermediate risk. **Pathologic features that should prompt lymphadenectomy in patients with pT1 penile carcinoma include high-grade histology, nodular growth pattern, or the presence of lymphovascular invasion.** Patients with low-grade T1 disease with superficial growth patterns and no lymphovascular invasion should be considered as having an intermediate risk of metastasis. Patients in the risk group should be considered for prophylactic lymphadenectomy because they have a 50% to 70% risk of nodal metastasis (Fig. 18.2). Patients who do not undergo a prophylactic lymphadenectomy should have very close and frequent follow-up in order to prompt immediate lymphadenectomy at the first indication of adenopathy (Table 18.8).

TABLE 18.7 Risk of Nodal Involvement

Stage or Grade of Primary Tumor	Risk of Nodal Involvement
Tis, Ta	Low risk, < 16% inguinal nodes positive
T1	Intermediate risk, 5%–20% inguinal nodes positive[a]
T2	High risk, average 59% with nodal involvement regardless of groin exam
High grade (3 and 4)	High risk

[a]Risk increases with Grade 2 histology.

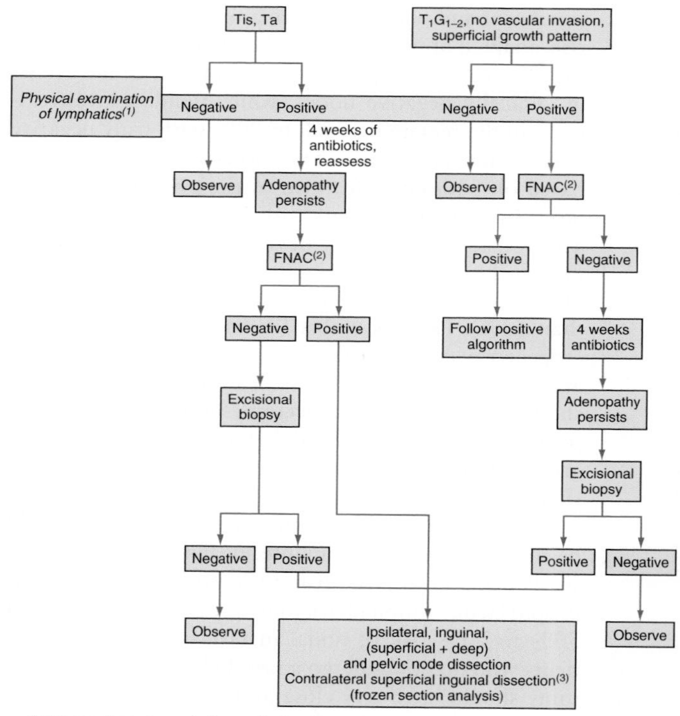

FIGURE 18.1 Management of the inguinal basins in low- and intermediate risk patients. (From Pettaway CA, Lance RS, Davis JW. Tumors of the penis. In: Wein AJ, ed. *Campbell-Walsh Urology*. 10th ed. Philadelphia: Saunders Elsevier; 2011.)

Patients with clinically negative nodes but at high risk of metastasis by primary tumor characteristics may be considered for additional surgical staging procedures including dynamic sentinel lymph node biopsy (SLNB) or superficial ILND with frozen section analysis. It should be noted that FNA has insufficient sensitivity when nodes are nonpalpable and should not be considered reassuring in this patient population. Similarly,

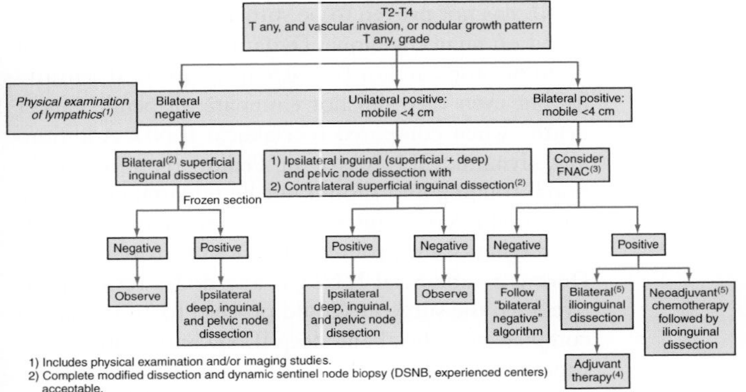

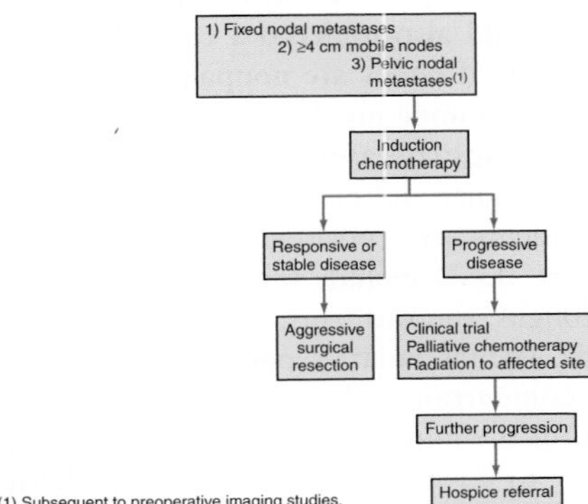

FIGURE 18.2 Management of the inguinal basins in high-risk patients. (From Pettaway CA, Lance RS, Davis JW. Tumors of the penis. In: Wein AJ, ed. *Campbell-Walsh Urology*. 10th ed. Philadelphia: Saunders Elsevier; 2011.)

TABLE 18.8 Management of Groins by Clinical Stage

Tumor	Treatment
Tis, Ta, T1a	Close surveillance of groins
T1b, T2, any high grade	Surgical staging of groins

SLNB has not proven to be sufficiently sensitive when based on anatomy alone. Dynamic SLNB with aid of a radioisotope and/or blue dye has improved sensitivity but even then did not eliminate all penile cancer deaths when compared to classical ILND. Additionally, dynamic SLNB is a procedure requiring additional training and should not be undertaken outside advanced referral centers. The gold standard for surgical staging of the groins is ILND with frozen section. During a superficial ILND, if any nodes return positive, then the surgeon should proceed to an ipsilateral complete superficial and deep ILND and contralateral superficial ILND.

3) **Surgical considerations for extent of lymphadenectomy: Patients with palpable lymph nodes should undergo both superficial and deep ILND on the ipsilateral side. These patients should also undergo a contralateral superficial ILND, even if nodes are nonpalpable, because contralateral inguinal node involvement may be present in 50% of patients.** Ipsilateral pelvic lymphadenectomy adds minimal morbidity and provides useful staging information in patients with positive lymph nodes. The boundaries of the ILND include the inguinal ligament, the adductor longus, the sartorius, and the base of the femoral triangle. The fascia lata separates the superficial from the deep compartment. The sartorius muscle may be detached from the anterior superior iliac spine and rotated medially to cover the femoral vessels. Alternatively, gracilis or rectus abdominis flaps may be used to fill large defects after resecting large masses, thus preventing vessel erosion and skin necrosis.

The superficial ILND carries lower morbidity than the deep dissection given that the saphenous vein is more commonly preserved, the femoral vessels remain covered, and no muscular flap is required for reconstruction. Contemporary series shows that robotic or laparoscopic approach to this dissection may be performed with similar outcomes and potentially substantial improvement in perioperative morbidity.

A pelvic lymphadenectomy should be considered for patients with > 1 positive node on frozen section or any single node > 3.5 cm, or extranodal extension positive on prior pathology. Pelvic lymphadenectomy does not provide significant survival benefit and is primarily a tool for staging. If pelvic lymphadenopathy is suspected or evident prior to treatment of the primary tumor, the patient should be referred for neoadjuvant chemotherapy. If the nodes are identified on surgical pathology, the patient should be referred for adjuvant chemotherapy.

4) **Surgical treatment of inguinal nodes by groin exam** (Table 18.9)

h. **Advanced disease**

Patients who present with bulky adenopathy and/or unresectable primary tumors should be considered for neoadjuvant chemotherapy or chemoradiotherapy followed by surgical consolidation if their disease is stable or responds well to systemic therapy. Per NCCN Penile Cancer Guidelines 2020, the ideal chemotherapy regimen consists of paclitaxel, ifosfamide, and cisplatin ("TIP"). Response rate in this group is approximately 50%. As stated previously, patients with poor pathologic features

TABLE 18.9 Management of Groins by Clinical Nodal Status

Groin Exam	Surgical Intervention
Palpable bilateral groin adenopathy	Bilateral superficial and deep inguinal node dissection
Palpable unilateral groin adenopathy	Superficial and deep inguinal node dissection on palpable groin, superficial node dissection on contralateral groin with intraoperative frozen section. If positive, proceed to deep inguinal node dissection.
Nonpalpable nodes	Intervention based on primary tumor pathology, see above section.
Delayed palpable nodes after primary treatment	Treat based on laterality as above

after lymphadenectomy (extranodal extension, two or more positive nodes, bilateral inguinal metastases, or positive pelvic nodes) should be considered for systemic chemotherapy in the adjuvant setting.

i. **Surveillance**

Surveillance strategies should be tailored to the individual patient's risk of recurrence, varying by the pathologic characteristics of the primary tumor and the treatment employed. Men at a higher risk for locoregional recurrence should have more rigorous follow-up, especially those treated with minimally invasive or organ-sparing techniques. So too should patients with clinically negative inguinal lymph nodes who are managed without lymphadenectomy despite high-risk primary tumors (pT2-3, high-grade T1, vascular invasion) and those with lymph node metastases after lymphadenectomy be followed up carefully. Good candidates for less stringent surveillance schedules include patients with low-risk primary tumors (pTis, pTa, and low-grade pT1) and those with negative inguinal nodes after lymphadenectomy whose primary tumors were managed with partial or total penectomy.

NCCN SURVEILLANCE RECOMMENDATIONS BY TREATMENT AND STAGE

Treatment of Primary Lesion	Clinical Exam
Topical or organ sparing	• Years 1–2, every 3 months • Years 3–5, every 6 months • Years 5–10, annually
Partial or total penectomy	• Years 1–2, every 6 months • Years 3–5, annually

Nodal Stage	Clinical Exam	Imaging
Nx	• Years 1–2, every 3 months • Years 3–5, every 6 months	

Nodal Stage	Clinical Exam	Imaging
N0–N1	• Years 1–2, every 6 months • Years 3–5, annually	
N2–N3	• Years 1–2, every 3–6 months • Years 3–5, every 6–12 months	• Year 1: Chest CT or XR every 6 months AND CT abdomen/pelvis every 3 months • Year 2: Chest CT or XR every 6 months AND CT abdomen/pelvis every 6 months

CLINICAL PEARLS

1. Overall survival in penile cancer is primarily predicted by lymph node involvement.
2. Histology and T stage should be used to guide options for treatment of primary lesions.
3. Careful surgical staging of the groins in a risk-adjusted manner is key to preventing deaths from penile cancer while limiting morbidity from lymphadenectomy.

Self-Assessment Questions

1. *Which HPV subtypes are associated with penile carcinoma? What percent of penile cancers are thought to be associated with HPV infection?*
2. *Which pathologic features of a penile tumor places a patient with nonpalpable lymph nodes at high risk for inguinal metastasis? How should they best be managed?*
3. *What is the appropriate sequence for surgically evaluating clinically negative groins? How are patients surveilled based on their nodal stage?*

Urethral Cancer

GENERAL CONSIDERATIONS

Primary urethral cancer is a rare diagnosis in the United States, representing less than 1% of GU malignancies. Between 1973 and 2002, the annual age-adjusted incidence rates were 4.3 and 1.5 per million for men and women, respectively. While there is not a recently published incidence rate for only primary urethral cancer, there is an estimated 3970 new cases and 1010 deaths of primary cancers of the ureter and other urinary organs excluding the bladder, kidney, and renal pelvis in 2020. This cancer can occur in patients of all ages with an incidence that increases to 32 and 9.5 per million in men and women, respectively, from ages 75 to 84. In the United States, population data suggest urethral carcinoma is more common among Black. Current management of this rare disease is based on sparse evidence that is limited to case series and several population-based database studies. Much of the treatment is also extrapolated from the bladder and penile cancer literature.

1. **Benign lesions of the urethra**
   a. **Leiomyoma:** A leiomyoma of the urethra is a tumor of the periurethral smooth muscle and is more common in women than in men. These tumors can present as a palpable mass of the anterior vagina, irritative voiding symptoms, or recurrent urinary tract infection (UTI). **Leiomyomas can be hormone sensitive, changing with the menstrual cycle or pregnancy.** They are best evaluated with MRI or ultrasound for surgical planning. The choice between transvaginal excision or transurethral resection (TUR) is made based on location and depth. Once resected, recurrence is rare.
   b. **Hemangioma:** Hemangiomas of the urethra are a finding more common in men than women. Like other hemangiomas, these tumors are benign vascular tumors made up of nests of thin-walled aberrant vessels. They rarely affect the urethra, but when they do, **hemangiomas can be a cause of gross hematuria or hematospermia.** If found in the anterior urethra, the patient tends to be a young male in the third decade of life with intermittent hematuria, bloody urethral discharge, or hematospermia. Posterior hemangiomas, on the other hand, tend to affect older men and present with postejaculatory hematuria or hematospermia, with the lesion often found between the verumontanum and the external sphincter. The diagnosis can be confirmed via cystourethroscopy, though an MRI should be obtained to evaluate depth. Superficial hemangiomas are amenable to TUR, whereas deeper or more extensive lesions may require excision and urethroplasty.

c. **Fibroepithelial polyp:** Fibroepithelial polyp is a congenital tumor of connective tissue and smooth muscle. **This entity is more common in males than females and can affect both the upper and lower urinary tracts.** The most common symptoms are urinary obstruction, restricted stream, dysuria, and hematuria. When involving the urethra these tumors typically present in the first decade of life given the propensity to cause obstruction and their congenital nature. These can be safely treated endoscopically.

2. **Male urethral cancer**
   a. **Epidemiology:** As noted in the introduction, primary cancer of the urethra is exceedingly rare. **Known associations include history of sexually transmitted diseases, history of urethritis, history of stricture, and HPV 16 infection.** Patients often present with a palpable urethral mass, urethral bleeding, or obstructive voiding symptoms due to the mass effect of the lesion. Due to the rarity of the disease, data informing treatment recommendations and prognosis are based on small series and expert opinion. Of note, primary carcinoma of the prostatic urethra is a unique entity but it too is exceedingly rare. Rather, a patient with evidence of prostatic urethral carcinoma must undergo a thorough evaluation of the bladder and upper tracts looking for a synchronous source of disease. Diagnostic biopsies of the prostatic urethra are not commonplace during the workup of bladder cancer, but involvement of the prostatic urethra is seen in 20%–40% of pathologic specimens after radical cystectomy performed for urothelial malignancy.
   b. **Pathology:** There are several subtypes of urethral cancer including urothelial carcinoma (formerly transitional cell carcinoma), SCC, and adenocarcinoma. Per the NCCN 2020 urethral cancer guidelines, SCC is the most common histologic subtype of primary urethral carcinoma. Melanoma and sarcoma of the urethra have also been described in case reports. **The most common site of involvement is the bulbomembranous urethra, with 60% of tumors occurring here, whereas 30% of tumors are found in the penile urethra.** Importantly, the commonality of the different histologies varies by location of the tumor. Tumors of the prostatic urethra tend to be urothelial carcinoma. The

TABLE 18.10 Grading of Urethral Cancer

Urothelial Carcinoma	Low grade High grade
Squamous Cell Carcinoma, Adenocarcinoma	
Gx	Grade cannot be assessed
G1	Well differentiated
G2	Moderately differentiated
G3	Poorly differentiated

further distal in the urethra, the more prevalent SCC becomes. Thus, penile and bulbomembranous urethral tumors tend to more commonly be SCC, or even more rarely, adenocarcinoma. Histologic grading is stratified based on level of differentiation and varies based on subtype (Table 18.10).

c. **Lymphatic drainage:** Lymphatic drainage varies based on the location of the primary tumor. **Anterior lesions drain to the superficial and deep inguinal nodes, and sometimes to the external iliac nodes. Posterior lesions drain to the pelvic chains.** Hematogenous spread of urethral cancer is rare and only seen in advanced disease. In this clinical scenario, palpable nodes at presentation are usually indicative of metastasis. In fact, 10%–20% of patients will have positive nodes at presentation, and 5%–20% will have metastatic disease at presentation. The metastatic pattern for urethral cancer is usually regional nodal involvement, followed by distant nodal involvement or bone, liver, or lung metastases.

d. **Diagnosis:** When urethral cancer is suspected, patients should undergo an exam under anesthesia and cystoscopy, with biopsies obtained either by TUR, cold cup biopsy, or FNA. **Urine cytology can be useful in identifying urothelial carcinoma, but performs poorly when the tumor is low-grade, SCC, or adenocarcinoma, and thus is not routinely relied upon.** MRI pelvis should be obtained to evaluate for depth of invasion and provides the best characterization of the primary lesion. These authors recommend securing the patient's penis with tape prior to the MRI to prevent motion artifact. To rule out distant metastases, a CT chest/abdomen/pelvis with contrast should be obtained.

e. **Staging:**
Primary Tumor (T) Male and Female (Tables 18.11 to 18.15)

f. **Prognosis:** The prognosis for urethral cancer varies widely based on several factors including grade, stage, location of primary tumor, and histologic subtype. Five-year cancer-specific survival is estimated to be 50%–70%, with 5-year

TABLE 18.11 Urothelial Carcinoma of the Prostate Staging

Tx	Primary tumor cannot be assessed
T0	No evidence of primary tumor
Ta	Noninvasive papillary carcinoma
Tis	Carcinoma in situ
T1	Tumor invades subepithelial connective tissue
T2	Tumor invades any of the following: corpus spongiosum, periurethral muscle
T3	Tumor invades any of the following: corpus cavernosum, anterior vagina
T4	Tumor invades adjacent organs (bladder, etc.)

TABLE 18.12 Urethral Cancer Staging

Tis	Carcinoma in situ involving prostatic urethra or prostatic ducts without stromal invasion
T1	Tumor invades urethral subepithelial connective tissue immediately underlying the urothelium
T2	Tumor invades the prostatic stroma surrounding ducts either by direct extension from the urothelial surface or by invasion from prostatic ducts
T3	Tumor invades periprostatic fat
T4	Tumor invades adjacent organs (bladder, rectum, etc.)

TABLE 18.13 Urethral Cancer Nodal Staging

Nx	Nodes cannot be assessed
N0	No positive lymph nodes
N1	Single regional lymph node metastasis in the inguinal region, true pelvis,[a] or presacral region
N2	Multiple regional lymph node metastases in the inguinal region or true pelvis,[a] or presacral region

[a]True pelvis: perivesical, obturator, internal and external iliac chains.

TABLE 18.14 Urethral Cancer Metastasis Staging

M0	No distant metastasis
M1	Distant metastasis

TABLE 18.15 Urethral Cancer Staging

Stage	T	N	M
Stage 0is	Tis	N0	M0
Stage 0a	Ta	N0	M0
Stage I	T1	N0	M0
Stage II	T2	N0	M0
Stage III	T1	N1	M0
	T2	N1	M0
	T3	N0	M0
	T3	N1	M0
Stage IV	T4	N0	M0
	T4	N1	M0
	Any T	N2	M0
	Any T	Any N	M1

overall survival around 40%–50%. Again, these estimates vary based on tumor location, with **distal tumors often curable and 5-year survival for bulbar tumors as low as 20%–30%. Adenocarcinoma of the urethra is the most favorable subtype.** Patients can be counseled that recurrence is common at nearly 50%, and they will require thorough long-term surveillance (Table 18.16).

g. **Treatment:** Generally, surgical treatment should include complete resection of the primary tumor with negative margins. Classically, a 1-cm margin was recommended, but **data suggest a 5-mm margin provides sufficient control.** In patients with a T2 or higher primary lesion, neoadjuvant chemotherapy should be considered. Treatment recommendations are based on T stage, location, and patient gender as can be seen in Table 18.17.

h. **Surgical management by location**

1) **Male anterior urethra: pendulous and fossa navicularis**

Tumors involving the male anterior urethra carry better prognostic factors, **can be curable with resection**

TABLE 18.16 Presentation Rates of Urethral Cancer

Grade	Percentage
Low stage (0, I, II)	83%
High stage (III, IV)	36%
Location	
Pendulous	69%–72%
Bulbar	26%–36%
Prostate-superficial	67%–74%
Prostate-stroma	36%

TABLE 18.17 Treatment Options by Stage and Location

Tumor Stage and Location	Treatment Options
Tis, Ta, T1 (any location)	• Repeat TUR • Intraurethral BCG or chemotherapy
Male T2 anterior	• Partial urethrectomy, consider partial penectomy • If margins positive, chemotherapy vs repeat resection
Male T2 posterior	• Urethrectomy, consider radical cystectomy
Male prostatic	• Aggressive TURP followed by BCG • Consider radical cystectomy if disease progresses
Mucosal	• TURP + BCG
Ductal or acinar	• TURP + BCG *or* • Radical cystectomy, ± urethrectomy
Stromal	• Radical cystectomy ± urethrectomy, consider neoadjuvant chemotherapy
≥ T3	
Node negative	• Chemoradiotherapy, consider consolidative surgery • Neoadjuvant chemotherapy with consolidative surgery or radiation therapy • Radiation alone
Node positive	• Chemoradiotherapy, consider consolidative surgery • Systemic therapy alone

BCG, Bacille Calmette-Guérin; *TUR*, transurethral resection. *TURP*, transurethral resection of the prostate.

alone, and can sometimes be managed with organ-sparing techniques. Primary surgical management strategies include TUR, distal urethrectomy with or without partial penectomy, or total urethrectomy with perineal urethrostomy. If a partial approach is pursued, serial intraoperative frozen sections should be obtained with the goal of at least a 5-mm negative margin. As previously stated, **there is no consensus support for a prophylactic ILND** in this patient population. Neoadjuvant chemotherapy is recommended for those with clinically positive groins, and in certain patients with increased risk of poor surgical outcomes, primary chemoradiotherapy may be advisable. In those treated with primary chemoradiotherapy 79% demonstrated a response, however, nearly a third of those who responded progressed and a cohort of those were not able to be salvaged. **Primary radiotherapy is not recommended unless the patient refuses surgery or the stage is advanced.** If radiation is pursued, prophylactic radiation to the groins is recommended.

2) **Male posterior urethra: bulbar and membranous urethra**
Given the deep location of these tumors, they often present at a more advanced tumor stage than those in the anterior urethra, and thus are less amenable to organ-sparing surgical techniques. Lesions that are small or low stage may be managed with thorough TUR or excision and primary anastomosis. As with bladder cancer, if the primary tumor is addressed with TUR, a second TUR is recommended for complete staging. This carries significant urethral stricture risk. The most aggressive surgical management for these tumors includes radical cystoprostatectomy with total penectomy in an en bloc fashion, as well as pelvic lymphadenectomy. Neoadjuvant chemotherapy is recommended in T3 tumors and those involving the prostatic stroma. Even in advanced patients, median survival for those who received neoadjuvant chemotherapy and aggressive surgery was 46 months. If the tumor is invading the pelvic

floor musculature or the inferior pubic rami, significant reconstruction may be undertaken with the assistance of orthopedic and plastic surgeons. As mentioned for anterior tumors, **primary radiotherapy is not recommended but can be useful for treatment of positive surgical margins or recurrence.**

3) **Male posterior urethra: prostatic urethra**

Involvement of the prostatic urethra was once considered automatic T4 disease and required radical cystoprostatectomy. However, more recent data suggest that **endoscopic management is a reasonable first line, with radical cystectomy still supported as an option.** As would be expected, **aggressive transurethral resection of the prostate (TURP) improves treatment response** both by removing involved tissue and increasing surface area exposed to intravesical bacille Calmette-Guérin (BCG). Superficial mucosal disease is best managed endoscopically, as is ductal or acinar disease, though the latter diagnosis carries a higher risk of recurrence and progression and thus requires close follow-up with repeat biopsies of the prostatic urethra during surveillance cystoscopy. **Stromal invasion requires aggressive treatment similar to muscle invasive bladder cancer (MIBC) with radical cystoprostatectomy and consideration of adjuvant or neoadjuvant chemotherapy.**

3. Female urethral cancer

a. **Epidemiology: Primary malignancy of the female urethra is exceedingly rare**, with an incidence of only 1.5 cases per million women per year diagnosed in the United States. However, urethral involvement can be seen in 8%–13% of pathologic radical cystectomy specimens removed during the treatment of bladder cancer. Factors associated with increased risk of developing primary female urethral cancer include age, African American ethnicity, HPV, chronic irritation, urethral diverticulum. In fact, 6% of urethral diverticulae are found to have malignant involvement. **Nearly all female urethral cancers present symptomatically, though the symptoms of lower urinary tract symptoms (LUTS), hematuria, and urethral spotting are all relatively common and more likely due to nonmalignant etiologies.** A high suspicion for urethral cancer must be maintained during workup of these patients. Urethral or vaginal mass can also be seen at presentation and is more obvious but also often more advanced.

b. **Anatomy, lymphatic drainage, pathology:** Although the female urethra is only 4 cm long on average, there are histologic and anatomic divisions that affect diagnosis and management of female urethral malignancy. Like the male urethra, the female urethral has a posterior and anterior portion. **The distal third is considered the anterior segment and is lined with stratified squamous epithelium. The proximal two-thirds is considered the posterior segment and transitions from stratified squamous to urothelium halfway through.** The differences in mucosal histology account for the subtypes of female urethral cancer, with urothelial cancer arising only from the portion lined with urothelium and SCC or adenocarcinoma arising from the squamous portion. The incidences of each of these histologic subtypes are similar (Table 18.18). These boundaries also dictate lymphatic drainage, with the anterior segment draining to the inguinal nodes and the posterior segment draining to the pelvic nodes. **This is the same pattern as lymphatic drainage of the male urethra.** Urethral sarcoma, small cell carcinoma, melanoma, and lymphoma are case reportable occurrences.

c. **Diagnosis:** As with other GU malignancies, thorough physical exam and cross-sectional imaging are the mainstays of diagnosis. Vaginal involvement should be evaluated with a thorough bimanual exam, and inguinal lymphadenopathy should be assessed. Tissue is most commonly obtained via cystoscopy and TUR, though a transvaginal approach can be taken if needed. MRI is preferred over CT to assess local soft tissue extension while also evaluating pelvic lymph

TABLE 18.18 Female Urethral Cancer Histology by Location

Histology	Anatomic Origin	Incidence
Urothelial	Proximal 1/3	28%–45%
Squamous	Distal 2/3	19%–29%
Adenocarcinoma	Distal 2/3	28%–30%

TABLE 18.19 Female Urethral Cancer Stage at Presentation

Stage at Presentation	Percentage
Locally advanced	30%–50%
Palpable inguinal nodes	20%
Distant metastases	10%–20%

TABLE 18.20 Female Urethral Cancer Survival

Location	5-Year Survival
Distal	71%
Proximal	48%
Pan-urethral	24%
Stage	
II or less	67%
III	53%
IV	17%
Size	
< 2 cm	89%
2–4 cm	36%
4 cm	19%

nodes. Chest imaging is appropriate, as is bone scan if there is concern from the history for possible osseous metastases.

d. **Staging:** Women tend to present with more advanced and higher grade disease than their male counterparts, potentially due to the rare nature of female urethral cancer and its low likelihood on differential diagnoses (Table 18.19). **Staging is the same as male urethral cancer. Palpable nodes are nearly always cancerous in females. Most common sites of distant metastasis are the lung, bone, and brain.**

e. **Prognosis: Prognosis is determined primarily by location and stage at diagnosis (Table 18.20).** Squamous histology may be associated with better prognosis, but data are limited.

f. **Management by location**

1) **Female urethra: anterior**

Anterior tumors can be treated with TUR, laser ablation, primary radiation, or partial urethrectomy, though the latter carries a risk of stress urinary incontinence. **More conservative management strategies carry a higher risk of recurrence.** If there is no bladder involvement and the tumor is nonurothelial, histology, radical urethrectomy with bladder neck closure and catheterizable channel could be considered.

2) **Female urethra: posterior**

Malignancy of the female posterior urethra is considerably more aggressive and requires equally aggressive management. Neither surgery nor radiation is recommended as monotherapy. **Anterior exenteration with excision of any involved external genitalia, and even pubectomy if necessary, is the standard of care, with benefit seen in combination with radiation and chemotherapy.** Frozen section analysis should be used intraoperatively to determine success of wide periurethral excision. Pelvic lymph node dissection is usually completed during exenteration, though pelvic nodal involvement is an exceedingly poor prognostic factor and a survival benefit of the nodal dissection has not been demonstrated.

3) **Nodal management:** Palpable inguinal nodes in female patients require the same treatment as in males. Options include any combination of chemotherapy, radiation, and surgical excision. There are no additional surgical considerations for female inguinal node dissection compared to male.

There is no evidence to support prophylactic inguinal node dissection in patient without palpable adenopathy of the groin; however, if the patient is opting for radiation therapy of the primary tumor, prophylactic radiation to the groins may be considered. Inguinal node recurrence can be seen in up to 20% of patients with clinically negative nodes at presentation and **groin exam must be part of surveillance in these patients.**

4) **Metastatic disease: Neoadjuvant systemic chemotherapy followed by consolidative surgery should be considered for patients with distant metastases.** The histology of the primary tumor guides choice of chemotherapeutic regimen.

❋ CLINICAL PEARLS

1. Urethral cancer is similar to bladder cancer and can be managed conservatively for superficial lesion but can require aggressive surgical resection to control if invasive.
2. Distal tumors can be managed with organ-sparing techniques. Proximal urethral and prostatic urethral primaries often present at later stages and are harder to surveil, often requiring more significant surgical control, neoadjuvant chemotherapy, and close follow-up.

Self-Assessment Question

1. *Describe the evaluation of carcinoma of the prostatic urethra. Is this entity more likely to be a primary urethral tumor or evidence of undiagnosed bladder cancer? Does management of prostatic urethral carcinoma always require cystectomy? Why or why not?*

CHAPTER 19

Radiation Therapy

Michael J. LaRiviere, MD, and Neha Vapiwala, MD

In light of excellent disease control achievable with a variety of different treatment modalities, the optimal role of radiation in the curative and palliative management of genitourinary malignancies is one of the more high-profile topics in clinical oncology. Radiation may be used alone as curative treatment of some cancers, as an adjuvant to surgery, or in combination with systemic or other chemotherapy. It is also used as salvage local therapy for disease recurrence in the postoperative setting or as a palliative therapy to alleviate symptoms in patients with advanced or metastatic disease. The continued rapid advancement in radiation technology has not only provided new tools to further improve the therapeutic index but has also raised important questions regarding its uses. Appropriate utilization of radiation requires knowledge of its mechanisms and techniques to fully understand the potential and the limitations of this modality.

X-rays, gamma rays, electrons, and **protons** are types of electromagnetic energy used to treat cancer. First discovered in 1895 by Wilhelm Röntgen, x-rays were rapidly put to use to treat malignancy. In March 1896, Emil Grubbe, a 21-year-old medical student, irradiated the chest wall of a woman with relapsed breast cancer and was the first to document a local response with radiation. In the early 1900s with the discovery of radium, tumors were implanted with gold wires infused with radium to deliver more focal radiation therapy. Decades later, with the advent of linear accelerators, cyclotrons, and complex computer algorithms, radiation dose can be conformed and adapted to "wrap around" the targeted structure and account for internal motion, all while avoiding critical normal tissues. Some forms of radiation can even be engineered to stop on a dime.

Physics

Gamma rays are radiation produced by the decay of radioactive isotopes, either natural or man-made, whereas x-rays, or **photons,** are artificially produced when charged particles strike a target. Photons are typically produced in a **linear accelerator** in which electrons are accelerated to hit a tungsten target to emit the photons. When that tungsten target is removed from the path of the beam, **electron** beams are generated; funnel-like applicators and collimators can be inserted to help shape the beam. Gamma rays have well-defined energies characteristic of the isotope that emits them, whereas x-rays have a broader spectrum that is determined by the energy of the machine that produced them. **Protons** are heavy charged particles that are accelerated to strike a target and that deliver their energy at a specific point in the tissue. Radiation dose delivered to the body is expressed in gray (**Gy**) or for protons in Gy (relative biologic effectiveness), abbreviated **Gy(RBE)**.

For photons, the energy of electromagnetic radiation determines the ability of radiation to penetrate tissue, with higher energies allowing deeper penetration. Higher energies scatter their radiation dose in a more forward direction. In high-energy machines, the maximum dose is deposited below the skin surface. For this reason, a low-energy machine operating at peak energy of 140,000 V would be preferable in treating superficial tumors such as skin cancer because the maximum dose is deposited in the skin, and the dose decreases exponentially to less than 25% of the maximum dose at a depth of 4 cm. For tumors deeper in the body, a more penetrating beam from a linear accelerator, such as one operating at a peak energy of 10 to 15 million volts (10–15 MV) is preferable. A 15-MV beam deposits its maximum energy at a depth of 2.8 cm and is still able to deliver 50% of its maximum dose at a depth of 20 cm. Unlike the higher-energy photons, electrons deposit their maximum dose at or near the surface, penetrate to a predictable depth with a relatively constant dose, and then decrease rapidly. Protons, on the other hand, deliver their energy at the end of their **Bragg peak**. Like photons, the ability of the proton beam to penetrate deeper in the body depends on its energy. The main difference, however, lies in the exit dose. Because photons continue to deliver energy over a range, tissues beyond the target will also receive dose from photon irradiation.

Because almost all of the energy in protons is delivered at the end of the Bragg peak, virtually no dose is delivered to tissues beyond that point.

In some situations, it is preferable to deliver radiation to the tumor from an internal source. This technique is known as **brachytherapy**, meaning short-distance therapy. Radiation dose is determined by the ability of the radiation to penetrate tissue and the distance from the source of the radiation. Like visible light, the intensity of the radiation decreases in proportion to the square of the distance from the source ($1/d^2$). Because doubling the distance from the source of radiation will decrease the intensity by 75% and tripling the distance will decrease the intensity by 89%, it is reasonable to consider placing the source of radiation within the tumor to minimize the dose that would be delivered to the surrounding normal tissue.

Radioactive **isotopes** produce radiation with a decreasing dose rate as time passes, a process known as radioactive decay. Every isotope has a **half-life**, defined as the time required for the dose rate to decrease by 50%. Depending on the half-life, certain isotopes are used for either **high-dose rate (HDR) brachytherapy** or **low-dose rate (LDR) brachytherapy**. For HDR, an applicator or catheter is inserted into the target structure, and the radioactive isotope is inserted for a specific amount of time (usually a few minutes) and then removed. The procedure can be repeated as often as needed to deliver the adequate total dose. In LDR, the isotope is left in the applicator for several hours to days or may be inserted directly into the target organ and left there permanently.

Radiobiology

Radiation causes its effects in tissue by producing ionizations within the cell. The target in cells is the DNA molecule, and the ionizations will produce breaks in the DNA strand. Nonmalignant, healthy cells can repair this damage if it is confined to a single strand because the opposite strand serves as a template for repair. However, if two strand breaks occur on opposite chains in close proximity, the two ends of the chromosome may drift apart. These fragmented chromosomes may adhere to other chromosomes or they may sort out randomly when the cell divides, resulting in the daughter cells having critical segments of

DNA missing or having excess and unregulated copies of other genes, either of which may be fatal to the cell. Thus the damaged cells are observed to undergo a mitotic death; the lethal effect of radiation is not expressed until the cell replicates.

Radiobiologic research is ongoing to identify factors that affect the survival of cells and methods to selectively increase radiation effects on tumor cells. The easiest method to assay the effect of radiation is to deliver a dose of radiation to a suspension of single cells and then measure the percentage of surviving cells. The technique uses a suspension with a known concentration of cells. A sample is placed on a culture plate and the colonies are counted. At the same time a similar-sized sample is radiated and plated and the number of colonies counted. The ratio of the number of colonies developing on the two plates is the surviving fraction.

Because a Gy represents a specific amount of energy transferred to tissue, each Gy in theory should have an equal physical effect on the cell. However, the biologic effect is less for the first Gy than it is for the 101st Gy, suggesting that cells are capable of accumulating a certain amount of damage that is not lethal. Interestingly, if the radiation dose is split up and delivered over several **fractions** with time between fractions for cells to repair the damage, each fraction of radiation will kill the same proportion of the surviving cells. If the cells are allowed to completely repair the damage from the first dose, the second dose of radiation will have the same effect on the surviving cells as it would have if they had never been radiated the first time. This effect demonstrates the importance of uninterrupted radiation treatments. In vitro studies have shown normal cells to repair radiation-induced damage more efficiently than tumor cells, and attempts to deliver two doses of radiation per day, known as **hyperfractionation,** may increase the efficacy of treatment.

Oxygen is known to enhance the effects of radiation both in vivo and in vitro. Cells are more sensitive when radiated under oxygenated conditions than when they are hypoxic. Normal tissues are always oxygenated, but experimental measurements in tumors have shown that these cells pile up around a capillary and consume the available oxygen, limiting diffusion into the deeper tissues. This scenario results in well-oxygenated, relatively sensitive cells adjacent to the capillary and necrotic material at a distance away from the capillary. Between these two areas is a region of viable but hypoxic cells that are more resistant to radiation. In vitro studies show that hypoxic cells require 1.5 to 3 times as much radiation to achieve the same cell kill.

Current efforts are being taken to develop substances that act like oxygen in cells but are not metabolized like oxygen. Ideally, these substances will help to deal with the problem of hypoxic tumor cells without affecting the sensitivity of normal cells. In vitro work showed that these compounds, known as **radiosensitizers,** sensitized hypoxic tumor cells to the effects of radiation. However, clinical trials were limited by toxicity. Similarly, efforts to develop drugs that protect normal cells from the effects of radiation are underway. Although these trials also have failed to show in vivo benefit, efforts continue to develop a new generation of sensitizers and protectors. More importantly, chemotherapy and hormonal therapies have been observed to affect tumor sensitivity in vivo, and these agents form the basis of many current combined modality trials.

Treatment Planning

The delivery of radiation to a tumor requires a physician to perform five functions: (1) identify and locate the structures to be treated, (2) identify those adjacent structures that need to be protected, (3) prescribe the appropriate dose of radiation for the tumor based on its size and histology, (4) consider the tolerance of tissue within the target that may be affected by treatment, and (5) consider the tolerance of tissues between the skin and the target (transit volume). Although a complex but solvable problem, most clinical situations require some compromise on one or more issues. The clinician must select those compromises that will minimize effects on normal tissue while maximizing the probability of tumor control, known as the **therapeutic ratio.**

Modern equipment and computer software allow for sophisticated **three-dimensional conformal radiation treatment** (3D-CRT) and **intensity-modulated radiation therapy** (IMRT). Both of these techniques have become the standard of care in most radiation oncology centers. Patients undergo computed tomography (CT)–based simulation in which a series of axial images are obtained of the target and the adjacent critical structures. Often fiducial markers are placed prior to simulation in the target organ to improve target localization during the treatments. The target or targets, depending on other areas at risk for tumor involvement, bony structures, and sensitive normal tissues, are defined on the CT imaging. Today's treatment machines are able to deliver radiation from a wide range of angles to specifically shape dose intensities to conform around the target.

For example, in the treatment of prostate cancer, newer techniques using IMRT can reduce the dose exposure to normal tissues and allow for higher doses to be delivered to the prostate without increased complications. Computers are used to plan the delivery of radiation using several smaller radiation fields, known as **beamlets,** from different beam directions. Each beamlet treats only a portion of the prostate, but when the dose intensity from all of the beamlets are added together, the entire prostate receives the full dose with slight inhomogeneity, while reducing the volume of normal tissue receiving a high dose. Although the part or the entire target receives the maximal dose, a larger volume of normal tissue is exposed to a small amount of radiation. Fig. 19.e1A–D shows the dose distribution around the target and the nearby organs. Because of the decreased exposure to normal tissues, higher and more effective doses can be delivered to the target with patients experiencing fewer side effects. As with conventional radiation delivery techniques, patient positioning is extremely critical in the delivery of IMRT; these techniques require consistent localization and patient positioning to allow tighter margins and potentially deliver higher doses. Immobilization casts or molds, rectal balloons, rectal spacers, and fiducial markers are all tools used to assist in proper targeting of the radiation to the desired location. Monitoring the target position before each radiation treatment is known as **image-guided radiation therapy (IGRT)**, and this is typically accomplished using kilovoltage-range x-rays (similar to diagnostic x-rays) or cone-beam computed tomography (CBCT) scans. Most techniques focus on patient alignment and target localization just prior to treatment delivery using IGRT. However, the prostate often moves during the radiation treatment itself because of physiologic reasons, such as gas in the rectum; thus there is a risk that the targeted prostate may move out of the irradiated area during the radiation delivery. To combat this intrafraction movement, fiducial markers fitted with transponder technology can be implanted transrectally into the prostate. These beacons, each about the size of a rice grain, communicate with the treating therapist's console and allow 3D tracking of the prostate position in real time. The radiation beams can be adjusted accordingly.

IMRT and IGRT, along with advances in computer-based treatment planning, have allowed for higher doses per day to be delivered as neighboring organs at risk can be better avoided. Because fewer total fractions are delivered, but a similar biologically effective dose is achieved, this technique is called **hypofractionation**. Multiple randomized controlled trials have demonstrated similar rates of prostate cancer control using treatments that are delivered over as few as 4–5.5 weeks, rather than the 8–9 weeks required with conventionally fractionated radiation. With only modestly increased rates of gastrointestinal or genitourinary toxicities, hypofractionated regimens are now considered standard of care for many prostate cancer patients.

Stereotactic body radiotherapy (SBRT) is an example of extreme hypofractionation: very large radiation doses are delivered over 5 or fewer *days* using the most advanced IMRT and IGRT techniques. SBRT is technically demanding, requiring equipment capable of delivering ablative doses of radiation to tolerances on the order of millimeters, precise patient immobilization and target localization, and radiation oncologist and radiation physicist expertise. Because such high doses of radiation are delivered, SBRT carries risks of severe, high-grade toxicities, but these toxicities are rare in experienced hands using advanced equipment in high-volume centers. Generally, the safe delivery of SBRT is well tolerated by patients and is an emerging treatment option for selected prostate cancers. In prostate and other cancers with a limited number of metastases, known as **oligometastatic** or **oligoprogressive** disease, SBRT is seeing increased use as an ablative treatment to extirpate these metastases, a concept analogous to metastatectomy.

In the 1930s, particle accelerators were developed that could accelerate heavier particles such as protons. It was not until 1954 that protons were put to use in the treatment of cancer at the Lawrence Berkeley National Laboratory. Since then, multiple facilities offering proton therapy have sprouted throughout Europe, Asia, and the United States. The physical advantages of proton therapy over standard photons are that proton beams have a maximal peak dose (known as the Bragg peak) that can be delivered to a specific location in the body, and have essentially no exit dose beyond the Bragg peak. These characteristics may allow more sparing of the tissues outside of the target volume than is

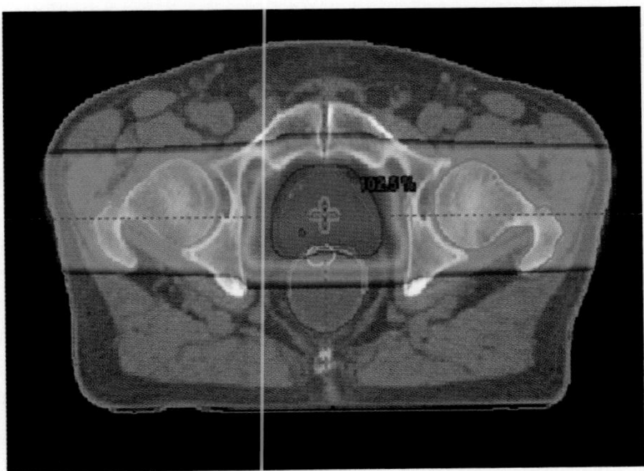

FIGURE 19.1 Radiation treatment plan of prostate using opposed proton fields. Virtually no dose enters or exits through the rectum or bladder.

possible with IMRT or IGRT techniques. Fig. 19.1 shows a transaxial slice of a prostate being treated with two opposing proton beams. Each beam delivers virtually no dose beyond the distal edge of the target structure. Studies have shown modest improvements in bladder and rectal toxicity rates with proton therapy. However, no randomized data that compare outcomes for patients treated with IMRT and proton therapy for prostate cancer have been reported. To that end, the phase III, randomized PARTIQoL trial is testing proton therapy versus photon IMRT for low- and intermediate-risk prostate cancer. With a target enrollment of 400 patients, this trial is ongoing and estimated to complete at the end of 2026. Its primary endpoint is 2-year bowel toxicity, with secondary endpoints related to quality of life, cost effectiveness, survival, and second malignancy. Also ongoing is the nonrandomized COMPPARE trial testing photon IMRT, conventionally fractionated proton therapy, and hypofractionated proton therapy. With a primary endpoint of 2-year bowel, urinary, and sexual toxicity, this trial is estimated to be complete in 2023. Until recently, the cost of building and maintaining a proton facility was prohibitively expensive, on the order of \$100–\$300 million, with operating costs of \$15–\$25 million per year. However, the past decade has seen the emergence of more single-room proton centers, with initial costs closer to $40 million. While this is still an order of magnitude greater than the approximately $5 million cost of a modern photon linear accelerator, it does put protons within reach of more centers, as evidenced by the increasing number of proton units in the United States.

An alternative method is to deliver the radiation from within the tumor using interstitial radiation, or brachytherapy. LDR permanent implants in prostate cancer typically use radioactive seeds containing iodine or palladium isotopes. The patient is taken to the operating room, where epidural, spinal, or general anesthesia is administered and the patient is placed in the lithotomy position. Using transrectal ultrasound guidance, hollow needles are placed through the perineum into the prostate, and the radioactive seeds are deposited interstitially. The needles are removed after the procedure. Seed positions within the prostate are determined prior to the procedure using reconstructed images from sophisticated CT, magnetic resonance imaging (MRI), and/or ultrasound planning equipment. Intraoperative planning can also be accomplished with the assistance of a physicist in the operating room, allowing for real-time modification of the treatment plan at the time of the procedure to ensure accurate placement of seeds. After the procedure, reimaging confirms seed placement, and the quality of the implant can be judged. Fig. 19.e2A shows axial slices through the prostate demonstrating the placement of seeds in the prostate. Fig. 19.e2B shows a 3D reconstruction of the prostate obtained from the postimplant CT scan demonstrating radioactive dose clouds from the seeds within the prostate. Although the implant delivers lower doses to the periprostatic tissues, substantially higher doses are delivered to the interior of the prostate.

As with LDR brachytherapy, in HDR brachytherapy the patient is sedated and anesthetized, after which hollow catheters are inserted percutaneously through the perineum into the prostate. A radiation plan is designed based on the 3D rendering of the prostate, rectum, urethra, bladder, and catheters through which the radioactive sources will travel, with a goal of emitting adequate dose throughout the prostate gland from the designated positions. The radiation oncologist can preferentially deliver a higher dose to certain parts of the organ, while sparing critical areas such as tissue surrounding the urethra. Images of HDR brachytherapy of the prostate are shown in Fig. 19.e3A–C.

Because many prostate tumors have some degree of extracapsular extension (ECE), the reduced periprostatic dose may not effectively treat the tumor volume. Patients with very large prostate glands may have anatomical constraints because of the pelvic bones (i.e., pubic arch interference) that could limit placement of the needles or applicators. However, with appropriate intraoperative positioning techniques, many larger prostates can be implanted. With HDR brachytherapy, radiation doses can be delivered beyond 3 mm, which is the distance from the capsule that 90% of microscopic ECE extends. Furthermore, Merrick et al. demonstrated that prostates greater than 60 cc had no greater risk of postimplant obstruction.

Clinical Radiation Oncology

RENAL PELVIC AND URETERAL CARCINOMA

While the use of radiation in the treatment of patients following resection is generally not indicated, the role of radiation for renal cancers is currently evolving with ongoing studies looking at SBRT for oligometastases or oligoprogressive metastases. Among patients with tumor transgressing the renal capsule, the risk of local recurrence is high. Rafla et al. reviewed their experience and found an apparent benefit to the use of adjuvant radiation therapy for patients with involvement of the renal capsule (T3). Among patients receiving adjuvant radiation, the 5-year survival was 57% compared to 28% for patients treated with surgery alone. It is presumed that the improved survival was related to the reduced incidence of local recurrence, although this finding could not be documented because these patients were treated in the pre-CT era. In contrast, subsequent trials reported by Finney et al. and Kjaer et al. found no benefit with adjuvant radiation. The results of the Finney trial although limited by the small number of patients, demonstrated an 8% treatment-related mortality as a result of liver injury in the radiation arm. The results reported by Kjaer are clouded by the registration of node-positive patients in whom Rafla demonstrated no benefit. This study also was complicated by the fact that 16% of the patients randomized to radiation did not receive radiation and those patients who were treated experienced a 44% incidence of major toxicity. Both Finney and Kjaer used anterior and posterior fields, and the toxicity occurred in patients with right-sided tumors. In such cases, large parts of the liver were treated to 45 Gy, which is well above liver tolerance. Because many tumors today are found incidentally at the time of a diagnostic CT scan for other reasons, it is not clear that these patients have the same prognosis after surgery as patients in these older studies who presented with hematuria, mass, or other more advanced findings. Given the potential serious side effects and little data demonstrating a benefit, radiation has historically not been indicated in the adjuvant setting for renal cell cancers. However, more recent data from the International Radiosurgery Oncology Consortium for Kidney (IROCK) have reported 97.8% 4-year local control using SBRT in the definitive treatment of renal cell carcinoma, as an alternative to surgery. Importantly, this highly conformal technique yielded a favorable toxicity profile, with only 39% of patients experiencing any toxicity; only three patients experienced a grade 3–4 toxicity. Therefore, although surgery remains the standard of care, SBRT may emerge as an alternative for patients whose medical comorbidities preclude surgery.

Radiation is often used for *metastatic* renal cell carcinoma to palliate bleeding, pain, or neurologic symptoms related to spinal or central nervous system (CNS) involvement. These tumors have traditionally been thought to be radioresistant, arguing for surgical excision of limited metastatic disease. In a review of their experiences, Onufrey and Halpern reported that although these tumors tended to respond slowly and did not seem to respond to higher doses of radiation, patients still achieved good palliation of symptoms in most cases. Zelefsky et al., Yamada et al., and Siva et al. (reporting the aforementioned IROCK results) have demonstrated that renal cell carcinomas respond to higher hypofractionated radiation doses in the range of those typically used with SBRT. A growing body of retrospective evidence supports the relatively high rates of durable local control achieved with SBRT, and this technique sees an increasing use with oligometastatic or oligoprogressive renal cell carcinoma.

Data are very limited on the use of radiation to manage tumors in the renal pelvis and ureter. The rationale that supports the use of radiation is based on the anatomy of the retroperitoneum as it affects the surgical resection. Tumors of the renal pelvis and ureter are resected with wide proximal and distal margins. Because these tumors are frequently multifocal and can spread along the urothelium, the resection includes the kidney and a generous bladder cuff. The radial margin, however, is more problematic, and radiation may be indicated to sterilize any tumor in this region. The thin wall of the ureter is the only barrier to lateral spread of the tumor, and the surgeon is limited in the ability to laterally extend the dissection. No additional barriers for tumor spread in the retroperitoneum exist. There have been no recent reports of the use of radiation in the postoperative setting, but an older report from the University of Texas MD Anderson Cancer Center described 8 out of 58 patients who underwent nephroureterectomy for transitional cell carcinoma who were thought to have a high risk for local recurrence. The proximal and distal margins of resection were negative, but because of the thin wall of the ureter and the transmural extension of the tumor, there was concern that the radial margin may not have been adequate. These eight patients received 40 to 60 Gy of radiation to the ureteral bed with no major morbidity reported, although most of the patients developed anorexia, nausea, and diarrhea. Four of the eight patients died with a tumor, but only one of these patients had a recurrence of a tumor in the retroperitoneum. Extrapolating these findings to tumors in the renal pelvis would suggest that patients with transitional cell carcinomas lower in the pelvis or extending into perinephric fat may benefit from adjuvant radiation, though this approach would require a multidisciplinary discussion with a medical oncologist, as national guidelines support the use of systemic therapy, rather than adjuvant radiation, in this setting. Ultimately, except in rare circumstances, radiation in this setting is not typically done.

BLADDER CARCINOMA

Radiation in the management of bladder cancer can be an effective treatment option. Although radical cystectomy is the standard approach for most patients, postoperative radiotherapy may be indicated in patients at high risk of locoregional recurrence, and definitive chemoradiation may be used in place of radical cystectomy for medically or surgically inoperable patients, as well as for a highly selected subset of operable patients. Historically, radiation was initially used prior to surgery to increase the probability of successful cystectomy, but this is not standard in the modern era.

In the United States and Europe, there has been an interest in chemosensitized radiation in treating a number of tumors based on the theories advanced by Steele and Peckham. Chemotherapy can reduce the tumor burden so that radiation may deal more effectively with the residual tumor. Similarly, spatial cooperation may allow the radiation to deal effectively with the bladder tumor, whereas systemic chemotherapy may treat subclinical metastatic disease.

The National Bladder Cancer Cooperative Group (NBCCG) in the United States and the group in Innsbruck, Austria, sponsored trials delivering cisplatin on days 1, 22, and 43 of radiation following transurethral resection of bladder tumor (TURBT) with reevaluation after 40 Gy had been delivered. Patients with less than visual complete responses after 40 Gy were sent to cystectomy because researchers found it was unlikely that these patients would achieve a complete response with an additional 20 to 25 Gy. Among patients with complete responses or only positive cytology who received an additional 20 to 25 Gy, the 2-year relapse-free survivals were 68% and 53% in the Innsbruck and NBCCG trials, respectively. In an effort to improve the results with conservative surgery and chemosensitized radiation, the NBCCG and Radiation Therapy Oncology Group (RTOG) began a joint trial delivering two cycles of methotrexate, vinblastine, and cisplatin (MVC) prior to radiation-cisplatin therapy. The 4-year survival with bladder conservation was 44% and the overall survival was 62%. A subsequent trial randomized patients to neoadjuvant chemotherapy prior to chemosensitized radiation versus immediate chemosensitized radiation; no benefit to the neoadjuvant therapy was observed.

To evaluate the role of definitive radiation therapy for bladder cancer, Shipley and colleagues prospectively studied 190 patients with muscle-invasive T2-4a bladder cancers. After maximal TURBT, patients were treated with 40 Gy to bladder with chemotherapy and then reevaluated by repeated biopsy and urine cytology. The tumor response guided subsequent therapy. Patients with a complete response or who were medically unfit for cystectomy received additional radiation to a total dose of 64 to 65 Gy. Patients without a complete response underwent radical cystectomy. A total of 66 patients (35%) ultimately underwent radical cystectomy. In all, 60% of patients treated with chemoradiation alone had long-term control of their bladder cancer. Superficial disease recurred in the bladder in 24 patients; in most cases, it was managed conservatively by means of further resection and/or intravesical chemotherapy. Muscle-invasive recurrence developed in 16%. The 10-year cause-specific survival rates were 60% overall and 45% with an intact bladder. These findings suggest further study with dose escalation or more radiosensitizing chemotherapy is warranted for bladder preservation in bladder cancer. A recent report from Azuma et al. from Japan demonstrated over 70% complete responses in patients with locally advanced bladder cancer with the use of a balloon-occluded arterial infusion of cisplatin and gemcitabine with concomitant hemodialysis and concurrent radiation therapy.

In the postoperative setting, adjuvant radiation may be indicated in patients at high risk of locoregional recurrence. To identify which features would select those patients who would most benefit from adjuvant radiation, Christodouleas et al. developed risk classifications based on retrospective data, refining these classifications based on patients enrolled in the SWOG-8710 randomized controlled trial. High-risk patients who would most benefit from adjuvant radiation were defined as those with at least pathologic T3 (perivesical soft tissue-invasive) disease plus either positive margins or fewer than 10 lymph nodes dissected. Without adjuvant radiation, these patients were at risk of 5-year locoregional failure in excess of 40%. Even intermediate-risk patients, defined as those with at least pT3 cancer but negative margins and at least 10 nodes removed, saw a locoregional recurrence rate of nearly 20% without radiation, as compared to 8% among low-risk patients. Likewise, an Egyptian randomized trial assessed patients with transitional cell or urothelial carcinoma as well as squamous cell carcinoma (which is less common in the United States) bladder cancer. These postoperative, margin-negative patients were required to have at least pT3b, grade 3, or node-positive disease. Among these patients at high risk of pelvic failure, postoperative radiation and chemotherapy yielded a 2-year locoregional recurrence-free survival of 96%, as compared to just 69% with adjuvant chemotherapy alone.

In the modern era, bladder preservation with definitive chemoradiation is reserved for highly selected patients, as surgical techniques have significantly improved continent diversions and allow for better quality of life by preserving normal voiding function and potency in men. Women and some men will intermittently catheterize an internal reservoir, which is much easier than maintaining an external appliance. Appropriate candidates for chemoradiation-based bladder preservation include medically or surgically inoperable patients, as well as operable patients who meet the following criteria: (1) clinical T2 (muscle-invasive) to T3a (microscopic perivesical soft tissue-invasive) disease; (2) unifocal cancer that is (3) < 5 cm in maximum diameter; (4) no extensive carcinoma in situ; (5) visibly complete TURBT; (6) no ureteral obstruction, (7) no hydronephrosis, and (8) good bladder function ("a bladder worth preserving"). It is estimated that fewer than 15% of operable bladder cancer patients meet these criteria. For these highly selected patients, the decision to proceed with radical cystectomy or bladder preservation requires individualized, shared decision-making that takes into account patient age and comorbidities—with younger, fitter patients generally comprising more appropriate surgical candidates—as well as institutional surgical and radiation oncology expertise. The morbidity of cystectomy and definitive radiotherapy have been compared, albeit among patients treated prior to 1995 with less advanced radiation and surgical techniques. This analysis reported sexual dissatisfaction and erectile dysfunction in 36% and 75% of patients treated with definitive radiation versus 67% and 92% after cystectomy, respectively. On the other hand, gastrointestinal toxicity was seen in 32% of patients treated with radiation versus 24% with cystectomy. In more modern series, reported toxicities of definitive chemoradiation include mild urinary frequency, erectile dysfunction, leakage generally not requiring the use of pads, and more rarely, proctitis and diarrhea. Although pain has been reported, palliative cystectomy for radiation-related symptoms is required in only 0%–2% of patients.

PROSTATE CANCER

With the advent of prostate-specific antigen (PSA) screening, the incidence of prostate cancer is now reported to be over 190,000 new cases per year. Many of these tumors may not be clinically significant because a high prevalence of occult prostate cancer is found incidentally in autopsy series. Thus screening asymptomatic men with no clinical signs of prostate cancer is also controversial.

Nonetheless, it remains difficult to reliably distinguish men with incidental tumors from those with clinically significant cancer, and the number of deaths from prostate cancer in the United States still stands at over 30,000 per year.

The critical elements in evaluating a man with prostate cancer require that the clinician estimate the annual risk of distant, metastatic spread, and cancer-related mortality, as well as the annual non–prostate cancer–related mortality risk for the individual. In completing an ad hoc risk-benefit analysis, it is necessary to factor into the equation any conditions that may increase the risk of radiation-related morbidity, including prior abdominal surgeries, any history of peritonitis or pelvic inflammatory conditions, such as Crohn disease or ulcerative colitis, or a history of diverticulitis.

It is necessary to have the proper equipment to deliver radiation for prostate cancer. CT-based treatment planning, IMRT, and escalation of the dose to the prostate past 70 Gy have become standard at modern radiation oncology centers. Proton therapy centers are increasing in number throughout the United States, but proton therapy's superiority over IMRT is still being tested in the PARTIQoL and COMPPARE trials. Accurate localization and patient and target immobilization techniques have become more crucial given the high dose delivered by advanced radiation treatment methods.

Radiation doses to target structures are limited by nearby critical normal structures. Prior to CT-based planning, the bladder and rectum could only be visualized by the insertion of contrast material into these organs and visualizing on radiographs. Radiation treatment plans often erred on the side of underdosing the prostate to avoid long-term toxicity or morbidity. With the advent of CT-based planning, the radiation oncologist can outline the prostate, bladder, rectum, and femoral heads to generate 3D models of each organ. Computer-assisted planning allows various shapes of beams to be generated, each of which helps to conform the dose to the target while minimizing doses to the bladder and rectum. With IMRT and sophisticated planning software, radiation oncologists have been escalating the dose delivered to the prostate as their ability to spare the critical organs continues to improve.

A radiation treatment plan must be evaluated by the radiation oncologist to determine if certain dose constraints are met. The

RTOG has published a series of recommended dose constraints on critical organs, namely the rectum, bladder, femoral heads, and penile bulb that should have minimal morbidity to prostate cancer patients. Careful examination of the **dose volume histogram (DVH)** for each treatment plan will ensure these constraints are met and patients will be treated safely. Fig. 19.2 shows the DVH for the prostate, bladder, and rectum of a patient being treated for prostate cancer. A dose of 86.4 Gy was prescribed to the prostate and seminal vesicles plus a small margin; 95% of entire target volume received a minimum dose of 84 Gy, but a small fraction of the prostate received higher doses. The mean dose through the prostate is fairly homogenous. Likewise, similar histograms for the rectum and bladder demonstrate the maximum and minimum doses delivered to each organ. Whereas a small volume of rectum will tolerate high doses of radiation, the graph shows that most

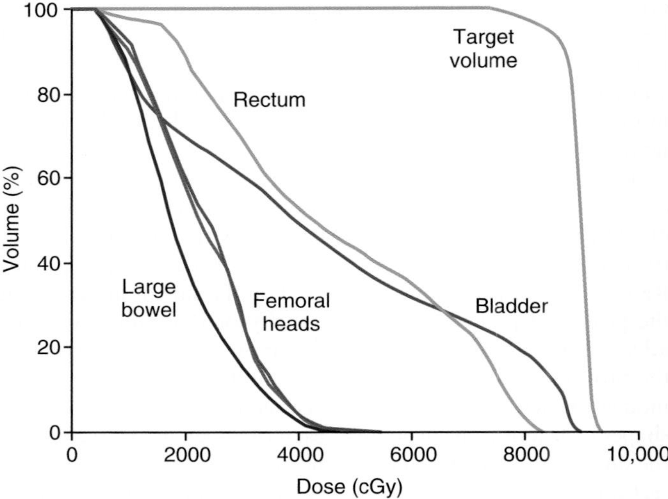

FIGURE 19.2 Dose volume histogram (DVH) demonstrating the dose delivered to the target organ (prostate and proximal seminal vesicles) and organs at risk (bladder, rectum, large bowel, and femoral heads) is shown. The goal in evaluating radiation treatment plans is to maximize the dose to the maximum volume of the target while minimizing the dose to normal structures. *cGy*, Centigray.

of the rectum receives a much lower dose. In this histogram 50% of the rectum received less than 45 Gy.

The maximum radiation dose tolerated by the prostate continues to be evaluated. Although some centers use doses of 74 to 81 Gy, others such as Memorial Sloan-Kettering and the University of Michigan explored doses of 84 to 91 Gy, utilizing the concept of dose escalation. Between October 1988 and December 1998, Zelefsky et al. treated more than 1000 patients with clinical stages T1c-T3 prostate cancer with either 64.8 to 70.2 Gy or 75.6 to 86.4 Gy. Five-year actuarial PSA relapse-free survival was significantly improved with the higher dose. However, questions remained, including whether PSA control would improve overall survival, and whether the improved PSA control outweighs the higher toxicity observed with the higher doses. Combining external beam radiotherapy and interstitial brachytherapy has also been explored to escalate doses to the prostate. Morris et al. reported the results of the ASCENDE-RT randomized controlled trial that exploited highly conformal interstitial brachytherapy to deliver a 125-Gy boost to an external beam radiation dose of 46 Gy, yielding a biochemical control advantage at 9 years, again at the expense of increased early and late genitourinary toxicity.

When external beam radiation alone is used, 60 Gy over 4 weeks or 70 Gy over 5.5 weeks is the standard hypofractionated regimen that is appropriate for many patients. These doses are biologically equivalent to conventionally fractionated regimens of 74 Gy over 7.5 weeks and 73.8 Gy over 8 weeks, respectively, and have been shown in randomized controlled trials to have similar rates of cancer control with only modestly increased gastrointestinal or genitourinary toxicity. These hypofractionated regimens are now considered standard and are preferred by national guidelines and multiple professional societies for many patients with prostate cancer. SBRT is an emerging technique for appropriately selected prostate cancer patients, generally those with low- or favorable intermediate-risk disease. A total dose of 35–36.25 Gy delivered over 5 days is mathematically biologically equivalent to 85 Gy given in conventionally fractionated daily doses over 8.5 weeks. Although early cancer control and toxicity reports are favorable, SBRT has more limited follow-up data than conventionally and moderately hypofractionated radiation, and SBRT has not been directly compared with these techniques in a randomized controlled trial.

In comparing the results from different series, it is necessary to compare the definitions of tumor control and treatment-related morbidity. Following surgery, PSA should be undetectable because all prostatic tissue has been theoretically removed. However, following radiation the residual normal prostate epithelium will continue to produce PSA. The latest consensus from the **American Society of Therapeutic Radiology Oncology (ASTRO)** is nadir PSA following radiation plus 2 ng/mL defines treatment failure. Often following radiation, a PSA bounce is observed. A **PSA bounce** is a temporary PSA rise after the initial postradiation PSA drop. The etiology is not clear, but this occurs about 18 months (range 6 to 36 months) after radiation. If the clinician is too sensitive to the results of the serum PSA, the risk of recurrence may be overestimated.

Grading of radiation-induced side effects is also subject to a lack of uniformity. Individuals who have had radiation may develop painless rectal bleeding, and proctoscopy often reveals mucosal atrophy and telangiectasias. Many physicians would score this effect as a minimal or grade 1 toxicity (not requiring intervention), whereas others would score it as grade 2 toxicity because they may have a lower threshold to recommend symptomatic treatment. Some studies have also considered rectal hemorrhage requiring transfusion or laser ablation of the anterior rectal wall grade 2 toxicity, whereas others consider it grade 4 (life-threatening) toxicity. Similarly, men who advise their physicians that they are able to obtain partial erections may be considered by some physicians to be potent, although they are not able to achieve penetration. Others require that men be able to sustain an erection and reach orgasm. Thus specialized symptom inventories for prostate cancer may provide more nuance than the Common Terminology Criteria for Adverse Events (CTCAE) used in different cancer types across the body.

Furthermore, controversy in the treatment of prostate cancer exists over the definition of the target volume. Many institutions will deliver a dose of 45 Gy to the obturator, hypogastric, external iliac, and common iliac lymph nodes and boost the prostate to the final total dose of greater than 76 Gy. Others will treat the prostate only, with or without part or all of the seminal vesicles.

Debate continues on the benefits of pelvic nodal irradiation. Roach et al. reported on data from the RTOG 9413 trial in which patients with an estimated greater than 15% risk of lymph nodal involvement were treated to the pelvic nodal areas or to the prostate only. Although rectal toxicity in the pelvic irradiation arm was slightly higher, there was an improved progression-free survival at 7 years of follow-up (40% versus 27%) with pelvic radiation. IMRT is now routinely used to treat the pelvic nodes and spare bowel toxicity, with a volume of 1–2 cm around the iliac vessels expanded during the simulation and targeted for treatment. Recently, Pollack et al. presented an abstract of the RTOG 0534/SPPORT trial, which compared postoperative salvage radiotherapy to the prostate bed, prostate bed radiation plus short-term hormone therapy, and prostate bed plus lymph node radiation and short-term hormone therapy. The highest 5-year freedom from progression, 89%, was seen in the third arm, suggesting that if these differences persist when the final manuscript is published, there may be an additive benefit of both the hormone therapy and nodal radiation to prostate bed radiation alone in these higher-risk postoperative salvage patients.

Treatment to only the prostate gland for low-risk disease or after pelvic irradiation encompasses the prostate as defined by treatment planning CT scan, the proximal prostatic urethra, and some portion of the seminal vesicles. Some clinicians will include the entire seminal vesicles in the treatment volume, whereas others will spare them if no clinical concern of invasion exists. Occult seminal vesicle involvement occurs in 20% to 30% of men with stage T2 prostate cancer and in approximately 50% to 70% of men with T3-T4 prostate cancer. If this portion of the tumor is not treated, then the cancer cannot be cured; but when the seminal vesicles are included, the amount of rectum in the treatment field will increase and cause additional morbidity. To address this, pretreatment MRI is extremely sensitive in detecting extent of disease for both ECE and seminal vesicle invasion.

Although node-positive prostate cancer has become less frequent in the modern era of community screening, controversy remains over the treatment of node-positive disease. Because these patients have such a high rate of distant metastases, oncologists historically may have recommended against local therapy. However, a review of the results in patients with conservatively treated prostate cancer shows a significant risk of bladder outlet obstruction, bladder invasion, hemorrhage, and pain, which may be prevented with radiation. Furthermore, radiation may offer the opportunity to "debulk" the tumor, leaving a smaller tumor burden to be treated by hormone therapy. Moreover, data from the randomized HORRAD and STAMPEDE trials suggest that among men with metastatic prostate cancer with low volume or limited metastases, treating the prostate with radiation may actually prolong overall survival. Therefore radiation therapy should be considered in patients with advanced disease who are at risk for local progression that may lead to significant morbidity of their cancer.

Men with earlier-stage prostate cancer can choose among three accepted treatments: radical prostatectomy, external beam radiation, or interstitial therapy. For men with shorter life expectancies, significant medical comorbidities, or lower risk disease, active surveillance is a fourth option: the ProtecT trial, reported by Hamdy et al., randomized 82,429 men with primarily low-risk prostate cancer to radical prostatectomy, non–dose-escalated radiation plus short-term hormone therapy, and active surveillance. Ten-year outcomes found no difference in overall survival, with a 3% increased absolute risk of developing distant metastases among men who started with active surveillance. Ultimately, about half of men who started with active surveillance ultimately required treatment, but they were at least able to defer the toxicities associated with surgery or radiotherapy. Notably, Donovan et al. published a companion paper with 6-year patient-reported outcomes for surgery, radiation plus short-term hormone therapy, and active surveillance. Long-term erectile function is similar whether patients undergo surgery or radiation, but key differences in toxicities include proctitis and irritative urinary symptoms that are associated with radiation versus leakage that is associated with surgery. Ultimately, patients, urologists, and radiation oncologists engage in shared decision-making to select the management approach whose toxicity profile is most aligned with the patient's preferences.

In reviewing a large series of men, most physicians divide patients into three groups. The group with a low risk of recurrence within 5 years consists of men with tumors confined to less than one half of one lobe of the gland, PSA less than 10 ng/mL, and a

Gleason score less than 6. The intermediate-risk group has tumors greater than one half of one lobe of the gland but not involving the other lobe, PSA between 10 and 20 ng/mL, or a Gleason score of 7. The high-risk group has tumors involving both lobes of the gland, ECE, seminal vesicle invasion, a PSA greater than 20 ng/mL, or a Gleason score greater than 8. In one analysis comparing the aforementioned three treatments in these three risk groups, D'Amico found no difference in the relative risk of recurrence between the treatments in the low-risk population. Among intermediate- and high-risk patients there was a threefold higher risk of recurrence among men undergoing interstitial radiation therapy when compared to external beam radiation or surgery, although the difference disappeared in the intermediate-risk group when men were treated with 6 months of androgen deprivation therapy in addition to the implant. In fact, in this intermediate-risk group of patients, D'Amico demonstrated a 10% overall survival benefit at 5 years with the addition of 6 months of androgen deprivation therapy to external beam radiation. Among men with high-risk cancers, the risk of recurrence was greater than 65% in all of the treatment groups, but the recurrences occurred earlier after interstitial therapy than with surgery or external beam radiation. These results suggest that local treatment is not adequate in patients with higher-risk disease and that possibly combining local therapies with androgen deprivation or introducing new therapies such as cytotoxic chemotherapy, higher radiation doses, or more extensive surgery would benefit this population.

There is a spectrum of androgen sensitivity in prostate tumors at diagnosis, and hormonal therapy exposure may select the androgen-independent population to proliferate while the more androgen-dependent population involutes and enters an extended G_0 state or undergoes apoptosis. In men with locally advanced, nonmetastatic prostate cancer treated with deferred therapy and androgen deprivation at the time of symptomatic progression, the median time to develop a hormone-resistant tumor was 48 months, whereas men treated with immediate androgen deprivation did not develop a hormone-independent tumor until a median of 84 months after diagnosis. These findings argue for earlier intervention at the time of diagnosis. The most common sites of progression when androgen resistance develops are at sites of previous disease. Therefore at the University of Pennsylvania, men at high risk are treated with concurrent hormone therapy and radiation to address both the pelvic tumor and occult distant metastatic disease. In a series of 80 patients with a median follow-up of 5 years, the 12-year cancer-specific survival was 90% and the biochemical relapse-free survival was 57%.

The use of combined hormonal and radiation therapy has been prospectively studied in multiple trials. The earliest study from MD Anderson demonstrated comparable 10-year survival among men with T3 tumors treated with radiation, including radiation to the pelvic lymph nodes, with or without lifelong adjuvant diethylstilbestrol (DES) 5 mg/day. A review of these results found an excess of cardiovascular deaths in the hormone group and an excess of cancer-related deaths in the control group. Two subsequent RTOG trials randomized men to radiation with or without hormone therapy and found that the hormones prolonged disease-free survival. One study treated men with 4 months of androgen deprivation therapy using a luteinizing hormone-releasing hormone (LHRH) agonist delivering 2 months of therapy before starting radiation and completing treatment with the end of radiation. The second study began radiation concurrently with the LHRH agonist and continued the therapy indefinitely. The median duration of hormone therapy in this group was 24 months. In a recent analysis of the results of these two trials, there appeared to be a small advantage favoring the longer course of therapy, although the results are not conclusive because of slight differences in the eligibility for the two studies. Most of the patients in both studies had T3N0 tumors, but patients with involved lymph nodes, positive margins following radical prostatectomy, and high-grade tumors were eligible for the study with indefinite hormone therapy.

Bolla et al. reported a European randomized trial comparing radiation and 3 years of hormone therapy to radiation alone. The authors demonstrated a survival benefit, with a 5-year overall survival of 79% in the patients receiving radiation and hormones versus 62% in men treated with radiation alone. Most of these men had T3N0 disease based on CT scan, lymphangiogram, or node sampling, although approximately 10% of the patients on each arm had T3 World Health Organization (WHO) grade 3 tumors. Published literature and current practice trends generally support the use of androgen deprivation in primary Gleason score

4 intermediate- and high-risk patients. For patients in the intermediate-risk group, a course of 6 months of androgen deprivation is usually given. Longer courses of androgen deprivation of 2 to 3 years are generally prescribed for patients falling in the high-risk categories. Side effects from androgen deprivation, which include impotence, hot flashes, and anemia, should be discussed with patients before they are placed on long-term androgen deprivation. Furthermore, long-term androgen deprivation may increase cardiovascular risks; so the duration of hormonal treatments should be specifically tailored to the individual patient. In light of this and other toxicities, multiple randomized controlled trials have sought to determine the optimal duration of hormone therapy. While Bolla et al., Lawton et al., and Zapatero et al. reported on trials that found an overall survival advantage with 28–36 months of hormone therapy when compared with short-term, 4–6 months of androgen deprivation; Nabid et al. found no overall or disease-specific survival advantage with 36 versus 18 months of hormone therapy, although Denham et al. found that 18 months was superior to 6 months. Across trials, these advantages were more pronounced in high-risk, in contrast to intermediate-risk, prostate cancer patients. Thus national guidelines support the use of 18–36 months of hormone therapy in high-risk patients, 4–6 months in unfavorable intermediate-risk patients, and omission of hormone therapy in favorable intermediate- and low-risk patients.

A number of centers have reported that men in the intermediate-risk group appear to have a longer biochemical disease-free survival with higher doses of radiation and the higher doses may be a substitute for the addition of hormonal therapy. Hanks initially reported in a retrospective review that the **biochemical no evidence of disease (bNED) survival** (i.e., PSA control) was better with doses greater than 76 Gy than with doses less than 70 Gy. Numerous subsequent studies have compared different doses of radiation therapy, and centers continue to **dose escalate** with newer radiation techniques. Treating the prostate to a minimum of 75 Gy has become standard, and some institutions are trying to push the dose to as high as 91 Gy. Whether these higher doses result in better tumor control or improved survival remains to be seen.

Patients who undergo prostatectomy for their prostate cancer must continue to be monitored. Theoretically, PSA levels in these patients should be undetectable. However, for patients with rising PSA after prostatectomy, radiation has been shown to salvage almost 50% of these patients. This scenario should not be confused with adjuvant radiation therapy following prostatectomy in the event of adverse pathologic features (discussed later). An estimated 25% to 33% of patients who undergo radical surgery will unfortunately have biochemical failures. Retrospective studies have demonstrated that patients with favorable characteristics of PSA doubling time of greater than 10 months, positive margins on pathological review, a Gleason score of 4 to 7, and a presalvage radiation PSA of less than 2 ng/mL had a 4-year progression-free probability of close to 70%; alternatively, the presence of these factors reduced this figure to below 20%.

Patients who are at high risk for local recurrence after prostatectomy should be evaluated for adjuvant radiation. These risk factors include the presence of ECE, seminal vesicle involvement, and positive surgical margins. Three postoperative phase 3 randomized trials each demonstrated improved biochemical progression-free survival or metastasis-free survival for patients with high-risk features who received radiation in the adjuvant setting. The SWOG92 08794 study, in particular, specifically demonstrated an improvement in *overall survival* from 49% to 58% at 12.7 years in these high-risk patients who received adjuvant radiation compared to observation after radical prostatectomy. Patients with detectable PSA after prostatectomy should be offered radiation in the salvage setting.

Toxicity from salvage and adjuvant radiation is increased compared to patients treated with radiation alone. Urinary incontinence is often an issue immediately following prostatectomy, and these symptoms usually stabilize after radiation. Therefore it is suggested to wait until incontinence has resolved or achieved maximal improvement before initiating radiation.

TESTICULAR CANCER

The role of radiation in managing testicular tumors is limited to the management of seminoma. Data show efficacy for radiation in clinical stage I nonseminomatous germ cell tumors, but the necessary dose and the associated toxicity suggest that these patients are better managed with comprehensive staging and close observation or chemotherapy if indicated. Radiation should be considered for adjuvant treatment for seminomas because of the unique sensitivity of these germ cell tumors to radiation. Almost all cells need to divide to express the lethal effects of radiation; seminoma cells undergo an intermitotic death because of their inability to accumulate and repair sublethal damage. Because of this characteristic, there is no shoulder on the cell survival curve, rendering seminomas exquisitely radiosensitive.

Staging of seminomas requires chest radiography to rule out metastatic disease, serum alpha-fetoprotein (AFP) and beta-human chorionic gonadotropin, and abdominal CT scan. Men who have not completed their family should consider a semen analysis because 10% of newly diagnosed seminoma patients are infertile, and an estimate of fertility is needed to counsel a patient concerning the effects of treatment on fertility. The use of chest CT is limited to patients with disease beyond the testicle because the incidence of distant metastases in patients with stage I disease is small, as evidenced by the less than 5% relapse rate among patients treated with adjuvant radiation.

The treatment of stage I seminoma has evolved following reports by Duchesne and Thomas that in patients followed without adjuvant therapy after orchiectomy, the risk of recurrence is less than 20%. For men willing to undergo close follow-up with CT scanning and chest x-ray for 5 years, observation may be an option with the understanding that they may need higher doses of salvage radiation or chemotherapy if they relapse. Because younger men comprise the largest group with this cancer, preservation of fertility is an issue when radiotherapy is used, and steps are taken to minimize the scattered radiation to the opposite testicle. However, many men elect surveillance and avoid radiation and its low but not insignificant risk of causing a secondary malignancy. Because of its ability to substantially reduce the volume of irradiated normal tissue, proton therapy is being explored as an approach to potentially reduce late effects, including second cancers. More broadly, in an effort to further reduce the dose to the pelvis using conventional photon-based radiotherapy, Fossa et al. have reported the results of a randomized trial with treatment to the paraaortic lymph nodes and renal hilum versus the same field plus the common and external iliac nodes. Fig. 19.3 shows radiation treatment fields for treatment of the paraaortic lymph nodes. Because most of the scattered

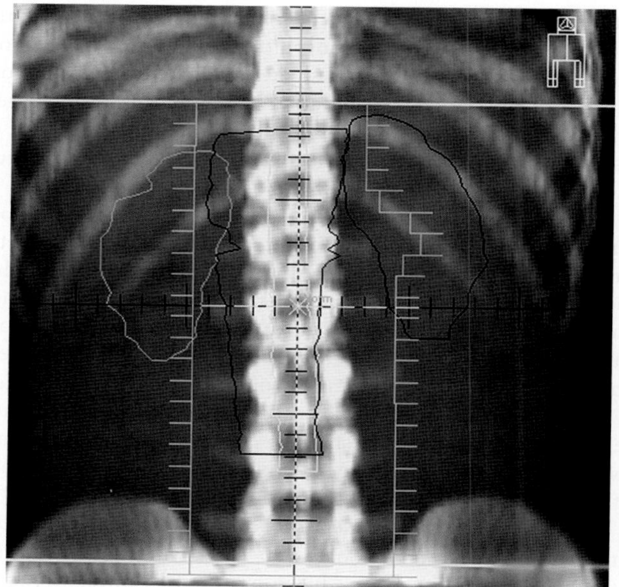

FIGURE 19.3 Radiation treatment fields to treat the paraaortic lymph nodes in patients with seminomas. The left and right kidneys are outlined to block excess dose to these structures.

dose to the testicle comes from the pelvic portion of the field, eliminating this substantially reduces the dose to the testicle and the risks of treatment-related infertility. The incidence of azoospermia was reduced from 30% in the group treated to the iliac region to 11% in the group treated to the paraaortic nodes only. The 11% figure is identical to the risk of primary infertility with no adjuvant therapy in men with a history of seminoma. Doses as low as 20 Gy may be used to treat seminomas, reducing the risk of retroperitoneal recurrence from 15% to 20% to less than 5% with a more favorable toxicity profile than the higher doses historically used.

Patients with stage II seminomas comprise a heterogeneous group including patients with retroperitoneal nodes measuring between less than 1 cm to greater than 5 cm. Patients with nodes smaller than 3 cm are generally treated with radiation fields similar to those used to treat a stage I tumor with the inclusion of the external and common iliac nodes. After a dose of 20–25.5 Gy is delivered, the initially involved nodal areas are boosted to a total dose of 30–36 Gy. Relapse-free survival rates approach 80%–90%. Acute and long-term toxicity is the limiting factor with radiation therapy. Abdominal radiation to a dose of 36 Gy can cause toxicity to organs of the gastrointestinal and genitourinary tracts, as well as fibrosis that increases the risk of bowel obstruction and potentially complicates future surgery that might be necessary in these relatively young men. Like radiation, bleomycin, etoposide, and cisplatin chemotherapy carry risks of infertility and second cancers. Yet the unique toxicities of these chemotherapies include a risk of pulmonary fibrosis, peripheral neuropathy, renal dysfunction, ototoxicity, and heart disease. For patients with stage II disease and non-bulky lymph nodes smaller than 3 cm, it appears that radiotherapy- and chemotherapy-based approaches have similar overall and disease-free survival benefits, and therefore treatment should be individualized. For patients with stage II seminoma and bulky nodal disease greater than 3 cm, chemotherapy is preferred, as relapse-free survival with radiotherapy is unacceptably low. Likewise, there is little modern experience with radiation for stage III and IV seminoma, and the available data suggest that these patients are better treated with chemotherapy. It should be noted that a history of seminoma in one testicle puts the patient at risk for seminoma in the other testicle, and these patients should be carefully monitored for their lifetime. Emerging radiation techniques in the treatment of stage I-II seminoma includes the use of proton therapy to reduce the dose of radiation outside of the nodal targets, potentially sparing anterior gastrointestinal and genitourinary organs and theoretically reducing the risk of second malignancy.

PENILE AND URETHRAL CANCERS

Squamous cell carcinoma of the penis is rare in the United States and is more prevalent in other countries. Surgery is an option for many patients, but radiation offers an organ-sparing approach for selected patients. Although penectomy is associated with better local control, a meta-analysis has shown similar 5-year overall survival, approximately 75%, whether penectomy or radiotherapy is used. Before radiation is administered, circumcision should be performed if the penis is not already circumcised. Superficial lesions can be treated with either external radiation or interstitial radiation using radium needles or iridium seeds in catheters. It is frequently necessary to treat the superficial inguinal nodes because 50% of men will have palpable adenopathy and the risk of occult involvement of nodes is high in men with poorly differentiated cancers or tumors of the glans. If a patient is treated with external radiation, he may most easily be treated with an en face electron beam to treat the penis and the lymph nodes (which can lie at a depth of 5 cm below the skin). However, this beam arrangement results in significant toxicity, and with CT planning, IMRT may offer a better radiation dose distribution. A dose of 45 to 50 Gy is generally prescribed to treat clinically uninvolved skin and lymph nodes, but the primary tumor and areas of gross disease need to be treated to a dose of 65 to 70 Gy. Morbidity of radiation to this area includes moist desquamation of the penis and scrotum with accompanying edema, often lasting 8 to 12 weeks after radiation. Nodal dissection increases the frequency and severity of edema. For small, low-grade tumors (less than 2 cm) of the shaft of the penis, the risk of nodal involvement is low, and these patients may be treated with interstitial radiation to the local area only.

Historically, small series reported that while definitive radiation was effective in controlling the tumor, this came with substantial morbidity. More recent series using HDR brachytherapy have reported long-term penis preservation rates of 67%–87%, with local control on the order of 71%–93%. Key toxicities include acute dermatitis, long-term cosmetic changes, necrosis, and meatal or urethral stenosis that may require dilation or catheterization. Nonetheless, physicians and patients may be willing to accept these toxicities when weighed against the alternative of up-front penectomy. Limited data likewise support the use of radiation for organ preservation in selected urethral cancers, although these treatments come with an up to 20% complication rate with such toxicities as urethral stricture, fibrosis, and chronic edema of the penis. Limited data support the use of concurrent chemoradiation for selected urethral cancers, but for penile cancer, it remains to be determined whether radiation and chemotherapy may be combined to reduce the risk of distant metastases and to allow lower doses of radiation to be used to minimize morbidity.

Summary

Extensive experience with radiation in the treatment of genitourinary tumors demonstrates that it is an effective treatment for selected patients. External and interstitial radiation, in some cases with hormone therapy, is an effective alternative to radical prostatectomy for prostate cancer. Likewise, radiotherapy is an alternative to penectomy for selected penile cancer patients. Radiation with concurrent chemotherapy is an alternative to radical cystectomy in selected operable bladder cancer patients, as well as those who are medically or surgically inoperable.

Treatment decisions must be individualized based on the clinical findings and patient preferences. Although the incidence of urinary incontinence following radical prostatectomy may range from 1% to 30%, the incidence of proctitis following radiation may range from 3% to 20% following radiation. In facilities with state-of-the-art equipment and physicians with specialized skills, it may be difficult to recommend one treatment over another, whereas in other facilities, one department may have special abilities that would support a treatment preference based on institutional experience.

It is likewise necessary to consider the working relationship between the departments of Urology and Radiation Oncology within each institution. For instance, even though chemosensitized radiation may be equivalent to radical cystectomy, it may not be desirable to pursue a course of bladder conservation if the urologist does not believe that a salvage cystectomy is possible after radiation.

Because there may be alternatives that are similarly effective, it is important to avoid confusing patients with conflicting claims of superior results. Patients should be presented with all alternatives for treatment and encouraged to select the treatment that will produce the most desirable results and the most acceptable morbidity risks.

CLINICAL PEARLS

1. Radiation doses above 76 Gy can be safely prescribed to the prostate and seminal vesicles without significant toxicity using modern radiation technologies.
2. Moderately hypofractionated radiation, to doses of 70 Gy in 28 fractions or 60 Gy in 20 fractions, is now standard for many patients with prostate cancer.
3. Patients with rising PSA after radical prostatectomy should be referred for salvage radiation therapy.
4. Bladder cancer patients who are not surgical candidates should be offered definitive chemoradiation as an alternative to cystectomy.

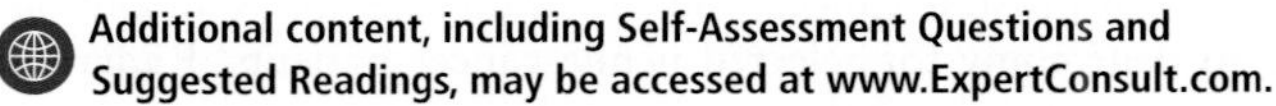

Additional content, including Self-Assessment Questions and Suggested Readings, may be accessed at www.ExpertConsult.com.

Laparoscopic Surgical Anatomy, Laparoscopy, and Robotic-Assisted Laparoscopic Surgery

Kiran Sury, MD, and Phillip Mucksavage, MD

Introduction

When Georg Kelling performed the first diagnostic laparoscopy on a dog in 1901, it is unlikely he understood the full ramifications of his innovative technique. Over a century later, the laparoscopic approach provides equivalent efficacy for many upper and lower urinary tract surgeries and has a distinct advantage over open techniques in terms of postoperative pain, cosmesis, recovery, and length of stay. Urologists have been quick to incorporate robotic assistance as well, to the point that minimally invasive surgery has become the gold standard for many urologic procedures. A thorough knowledge of the basics of laparoscopy and laparoscopic anatomy is essential for any practicing urologic surgeon.

Patient Selection

The indications for laparoscopic surgery continue to expand, and now include partial and radical nephrectomy, nephroureterectomy, pyeloplasty, adrenalectomy, prostatectomy, cystectomy with diversion, and retroperitoneal or pelvic lymphadenectomy. In choosing patients for laparoscopic surgery, absolute and relative contraindications must be considered. Absolute contraindications to laparoscopic surgery, such as uncorrected coagulopathy or severe cardiopulmonary disease, are no different than for open alternatives. Relative contraindications take into consideration the patient's ability to tolerate insufflation and laparoscopic instruments. As the skill and comfort level of the surgeon increases, even patients with relative contraindications may be appropriate candidates for minimally invasive surgery.

RELATIVE CONTRAINDICATIONS

Chronic Obstructive Pulmonary Disease

Typically, the abdomen is insufflated using carbon dioxide (CO_2), which is absorbed into the bloodstream. In patients with normal pulmonary function, this excess CO_2 is easily exhaled. Patients with chronic obstructive pulmonary disease (COPD) have impaired ventilation, however, and are at higher risk of developing hypercarbia or CO_2 narcosis. These patients benefit from lowering intraabdominal insufflation pressure to 10 to 12 mm Hg and are candidates for helium insufflation, though this gas is rarely used. They will also benefit postoperatively from increased pulmonary toilet and judicious use of narcotics.

Pregnancy

Despite known physiologic changes during pregnancy, laparoscopy has been shown to be safe and effective. In fact, laparoscopic cholecystectomy and appendectomy are considered the standard of care during pregnancy. While it is always preferable to defer elective surgeries to the postpartum period, they can be performed antepartum with careful fetal monitoring and modifications to the standard technique. Low pneumoperitoneum (12 mm Hg or less) and left-sided positioning (to increase venous return) can minimize placental ischemia and reduce the risk of cardiopulmonary compromise.

Obesity

Obesity (defined as a BMI > 30) was previously believed to be a relative contraindication to laparoscopic urologic surgery. Challenges include distortion of normal anatomy during trocar placement and higher operative time when compared to a lean population. Conversion rates and complications, however, are equivalent when comparing obese to normal weight patients. Among obese patients, studies have shown that the laparoscopic approach results in equivalent or lower operative time, blood loss, and length of hospital stay. Given the comorbidities and complications of wound healing that arise with obesity, this patient population may derive maximum benefit from minimally invasive surgery.

Prior Abdominal Surgery

Prior abdominal surgery or trauma may lead to intraabdominal adhesions, which can make obtaining laparoscopic access and insufflation more challenging. However, after safely obtaining access (discussed later), a laparoscopic lysis of adhesions (LOA) can be done efficiently and safely provided the surgeon is familiar with the technique. Laparoscopic LOA has been shown to confer a quicker recovery of bowel function and fewer wound complications when compared with open LOA. Minimally invasive retroperitoneal or extraperitoneal approaches can also be utilized to avoid the need for a LOA altogether.

Patient Positioning

RENAL SURGERY

Transperitoneal Approach

First, a nasogastric/orogastric tube and Foley catheter should be placed to ensure decompression of the stomach and bladder. The patient is then positioned in a modified 30- to 45-degree flank position (lateral decubitus) with the operative side up, and the break of the bed between the 12th rib and the anterior superior iliac spine. The lower leg should be flexed at the knee, and the upper leg should be straight, taking care to pad pressure points at the hips, knees, and ankles. An arm board is placed on the side of the bed to which the patient is facing, and the lower arm should be placed palm up in a natural position with an axillary roll to prevent brachial plexus injury. The upper arm may be flexed gently and placed over the chest or secured in parallel with the patient's body. Patients may be secured to the bed using straps or tape. At this point, a "test roll" should be performed with operative personnel on both sides of the bed to ensure that the patient is properly secured. The table can then be flexed slightly, and the anesthesia team should properly bolster the patient's head so it remains level with the rest of the spine. Once the desired position is attained, the patient may be prepped (Fig. 20.1).

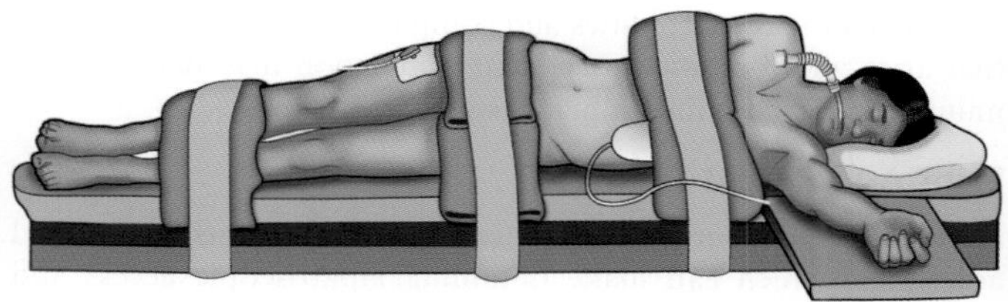

FIGURE 20.1 Positioning for renal surgery.

Retroperitoneal Approach

Retroperitoneal renal surgery requires the patient to be placed in a full flank position, and the table should be flexed as much as possible to facilitate retroperitoneal dissection. The patient's ventral surface should be more towards the midline, rather than the edge of the bed.

Robotic-Assisted Laparoscopic Prostatectomy

This section will focus on robot-assisted laparoscopic prostatectomy (RALP). Positioning for pure laparoscopic prostatectomy is similar.

The patient should be placed in a low lithotomy position to allow for the robot to be positioned between the patient's lower extremities. Alternatively, split leg positioners may be used. The patient's buttocks are brought to the end of the table, and the weight of the leg should be on the patient's heel, which should be padded. If the robotic model in use allows side-docking, supine positioning will suffice. The arms can be placed on either side and tucked, with the palms oriented so the thumbs are anterior. The elbows should be padded, and a strap should be placed over the patient's chest. After access is obtained the patient will be placed in extreme Trendelenburg to allow gravity to retract intraabdominal contents cranially, so the strap needs to be secure. However, a hand should still fit between the strap and the patient's body to allow for adequate chest wall excursion. The nasogastric/orogastric tube can be placed prior to prepping, but the Foley catheter should be kept sterile and placed after prepping, as it will be manipulated during the case.

Other Pelvic and Upper Tract Surgery

Other laparoscopic urologic surgery positioning may be adapted from that given earlier. For instance, robot-assisted and pure laparoscopic cystectomy or ureterectomy and reimplantation can be done from the same positioning as a RALP, and robot-assisted and pure laparoscopic upper urinary tract surgery can be done from the same positioning as laparoscopic renal surgery (i.e., pyeloplasty can be done from the same positioning as transperitoneal laparoscopic renal surgery). For a combined upper and lower tract case such as nephroureterectomy with bladder cuff, the patient can be positioned in low lithotomy with a bump under the ipsilateral side to create a modified "lazy" flank position. This will facilitate access to the upper abdomen and pelvis (though the robot may need to be redocked during the case).

Access

Obtaining access to the peritoneal cavity is done primarily via two techniques, Veress (closed) or Hasson (open). Multiple reviews and meta-analyses have shown both to be safe and effective means of access and insufflation. The surgeon should choose the technique with which they are most comfortable.

CLOSED (VERESS) ACCESS

The Veress needle has a spring-loaded inner sheath that retracts when the needle engages tissue as it moves through the abdominal wall. After passing into the peritoneal cavity, the sheath deploys and guards the needle tip. This greatly decreases the likelihood of injury to intraabdominal vessels and viscera.

The needle should be inserted perpendicularly to the skin, usually at either the umbilicus or Palmer's point (subcostal at the midclavicular line). Three "clicks" are heard/palpated when the needle passes through the successive layers of the anterior abdominal wall: skin, anterior rectus sheath, and posterior rectus sheath/peritoneum. Once the third "click" is noted, the needle is held stable, and a syringe is used to aspirate. Succus or blood indicates a bowel or vascular injury. Should this occur, the needle should be kept in place and an alternate puncture site chosen with a new needle. After the initial aspiration, irrigation and aspiration should be repeated with 2 mL of saline. If the needle is correctly located, it will aspirate easily and the saline will quickly drop into the peritoneal space.

The needle can then be connected to insufflation as the transduced pressure is monitored. Initial insufflation pressure should read less than 10 mm Hg. If the needle is pushed against an intraabdominal viscus, pressure may be elevated. In this circumstance, pressure may be reduced by retracting the abdominal pannus up and away from this viscus. In very obese patients, the weight of the abdominal wall may cause increased initial pressures, which will decrease with continued insufflation. If the abdomen is not uniformly insufflated or the pressure persists greater than 10 mm Hg, the needle is in the preperitoneal space and needs to be advanced.

Once insufflation reaches the preset pressure (usually 15 mm Hg), the primary trocar can then be advanced. The laparoscope is then introduced to survey the abdomen for anatomic variations, adhesions, and damage to viscera or vessels from the Veress needle. The remaining trocars can then be placed under direct visualization. The Veress needle is removed, and the insufflation tubing is connected to the camera trocar.

OPEN (HASSON) ACCESS

The Hasson technique involves a 12-mm or smaller incision, usually at the umbilicus. The layers of the abdominal wall are carefully dissected until the peritoneal cavity is reached, as confirmed by direct visualization and digital insertion. A Hasson or balloon trocar is then inserted and sutured to the fascia to prevent dislodgement (these sutures can be used to close the fascial defect at the end of the case). Insufflation is then connected to this trocar, and the abdomen can be surveyed prior to placement of further ports. The Hasson technique is often favored in children and pregnant patients. It is used for retroperitoneal and extraperitoneal approaches as well.

DIRECT ACCESS AND TROCAR TYPES

Direct trocar access is a possible alternative for the well-selected patient with low suspicion for adhesions. A primary trocar is advanced into the abdomen through an umbilical incision without prior Veress insufflation. Strong upward traction, rather than pneumoperitoneum, is used to separate the skin from the viscera below. After the primary trocar is placed, insufflation is connected, the camera is introduced, and subsequent ports are placed under direct vision. This blind technique significantly reduces the time needed to gain abdominal access. In the hands of an experienced surgeon, it has been shown to have a lower rate of failed entry when compared to the Veress technique, without any demonstrated significant increase in bowel or vascular injury.

Bladed trocars have been widely replaced by blunt trocars that spread, rather than cut through, the layers of the abdominal wall. This reduces the risk of port site bleeding and visceral injury. Further advancements include radially expanding and optical trocars. Radially expanding trocars penetrate the abdomen with a small gauge needle surrounded by a polymer sleeve. The needle is removed, and a larger blunt obturator is placed through the sleeve to expand the tract. This allows for a smaller skin incision and obviates the need to close fascia. Optical trocars have an obturator with clear plastic tip that allows visualization of the abdominal layers as the primary trocar is passed into the abdomen. Surgeons may use their preferred device, as meta-analyses of laparoscopic access have yet to identify one method as superior to the others.

Physiologic Changes of Pneumoperitoneum

Pneumoperitoneum is traditionally obtained using CO_2 gas maintained at an intraabdominal pressure (IAP) of 15 mm Hg. This can be lowered as needed (i.e., pregnancy) or raised briefly to assist in hemostasis or increase working space. However, animal studies have shown that prolonged increase of IAP to 20 mm Hg can result in impaired renal, cardiac, and pulmonary function.

CARDIOVASCULAR EFFECTS

The overall effect of pneumoperitoneum produces no net change in cardiac output. Pneumoperitoneum compresses the vasculature, causing increased peripheral vascular resistance and decreased peripheral venous return. The heart rate increases in response, and cardiac output remains the same. However, the increased sympathetic response and acidosis from hypercarbia leaves patients more susceptible to arrhythmias.

PULMONARY EFFECTS

The increased IAP from pneumoperitoneum is transmitted to the thoracic cavity, causing decreased compliance and elevated peak and mean airway pressures. The CO_2 used for insufflation is absorbed, causing hypercarbia and acidosis, which are poorly tolerated by patients with COPD or other pulmonary compromise. Arterial blood gases may be used to measure CO_2 levels in this patient population. If hypercarbia develops, decreasing the IAP to 10 mm Hg and/or changing the insufflation gas to helium can reduce this effect. The steep Trendelenburg positioning used for robot-assisted pelvic surgeries further reduces chest wall compliance and impairs O_2 exchange. Close coordination with anesthesia is of critical importance. In this situation, compliance can often be improved by increasing respiratory rate and tidal volume.

RENAL EFFECTS

Renal parenchymal compression and decreased renal blood flow from pneumoperitoneum cause a temporary decrease in urine output that can persist for several hours postoperatively. Studies have shown intraoperative oliguria is not predictive of acute kidney injury. It is important to make anesthesia and the peri-operative staff aware that this will normalize with time. Otherwise, over-resuscitation can lead to edema and respiratory compromise.

Trocar Placement

Stylistic differences exist among laparoscopic surgeons regarding trocar placement. We provide a description for effective trocar placement that can be adapted per surgeon preference and patient anatomic variation.

The camera can be placed via the initial access trocar or through a secondary trocar, depending on the procedure and location of initial trocar placement. In general, the camera should face the same direction as the surgeon's instruments, so the surgeon does not have to mentally reverse the laparoscopic image. Trocars should be placed in a position that the surgeon finds ergonomically acceptable and should be placed 7 to 10 cm away from one another to prevent arm clashing. During robotic surgery, a minimal distance of 8 cm is needed between robotic arms to limit intraoperative collisions.

TRANSPERITONEAL RENAL SURGERY

The initial trocar placement (5 or 12 mm) is halfway between the anterior superior iliac spine (ASIS) and umbilicus, just lateral to the rectus muscle. A second trocar (5 or 12 mm, dilating) is placed in line with the first trocar, but approximately 2 to 3 fingerbreadths below the costal margin. The third trocar (5 or 12 mm) is placed in the midline, just lateral to the umbilicus, midway between the first and second trocars. The third trocar is the camera port. Additional trocars can be placed as seen fit. Often, a fourth trocar is placed lateral to the most inferior trocar and used to help retract the kidney. For obese patients, the umbilicus is a less useful landmark and ports are shifted laterally. For right-sided renal surgeries, a 5-mm trocar can be placed immediately below the xiphoid process to accommodate a self-retaining retractor to retract the liver cranially (Fig. 20.2).

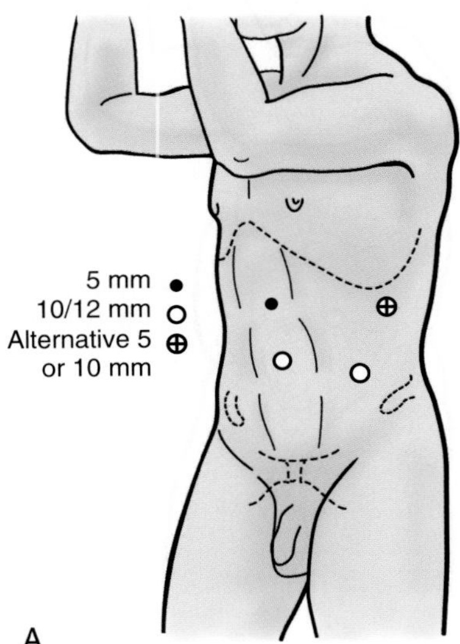

FIGURE 20.2 Port placement for transperitoneal renal surgery. (A) Left renal surgery. *Continued*

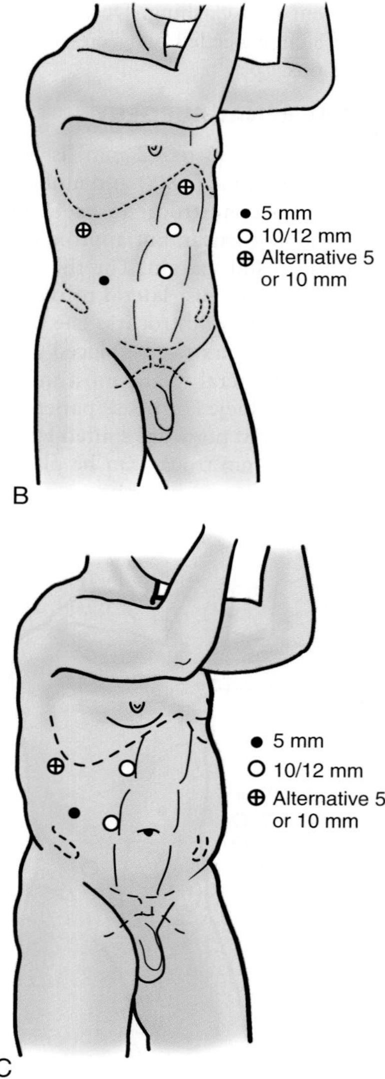

FIGURE 20.2, cont'd (B) Right renal surgery. (C) Right renal surgery, modified for the obese patient. (From Partin AW, Peters CA, Kavoussi LR, et al. *Campbell-Walsh-Wein Urology*. 12th ed. Philadelphia: Saunders; 2020:102, 2279-2308.e5.)

RETROPERITONEAL RENAL SURGERY

While transperitoneal renal surgery access can be obtained via an open or closed technique, retroperitoneal renal surgery access is uniformly performed via an open technique. After positioning, as previously described, a 2-cm incision is made below the 12th rib along the posterior axillary line, and the retroperitoneal space is accessed by a combination of sharp and blunt dissection. The lower pole of the kidney can be palpated, and retroperitoneal fat is visualized. A balloon dilator is used to expand the retroperitoneal space to approximately 800 mL. A secondary trocar is then placed lateral to the paraspinous muscle at the costovertebral angle. Via this trocar, the peritoneum is swept forward and medially to allow space a third trocar. This is placed anteriorly to the primary access site along the same line as the first two trocars (Fig. 20.3). Adjustments for obesity are not necessary during retroperitoneal surgery.

HAND-ASSISTED LAPAROSCOPIC RENAL SURGERY

Access may be attained via an open or closed approach. Alternatively, the hand port itself can be used to insufflate the abdomen. The hand port is usually placed in a periumbilical location, and the incision is made commensurate with the surgeon's glove size (i.e., a size 7 glove should make a 7-cm initial incision). Additional trocars can then be placed under direct vision or using the surgeon's hand to safely guide the trocar into position.

PROSTATECTOMY

Three robotic arms are classically used, with one camera trocar and two assistant ports. The symphysis pubis is marked after insufflation, and the 12-mm camera port is placed one fingerbreadth above the umbilicus. An 8-mm port is then placed on either side of the umbilicus, at a level of 14 to 15 cm from the superior aspect of the pubic symphysis, and 7 to 8 cm from the camera port to allow for full range of motion. These ports will dock the working robotic arms, usually bipolar forceps and monopolar scissors. Two more ports are then placed laterally, another 8 cm apart, in mirror image of each other. The rightmost port will be 8 mm for the third robotic arm for retraction, and the leftmost port will be a 12-mm assistant port, with an AirSeal

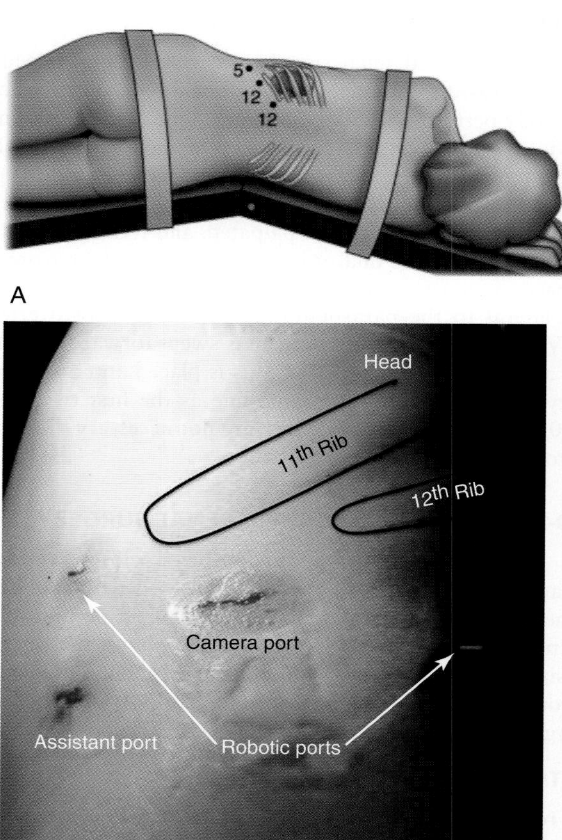

FIGURE 20.3 Port placement for retroperitoneal renal surgery. (A) Left Retroperitoneal renal ports. (B) Port placement seen on actual patient.

to maintain constant pressure. Another 5-mm assistant port for suction is placed at a 45-degree angle cranial and lateral to the camera port (Fig. 20.4). The assistant ports and third arm may be swapped based on surgeon preference. This configuration can be adapted for other pelvic surgeries. For patients with a hostile abdomen, an extraperitoneal approach may be favorable. An

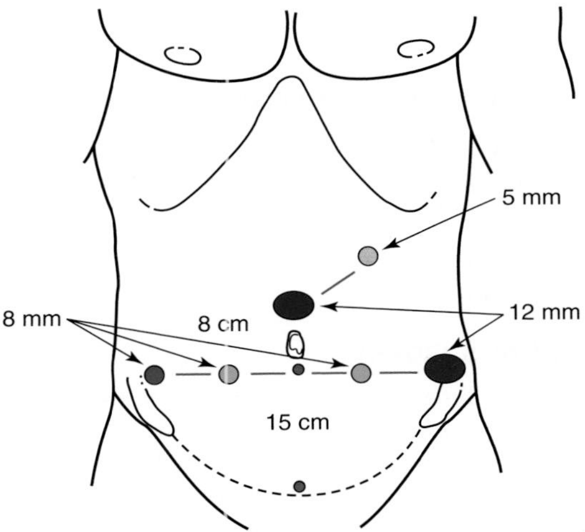

FIGURE 20.4 Port placement for robotic-assisted laparoscopic prostatectomy.

incision is made below the umbilicus, and dissection is carried down to the posterior rectus sheath. A trocar with balloon dilator is then used to develop the space of Retzius under direct vision. Secondary ports may be placed as given earlier, being mindful of the reduced working space.

Laparoendoscopic Single-Site Surgery

As surgeons continue to optimize laparoscopic technique and reduce patient discomfort, single-site surgery is becoming more available. Rather than placing multiple 0.5 to 1.2 cm ports, a single 2.5-cm incision is made at the umbilicus. Skin flaps are raised, and multiple ports can be placed in proximity. Various companies sell devices that combine the ports and valves into one trocar. Robotic manufacturers also offer a single port system, with curved instruments to accommodate the reduced working space and minimize clash. Often a second 5-mm incision is needed for an assistant port. While there are no long-term data on outcomes, some patients may prefer single-site surgery from a cosmesis standpoint. Anatomy remains the same, and surgical steps are as outlined below.

OTHER UPPER TRACT AND PELVIC SURGERIES

Port placement for other upper urinary tract procedures and pelvic surgery may be adapted from the above port descriptions for renal and prostate surgery.

Surgical Anatomy of the Upper Urinary Tract

RIGHT RENAL SURGERY

Renal anatomy differs based on laterality. On the right, the liver will immediately come into view and typically drapes over the upper pole of the kidney. The colon is identified and reflected medially after incision of the white line of Toldt membrane (Fig. 20.5). Dissection is continued inferiorly, directly on top of Gerota's fascia, ideally in the avascular field between the perirenal and mesenteric fat. Once the colon is adequately reflected and mesenteric fat is swept medially, the psoas muscle will come into view posterior and inferior to the kidney. Overlying the psoas muscle will be the genitofemoral nerve and psoas tendon. The gonadal vein and ureter are identified medial to the psoas muscle and kidney (Fig. 20.6).

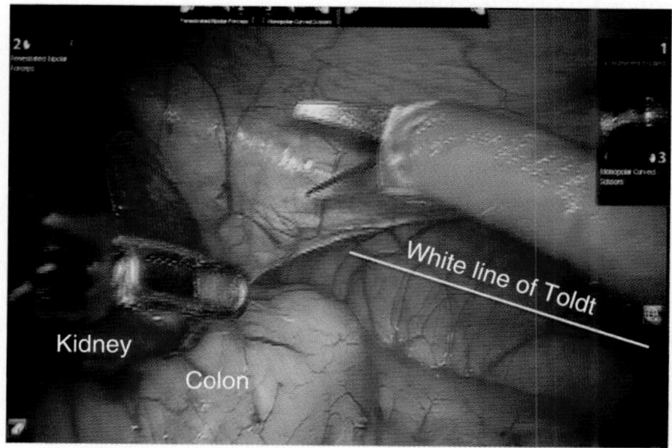

FIGURE 20.5 Incision of the white line of Toldt membrane.

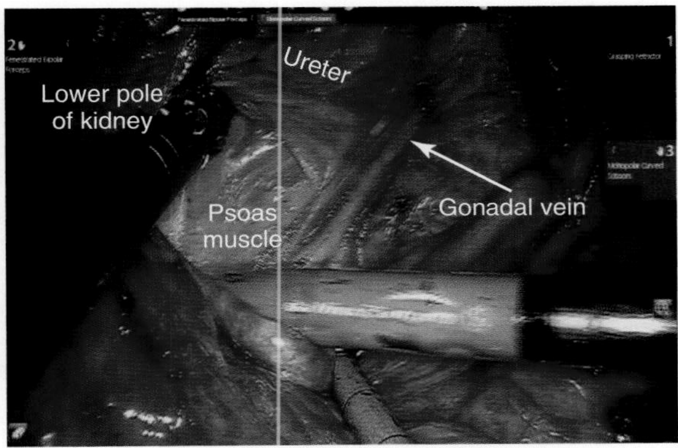

FIGURE 20.6 Gonadal vein and ureter.

The gonadal vein is often encountered first, and the ureter is found just medial and inferior to the vein. Subsequently, the ureter and gonadal vein can be traced cranially and used as a road map to the renal hilum.

In the region of the kidney itself, after the colon is reflected medially, the duodenum will be draped over the kidney and must be reflected medially as well (also known as Kocherization) to gain access to the hilum. The next major structure encountered, oriented on a horizontal plane, is the inferior vena cava (IVC). From caudal to cranial (or left to right, if the IVC is the lower horizon), a careful dissection along the IVC reveals the insertion of the gonadal vein, the main renal vein, and the adrenal vein. Most commonly, the renal artery lies directly superior and posterior to the renal vein (Fig. 20.7). Often the ureter can be mobilized and used to lift the kidney upward to facilitate hilar dissection. Once the main hilar structures have been divided, the adrenal gland can be accessed just medial to the upper pole of the kidney. The adrenal vein drains directly into the IVC and must be clearly identified if the adrenal gland is to be resected (Fig. 20.8). Due to its short size and direct drainage into the IVC, rapid exsanguination can occur if the right adrenal vein is accidentally torn during dissection. This has earned this diminutive vein the nickname "the vein of death."

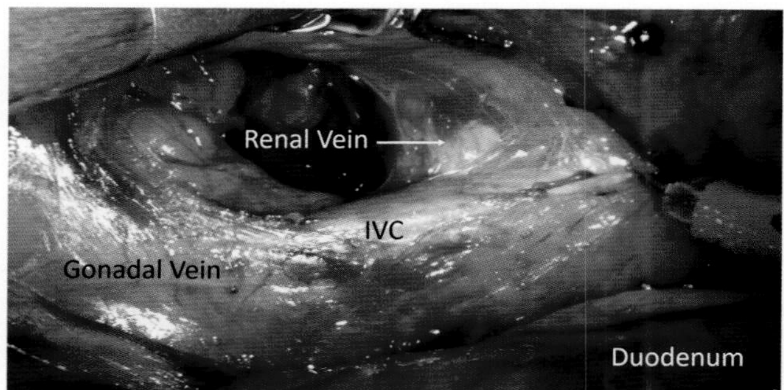

FIGURE 20.7 Right renal venous anatomy. *IVC*, Inferior vena cava.

LEFT RENAL SURGERY

On the left side, the spleen lies anterior and superior to the kidney. Left colon mobilization begins with division of the splenocolic ligaments that adhere the colon to the abdominal wall just inferior to the spleen. Releasing the splenorenal ligament, which contains the tail of the pancreas and splenic vessels, can help

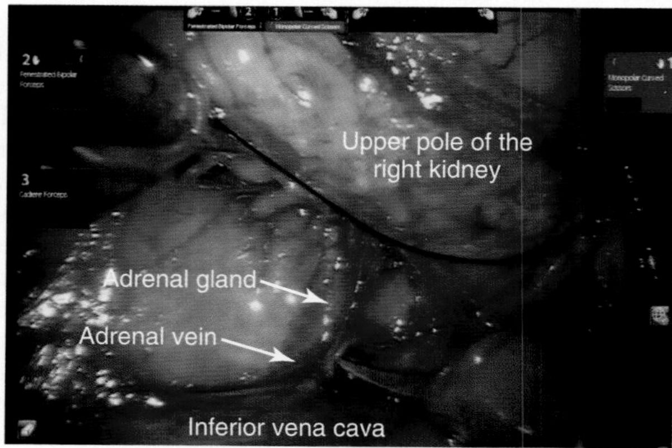

FIGURE 20.8 Right adrenal vein.

further visualize the hilum. Landmarks on the left mirror those on the right. Instead of the IVC, the aorta will be the dominant structure crossing horizontally across the bottom of the dissection field. The gonadal vein is more useful on the left, as it can be traced to its insertion into the renal vein. As the hilum is approached along the course of the gonadal vein, it is also important to remember the venous tributaries of the left renal vein. The adrenal vein, the ascending lumbar vein, and the gonadal vein all consistently drain into the renal vein (Fig. 20.9). If performing an adrenalectomy alone, the adrenal vein (much longer on the left) is ligated and the adrenal is easily dissected off the anteromedial surface of the kidney. Adrenal arterial supply comes from the aorta and the ipsilateral inferior phrenic artery and renal arteries.

RETROPERITONEAL RENAL SURGERY

The challenge of retroperitoneal renal surgery comes from the lack of working space and unfamiliarity of the anatomy when viewed from behind. Maintaining the proper anatomic landmarks is crucial to avoid catastrophic mistakes. The approach is similar on the left and right side. If the initial expansion balloon is positioned directly on the posterior surface of the psoas

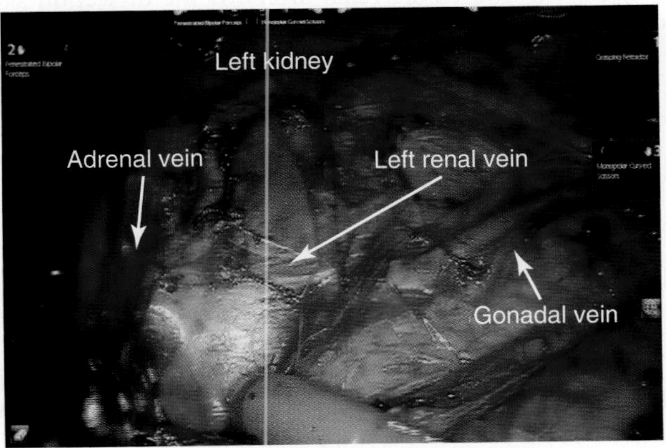

FIGURE 20.9 Left renal venous anatomy.

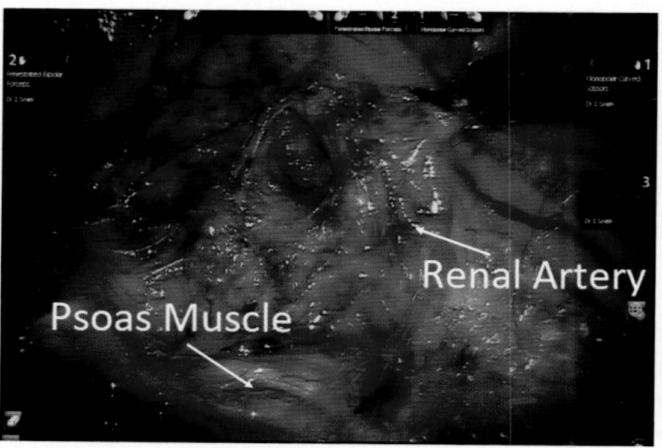

FIGURE 20.10 Retroperitoneal renal anatomy. The kidney is elevated towards the top of the picture.

muscle, the kidney (still encased in Gerota's fascia) will remain attached to the peritoneum and anterior structures and be "above" the surgeon throughout most of the case. It is most helpful to keep the psoas muscle as the "floor" of the screen. Once the retroperitoneal space is developed, an incision into Gerota's fascia is made 2 cm above and parallel to the psoas muscle. This incision is widened, and pulsations in the perirenal fat should lead to the renal artery. If the dissection skews lower, too close to the muscle, it can continue directly under the great vessels and lead to injuries of the contralateral kidney. If the proper plane is maintained, the renal vessels should appear directly in front of the surgeon, since the camera port is placed almost at the level of the hilum. The renal vein will lie directly behind the artery in this approach (Fig. 20.10).

Surgical Anatomy of the Lower Urinary Tract

As described in the previous section on positioning, the patient will be supine in steep Trendelenburg, which allows gravity to retract the bowels to the upper abdomen. The medial umbilical ligaments and the internal inguinal rings form the initial landmarks (Fig. 20.11). The rectum dives caudally, with the rectovesical pouch just posterior to the tip of the Foley balloon, anterior to the rectum.

During radical prostatectomy, the bladder is dropped by incising the peritoneum across both medial umbilical ligaments, which opens the pre-vesical space of Retzius. Blunt dissection in this space will reach the pubic symphysis. Superficial fat overlying the prostate and bladder can be mobilized to visualize the puboprostatic ligaments, with the endopelvic fascia spreading laterally. The superficial venous complex of the prostate will run midline and is easily controlled with bipolar electrocautery (Fig. 20.12).

The endopelvic fascia is then incised from the base of the prostate to the puboprostatic ligaments, revealing the levator muscles below. These muscles are gently separated from the lateral borders of the prostate. The fine fibers at the apex of the prostate are very prone to bleeding. The puboprostatic ligaments are then sharply divided, and the midline deep dorsal venous complex is ligated via suture or laparoscopic stapler (Fig. 20.13).

Removal of excess periprostatic fat will aid in visualization of the vesicoprostatic junction. The assistant can advance and retract the Foley catheter to help delineate the bladder neck. Dissection in the proper plane will reveal a clear distinction between the smooth prostate capsule and detrusor fibers. When the Foley catheter is visualized, the balloon is deflated and the catheter is

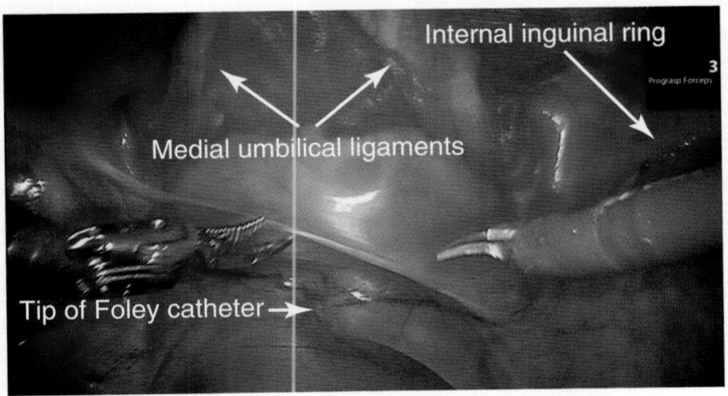

FIGURE 20.11 Initial image for robotic prostatectomy.

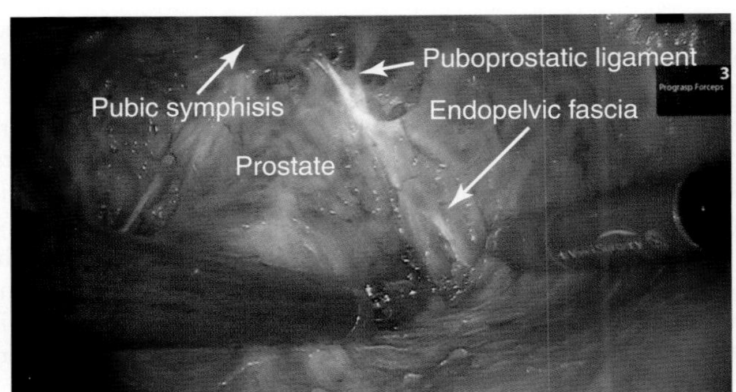

FIGURE 20.12 Endopelvic fascia.

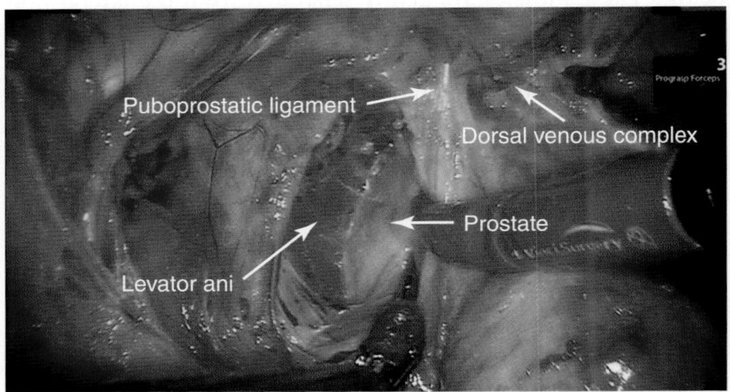

FIGURE 20.13 Incision of endopelvic fascia.

grasped and used for upward traction by the third robotic arm (Fig. 20.14). As the posterior bladder neck is transected, the vas deferens and seminal vesicles will come into view. When they are dissected free, Denonvilliers' fascia is identified and incised and the space between the rectum and prostate is developed. If this plane is taken posteriorly and toward the apex of the prostate, only the prostatic pedicles remain as lateral attachments (Fig. 20.15).

The neurovascular bundles run along the posterior-lateral aspects of the prostate, deep to the prostatic fascia and lateral to

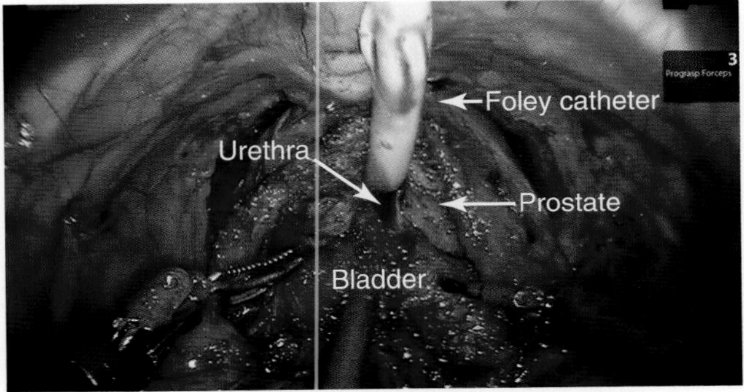

FIGURE 20.14 Dissection of bladder neck and prostate.

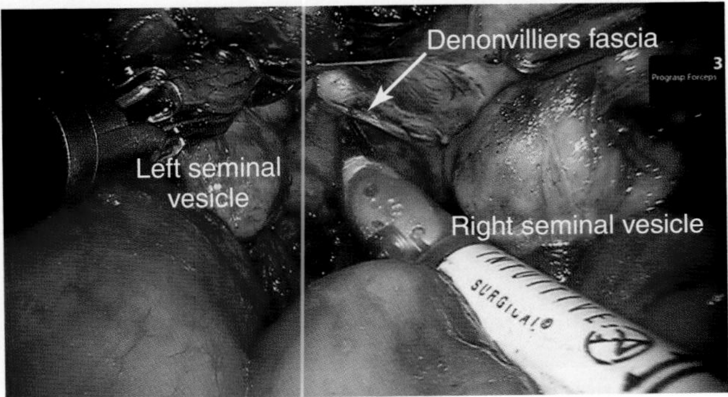

FIGURE 20.15 Denonvilliers fascia.

the prostatic pedicles. They can be released from the prostate by incising the lateral prostatic fascia and sweeping it away from the prostatic capsule with minimal electrocautery (Fig. 20.16). This is important when attempting a nerve-sparing operation. The pedicles are then clipped and divided to free the base of the prostate. The apex of the prostate is contiguous with the striated urethral sphincter. When the dorsal venous complex is incised, the urethra will appear as longitudinal muscle fibers extending into the prostate. Incision of the urethra will complete the prostatic dissection (Fig. 20.17).

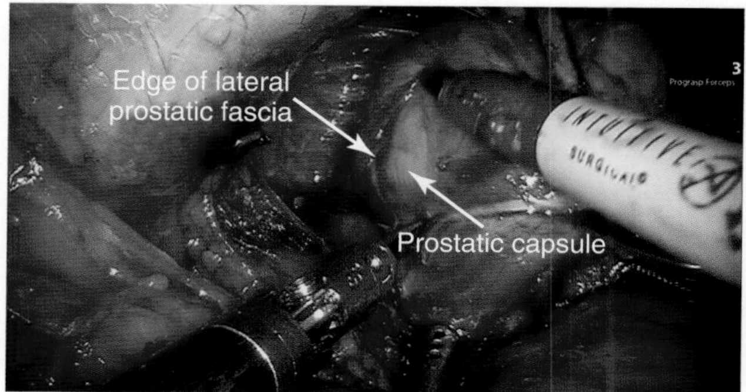

FIGURE 20.16 Release of neurovascular bundle.

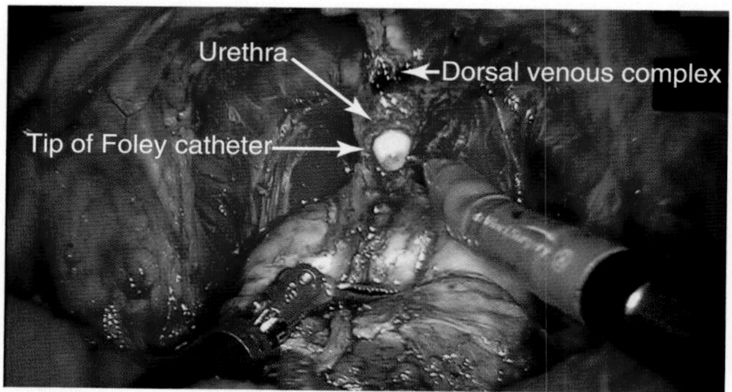

FIGURE 20.17 Dissection of apex of the prostate.

Some surgeons prefer to begin with a posterior approach, with an incision in the rectovesical pouch and dissection of the vas deferens and seminal vesicles while the bladder is still tethered to the anterior abdominal wall. For Retzius-sparing surgery, this dissection is carried laterally to the pedicles and continued anteriorly, such that the bladder is never dropped and remains suspended in its original anatomic location. During a radical cystoprostatectomy, ligation of the major branches of the internal iliac artery (superior vesical artery and posterior pedicle of the bladder) and complete division of the peritoneum along the inferior peritoneal fold of the rectovesical pouch will allow posterior dissection of the bladder and prostate away from the rectum. Anterior dissection can then be performed as previously described.

Complications

Complications are inevitable with any surgical procedure, and laparoscopic surgery is no different. Injuries are possible at any step of the operation and can vary from temporary nerve paralysis to lethal damage of a major vessel. Here we describe the more common complications of laparoscopic surgery and techniques that may reduce their occurrence.

NEUROMUSCULAR INJURIES

Neuromuscular injuries can largely be prevented by careful attention to detail during patient positioning. As described in the positioning section, padding of pressure points and limiting joint flexion and extension to within the normal range of motion will reduce postoperative discomfort. During lateral positioning, the term "axillary roll" is a misnomer. Padding should be placed under the chest, not the axilla, so as to lift the brachial plexus and prevent compression injury. During lithotomy positioning, padding the lateral surface of the leg and confirming that the weight of the leg lies on the heel prevents peroneal nerve injuries. Lower leg compartment syndrome is also possible when patients are placed in the lithotomy position for an extended amount of time. Lowering the legs every 2 hours can avoid this complication.

Rhabdomyolysis can also occur with patients in the flank or lithotomy position, especially with prolonged operative times. This complication is more common in males (who tend to have more muscle mass) and the obese (compression from the excess body mass increases muscle ischemia). Urine may be tea-colored, and a urine dipstick will be positive for blood but negative for red blood cells. Protein may not be present initially, as proteinuria does not develop until the renal tubules are damaged. Hydration and close monitoring of electrolyte balance are usually enough to overcome mild kidney injury, but dialysis may be needed in cases of acute renal failure.

VASCULAR INJURIES DURING ENTRY

Fortunately, the incidence of major vascular injury during entry is exceedingly low, often cited as roughly 0.2%. If blood is aspirated after Veress needle placement, the needle should not be removed. Instead, a second Veress should be placed elsewhere with the intention of evaluating the location of the first Veress placement. Similarly, if blood fills the initial trocar, it should be kept in place. A laparotomy will be required to repair the vascular injury. More commonly, injury occurs to non-major vessels such as the epigastrics. These can be avoided by placing initial trocars either directly midline or at least 6 cm lateral. If the patient is thin, transillumination with the laparoscopic camera can highlight the vessels running along the anterior abdominal wall.

BOWEL INJURIES

Bowel injury during minimally invasive surgery has a similarly low incidence, with a urology-focused series finding an incidence of 0.75%. Unlike vascular injuries, which are usually readily apparent, almost half of all bowel injuries are unrecognized at the time of surgery. These injuries are most often due to electrocautery, which causes thermal injuries that do not present until 1 to 2 days postoperatively. Symptoms include abdominal pain, diarrhea, and extreme pain at a single trocar site without erythema or purulence. Labs may show a paradoxical leukopenia, instead of the usual postoperative leukocytosis. Computed tomography (CT) with oral contrast is the best diagnostic study to reveal the injury.

If a bowel injury is recognized intraoperatively, there are several treatment options based on severity. If the injury is secondary to Veress needle placement only, no formal repair is needed. Full thickness injury from errant trocar placement requires resection and anastomosis, often with the aid of general surgery colleagues. Thermal injury may be repaired with interrupted sutures. These must be followed postoperatively, as delayed cell necrosis can result in serosal breakdown and further bowel perforation.

CO_2 EMBOLISM

CO_2 embolism can occur at any time during laparoscopic surgery. It presents with a sudden drop in end-tidal CO_2 and collapse of the other cardiovascular parameters. Monitors will show an elevated central venous pressure, and anesthesia may be able to appreciate a "millwheel" heart murmur on exam. Management includes immediate desufflation, application of 100% oxygen, and Trendelenburg positioning with the right side up (left lateral decubitus). Theoretically this should trap any gas emboli in the right atrium for subsequent aspiration via central venous catheter. There is not much a surgeon can do to prevent this dreaded complication, though if blood is aspirated on initial Veress placement, insufflation through that needle should not be performed.

CLINICAL PEARLS

1. When using the Veress insufflation technique, initial pressure should remain less than 10 mm Hg if truly in the intraperitoneal space.
2. Insufflation causes intraoperative oliguria that resolves without the need for excess hydration.
3. Bowel injury secondary to electrocautery can present days after surgery with leukopenia and isolated port site tenderness.

Additional content, including Self-Assessment Questions and Suggested Readings, may be accessed at www.ExpertConsult.com.

Male Sexual Dysfunction

Hailiu Yang, MD, Zachary Winnegrad, MD,
Daisy Obiora, MD, and Allen D. Seftel, MD

Introduction

Laumann and colleagues from the University of Chicago reported a comprehensive study of male sexual dysfunction in 1992. The three most common male sexual dysfunctions identified were decreased libido, erectile dysfunction (ED), and ejaculatory dysfunction (EJD). The study cohort was men aged 18 to 59. Premature ejaculation (PE), a subtype of EJD, was the most common of all the male sexual dysfunctions. Sexual dysfunction was assesed in women as well, and was noted to be more prevalent in women (43%) versus men (31%) and was associated with age and educational attainment.

In a follow-up study, Lindau and colleagues, also from the University of Chicago, conducted a large population survey. They reported the prevalence of sexual activity, behaviors, and problems in a national probability sample of 3005 US adults (1550 women and 1455 men) 57 to 85 years of age and described the association of these variables with age and health status. Among men, the most prevalent sexual problem was erectile difficulties (37%). Fourteen percent of all men reported using medication or supplements to improve sexual function. Men and women who rated their health as being poor were less likely to be sexually active and, among respondents who were sexually active, were more likely to report sexual problems.

Thus, there seem to be two subgroups of men with specific sexual issues based on their age. The predominant problem for the younger cohort is PE, whereas for the older cohort it is ED.

In spite of these seemingly clear age-related divisions, clinically the waters have become a bit muddied. Data suggest that male ED that is vasculogenic in origin may start as early the fourth decade and that ED is related to garden-variety vascular risk factors such as hypertension, hyperlipidemia, and diabetes.

Remarkably, ED that starts in the fourth decade may also be a strong predictor of future cardiovascular disease (CVD). From January 1, 1996, to December 31, 2005, a Mayo Clinic group (Inman 2009) biennially screened a random sample of 1402 community-dwelling men with regular sexual partners and without known coronary artery disease (CAD) for the presence of ED. The prevalence of ED was 2% for men aged 40 to 49 years, 6% for men aged 50 to 59 years, 17% for men aged 60 to 69 years, and 39% for men aged 70 years or older. The CAD incidence densities per 1000 person-years for men without ED in each age group were 0.94 (40–49 years), 5.09 (50–59 years), 10.72 (60–69 years), and 23.30 (70 years or older). For men with ED, the incidence densities of CAD for each age group were 48.52 (40–49 years), 27.15 (50–59 years), 23.97 (60–69 years), and 29.63 (70 years or older). These authors concluded that ED and CAD may be differing manifestations of a common underlying vascular pathology. When ED occurs in a younger man, it is associated with a marked increase in the risk of future cardiac events, whereas in older men, ED appears to be of lesser prognostic importance. Importantly, these researchers concluded that young men with ED may be ideal candidates for cardiovascular risk-factor screening and medical intervention.

To complicate the issue a bit further, ED and male benign prostatic hyperplasia/lower urinary tract symptoms (BPH/LUTS) have now been linked both epidemiologically and pathophysiologically, adding importance to querying for BPH/LUTS in men with sexual dysfunction, particularly ED.

Thus, ED is no longer easily subdivided by age into distinct groups. Significant age-related overlap exists because the importance of ED detection in the younger male appears to have prognostic importance for both BPH symptoms and CVD.

This backdrop now serves as the foundation for a discussion of male sexual function and dysfunction with the hope of providing some clarity and guidance to a formerly simple disease process that has now become a bit more complex.

Peyronie's Disease

Peyronie's disease (PD) is an acquired penile deformity that manifests during a penile erection (curvature, indentation, hourglass deformity, or shortening). The condition usually presents with palpable induration (plaque) in the penis with or without painful erection. The symptomatic incidence of PD has been estimated at 1%, though recent evidence suggests that this is a significant underestimate of the true disease burden. DiBenetti et al. in 2012 estimated the number of patients with diagnosed PD to be 0.5%, while 13% were likely to have PD based on a questionnaire of their symptoms. Stuntz et al. in 2016 estimated 0.7% of patients with PD while 11% were probable cases of PD. These results illustrate the need to raise awareness of this disease process. A survey of 152 primary care physicians (PCPs) and 98 urologists found that both urologists and, to a greater extent, PCPs underestimate the prevalence of PD and the rate of ED in patients with PD. They also overestimate the rate of spontaneous resolution. In addition, 44% of PCPs and 17% of urologists reported that they do not examine the penis as part of a routine physical, which the authors note is a missed opportunity to allow a patient to bring up any concerns he might have.

PD has also been reported to occur in association with Dupuytren contractures, plantar fascial contractures, tympanosclerosis, trauma, urethral instrumentation, diabetes, gout, Paget disease, and the use of beta-blockers. This condition may occur in a familial pattern.

BURDEN OF DISEASE

PD can cause significant psychological bother and distress and potentially strain sexual relationships. Anxiety and stress manifest in a variety of ways. In a survey of 92 men with diagnosed PD, 48% were classified as clinically depressed based on their scores on the Center for Epidemiological Studies Depression Scale. In an analysis of the prevalence of depression as a function of time since diagnosis, the percentage of PD patients with depression did not change significantly in patients with PD for less than 18 months versus those who have carried the diagnosis for more than 18 months, suggesting a lack of mental adjustment to the diagnosis of PD. Similarly, in a subset of patients who were assessed for depression at baseline and after 18 months, the percentage of patients with severe depression was not statistically different (21% versus 23%, respectively).

In addition to depression, men with PD also experience problems with psychosocial and sexual function. In interviews, patients with PD indicated that problems with functioning typically fall into one or more of four domains: (1) physical appearance and self-image, (2) sexual function and performance, (3) PD-related pain and discomfort, and (4) social stigmatization and isolation. While men with PD varied in the type and intensity of their subjective reactions to this condition, the major themes and patterns of response were consistent across groups. A questionnaire survey of men with PD also revealed a high prevalence of emotional and relationship problems.

PATHOGENESIS

PD is thought to be a wound-healing disorder within the penis characterized by formation of a fibrous, inelastic plaque, predominantly of collagen, on the tunica albuginea, the fibrous sheath surrounding the corpora cavernosa of the penis. The formation of fibrotic plaque or plaques results in penile deformities during erection including curvature, shortening, narrowing (hourglass), and bending (hinge effect). The degree to which PD limits sexual performance varies, depending on the angle and orientation of the penile curvature. Patients with mild curvature may feel slight discomfort during penetration, whereas patients with more severe curvature may be incapable of intercourse. Interestingly, some evidence suggests that the degree of curvature deformity does not directly correlate with the severity of the psychosocial bother of the disease. Men with lesser degrees of curvature may be as bothered as men with more severe deformities. The symptoms of PD are frequently accompanied by varying degrees of ED. Pain may or may not be correlated with the development of penile curvature.

PD represents localized aberration of the wound-healing process. The prerequisites for the development of PD in susceptible individuals include intercourse-related penile trauma, blunt penile trauma, bleeding within the tunica albuginea of the corpus cavernosum, clustering of fibrin and the inflammatory cells, and overexpression of cytokines and growth factors, which stimulate the production of more matrix proteins and inhibit the action of metalloproteinases. Growth factors such as TGF-beta are able to recruit more inflammatory cells and thus form a vicious cycle. The outcome is a prolonged inflammatory process in a matrix of excessive but disorganized elastic and collagen fibers resulting in focal loss of elasticity of the tunica albuginea. Furthermore, PD has been commonly associated with ED. The factors that contribute to ED are severe penile deformity preventing intercourse, a flail penis, psychological distress or performance anxiety, and impaired penile vascular function. It has also been proposed that the reduced compliance of the tunica albuginea of the plaque prevents normal compression of these veins during erection.

CLINICAL PRESENTATION AND EVALUATION

Patients usually present in either the early or late phase of the disease process. A patient in the early phase typically presents with a nodule or plaque, painful erection, and/or penile deformity during erection. In the late phase a patient presents with a harder plaque, and stable penile deformity during erection and ED. The diagnosis is easily made with detailed medical and sexual history and physical examination. A detailed psychosexual history should also be obtained that includes penile rigidity during erection, shortening, induration, hourglass constriction, or pain with or without erection, and psychological impact of the disease.

Physical examination usually detects a well-defined penile plaque or an area of palpable induration located on the dorsal surface of the penis with a corresponding dorsal penile deformity. Lateral and ventral plaques are less common but result in more coital difficulty. Penile pain may be present with erection or during sexual intercourse. Spontaneous improvement in pain usually occurs within 6 months as the inflammation settles.

Penile ultrasonography is useful in identifying the number and site of the plaques and calcification. Additionally, penile injection with a vasoactive agent (i.e., prostaglandin) can be useful for formal evaluation of the degree and stability of curvature in the office setting. Per the recent American Urological Association (AUA) Peyronie's disease guideline by Nehra et al. in 2015, penile injection with a vasoactive agent with or without ultrasound is recommended for characterization prior to surgical treatment.

TREATMENT

The treatment of PD is typically conservative at the onset. Reassurance is all that is necessary in patients with a slight curvature (less than 10 degrees), minimal bother, and no ED. If treatment is required, patients can be managed medically or surgically.

The efficacy of medical management of PD is difficult to determine due to the lack of prospective studies, as noted by Nehra et al. (2015). Treatment is primarily aimed at correction of the penile deformity and curvature. Medical therapies include systemic agents and local or intralesional injections. Oral systemic agents include potassium aminobenzoate, tamoxifen, acetyl-L-carnitine, colchicine, and vitamin E. Due to the lack of quality evidence, the AUA guidelines, noted by Nehra et al. (2015), currently do not recommend any oral treatment for PD, with the exception of nonsteroidal antiinflammatory drugs (NSAIDS) for pain.

Many intralesional therapies for PD have been used, including injection of calcium channel blockers (such as verapamil), steroids, and interferon. The use of collagenase Clostridium histolyticum (CCH) as an intralesional agent has been subjected to a number of double-blind placebo-controlled protocols that have demonstrated good efficacy. In a phase 3 double-blinded, placebo-controlled randomized trial (IMPRESS I and II), CCH injection with modeling was shown to reduce penile curvature by 17 degrees or 34% compared to 9.3% in the placebo group. The treatment group also had decreased bother compared to the placebo group. As a result of these studies, CCH is now Food and Drug Administration (FDA)–approved for the treatment of PD. The treatment protocol is up to eight injections of 0.58 mg CCH, two injections per cycle separated by approximately 24 to 72 hours. Modeling was performed after each injection and recommended to patients between treatment sessions. Note that CCH should only be used on patients with 30 to 90 degrees of stable deformity in the absence of calcified plaques, hourglass deformity, ventral curvature, and curvature > 90 degrees. Anyone using CCH should be warned regarding the rare risk of penile fracture, which requires urgent surgical exploration.

Mechanical devices for the treatment of PD, such as the vacuum erection device or devices for penile traction, have not been adequately studied.

Penile low-intensity extracorporeal shockwave therapy (Li-ESWT) is a novel treatment for both ED and PD that has recently gained significant popularity. In terms of PD treatment, multiple randomized controlled trials of Li-ESWT show lack of significant efficacy. Thus, the only current, true indication for penile LI-ESWT treatment may be penile pain, which may resolve over time without any treatment.

Surgical treatment is an option for all patients with PD, including those with severe penile curvature or narrowing that interferes with sexual intercourse. Penile surgery should be delayed until the disease has stabilized, typically 6 to 18 months after onset. Detailed evaluation of penile vascular and erectile function (EF) is highly recommended before surgical intervention. This can be performed by penile ultrasound with concurrent injection of a vasoactive agent to induce an erection. Patients will need thorough counseling with respect to the expected outcomes and possible side effects of surgery. Historically, penile implants were the only therapeutic option for patients with severe curvature with or without preserved EF. However with recent developments, surgical reconstruction is generally divided into three categories: tunical shortening procedures, tunical lengthening procedures, and prosthetic procedures.

Tunical shortening procedures are performed on the convex side of the penis opposite the penile plaque. Shortening procedures are most appropriate for patients with good EF, adequate penile length, and no penile narrowing or hourglass type of deformity. The technique of elliptical excision of the tunica to treat PD was introduced by Pryor and Fitzpatrick in 1979. In a review of 359 men operated on between 1977 and 1992, 82% regained the ability to have intercourse. Complications reported after the Nesbit procedure include penile shortening, ED, penile hematoma, penile narrowing or indentation, urethral injury, herniation, suture granuloma, glans numbness, and phimosis. Other modifications include the Yachia procedure. Instead of removing an ellipse of tunica, a long longitudinal or multiple smaller longitudinal incisions are made in the tunica albuginea and are then closed horizontally in a Heineke-Mikulicz fashion to correct the angle of penile curvature.

Tunical lengthening procedures involve lengthening the curved, shortened side in an attempt to straighten the penis; this is performed by incising or excising the plaque on the short side of the penis and placing a graft to cover the defect. Lengthening procedures are indicated in patients with severe penile curvature or narrowing or hourglass deformities. Historically, tunical grafting procedures met with limited success. The introduction of dermal grafts has changed the surgical success rates. Many autologous grafts (temporalis fascia, dura mater, tunica vaginalis, and saphenous vein), cadaveric tissue (dermis, fascia, pericardium, or porcine small intestine submucosa), and synthetic materials (polyester and polytetrafluoroethylene, collagen fleece) have subsequently been used with varying results. Excision of the plaque has been the standard approach. However, the pathological process of PD often extends far beyond the plaque and removing a large area of tunica albuginea may impair EF. Successful straightening is accomplished in 75% to 95% of the patients in published series, with 5% to 13% of potent men complaining of a decrease in EF after surgery. Thus, some surgeons have moved away from plaque excision and have moved to plaque incision with placement of a graft. Prospective studies comparing the two techniques remain lacking in the current body of literature.

The use of a penile prosthesis in patients with PD is reserved for those with severe curvature with or without ED that has not responded to medical management. Excellent results have been reported in the literature. Adjunct procedures during prosthesis placement include incising or excising the plaque during prosthesis placement, with placement of a graft, or with penile modeling. In most patients with mild to moderate curvature, insertion of a penile prosthesis tends to straighten the penis, with no additional procedures necessary. A recent review by Raheem and Hsieh reported satisfactory curvature correction rate of 4% to 71% with prosthetic placement alone, and 60% to 71% of patients requiring additional maneuvers at the time of prosthetic placement. Patient satisfaction rates were noted to be between 48% and 100% in a pooled group or retrospective and prospective studies.

Physiology of Sexual Function

ERECTION

Complex interactions between physiologic, neuroendocrine, vascular mechanisms, and psychogenic interplay produce penile erections. This is often following sexual stimulation that triggers a cascade of events. In essence, erections are neurovascular phenomena combining neurotransmission and vascular biologic responses.

A release of neurotransmitters results in smooth muscle relaxation in both penile erectile tissue and the penile arterial walls. This transforms the penile vasculature and erectile tissues from a contracted, minimally perfused state to a relaxed, blood engorged state.

1. Functional anatomy of the penis
   a. Corporal bodies

PENILE ANATOMY (Fig. 21.e1)

The penis is composed of three cylindrical structures: the paired corpora cavernosa and the corpus spongiosum. The corpora cavernosa comprise two spongy, paired cylinders contained in the thick envelope of the tunica albuginea. This is covered by a loose subcutaneous layer underlying the skin. The tunica affords great flexibility, rigidity, and tissue strength to the penis. Between the layers of tunica run the emissary veins which are compressed during erection to ensure high-pressure rigidity. In the ventral groove of the tunica albuginea between the 5 o'clock and 7 o'clock position the outer layer is absent leaving this area most vulnerable to penile prostheses extrusion. Each corpora cavernosum houses a network of endothelial-lined sinusoids within a trabecula of smooth muscle. An incomplete septum between both erectile bodies allows passage of blood from one side to the other. The terminal cavernous nerves and helicine arteries are intimately associated with the smooth muscle. In the flaccid state, the blood slowly diffuses from the central to the peripheral sinusoids. During erection, the rapid entry of arterial blood through the central and the peripheral sinusoids expand and fill the cavernosa, producing an increase in pressure and a firm erection (Fig. 21.e2).

The corpus spongiosum covers the urethra and expands distally to form the glans penis. The spongiosum is covered with only one layer of tunica albuginea, allowing low pressure during erection. The glans penis has a high concentration of nerve receptors to provide sensory input to facilitate erection and enhance pleasure.

In cavernosal tissue, nitric oxide (NO) is accepted as the principal neurotransmitter responsible for erectile response (Fig. 21.e3). With sexual arousal, NO synthase converts L-arginine and oxygen to NO. NO is also released from nonadrenergic-noncholinergic (NANC) nerves and endothelial cells to cause an increase in the production of cyclic guanosine monophosphate (cGMP), a second messenger that activates protein kinase G. NO enters into the target cell and binds to guanylate cyclase, launching a signaling pathway which ultimately produces penile cavernosal smooth muscle relaxation via formation of cGMP. This leads to the opening of potassium channels and the closing of calcium channels resulting in a drop in cytosolic-free calcium. This drop in calcium is the direct cause of arterial and cavernous smooth muscle relaxation, culminating in increased penile blood flow and rigidity. The erection is further enhanced by the compression of the emissary veins between the layers of the tunica upon corporal engorgement, preventing the outflow of blood. Downregulation of components of this pathway is thought to be central to the pathophysiology of many forms of ED.

Cyclic nucleotide levels are determined by both synthesis, through the activities of guanylate cyclase on 5'-guanosine triphosphate (GTP), and enzymatic degradation, through the activity of phosphodiesterases (PDEs). Penile detumescence partly results from an increase in phosphodiesterase inhibitor type 5 (PDE-5) activity, which breaks down cGMP. The smooth muscle regains its contractile tone when cGMP is degraded by PDE-5. Competitive inhibition of the action of PDE-5 can be accomplished by a class of drugs known as PDE-5 inhibitors. These drugs prevent the degradation of cGMP, allowing cGMP to act longer and produce an erection of better quality and longer duration. Some examples include sildenafil, vardenafil, and tadalafil which can all be used to enhance EF.

Ejaculatory Dysfunction

EJD is subdivided into retrograde ejaculation, delayed ejaculation, anejaculation, and premature or rapid ejaculation. Retrograde ejaculation occurs when the bladder neck does not close as the seminal fluid or ejaculate reaches the prostatic urethra. Thus, this fluid enters the bladder instead of expulsion outside the body. Delayed ejaculation can be due to a dysfunctional nervous system, such as seen in diabetes or other neurological conditions that dampen the neurologic impulses. It may also be due to psychogenic causes. Psychologically, one theory is that the male is "punishing" his partner by not ejaculating. This condition can be so severe that electroejaculation or sperm aspiration may be required to procure sperm for fertility. The same holds true of anejaculation.

Rapid ejaculation or PE is somewhat enigmatic. In the animal kingdom, rapid ejaculation is the rule as the animal wishes to mate quickly to avoid predators. Humans however have different motivational issues for intercourse. In light of this, the definition of rapid is not as clear. The historical definition of PE is ejaculation outside the vagina or just upon entrance, within 1 to 2 minutes of an erection. The newly proposed definition of lifelong PE in heterosexual men is ejaculation occurring within approximately 1 minute of vaginal penetration on 75% of occasions for at least 6 months. Acquired PE is a condition in which the man suddenly ejaculates rapidly after some incident or event, but was ejaculating "normally" prior to this event.

Normal ejaculatory times or latencies were described by Waldinger et al. The duration of ejaculation as measured by intravaginal ejaculation latency time (IELT) may help assess subjective complaints of PE and is usually determined by self-assessment with a stopwatch.

Waldinger's group investigated the IELT distribution in the general male population and the accuracy of IELT assessment by using a blinded timer device instead of a stopwatch. This was done to minimize potential interferences with the spontaneous and natural progression of intercourse. In a sample of 474 men from the Netherlands, Spain, the United Kingdom, Turkey, and the United States, the IELT was measured with a timer device for a duration of 4 weeks. Questionnaires were administered before and after the 4-week IELT assessments.

The data revealed that the IELT had a positively skewed distribution, with a geometric mean of 5.7 minutes and a median of 6 minutes (range: 0.1–52.1 minutes). Men from Turkey had the shortest median IELT (4.4 minutes). Men from the United Kingdom had the longest IELT (10 minutes). Circumcision and condom use had no significant impact on the median IELT. Subjects who were discontent with their latency time had slightly lower median IELT values of 5.2 minutes than the median of the population. These data were essential as they helped provide guidance on defining "normal" ejaculatory periods.

TREATMENT OF EJACULATORY DYSFUNCTION

Retrograde ejaculation can be treated with oral sympathomimetics taken within a few hours of sexual activity to aid in closure of the bladder neck. Delayed ejaculation and anejaculation are frequently caused by psychogenic issues and as such, can often be treated with appropriate psychotherapy.

PE or rapid ejaculation is best treated with a combination of psychotherapy and drug therapy. While there are no FDA-approved treatments for PE, topical anesthetics and antidepressive medications have been shown to be effective in randomized controlled trials. Topical lidocaine can be applied to numb penile sensation prior to intercourse, resulting in delayed ejaculation and improved sexual function. Various tricyclic antidepressants and serotonin reuptake inhibitors have known side effects of decreased libido and delayed ejaculation. These medications have been shown to be efficacious in the management of PE and include dapoxetine, paroxetine, clomipramine, imipramine, fluoxetine, sertraline, and citalopram. A list of the recommended dosing can be found on the AUA guideline (https://www.auanet.org/guidelines/premature-ejaculation-guideline). Patients with ED and acquired PE should be treated for ED prior to initiating therapy for PE. Psychosexual therapy as monotherapy, or combined with any of the aforementiokned therapies is often very useful and helpful.

PATHOPHYSIOLOGY OF ERECTILE DYSFUNCTION

Erectile dysfunction is defined as the inability of the male to achieve an erect penis as part of the overall multifaceted process of male sexual arousal. This definition is not limited to intercourse and gives equal importance to other aspects of male sexual behavior.

ERECTILE DYSFUNCTION PREVALENCE AND MEDICAL RISK FACTORS

It is estimated that at least 10 million to 20 million American men have ED. In the National Health and Social Life Survey, the prevalence of male sexual dysfunction was 31% in a population of approximately 1400 men aged 18 to 59 years. Hypogonadism (5%), ED (5%), and PE (21%) were the three most common male sexual dysfunctions in this study.

The Massachusetts Male Aging Study (MMAS), a large multidisciplinary epidemiologic survey, reported the results of self-reported ED in men between the ages of 40 and 70 years and categorized their ED as complete, moderate, minimal, or not impotent. Fifty-two percent of the sample reported some degree of

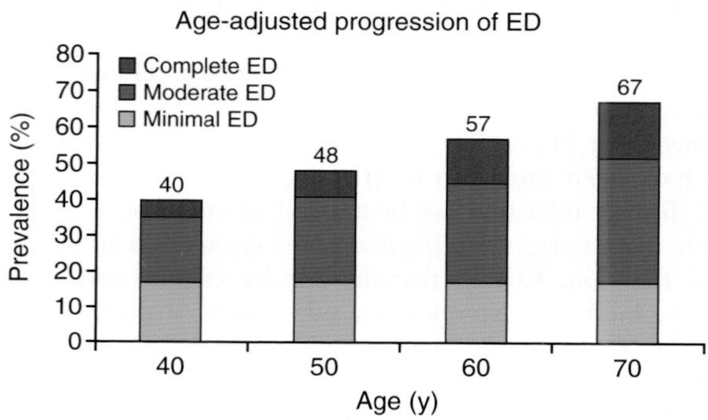

FIGURE 21.1 The landmark Massachusetts Male Aging Study (MMAS), a community-based observational study of nearly 3000 men, aged 40 to 70 years, clearly established that erectile dysfunction *(ED)* is highly prevalent, age related, and progressive. Subjects (n = 1290) were asked to respond to a sexual activity questionnaire characterizing their level of ED. Minimal ED was defined as "usually able to get or keep an erection"; moderate, as "sometimes able"; and complete, as "never able to get and keep an erection." Self-rated ED was reflected by higher frequency of erectile difficulty during intercourse, lower monthly rates of sexual activity and erection, and lower satisfaction with sex life and partner. In the MMAS study, 40% of men were estimated to have ED at age 40, but this increased to 67% at age 70. Age was the only variable that proved to be a statistically significant predictor of ED (*P* < .0001). (From Feldman HA, Goldstein I, Hatzichristou DG, et al. Impotence and its medical and psychosocial correlates: results of the Massachusetts Male Aging Study. *J Urol*. 1994;151:54-61. As reproduced with permission, courtesy TestosteroneUpdate.org/Causeducation.org.)

ED. This study demonstrated that ED is an age-dependent disorder. Between the ages of 40 and 70 years the probability of complete impotence tripled from 5.1% to 15%, moderate impotence doubled from 17% to 34%, and the probability of minimal impotence remained constant at about 17%. By the age of 70 years, only 32% of the sample reported no ED (Fig. 21.1).

In MMAS, cigarette smoking was a risk factor for total ED in men who had been treated for heart disease and hypertension and had untreated arthritis. After the data were adjusted for age, men treated for diabetes (28%), heart disease (39%), and hypertension (15%) had significantly higher probabilities of ED than the overall sample (9.6%). Men with an untreated ulcer (18%), untreated arthritis (15%), and an untreated allergy (12%) were also significantly more likely to develop ED.

The association between ED and hypertension, hyperlipidemia, diabetes mellitus (DM), and depression is documented in several studies. This evidence supports the fact that ED shares common risk factors with these four clinical conditions. Therefore, as a pathophysiologic event, ED can be viewed as a potential observable marker of these concurrent diseases and most importantly for CVD.

CLASSIFICATION OF ERECTILE DYSFUNCTION

1. Psychogenic ED

   Male sexual behavior is complex and depends on intrinsic and extrinsic factors including olfactory, somatosensory, and visceral signals. Most cases of ED have organic causes and less than one-third are purely psychogenic. Cortical regions of the brain including the hypothalamus and the hippocampus act as centers for integration of sensory stimuli and hormonal influences to initiate sexual behavior. These stimulatory or inhibitory signals act through spinal erection centers to control penile erection. Two mechanisms have been proposed for psychogenic ED: direct inhibition of the spinal erection center by the brain as an exaggeration of the normal suprasacral inhibition and excessive sympathetic outflow with elevated peripheral catecholamine levels resulting in increased penile vascular smooth muscle tone thereby preventing its necessary relaxation. Many psychological conditions such as performance anxiety, depression, stress, low self-esteem, and personality disorders can cause psychogenic ED.

2. Neurogenic

   Any pathology involving the brain, spinal cord, or peripheral nerves can cause ED. It has been estimated that 10% to 19% of ED is neurogenic. Onset of ED relating to the development of a neurological disability may suggest neurogenic cause for ED but does not exclude other causes of ED.

   Brain pathologies that may cause ED include temporal lobe epilepsy, hypothalamic pituitary disorders, Parkinson disease, stroke, tumors, and Alzheimer disease. Spinal cord injuries, multiple sclerosis, spina bifida, syringomyelia, multiple system atrophy, cord compression secondary to herniated disk, and Shy-Drager syndrome may also cause ED.

Peripheral autonomic nerve dysfunction is also associated with ED. This may be secondary to pelvic trauma, surgical procedures, or a systemic disease affecting peripheral nerves such as diabetes, uremia, amyloidosis, chronic alcoholism, scleroderma, vitamin B deficiency, systemic lupus erythematosus, or acquired immunodeficiency. Penile sensory nerves are essential for adequate EF. As such, decreased penile tactile sensitivity caused by systemic disease or aging may in turn induce ED.

3. Endocrine causes of erectile dysfunction
   a. Diabetes mellitus

      Diabetes is a very common cause of ED in the United States. Age, duration of diabetes, HbA1c level, smoking habits, hypertension, dyslipidemia, obesity, and sedentary lifestyle are independent risk factors for ED in patients with diabetes. ED in diabetic men is more common than retinopathy or nephropathy and is often mixed in etiology. This is usually as a result of existing comorbid conditions, psychological factors, and certain medications used in therapy of these conditions.

      Laboratory studies looking at the causes of diabetes-induced ED have demonstrated impaired cavernosal relaxation caused by altered smooth muscle function and NO dysfunction in diabetic animals (Zhang 2012). In animal models of type 1 and type 2 diabetes, endothelium-dependent vasodilation of cavernosal tissue is impaired because of decreased endothelial NOS (eNOS) expression and activity along with increased NO scavenging.

      Chronic hyperglycemia induces free-radical production which may have detrimental effect on NO-mediated cavernosal relaxation. This cavernosal hypercontractility is an underlying mechanism for ED in some animal models and may also result from increased sympathetic activation and intracellular contractile signaling of penile smooth muscle cells. Venoocclusive dysfunction has also been implicated in diabetic ED.

b. Hypogonadism

In healthy young men, serum testosterone levels range from 300 to 1050 ng/dL and decline with advancing age. The FDA defines hypogonadism as serum total testosterone level less than 300 ng/dL, but this level is controversial in the medical literature. The overall prevalence of hypogonadism in men aged 45 years or older is about 38%. Using a serum testosterone level of 325 ng/dL, approximately 12%, 20%, 30%, and 50% of men in their 50s, 60s, 70s, and 80s, respectively, are hypogonadal. Late-onset hypogonadism is a clinical and biochemical syndrome associated with an older age group. It is characterized by testosterone deficiency symptoms that decrease quality of life, along with a total T level of less than approximately 350 ng/dL.

Androgens play a critical role in the physiology of EF, but the underlying mechanism by which androgens regulate EF remains largely unclear. In preclinical studies, testosterone has been shown to potentially modulate central and peripheral mechanisms of penile erections. Androgen deficiency has been associated with cavernosal nerve atrophy that may be reversed with subsequent androgen supplementation. Nitrous oxide synthase (NOS) and vasoactive intestinal peptide (VIP) play a critical role in the relaxation of the cavernosal smooth muscle necessary for erections. It has been shown that reduced NOS expression was reversed with androgen administration. Androgen deficiency has also been shown to alter smooth muscle content and structure resulting in increased connective tissue deposition in the corpus cavernosum.

Primary hypogonadism (hypergonadotropic hypogonadism) causes ED as a result of decreased testosterone. It can be congenital as in Klinefelter syndrome or due to tumor, injury, radiation, surgery, or mumps orchitis. Decreased luteinizing hormone (LH) production from the pituitary causes hypogonadotropic hypogonadism and may result from injury, tumor, or conditions such as Kallmann, Prader-Willi, or Laurence-Moon syndromes.

Hyperprolactinemia may result from medication administration or from a pituitary adenoma. This can cause ED from the inhibition of gonadotropin-releasing hormone secretion from the elevated prolactin levels, ultimately resulting in low testosterone levels.

4. Vasculogenic

Any vascular disease can affect the penile blood supply and cause ED. ED and CVD share the same risk factors such as atherosclerosis, hypertension, hyperlipidemia, and cigarette smoking. Reports demonstrate that ED in men younger than 60 years of age is associated with a significant increase in the risk of future cardiac events when compared with men without ED. This may result from underlying endothelial dysfunction that exists in both ED and CVD.

Hyperlipidemia and high concentrations of low-density lipoprotein (LDL) are also associated with ED. In animal models, chronic hypercholesterolemia causes ED by decreasing endothelium-dependent relaxation of cavernosal smooth muscle. In rodents with cavernosal ischemia without hyperlipidemia, atherosclerotic ischemia is associated with ED secondary to decreased NOS activity and impaired endothelium-dependent and neurogenic NO-mediated relaxation of cavernosal tissue. Cigarette smoking increases oxidative stress, which causes downregulation of the NO/cGMP pathway, resulting in ED.

5. Drug-induced ED

Antihypertensive and psychotropic drugs are the most common medications associated with the development of ED. Nonspecific beta-blockers and thiazide diuretics are associated with a higher rate of ED. Psychotropic drugs, including antidepressants, antipsychotics, and anxiolytics, can affect sexual function by acting on the central nervous system (CNS). Of the antipsychotics, risperidone and olanzapine are associated with a higher rate of ED. The role of statins in the development of ED remains controversial.

Evaluation of Sexual Dysfunction

HISTORY

The diagnosis of ED can often be made by a detailed history alone. A thorough history should be the starting point of any evaluation of a patient presenting with the complaint of sexual dysfunction. Patients can assist in the diagnosis by completing a questionnaire, such as the International Index of Erectile Function (IIEF) or the Sexual Health Inventory for Men (SHIM), to assess EF before a medical interview even begins.

Medical History

The clinician should first determine the general health status of any patient presenting for evaluation of ED. This initial evaluation should include a detailed medical history of diagnoses and symptoms suggesting a diagnosis of diabetes, CAD, peripheral vascular disease, chronic renal insufficiency, depression, thyroid disorders, or hypogonadism.

A thorough medical history must also include a list of the patient's medications. Special attention should be paid to those which are known to be associated with ED and any medications that coincide temporarily with an onset or worsening of symptoms. Medications commonly associated with increased rates of ED include thiazide diuretics, nonselective beta-blockers, central alpha-blockers, antiandrogens, antipsychotics, antidepressants, and opiates. A history of tobacco or alcohol use, pelvic or perineal surgery, radiation and trauma, including frequent or long-distance cycling should be assessed. A family history of CVD should be ascertained.

Sexual History

The sexual history is the key portion of the evaluation. The success of this evaluation will be dependent both on the data gathered during the interview and the manner in which the interview is conducted. Frequently, these patients will be embarrassed or hesitant to discuss the details of their sexual dysfunction. A private setting and nonjudgmental manner can help put the patient at ease and foster a therapeutic physician-patient relationship.

The sexual history should first address the onset, duration, and extent of erectile symptoms to assess the degree of current function. Any alleviating or aggravating factors should be identified. These questions should help clarify the specific complaint and differentiate ED from other sexual dysfunction such as PE, lack of interest or arousal, or anorgasmia. The onset of symptoms can help differentiate organic and psychogenic ED; organic ED usually has a gradual progression of symptoms whereas psychogenic ED often has an acute onset of symptoms. The presence of erections at night or during masturbation can also help identify cases of nonorganic ED.

Psychosexual History

A social history inquiring about stressors at home or at work, financial or intrapersonal difficulties, activity level, and general happiness can help identify patients with depression or other nonorganic sources of low libido. Often psychogenic ED can coexist with organic ED. Identifying these patients and referring them to a mental health specialist can allow for concurrent treatment of their psychogenic and organic ED.

ED can represent an opportunity for the diagnosis of CVD or modification of CVD risk factors. Furthermore, patients with CVD may be at increased risk of acute cardiac events upon resumption of sexual activity. Therefore, an evaluation of exercise tolerance and cardiac risk stratification (Fig. 21.2) should be undertaken prior to the treatment of ED.

Patients should be divided into low-risk, high-risk, or indeterminate risk categories based on their CVD status. Patients in the low-risk category include those who can perform moderately intense exercise without symptoms. This group includes patients who have treated and controlled coronary disease, hypertension, congestive heart failure (New York Heart Association [NYHA] class I or II), or mild valvular disease. These patients may undergo elective cardiac evaluation but may safely be treated for ED without it. These patients can often be treated with restorative medications for ED.

High-risk patients should not be treated for ED without evaluation by a cardiologist and should be counseled to avoid sexual activity until they have been assessed. These patients include those with severe or uncontrolled cardiac conditions including but not limited to: angina, uncontrolled hypertension, heart failure (NYHA class IV), recent myocardial infarction, moderate-to-severe valvular disease, or poorly controlled arrhythmias.

Patients with intermediate risk should undergo exercise or chemical stress testing and be restratified to either low- or high-risk groups (see Fig. 21.2).

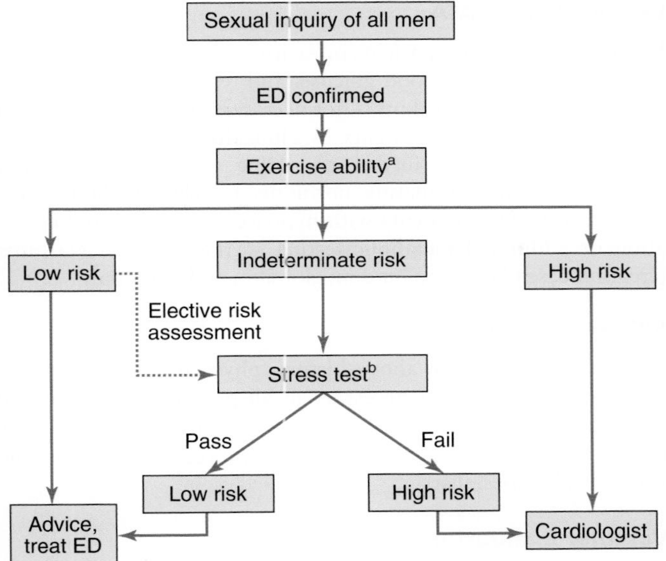

FIGURE 21.2 Management of erectile dysfunction *(ED)* in all men with ED, especially those with known cardiovascular disease. [a]Sexual activity is equivalent to walking 1 mile on a flat surface in 20 minutes or briskly climbing two flights of stairs in 10 seconds. [b]Sexual activity is equivalent to 4 minutes of the Bruce treadmill protocol. (From Nehra A, Jackson G, Miner M, et al. The Princeton III Consensus recommendations for the management of erectile dysfunction and cardiovascular disease. *Mayo Clin Proc.* 2012;87:766-778.)

PHYSICAL EXAM

The physical exam is a relatively straightforward part of the evaluation of a patient with ED. The exam should include a general assessment: vital signs, height, weight, and waist circumference. It should also include basic neurologic, vascular, heart, lung, and abdominal exams. The genitourinary portion of the exam should specifically examine the penis for abnormal curvature, plaques, lesions, and position of the urethra. The testicular exam should evaluate the size and texture of the testicles and rule out the presence of a mass. The rectal exam should be performed to evaluate the prostate for size, nodularity, sphincter tone, and the presence of a bulbocavernosus reflex.

LABORATORY DATA

Laboratory testing for patients presenting with ED should include a fasting lipid panel, blood glucose, and testosterone level (total or free). Additional workup is not necessary in every patient and should be ordered in patients as clinically appropriate. These optional tests include further endocrine evaluation (prolactin, estradiol, thyroid-stimulating hormone, follicle-stimulating hormone, LH, PSA) in patients with hypogonadism on initial evaluation or additional metabolic testing as the situation warrants (creatinine, sex hormone-binding globulin, and albumin).

SPECIAL STUDIES

Evaluation beyond the above history, physical, and basic laboratory evaluation is not necessary in all patients and should be ordered judiciously for patients in whom the results may alter treatment decisions. Usually, these tests are recommended by the sexual health specialist.

Vascular Evaluation

Vascular evaluation can be carried out to verify vasculogenic ED because the patient with vasculogenic ED without known CVD is thought to need CVD risk evaluation. Most likely, these men are in the low-risk arm of the decision-making algorithm for ED risk stratification and will go on to therapy for their ED.

Testing penile blood flow is particularly useful in younger patients without known CVD or in those with a history of trauma in whom abnormal penile hemodynamics are suspected. Evaluation of arterial inflow to the penis can be easily conducted using duplex ultrasonography while evaluation of venoocclusive function can be conducted by either penile duplex ultrasonography or dynamic infusion cavernosometry and cavernosography (DICC). Each of these modalities utilizes intracavernosal injection of a vasodilatory agent to induce an erection that is independent of neurologic or hormonal control. Patients should routinely be monitored following vasodilator injection to ensure that detumescence occurs with post-procedural intracavernosal vasoconstrictor administration.

Duplex Doppler ultrasonography is a noninvasive and cost-effective method of evaluating the penile vascular system and is preferred over traditional arteriography. The ultrasound is used to first evaluate the flaccid penis, confirming normal, homogenous-appearing cavernosa without evidence of plaques or fibrosis. The size and systolic flow within the intracavernosal arteries are also assessed. Intracavernosal injection with a single or a combination of vasoactive agents such as prostaglandin E1, phentolamine, or papaverine is conducted. Once erection has been achieved or at predetermined time points, a variety of parameters, including peak systolic velocity (PSV), end diastolic velocity (EDV), and resistive index (RI), are obtained. Decreased PSV indicates poor inflow, whereas elevated EDV or diminished RIs can indicate venous leak. The patient's self-reported degree of rigidity should be compared to his baseline level of rigidity because false-positive results can be caused by anxiety or embarrassment.

Penile arteriography is a more definitive modality for the evaluation of penile vasculature. Selective angiography of the internal pudendal artery can be undertaken to identify arterial occlusion leading to vasculogenic ED. This test should be considered in patients with abnormal duplex and a high suspicion for traumatic injury to the pudendal system (i.e., pelvic trauma, long-distance cyclists). Generally, arteriography should be reserved for patients who may undergo surgical penile revascularization.

While Doppler and arteriography provide useful information about vascular inflow, evaluation of venoocclusive dysfunction is often conducted with cavernosometry and cavernosography. The penile corpora are cannulated with two needles, one to infuse saline and the other to measure pressures. After injecting a vasodilator, saline is infused into the corpora cavernosa, and intracavernous pressure is monitored. A failure of the pressure to rise sufficiently or a rapid decline in the pressure upon stopping saline infusion may be indicative of a venoocclusive dysfunction. Cavernosography, or injection of contrast into the corpora at the end of the test, can rarely identify the source of venous leak. This test has fallen out of favor over time, as has surgical dorsal vein ligation procedure for the treatment of ED.

Neurologic Evaluation

The neurologic system is an important regulator of EF. As described previously, multiple pathways and centers within the central and peripheral nervous systems are involved in erection, ejaculation, and orgasm. Specific tests have been developed and studied to assess the afferent somatic sensory and autonomic function at the level of the penis. Other tests record the efferent system and conduction velocities, both centrally and peripherally in the pudendal nerve. The clinical utility of these tests remains in question and is the subject of ongoing research. Presently these tests are not recommended for routine use outside of a research setting.

Nocturnal Penile Tumescence Testing

NPT monitoring is the study of physiologic erectile capacity in men during rapid eye movement (REM) sleep. Monitoring devices are applied which measure the number, duration, tumescence (circumference), and rigidity of erections overnight. Classically NPT testing takes place in a sleep laboratory, with observers present to monitor patients and correlate erections with REM sleep. Portable devices for ambulatory NPT testing also exist and allow for a less expensive and less intrusive form of NPT testing. This does, however, carry a higher rate of false-positive tests because REM sleep is not confirmed in an ambulatory setting. NPT testing allows for a noninvasive form of erectile testing that can differentiate psychogenic and organic ED. NPT testing is no longer routinely used in the diagnosis of ED, and it is use is sporadic.

Cardiovascular Risk Assessment

In men with ED and no identified CVD, CV risk assessment is required. Incidentally, ED has a similar or greater predictive value for cardiovascular events than traditional risk factors including smoking, hyperlipidemia, and family history of myocardial infarction. Addition of ED to the Framingham Risk Score only modestly improved its 10-year predictive capacity for myocardial infarction or coronary death data in men enrolled in the MMAS. Other epidemiologic studies suggest that the predictive value of ED is quite strong in younger men. Indeed, in the Olmstead County Study in Minnesota, men 40 to 49 years of age with ED had a 50-fold higher incidence of new-incident CAD than those without ED. However, ED had less predictive value (fivefold increased risk) for CAD in men 70 years and older. Identification of ED, particularly in men less than 60 years old and those with diabetes, represents an important first step toward CVD risk detection and reduction.

Treatment

The AUA 2018 ED guideline represents a key shift in the paradigm of ED. Previous algorithms emphasized starting with less invasive measure prior to more invasive options. The new 2018 treatment algorithm emphasizes shared decision-making and presenting "all treatment modalities that are not contraindicated, regardless of invasiveness or irreversibility, as potential first-line treatments."

NONSURGICAL MANAGEMENT OF ERECTILE DYSFUNCTION

As previously discussed, ED has been defined by the National Institutes of Health (NIH) Consensus Development Panel on Impotence as the "inability of the male to attain and maintain erection of the penis to permit satisfactory sexual intercourse." Inherent in this definition is the subjective nature of erectile complaints. The expectations of normal EF may vary greatly among patients, and it is essential that the practitioner keep this in mind during the evaluation and management of ED. A widely accepted principle in the management of ED is the use of a goal-directed approach. Identifying satisfactory sexual function for an individual patient is an essential part of the treatment and can serve to limit and guide both diagnostic and therapeutic modalities.

LIFESTYLE

The association of ED with several systemic health conditions and lifestyle choices such as obesity, CVD, diabetes, hypercholesterolemia, metabolic syndrome, smoking, alcohol abuse, and other drug use is well known. For patients who are affected or at risk for these conditions lifestyle modification can be a valuable first step to treating ED. This therapeutic approach avoids the potential side effects of other therapies and provides the benefits of improving general health and improving risk factors for other diseases.

An interesting study examined weight reduction in obese men and revealed that the purposeful treatment of obesity objectively improved sexual function when compared to a nonintervention group. The study was conducted from 2000 to 2003 at a university hospital in Italy and was a randomized, single-blind trial of 110 obese men (body mass index [BMI] of 30 or more) aged 35 to 55 years. Participants had ED defined by a score of 21 or less on the IIEF without a history of diabetes, hypertension, or hyperlipidemia. The 55 men randomly assigned to the intervention group received detailed advice about how to achieve a loss of 10% or more of their total body weight by reducing caloric intake and increasing their level of physical activity. Men in the control group (n = 55) were given general information about healthy food choices and exercise. After 2 years, BMI decreased more in the intervention group, from a mean (SD) of 36.9 (2.5) to 31.2 (2.1), than in the control group, from 36.4 (2.3) to 35.7 (2.5) (*P*-value less than .001), as did serum concentrations of interleukin 6 ($P = .03$) and C-reactive protein ($P = .02$). The mean (SD) level of physical activity increased more in the intervention group, from 48 (10) to 195 (36) min/wk ($P < .001$), than in the control group, from 51 (9) to 84 (28) min/wk ($P < .001$). The mean (SD) IIEF score improved in the intervention group, from 13.9 (4.0) to 17 (5) ($P < .001$), but remained stable in the control group, from 13.5 (4.0) to 13.6 (4.1) ($P = .89$). Seventeen men in the intervention group and three in the control group reported an IIEF score of 22 or higher ($P = .001$). In multivariate analyses, changes in BMI ($P = .02$), physical activity ($P = .02$), and C-reactive protein ($P = .03$) were independently associated with changes in IIEF score. These data suggest that diet and weight loss can improve ED, but this must be a long-term commitment.

PSYCHOSEXUAL THERAPY

In patients in whom a psychogenic source of ED has been identified or is suspected, referral to a therapist, especially a sexual dysfunction specialist, should be recommended. Often psychosexual factors have some impact in ED, even for patients with an organic etiology. As such, these patients and their partners may also benefit from sexual counseling. Many psychotherapeutic options exist and are used by practitioners of various backgrounds.

TESTOSTERONE THERAPY

Testosterone therapy is indicated only for patients with a clinical presentation suggestive of hypogonadism and low serum testosterone levels. The AUA has recently issued a guideline on this topic. Bhasin (2021) has recently authored a comprehensive review of this topic.

The effectiveness of testosterone replacement should be monitored for clinical improvement using measured testosterone levels and discussions regarding symptom improvement. Supplementation should be stopped if clinical improvement does not occur after a defined period of time.

The goal of testosterone treatment is to increase serum testosterone levels to the mid-normal range for men 19 to 40 years of age. The increase in testosterone levels is usually associated with significantly increased sexual activity, significantly increased sexual desire, and an improvement in EF. Testosterone replacement also improves mood and lowers the severity of depressive symptoms (Snyder 2016).

Testosterone supplementation carries risks of short-term male infertility, dyslipidemia, erythrocytosis, acne, gynecomastia, worsening of obstructive sleep apnea, increased hematocrit, potential progression of prostate cancer, and increased platelet aggregation. Therefore, close monitoring is required for patients on supplemental testosterone. Patients should undergo routine DRE, PSA, CBC, and liver function testing.

Providers prescribing testosterone to elderly men with cardiovascular comorbidities should inform their patients of the potential risk of cardiovascular events (i.e., DVT, stroke, MI) while on testosterone. In 2014, the FDA issued a “black box” warning regarding the potential risk cardiovascular events in the use of testosterone for late-onset hypogonadism, resulting in thoughtful review of overall use (FDA, 2014). This FDA warning was based partly based on the TOM trial, a randomized controlled trial which was stopped early due to significantly higher risk of cardiovascular events in the treatment group and two retrospective studies showing similar results. However, several level-1 studies have since been completed showing no evidence of increased risk.

Time-honored testosterone replacement therapy includes daily topical gel application, daily cutaneous patch application, weekly or biweekly intramuscular injection, long-acting subcutaneous pellets, long-acting intramuscular injections, twice daily buccal application, intranasal spray. Recently an oral preparation has been introduced for daily use (Swerdloff).

PHARMACOLOGIC THERAPY FOR ERECTILE DYSFUNCTION

PDE-5 Inhibitors

PDE-5 inhibitors, by virtue of their safety, effectiveness, and ease of use, have revolutionized the treatment of ED in the United States and around the world. PDE-5 inhibitors have become first-line therapy for patients presenting with ED. Four PDE-5 inhibitors are commercially available in the United States: sildenafil, vardenafil, avanafil, and tadalafil. Sildenafil was introduced in 1998, vardenafil and tadalafil in 2003, and avanafil in 2012. Given the focus on goal-directed therapy for ED and the efficacy and simplicity of PDE-5 inhibitors, many patients are treated without an additional battery of diagnostic tests. However, costs of the medications often remain a barrier to treatment. Proliferation of web-based, nonprescription, PDE-5-inhibitor purchasing activity has increased over the past several years for a variety of reasons. Unfortunately, counterfeit pharmaceuticals are prevalent and readily available for purchase of online, exposing patients to potential risks.

Mechanistically, PDE-5 inhibitors prevent the breakdown of cGMP, thus potentiating endothelial and smooth muscle relaxation, allowing for increased arterial inflow to the cavernosa and promoting improved erections (Fig. 21.3). It is important to note that this effect potentiates NO-mediated vasorelaxation but does not produce erection without adequate sexual arousal and the initiation of NO release in the penis.

There are 11 types of PDE with a variety of functions throughout the body. PDE-5 is found primarily in penile smooth muscle, though it also exists in the vascular and gastrointestinal smooth muscle. The majority of the side effects of PDE-5 inhibitors result from cross-reactivity with PDE enzymes other than type 5 or the effect of PDE-5 inhibition.

The four different commercially available PDE-5 inhibitors all appear to be safe and effective. All appear to have equal efficacy in treating ED, and the limited comparative data that exist do not suggest the superiority of any one of these agents. All four drugs have been shown to be effective in a variety of patient populations and for various etiologies of ED. In general, the success rate of PDE-5 inhibitors in allowing patients to achieve erections

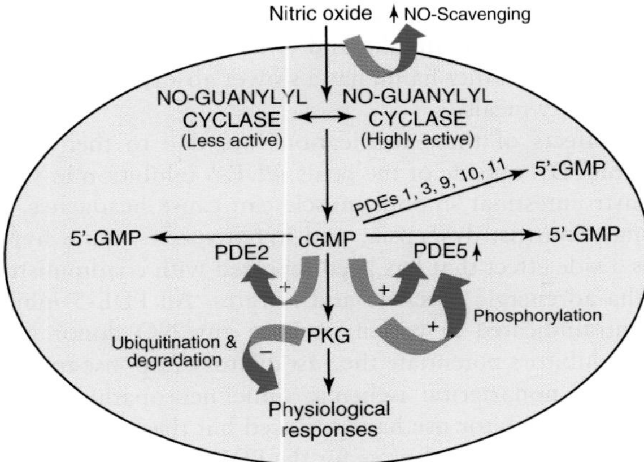

FIGURE 21.3 Negative feedback mechanisms that blunt or terminate nitric oxide *(NO)* and cyclic guanosine monophosphate *(cGMP)* signaling. cGMP signaling is blunted and/or terminated by multiple points of action that serve to decrease cGMP level by lowering NO-GC activity, activating cGMP-hydrolyzing phosphodiesterases *(PDEs)*, or decreasing levels of the proteins involved in the signaling. PDEs 1, 2, 3, 5, 9, 10, and 11 hydrolyze cGMP and are widespread throughout mammalian tissues. The activities of PDE-2 and PDE-5 can be further accelerated by allosteric cGMP binding and by phosphorylation for PDE-5. (Adapted in part from Francis SH, Corbin JD, and Bischoff E. Cyclic GMP-hydrolyzing phosphodiesterases. *Handb Exp Pharmacol.* 2009;191:367-408.)

suitable for sexual intercourse is approximately 70%, though the effectiveness is reduced in diabetic patients, patients with severe ED, and in patients who have undergone radical prostatectomy.

The four commercially available PDE-5 inhibitors have pharmacokinetic differences which have important consequences for their dosing. Sildenafil and vardenafil achieve peak plasma concentrations in approximately 1 hour and have half-lives of 3 to 5 hours, whereas tadalafil peaks in 2 hours and has a plasma half-life of approximately 18 hours. The longer half-life of tadalafil allows for once-daily dosing for continuous treatment, rather than the on-demand dosing that is necessary for sildenafil and vardenafil. Avanafil however has a much shorter onset of action with peak plasma levels noted at 30 to 45 minutes following administration and plasma half-life of 3 to 5 hours. Sildenafil, vardenafil, and avanafil should not be taken with fatty meals, as they are rapidly absorbed, and delayed gastric emptying caused by fatty meals can reduce the uptake and efficacy of these medications. Tadalafil, on the other hand, has a slower absorption and is unaffected by fatty meals.

Side effects of these medications are due to their systemic effects on PDE outside of the penis. PDE-5 inhibition in vascular and gastrointestinal smooth muscle can cause headaches, facial flushing, sinusitis, dyspepsia, and hypotension. Acute hypotension is a side effect that has been reported with coadministration of alpha-adrenergic blockers and nitrates. All PDE-5 inhibitors are contraindicated in patients taking any NO donor because PDE-5 inhibitors potentiate the vasodilatory response to nitrates. Reports of nonarteritic ischemic optic neuropathy associated with PDE-5-inhibitor use have surfaced but these reports remain rare. Avanafil is most selective for the PDE-5 isozyme and as such has fewer effects on tissues containing other PDE isozymes such as retina, systemic vasculature, and skeletal muscles.

Daily PDE-5 Inhibitors and Use of PDE-5 Inhibitors for Both BPH/LUTS and ED

As noted previously, tadalafil, like all PDE-5 inhibitors, is approved for therapeutic use in the United States, Europe, and many other countries. The recommended starting dose for as-needed use is 10 mg, decreasing to 5 mg and increasing to 20 mg if necessary. Food does not interfere with its absorption.

Tadalafil can also be used as daily therapy for ED. The starting dose is 2.5 mg and can be increased to 5 mg. A multicenter, double-blind and randomized controlled trial was conducted in a parallel group design to evaluate this. Two hundred and sixty-eight men were enrolled in a 1:2:2 ratio to placebo, 5 mg daily tadalafil, or 10 mg daily tadalafil for a 12-week period. Primary efficacy measures included changes in the IIEF Erectile Function domain (IIEF-EF), Sexual Encounter Profile diary questions 2 and 3 (SEP2: successful penetration, SEP3: successful completion of intercourse), and tolerability. Secondary measures included the percentage of patients at the conclusion of the study that reported improved EF resolution of ED (IIEF-EF score 26 to 30). For patient in the placebo, tadalafil 5 mg, and tadalafil 10 mg arms, changes from baseline after 12 weeks were, respectively, 0.9, 9.7, and 9.4 for IIEF-EF; 11.2, 36.5, and 39.4 for SEP2; and

13.2, 45.5, and 50.1 for SEP3. At the end point, 28.3%, 84.5%, and 84.6% reported improved erections, and 8.3%, 51.5%, and 50.5% reported resolution of ED, respectively. All comparisons between tadalafil and placebo were significant (P-value $< .001$). Adverse events that occurred in at least 5% of patients were dyspepsia, headache, back pain, upper abdominal pain, and myalgias; nine patients (3.4%) discontinued because of adverse events. Currently, only 2.5-mg and 5-mg dosing is approved for daily use in the United States. It is postulated that daily oral PDE-5-inhibitor use may prevent ED that is thought to occur due to normal aging and cell senescence.

Once-daily tadalafil 5 mg was recently approved by the FDA for daily use for the treatment of both BPH with LUTS and ED. Data suggest that tadalafil can improve LUTS in a similar manner to alpha-blockers without the alpha-blocker side effects, though there are the PDE-5 inhibitor side effects (Egerdie 2012, Oelke 2012).

The primary objective of the study by Oelke et al. was to compare the effect of tadalafil 5 mg once daily with placebo on BPH with LUTS. Given that the alpha-blocker tamsulosin is often a first-line treatment for BPH with LUTS, tamsulosin was included as an active control, with a secondary objective of comparing tamsulosin 0.4 mg once daily with placebo. This study was a double-blind, placebo and active-controlled, parallel-design trial conducted at 44 urology sites in Australia, Austria, Belgium, France, Germany, Greece, Italy, Mexico, the Netherlands, and Poland. Following screening (and a 4-week washout for BPH, overactive bladder, or ED drugs, as needed), participants began a 4-week single-blind placebo lead-in period, followed by randomization (1:1:1 ratio) to once-daily tadalafil 5 mg, tamsulosin 0.4 mg, or placebo for 12 weeks. The change from baseline to week 12 relative to placebo in total International Prostate Symptom Score (IPSS) was statistically significant for both tadalafil and tamsulosin ($P = .001$ and $P = .023$, respectively). Least squares mean (LS mean) plus or minus standard error (SE) differences in IPSS versus placebo were significant for both tadalafil and tamsulosin at 1 week (mIPSS: -1.5 ± 0.5; $P = .003$ and -1.5 ± 0.5; $P = .005$, respectively) and week 4 (-2.2 ± 0.6; $P < .001$ and -2.3 ± 0.6; $P < .001$, respectively). Based on prespecified subgroup analysis, there was no significant effect of previous alpha-blocker therapy with respect to changes in total IPSS ($P = .230$) (Fig. 21.4A,B).

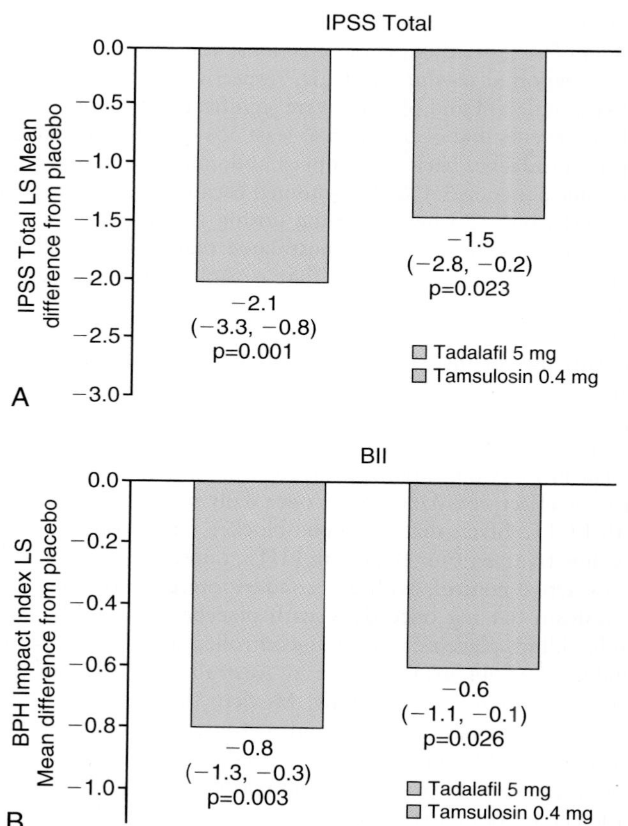

FIGURE 21.4 Differences from placebo in (A) total International Prostate Symptom Score *(IPSS)* and (B) Benign Prostatic Hyperplasia Impact Index *(BII)*. Numbers represent least squares *(LS)* mean treatment difference (95% confidence interval) versus placebo in the change from baseline to 12 weeks (last-observation-carried-forward) and corresponding *P* values from analysis of covariance. (From Oelke M, Giuliano F, Mirone V, et al. Monotherapy with tadalafil or tamsulosin similarly improved lower urinary tract symptoms suggestive of benign prostatic hyperplasia in an international, randomised, parallel, placebo-controlled clinical trial. *Eur Urol.* 2012;61:917-925.)

Additionally, tadalafil does not change the PSA at a 1-year time point (Donatucci 2011).

Sildenafil and vardenafil have also been reported to improve BPH/LUTS symptoms, but neither drug has cleared the FDA regulatory hurdles for the treatment of BPH/LUTS.

Intraurethral Agents

The intraurethral route for administration of vasoactive medications was initially developed in the mid-1990s as an alternative to intracavernosal injection. Alprostadil, a synthetic form of the naturally occurring prostaglandin E1 (PGE1), is inserted in pellet form into the urethra. It is absorbed by the mucosal lining of the urethra into the corpus spongiosum and corpora cavernosa, where it locally activates adenylate cyclase to produce cAMP and induce smooth muscle relaxation. Unlike PDE-5 inhibitors, alprostadil does initiate erections and does not require arousal for efficacy.

Intraurethral alprostadil is effective in 30% to 40% of patients and may ultimately help avoid the use of the more invasive intracavernous injections in this group. The efficacy of intraurethral alprostadil can be improved with use of local measures such as vacuum constriction, or with systemic therapy such as PDE-5 inhibitors. The side effects of an intraurethral suppository include local penile pain (approximately one-third of patients) and minor urethral bleeding, hypotension, dizziness, or priapism in less than 5% of patients.

Intracavernosal Injection

Intracavernosal injection of vasoactive agents for inducing erection was first discovered in the 1980s as the first effective medical therapy for ED, creating a paradigm shift in its treatment. Since then, understanding of the physiology of erection along with the introduction of intraurethral and oral systemic therapy have changed the management of ED. Nevertheless, injectable vasoactive agents are still commonly used in clinical practice today.

Alprostadil is the only FDA-approved intracavernosal injectable agent. This results in penile erection via the cAMP-mediated mechanism described previously. It is effective in creating an erection of sufficient rigidity for sexual intercourse in approximately 60% to 80% of cases with the side effect of penile pain in approximately 11% of patients.

Papaverine is a nonselective PDE inhibitor and was the first described agent for intracavernosal injection. It is less effective as a single agent than alprostadil and carries a higher rate of priapism and penile fibrosis. Consequently, it is no longer used as monotherapy for ED.

Phentolamine is an alpha-adrenergic antagonist that acts by inhibiting the postsynaptic alpha-1 receptor leading to relaxation of the penile vasculature. Unlike the other intracavernous agents, phentolamine has significant systemic side effects, including hypotension, tachycardia, gastrointestinal upset, and nasal congestion.

Each of the intracavernosal injectable agents carries a risk of priapism, hematoma, and penile fibrosis. Training and education regarding intracavernous injection should be provided in a monitored setting prior to self-injection, and patients naive to intracavernous injection should be observed for priapism. If priapism is detected in a timely fashion, it can usually be reversed with the injection of an alpha agonist.

Given the limited efficacy of individual intracavernous injection and the various side effects, administration of a combination of injectable agents has been developed. Because the mechanism of action varies for these different agents, combination therapy offers the possibility of synergistic function to improve efficacy in patients who have failed monotherapy. Additionally, this allows for use of lower doses of individual agents and may reduce side effects specific to certain agents. Commonly used combinations include Bi-mix (alprostadil and phentolamine), Tri-mix (alprostadil, papaverine, and phentolamine), and Quad-mix (alprostadil, phentolamine, papaverine and atropine), which have a reported efficacy of approximately 90% in achieving erection suitable for intercourse.

Vacuum Constriction Device

Vacuum constriction devices use external mechanical force to induce erection. An external negative pressure is created by a vacuum pump and applied to the penis, causing inflow of blood. Additionally, a constricting ring is applied to the base of the penis as a mechanical venoocclusive device, maintaining the erection. Most men report increased length, girth, and rigidity with the use of vacuum constriction, and the erection resembles a physiologic one, with engorgement of the entire penis including the glans and spongiosum. The disadvantages of this approach are limited time frame for erection (20 minutes maximum), penile pain and numbness, trapping of the ejaculation, discoloration and coolness of the penis, ecchymosis, and petechiae. The vacuum erection device remains a viable option for the select patient with ED.

Surgical Management of Erectile Dysfunction

Surgery is the oldest intervention for the management of ED, which can be offered at any point during the treatment pathway. Surgical therapy is indicated in patients who have traumatic injuries or structural deformities that do not improve with medical treatment alone but may be amenable to surgical intervention.

PENILE PROSTHESIS SURGERY

Penile implants were introduced in the 1970s and remain an important treatment option today. Penile implants are efficacious and provide excellent patient and partner satisfaction.

The ideal penile prosthesis is one that provides both complete flaccidity and the closest approximation of a normal erection.

1. Indications

   Implanted penile prostheses are usually used after failure of less invasive treatment options, including PDE-5 inhibitors, vacuum constriction devices, intraurethral injections, and intracavernosal injections. Patients may go directly to insertion of a penile prosthesis as a first-line treatment option. The decision to pursue penile prosthesis surgery should include the patient and partner when possible and the patient should be counseled regarding the different available prosthesis types, benefits, and disadvantages. Manual dexterity should be evaluated to ascertain whether an inflatable prosthesis is suitable. The patient should be adequately counseled regarding the realistic expectations of a penile prosthesis. As with intracavernosal injection, the erection produced using a penile prosthesis does not include the spongiosum or glans penis. Furthermore, the majority of penile prosthetic devices provide girth expansion only, without the increased length that accompanies natural erection. In light of this, the patient's erection may be of a shorter length than his previous, natural erection. Additionally, the sensitivity and ability to reach orgasm or ejaculate will not be affected by a penile prosthesis. A patient who is unable to reach orgasm or to ejaculate preoperatively will not regain that ability after penile implant insertion. It is also important to counsel the patient that infection of prosthetic material is a serious complication of the procedure, and infection will result in the need for reoperation.

Types of Prostheses

Penile prostheses can be divided into two general classes: inflatable and semirigid. Semirigid prostheses are made of one unit, either malleable or mechanical. Malleable prostheses have a silicone rod over a central metal core. Mechanical implants are made up of a series of stacked disks held together by a central cable. These semirigid prostheses have the advantage of being very simple, with a low rate of failure and without requiring a lot of dexterity to operate. However, they remain at a constant girth and rigidity, making them difficult to conceal. Furthermore, they cannot extend or enlarge, and may be too flexible during intercourse, often leaving patients unhappy with the quality of their erection.

Inflatable prostheses are composed of either two or three pieces. Three-piece inflatable implants include two corporal cylinders, a scrotal pump, and an abdominal reservoir. These implants come closest to the ideal prosthetic because they allow for girth expansion, elongation, and increased rigidity during intercourse, while also enabling easier concealment when flaccid. Additionally, as they are usually in a flaccid state, these devices put less pressure on the corpora and decrease the risk of device erosion. They are more complicated than semirigid devices and require a more complex procedure for their implantation.

Infection is the most dreaded complication of this procedure, and the use of perioperative broad-spectrum antibiotics is recommended. The duration of antibiotic prophylaxis post-operatively varies from surgeon to surgeon, and usually ranges from 1 to 7 days. The development of antibiotic impregnated devices has decreased the rate of infection but does not eliminate the need for systemic perioperative antibiotic prophylaxis. Infection occurs in less than 3% of cases, though this figure is higher for diabetics and patients with spinal cord injury. Prosthesis infection can occur at any time in the postoperative period and should always be considered in the differential diagnosis of a patient with persistent pain after implantation.

The advent of antibiotic coating of prosthesis components has significantly diminished the prosthesis infection rate. While the gold standard of therapy is to completely remove an infected prosthetic device, this conservative approach leads to fibrosis and shrinkage of the corpora and makes reoperation significantly more challenging. An alternative salvage operation has been described which involves the explant of the infected device, vigorous antimicrobial irrigation (i.e., Mulcahy protocol), and immediate replacement with a new device. This approach has been shown to be effective in greater than 75% of cases.

Mechanical complications are the most common, though rates have decreased since the 1970s with development of improved devices. Mechanical failure can be caused by leaks in the tubing, reservoir or cylinders, faulty connections, aneurysmal dilation of a cylinder, and pump malfunction. It is recommended that in the setting of a mechanical complication, the entire device be explanted and replaced as subclinical bacterial colonization is prevalent and may ultimately lead to device infection and persistent malfunction.

VASCULAR PROCEDURES

Revascularization of the penis for ED is an uncommon procedure and there are limited data regarding its efficacy. Proximal disease (aortoiliac or hypogastric) is rare and can be treated via bypass grafting, endarterectomy, or balloon angioplasty. Small vessel disease (pudendal, cavernosal, or penile arteries) can develop from atherosclerotic, traumatic, or idiopathic etiologies and may be treated by creating a direct anastomosis with the inferior epigastric artery to improve inflow. In all cases, proper patient selection is key. Arteriography is necessary to identify the anatomic defect and for preoperative planning. Limited data indicate that the highest success rates for penile revascularization are in young men with a traumatic etiology of pelvic penile arterial disease.

NOVEL TREATMENTS IN ERECTILE DYSFUNCTION

Low-intensity penile shockwave treatment (Li-ESWT) is a recently developed novel treatment for ED. It is described as a noninvasive therapy that is thought to induce vasculogenesis and reverse the underlying pathophysiology of ED. In 2012, Vardi et al. showed in a randomized, double-blind, placebo-controlled trial that 12 sessions of Li-ESWT resulted in a significant improvement in IIEF-EF domain score (6.7 vs 3.0; $P = .032$) and maximal postischemic penile blood flow (8.2 mL/min/dL vs 0.1). Since then, various studies have attempted to replicate these findings but with variable success. Some limitations, as described Yang and Seftel in 2019, include inconsistent long-term follow-up, lack of standardized therapy protocol, and the absence of cost-benefit analyses. Currently, the AUA 2018 ED guideline recommends that this treatment should only be used in the context of a clinical trial.

Additionally, some investigators are looking into penile stem cell injections as a potential therapy for ED. Various types of autologous stem cells have been reportedly used as a restorative treatment for ED. Despite promising results in animal studies, evidence for this treatment modality is limited to highly selective phase I and II human studies with small sample sizes and limited long-term data on safety and efficacy. According to the AUA 2018 treatment guideline for ED, this treatment is still considered experimental.

Platelet-rich plasma injections are also currently in the investigative stage. Treatment outside of a clinical investigation is not recommended by the AUA ED treatment guideline.

DIRECT-TO-CONSUMER WEBSITES FOR EVALUATION AND TREATMENT OF ERECTILE DYSFUNCTION

As ED has been increasingly identified in young men, direct-to-consumer (DTC) online marketing has become a prominent source of information and treatment for these men. These sites, including Hims, Roman, BlueChew, and HealthyMale, began proliferating in the early 2000s and, in recent years, have gained a significant foothold in the field of male sexual health treatment. Beyond the convenience that is offered by these sites, men may find the online option preferable to an in-person consultation due to fears of their complaints being dismissed by providers, not being offered treatment, or the embarrassment of discussing these issues. Many of these sites make a point of offering such features as discreet and convenient shipping, low monthly payments, and, of note, online consultation with a health care provider prior to prescription. Unsurprisingly, these sites have become a popular means for obtaining pharmaceutical treatment for ED.

A recent study revealed that the total number of unique, website quarterly visitors increased by 1,688% from 655,733 in the 4th quarter (Q4) 2017 to over 11 million in Q4 2019. In 2019, there were on average 4,971,674 visits to all sites combined each month. For the two largest sites (Hims and Roman), visitors predominantly reached the site via direct web address (27.3%) or search engine referral (27.3%).

These authors stated that the dramatic increase in visits to DTC prescribing sites that treat ED represents a major paradigm shift in ED care, and it is imperative that clinicians and researchers work to understand how patients utilize online telemedicine, the safety and efficacy of online management of ED, and the potential downstream implications of its widespread use.

While DTC websites and prescribing are attractive, office consultation identifies young men with significant comorbidities that would be missed by DTC platforms, which employ only questionnaires for health screening.

DTC platforms often present themselves as medical authorities without following AUA Guidelines and garner mostly positive press coverage. Patients engaging these platforms may falsely believe they are receiving adequate medical assessment. Urologists may do well to incorporate telemedicine to enfranchise young men with evidence-based evaluation.

Additional content, including Self-Assessment Questions and Suggested Readings, may be accessed at www.ExpertConsult.com.

Male Fertility and Sterility

Anisleidy Fombona, MD, and Puneet Masson, MD

Epidemiology

THE PROBLEM

1. Infertility affects approximately 15% of couples. It is defined as a couple's inability to achieve a pregnancy after **1 year of unprotected intercourse.**
2. Upon evaluation, **a male factor alone may be found in approximately 30% of couples,** and both a male and female factor in an additional 20%. Thus a male factor is involved in the infertility problem in approximately 50% of cases.
3. Compared to normal controls, men with abnormal semen analyses have a 2- to 20-fold increased risk of testicular malignancy.

Reproductive Anatomy and Physiology

EMBRYOLOGY

1. Genital organs are observed during the fifth gestational week and include an indifferent gonad, a mesonephric duct, and müllerian ducts.
2. The indifferent gonad forms from a thickening in the urogenital ridge near the mesonephros; germ cells migrate from the yolk sac to populate the urogenital ridge. These **primordial germ cells** are very closely related to **embryonic stem cells.**
3. Sexual differentiation of the embryo stems from the presence or absence of **testis-determining factor** (**TDF** or sex-determining region on Y [**SRY**]) located on the Y chromosome. This determines gonadal sex and forms the basis for sex-specific phenotypic development (Fig. 22.e1). Early embryonic genes that can modulate the influence of SRY include **WNT-4** and **DAX1**, both of which favor **female gonadal development.**

4. **Once gonadal sex is determined, Leydig cells make testosterone during the eighth week of gestation, which develops internal genitalia and promotes testis migration. Sertoli cells synthesize müllerian-inhibiting substance (MIS), which prevents müllerian duct from developing a uterus and fallopian tubes.**
5. Induced to form a testis, the gonad develops clustered cords of germ cells that converge to form the rete testis at the hilum of the testis. These **testis stem cells** serve as the renewing source of germ cells for spermatogenesis throughout life. To further underscore the relatedness of stem cells, human testicular stem cells can be "coaxed" into developing into cells virtually identical to **embryonic stem cells.**
6. Hormone production declines after the 12th week during which external genital development occurs (Fig. 22.e2).
7. The **mesonephric duct** forms the **ureter** in both sexes and regionally specializes to form the **vas deferens** and **epididymis** in the male, joining with the testis at the **ductuli efferentes** testis.
8. The **müllerian duct** develops into fallopian tubes, the uterus, and the upper portion of the vagina in the female; in the male this development is inhibited by an **MIS (müllerian-inhibiting factor[MIF])** produced by the primitive testis. Except for the **appendix testis** and **prostatic utricle**, regression is otherwise complete (Fig. 22.e2).
9. Late in gestation, the testis descends caudally along the posterior abdominal wall as a result of differential growth and through shortening of the **gubernaculum testis** within the scrotum under endocrine control. Descent into the scrotum is usually completed by birth, although it can still occur during the first year of life.

Gross Anatomy

1. The male reproductive system includes the following components: the testes and seminiferous tubules, efferent ductules and rete testis, epididymides, vasa deferentia, ejaculatory ducts, seminal vesicles, prostate, penis, and urethra.
2. From the standpoint of infertility, any consideration of anatomy must also include the hypothalamic-pituitary-gonadal axis (Fig. 22.e3).

Reproductive Hormonal Axis

EXTRAHYPOTHALAMIC CENTRAL NERVOUS SYSTEM

1. The extrahypothalamic central nervous system (CNS) exhibits a variety of stimulatory and inhibitory influences on fertility.
2. In humans, the effects of **stress** of both a physical and/or emotional nature are probably mediated through this system, but the mechanisms are unknown (Fig. 22.e4).

HYPOTHALAMUS: GONADOTROPIN-RELEASING HORMONE

1. The hypothalamus is responsible for production of gonadotropin-releasing hormone (**GnRH**), which is the primary releasing substance involved in male sexual function. To this day its only known function is to stimulate the secretion of luteinizing hormone (LH) and follicle-stimulating hormone (FSH).

PITUITARY GLAND

1. The anterior pituitary is the site of action of GnRH.
2. Both LH and FSH are glycopeptides with two molecular chains. They share a common alpha chain; specificity is determined by a unique beta chain.
3. LH and FSH are secreted in pulsatile manner. **Androgens and estrogens regulate LH secretion through negative feedback.** FSH is thought to have independence from GnRH because gonadal proteins, inhibin and activin, can affect its secretion, though it is also heavily regulated through negative-feedback loops from the secretion of androgens and estrogens.
4. The testes are the primary target for LH and FSH. No other target organs for these hormones have been found. **LH stimulates steroidogenesis within Leydig cells, and FSH stimulates seminiferous tubule growth and spermatogenesis at puberty.**

FEEDBACK MECHANISMS

GnRH, LH, and FSH are generally thought to be responsible for driving the production of testosterone and spermatozoa. Feedback mechanisms regulate the production and release of these substances (Fig. 22.e4).

1. LH regulation
   a. Testosterone and estradiol are the major **negative-feedback** substances that control the formation and release of LH. Normal testosterone production in men is around 5 g/day, and testosterone is metabolized into dihydrotestosterone (DHT) or estradiol.
   b. **Testosterone therefore regulates its own production** by acting on the pituitary and hypothalamus. This has implications for clinical care: **exogenous testosterone supplements will suppress both endogenous testosterone (through decreased LH) and sperm production (through decreased FSH).**
   c. **Estradiol is produced within the testicle and the liver upon conversion from testosterone (5-alpha-reductase).** It is found in smaller amounts within the blood stream (testosterone:estrogen ratio is typically 10:1) but is potent in action. The site of regulation is also at the level of the pituitary and hypothalamus.
2. FSH regulation
   a. In men, Sertoli cells produce **inhibin**, a two-subunit hormone in the transforming growth factor family, which has an inhibitory effect on pituitary FSH output. In contrast, **activin**, a glycoprotein formed as a homodimer of either inhibin chain, has a stimulatory effect on pituitary FSH. Neither inhibin nor activin affects pituitary LH release.
3. A variety of short feedback loops and other modulating substances more finely tune this system.

THE TESTES

- **Seminiferous tubules comprise the bulk** (80%) **of the testis mass** and are responsible for developing germ cells. Support cells include Sertoli cells, fibrocyte, and myoid cells.
- The **interstitium** between the **seminiferous tubules contains blood vessels, lymphatics, Leydig cells, mast cells, nerves.**
- **Arterial supply to the testis and epididymis comes from the internal spermatic artery, the vasal artery, and the cremasteric artery.**
  1. Seminiferous tubule: structural organization
     a. The tubules consist of long ducts lined by **Sertoli cells** that engulf and nurture developing germ cells.

b. Sertoli cells have membrane receptors that bind FSH, resulting in increased intracellular cyclic adenosine monophosphate (cAMP) and subsequent cytoskeletal reorganization for protein synthesis.
c. The primary secretion products from Sertoli cells include MIS in the fetus, androgen-binding protein (ABP), transferrin, and inhibin (a nonsteroidal glycoprotein) in the adult.
d. Sertoli cells regulate the tubule microenvironment. They govern fluid secretions into the lumen of the seminiferous tubules and partake in phagocytosis, steroid metabolism (in part), sperm production, and sperm movement through the tubule.
e. Sertoli cells are also mainly responsible for the **blood-testis barrier.** This anatomic barrier is surrounded by **myoid cells** and consists of the basement membrane and Sertoli cell **tight junctions**. These tight junctional complexes between Sertoli cells divide seminiferous tubule space into basal and adluminal compartments. This complex blood-testis barrier provides an **immunologically privileged site for mature spermatozoa** because these haploid cells harbor unique and specific antigens that are not otherwise recognized as "self" by the body's immune system.

2. Seminiferous tubules: spermatogenesis
   a. **LH, FSH, and testosterone are all required for normal spermatogenesis.**
   b. Sertoli cells, lining **250 m** of seminiferous tubules in the average testis, regulate the complex process of spermatogenesis.
   c. A variety of germ cell types exist, including **spermatogonia, primary spermatocytes, secondary spermatocytes, spermatids, and spermatozoa.** Spermatogonial cells are represented by three subpopulations: (1) dark spermatogonia, (2) pale spermatogonia, and (3) B spermatogonia.
   d. **Spermiogenesis is the maturation process of a spermatid to a spermatozoan.** It involves a proliferative phase, a meiotic phase, and a spermiogenesis phase. **Dark spermatogonia** function as quiescent diploid reserve and are active only during initial pubertal development and

after stem cell depletion from gonadotoxic exposure. **Pale spermatogonia** are mitotically active and serve as eternal progenitor cells. **Type B spermatogonia** are immediate precursors to primary spermatocytes and undergo two meiotic divisions to produce spermatids.

e. The process of spermatogenesis takes approximately **78 days** to complete. The average **daily output is 125 million spermatozoa,** which declines with age. A normal man makes about 1200 sperm for every heartbeat.

f. **Primary spermatocytes are the first germ cells to undergo meiosis, the resultant cell is the Sa spermatid. Spermatids mature into spermatozoa.**

g. **With paternal age, there are increases in sperm structural chromosomal abnormalities, autosomal-dominant mutations, and epigenetic alterations leading to disease in offspring.**

3. Interstitium: Leydig cells are responsible for the bulk of testicular steroid production. They differentiate from stem cell precursors under the influence of LH, human chorionic gonadotropin (hCG), and local paracrine factors such as insulin-like growth factor 1 (IGF1).
   a. LH stimulation results in the conversion of cholesterol to testosterone in a steroidogenic pathway.
   b. Testosterone diffuses into the plasma (**endocrine** function) or into the seminiferous tubule lumen (**paracrine** function). Testosterone peaks correspond to four developmental events: (1) development of fetal reproductive tract around 12–18 weeks of gestation, (2) neonatal "imprinting" of androgen-dependent target tissues, (3) masculinization at puberty, and (4) maintenance of growth and function of androgen-dependent organs in the adult.
   c. Depending on the target tissue, testosterone may be active by itself or may be reduced to **DHT** by the enzyme 5-alpha-reductase.

TESTICULAR TRANSPORT

1. As noted earlier, movement of developing germ cells from the basement membrane to the lumen and release into the lumen of the seminiferous tubules is controlled by Sertoli cells. **During**

early prenatal development, primordial germ cells migrate to gonadal ridge and associate with Sertoli cells. The failure of germ cells to migrate is thought to be a cause of extragonadal germ cell tumor and adult infertility resulting from azoospermia.

2. The movement of the spermatozoa from the testis to the epididymis is controlled by four factors:
   a. Fluid pressure generated within the seminiferous tubule
   b. Myoepithelial contractions of the seminiferous tubules
   c. Contraction of the tunica albuginea of the testis
   d. Cilia within and contraction of the wall of the efferent ductules

EPIDIDYMIS

The epididymis is a structure 3–4 cm in length with three histologically different regions (caput, corpus, and cauda).

1. Sperm maturation
   a. The chemical composition of the intraluminal fluid changes significantly in the three anatomic portions of the epididymis.
   b. A variety of sperm membrane changes in permeability and antigenicity occur during transport through epididymis.
   c. **Motility and fertilizing capacity** are gained during transport through the epididymis.
   d. Androgen effects on the epididymis are mediated mainly through DHT. Epididymal function is also influenced by temperature, which may explain how cryptorchidism and varicocele can affect male infertility.
   e. The final process of maturation, **sperm capacitation,** takes place after the sperm have been ejaculated and come in contact with the female reproductive tract. **Fertilizing capacity** lasts approximately **48 hours** within the external female genitalia, an important finding for counseling patients on the optimum frequency of sexual intercourse around the time of ovulation.
2. Transport and storage
   a. The spermatozoa traverse the length of the epididymis in **2–12 days.** Within the epididymis the principal mechanism responsible for transport is likely spontaneous rhythmic contraction of the contractile cells surrounding the epididymis.

b. **An average of 55–209 million sperm are present in each epididymis and half is stored in caudal region. Spermatozoa in the cauda are capable for progressive motility and are able to fertilize eggs**, which is important in harvesting sperm from the epididymis for in vitro fertilization (IVF) with intracytoplasmic sperm injection (ICSI).

VAS DEFERENS

The vas deferens is classically divided into five regions: (1) sheathless epididymal segment contained within the tunica vaginalis, (2) scrotal segment, (3) inguinal segment, (4) pelvic segment, and (5) ampulla. **It receives its blood supply from the deferential artery, a branch of the superior vesical artery.**

1. Sperm transport: Human vas exhibits spontaneously motility; fluid within can be propelled into the urethra by strong peristaltic contractions. The rapid transport is consistent with the vas having the highest muscle-to-lumen ratio (10:1) of any hollow viscus in the body.
2. At the time of **emission**, regular coordinated contractions of the tails of the epididymides and the vasa deferentia occur, mediated by the sympathetic nervous system, propelling sperm into the prostatic urethra. During **ejaculation**, somatic nervous system–stimulated rhythmic contractions of periurethral and pelvic floor muscles propel the sperm through the urethra in the presence of a closed bladder neck closure mediated by the sympathetic nervous system. Emission phase is coordinated through spinal ejaculatory generator **(T12-L2 region)**, and filling of the posterior urethra activates the urethral-muscular reflex activating the sacral spinal cord **(S2-S4)** initiating the expulsion phase of ejaculation.

SEMEN COMPOSITION

The bulk of seminal fluid originates from the accessory ducts, with the spermatozoa adding a small (less than 10%) amount to total volume.

1. Prostatic fluid
   a. The **prostatic fluid** is usually found in the first part of the ejaculate and contributes approximately **one-quarter of the total volume. This fluid is acidic (pH less than 6.5).**

b. Specific prostate products include liquefaction factors such as **prostate-specific antigen (PSA)**, zinc, citric acid, acid, phosphatase, and spermine. The latter substance, when oxidized to aldehydes, produces the characteristic odor of semen.

c. **PSA, a 33-kd molecular weight serum protease in the family of glandular kallikreins, serves to liquefy the coagulum** of human semen 5 to 20 minutes following ejaculation.

2. Seminal vesicle fluid

a. **The seminal vesicle fluid** is usually found in the second part of the ejaculate and contributes approximately **two-thirds of the total volume. This fluid is basic (pH greater than 7.0). Acidic ejaculate pH < 7.2 is associated with blockage or absence of seminal vesicles.**

b. Specific substances secreted by the seminal vesicles include coagulation factors, prostaglandins, and fructose. **Fructose** is measured on a semen analysis to investigate the diagnosis of ejaculatory duct obstruction (EDO).

Clinical Evaluation of the Subfertile Male

In 2020, the American Urological Association/American Society for Reproductive Medicine (AUA/ASRM) revised its guidelines for the diagnosis and treatment for male infertility. The specific goals of this evaluation include identification of the following:

1. Potentially correctable conditions
2. Irreversible conditions that are amenable to assisted reproductive technologies (ARTs) using the sperm of the male partner
3. Irreversible conditions that are not amenable to the aforementioned, and for which donor insemination or adoption is a possible option
4. Life- or health-threatening conditions that may underlie the infertility or associated medical comorbidities that require medical attention
5. Genetic abnormalities or lifestyle and age-related factors that may affect the health of the male patient or of offspring, particularly if ARTs are to be employed (Fig. 22.1)

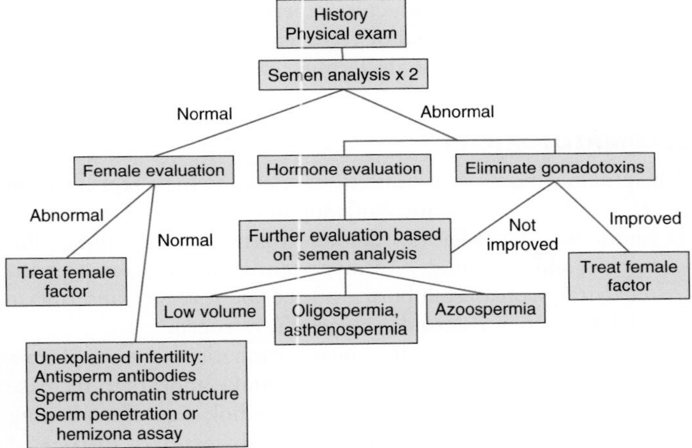

FIGURE 22.1 Algorithm for diagnostic evaluation of male-factor infertility. (From Turek PJ. Practical approaches to the diagnosis and management of male infertility. *Nat Clin Pract Urol*. 2005;2:226-238.)

ASSESSMENT

Timing of Evaluation

1. Generally, a fertility evaluation for male-factor infertility should take place after 1 year of trying to conceive naturally without success. However, there are additional circumstances that may prompt an earlier evaluation. They include:
   a. The presence of risk factors affecting male-factor infertility
   b. The presence of female fertility risk factors (i.e., advanced maternal age, etc.)
   c. The questioning of the fertility potential of the male (despite presence of a female fertility risk factor)

AUA/ASRM Guidelines Regarding Fertility

Both male and female partners should undergo concurrent assessment at the initial infertility evaluation. While the initial evaluation of the male should include a reproductive history and one or more semen analyses (SAs), men with abnormal semen parameters and/or suspected male infertility should be thoroughly evaluated by a male reproductive expert. Additionally, in couples with failed ART cycles and/or recurrent pregnancy loss (defined as ≥ 2 miscarriages), a male fertility evaluation should also be considered.

SPERMATOTOXICITY

A helpful mnemonic to ask questions related to male reproduction is *TICS* = Toxins, Infectious/Inflammatory, Childhood history.

1. Endocrine modulators: Antiandrogens—bicalutamide, flutamide, and nilutamide; Antihypertensive spironolactone, antiretroviral protease inhibitors, nucleoside reverse transcriptase inhibitors, corticosteroids, exogenous estrogen.
2. Recreational drugs: Studies suggest cannabis decreases plasma testosterone, heavy chronic alcohol intake appears to increase aromatization of testosterone to estradiol, cigarette smoking increases seminal oxidative stress and decreases metrics of sperm DNA quality.
3. Antipsychotics: Antagonism of dopamine, which causes loss of libido.
4. Opioids: Suppress LH release primarily through hypothalamic-mediated mechanisms and reduce testosterone synthesis.
5. Cytotoxic chemotherapeutics: Suppress briskly proliferating cells.
6. Antiinflammatory agents: Sulfasalazine is associated with oligoasthenospermia.
7. Radiation: Testes directly exposed to ionizing radiation suffer germ cell loss and Leydig cell dysfunction.
8. Childhood: Hydroceles and hernias repaired during childhood are associated with low incidence of complications causing vasal obstruction. Approximately half of men with torsion develop adverse spermatogenic effects with up to 11% developing antisperm antibodies.

FERTILITY HISTORY

1. Present fertility history
    a. Duration of infertility
    b. Contraceptive methods and duration used
    c. Length of time trying to conceive
    d. Number of pregnancies, including miscarriages and therapeutic abortions, which indicate the potential to conceive

2. Previous fertility history and relationships
   a. If the patient has attempted to conceive in the past, the duration and number of pregnancies should be determined.
   b. The duration and number of pregnancies conceived by the female partner should also be determined.
3. Sexual history
   a. Frequency of intercourse and masturbation: Overly frequent (daily) or infrequent (more than 48 hours apart around the time of ovulation) can adversely affect the couple's ability to conceive.
   b. Libido, potency, and sexual technique: A normal desire and ability to have intercourse is critical, and problems in these areas are often overlooked by clinicians. **Situational erectile dysfunction** (ED) caused by stress is common among couples trying to conceive and is easily treated with **phosphodiesterase inhibitors.**
   c. Ejaculation: This needs to occur deep within the vagina. Severe problems with **premature ejaculation, chordee, or severe hypospadias** may prevent proper deposition of sperm.
   d. **Dyspareunia** and the use of lubrication: Impaired natural vaginal lubrication can result in painful intercourse for either partner. Most lubricants are spermicidal.
   e. Understanding of the **ovulatory cycle:** It is important that the couple understand when ovulation occurs and have timed intercourse regularly during this time.
4. Genitourinary history
   a. Testicular descent: Bilateral **cryptorchidism** is associated with impaired spermatogenesis and fertility. With unilateral cryptorchidism, fertility potential slightly decreases.
   b. Sexual development and onset of puberty: **Delayed puberty** can indicate syndromes (e.g., Kallmann) or chromosomal issues (e.g., XXY).
   c. Infections: Venereal, nonvenereal, mumps (at the time of puberty or later), recent febrile illness, or other infectious problems that directly involve the genitalia or urogenital duct system may be associated with a significant scarring and subsequent fertility problems. Viral infections and other febrile illnesses not specifically involving the genitalia may also temporarily lower sperm counts.

   d. **Trauma or torsion:** Either condition may injure the duct system or result in ischemic damage to the seminiferous tubules.
   e. Exposure to chemicals: A variety of drugs and industrial compounds may be associated with abnormal semen analyses.
   f. Exposure to heat: Prolonged exposure to high temperatures may adversely affect spermatogenesis. **Hot tubs, hot baths, saunas, or steam rooms on a regular basis can be significant in this regard.**
   g. Exposure to radiation: Even small amounts of ionizing radiation, particularly that used for medical therapy, may destroy sperm-forming cells. **Spermatogonia are particularly radiosensitive.**
5. Previous infertility evaluation
   a. Patient: A history of previous semen analyses and medical or surgical treatment is certainly important for the etiology and prognosis of male infertility.
   b. Wife or partner: It is wise to understand the fertility potential of the partner (see Fig. 22.1). Conception involves two people and if for some physiologic or anatomic reason, an irreversible problem exists in the female partner, pregnancy is unlikely. The evaluation of each partner should be carried out simultaneously, and the male evaluation should be completed prior to invasive procedures on the female partner. **At least 1 year of maternal reproductive potential should exist for the best outcomes after male infertility treatment.**
6. Age
   a. Data indicate that advanced paternal age ($\geq$ 40) increases de novo intra- and intergenic germline mutations, sperm aneuploidy, structural chromosomal aberrations, sperm DNA fragmentation, birth defects, and genetically medicated conditions (e.g., chondrodysplasia, schizophrenia, autism) in offspring. Patients with advanced paternal age should be counseled on the low absolute risk (but high relative risk) of adverse health outcomes for their offspring.

GENERAL MEDICAL HISTORY

1. While most conditions causing male infertility do not lead to long-term medical consequences, **1% to 2% of men undergoing evaluation for infertility will have a significant underlying medical condition.** Infertile/subfertile men should be counseled

of the health risks association with abnormal sperm production. Additionally, these men with specific, identifiable causes of male infertility should be informed of relevant, associated health conditions.

a. Medical illnesses: Medical problems such as **diabetes** and **hypertension** or their pharmacologic treatments may adversely affect erectile and ejaculatory function and hence fertility.
b. Abnormal metabolism of sex steroids may be associated with various liver and renal diseases and interfere with the regulatory mechanisms of spermatogenesis. Rare medical illnesses such as **Young syndrome** (immotile cilia syndrome) and **Kartagener syndrome** (ciliary defect with situs inversus) can adversely affect fertility.

2. Surgical history
   a. Inguinal herniorrhaphy, particularly when performed on a young child and when performed bilaterally, may be associated with injury to the vas deferens in 1% to 2% of patients.
   b. Surgery on the ureter, bladder, bladder neck, or urethra may result in problems with emission and/or ejaculation.
   c. Retroperitoneal surgery and other major pelvic procedures may result in failure of emission and/or problems with retrograde ejaculation. Young males with nonseminomatous testis tumors are treated with retroperitoneal lymphadenectomy and subsequently have fertility problems caused by absent ejaculation either from failure of emission or from retrograde ejaculation. It appears that two to three cycles of adjuvant chemotherapy often given in lieu of retroperitoneal lymphadenectomy do not significantly impair male fertility.
3. Current and past medications
   a. A variety of drugs and chemotherapeutic agents may adversely affect sperm production and/or function. Adverse affects are usually reversible upon discontinuation (Box 22.1).
4. Occupation and habits
   a. Occupation and stress: The effects of daily stress on fertility are poorly quantified. **Severe, acute stress has been associated with decreases in ejaculate volume and sperm count.** While most patients inquire about stress, it is unlikely that they would change their job or lifestyle, making this problem difficult to

BOX 22.1 Drugs and Chemicals With Potential Adverse Fertility Effects

Alcohol
Alkylating agents (e.g., cyclophosphamide)
Arsenic
Aspirin (large doses)
Caffeine
Cimetidine
Colchicine
Dibromochloropropane (pesticide)
Diethylstilbestrol (DES)
Finasteride
Lead
Monoamine oxidase inhibitors
Marijuana
Medroxyprogesterone
Nicotine
Nitrofurantoin
Phenytoin
Spironolactone
Sulfasalazine
Testosterone

treat. Encouraging regular exercise, yoga, or acupuncture may help reduce stress.

b. The active ingredients in cigarettes, marijuana, coffee, tea, alcohol, and some naturopathic herbs have been demonstrated in laboratory studies to be potentially gonadotoxic. The susceptibility of individuals to these substances varies widely and is difficult to quantify.
c. Clinicians may discuss risk factors (i.e., lifestyle, medication usage, environmental exposures) associated with male infertility, and patients should be counseled that the current data on the majority of risk factors are limited.

5. Family history
   a. Sibling fertility status may identify familial conditions such as cystic fibrosis, genetic infertility due to Y chromosome deletions, and congenital adrenal hyperplasia.
   b. In utero exposure to **diethylstilbestrol (DES)** may result in testicular, epididymal, and penile anatomic abnormalities. Despite the finding of impaired semen quality in DES-exposed men, proof of decreased fertility is not obvious in extensive follow-up studies.

PHYSICAL EXAMINATION

1. General examination: This evaluates the patient's **body habitus** and secondary sexual characteristics. In particular, the pattern of hair distribution and **gynecomastia** can reflect endocrine disorders.
2. Obesity should be noted because substantial evidence associates it with reproductive dysfunction, such as elevated estradiol from peripheral conversion of testosterone, lower serum testosterone, lower sex hormone–binding globulin (SHBG).
3. Examination of the genitalia: Physicians should try to make the patient comfortable during examination, can consider asking partner to leave the examination room.
   a. Penis: The size of the penis and location of the meatus are important in assuring the delivery of spermatozoa proximal to the cervical os. Important to note phimosis, hypospadias/epispadias, and significant penile curvature.
   b. Testes: The **location, size, and consistency** of the testes should be noted. Testis size correlates with sperm production. Size can be assessed using calipers. **Normal length of a testicle in an adult is > 4.6 cm and a volume > 20 mL.**
   c. Epididymis: The epididymis should be examined for size and consistency. The **obstructed epididymis feels enlarged and firm.** The epididymis that is scarred from either trauma or chronic infection may be hard and irregular.
   d. Vasa deferentia: Each vas deferens should be palpable as a distinct, firm, cord-like structure in the scrotum. In **1% to 2% of infertile men, one or both vasa are not palpable in the scrotum, a condition termed congenital absence of the vas deferens (CAVD).**
   e. Spermatic cord: Examination of spermatic cord can tell you if the vas is palpable and the presence of a varicocele. **Unilateral absence of the vas deferens suggests the possibility of a complete lack of Wolffian ductal development on that side including renal agenesis.** If both vas are absent there is a high likelihood of a cystic fibrosis gene mutation.
   f. Inguinal region: The inguinal canals are palpated for hernias. In addition, the inguinal regions should be inspected to assess if previous surgery may have injured the vasa deferentia or testicular blood supply.

4. Rectal examination: Does not add a significant amount of information to the evaluation of the infertile man; if patient is apprehensive can be omitted. Seminal vesicles are not typically palpated; if palpable can represent ejaculatory ductal obstruction.

LABORATORY EVALUATION

1. **The three general laboratory assessments used are endocrine, semen analysis, and genomic assessment.**
2. **Testis biopsy is not indicated in the initial diagnostic evaluation of infertility.**

SEMEN ANALYSES

1. Collection: **A minimum of two semen analyses, ideally separated by 4 weeks, are needed to establish a baseline for a patient.** Two to five days of abstinence is optimal for assessing bulk seminal parameters. Sample should be evaluated within 1 hour of collection.
2. Minimal standards of adequacy: While there is no absolute measure of fertility on semen analysis, minimal standards of semen adequacy have been defined by the World Health Organization (Table 22.1).
3. Semen volume: Seminal hypovolemia can be due to anatomic factors (ejaculatory ductal obstruction or hypoplasia of prostate and seminal vesicles); functional factors such as retrograde ejaculation; neurologic conditions such as spinal cord

TABLE 22.1 World Health Organization Fifth Edition Normal Semen Parameter Reference Ranges

Variable	Cut-Off Value
Sperm volume	> 1.5 mL
Sperm concentration	> 15 million/mL
Total sperm count	> 39 million
Sperm progressive motility (A + B)	> 32%
Sperm morphology	> 4%
Sperm DNA fragmentation	< 30%
Nonsperm cells	< 1 million/mL

From World Health Organization. *WHO Laboratory Manual for the Examination and Processing of Human Semen*. 5th ed. Geneva: World Health Organization; 2010.

injury, diabetes mellitus (DM), multiple sclerosis (MS). Seminal hypervolemia is rare but described as > 5 mL; it is thought to dilute the sperm.

4. Sperm concentration: **Oligospermia or oligozoospermia refers to low sperm concentration.**
5. Sperm motility: **Asthenospermia describes low motility**, which is usually assessed within 30 minutes of liquefaction.
6. Sperm morphology: A large number of **abnormal sperm is termed teratospermia.** By assessing the dimensions and shape characteristics of the sperm head, midpiece, and tail, sperm can be classified as *normal* or abnormal. In the most recent strictest classification system (Kruger morphology), only 4% of sperm in the ejaculate are typically deemed normal. This number has been correlated with the success of egg fertilization in vitro. However, once the other parameters are within normal limits, abnormal sperm morphology has been shown to be of little value for couples pursuing natural conception or intrauterine insemination (IUI). Multiple meta-analyses have shown no difference in pregnancy and live birth rates for patients with a morphology ≥ 1% versus those with normal morphology when the rest of the parameters are within normal limits.
7. Tests of sperm function
    a. **Sperm chromatin assay:** The structure of sperm chromatin (the DNA-associated proteins) is independent of semen quality and can be measured by COMET and TUNEL assays and by flow cytometry after acid treatment and staining of sperm with a fluorescent marker. These tests assess the degree of DNA fragmentation and indirectly reflect the quality of sperm DNA integrity. In patients with failed ART cycles and/or recurrent pregnancy loss, DNA fragmentation testing should strongly be considered on the male partner's ejaculated sperm. If abnormal, there should be an evaluation to consider medically or surgically correctable causes of abnormal sperm DNA fragmentation (such as antidepressant use or presence of a genitourinary [GU] infection). Consideration should be given for using surgically extracted sperm for subsequent IVF cycles.
    b. **Antisperm antibodies:** A link between infertility and antisperm antibodies has been recognized for years. Enzyme-linked immunosorbent assay (ELISA) and immunobead binding assay

are two commonly used tests to detect antibodies on sperm. However, antisperm antibody testing should not be done in the initial evaluation of male infertility.

   c. **White blood cells:** Reproductive tract infections are a treatable cause of infertility and are often heralded by the presence of excessive white blood cells in the ejaculate (**pyospermia**). Special stains can distinguish white cells from immature germ cells, the latter of which are not pathologic. Patients with pyospermia should be evaluated for the presence of infection.

3. Additional physical parameters: Other properties are examined at the time of a routine semen analysis. These include:
   a. Color: The semen is generally grayish-white with an opalescent character.
   b. Coagulation: This occurs immediately after ejaculation.
   c. Liquefaction: This occurs 5 to 30 minutes following ejaculation. **PSA** is the serine protease responsible for this process.
   d. Viscosity: This parameter refers to the fluid consistency of the semen after coagulation and liquefaction have occurred. Viscosity is normal if it is possible to pour the semen in a drop-by-drop fashion.
   e. pH: The pH of semen is normally in the range of 7.2 to 8.0. A low pH implies absence or blockage of the seminal vesicles because the ejaculate consists entirely of acidic prostatic fluid.
   f. Fructose: As noted earlier, fructose is produced by the seminal vesicles. Semen fructose is examined in cases of azoospermia with low ejaculate volume (less than 1.5 mL). Absence of fructose in semen suggests absence of the vasa deferentia and seminal vesicles, EDO, or dysfunction of the seminal vesicles.

ENDOCRINE EVALUATION

1. **Normal testosterone level in men is ≥ 300 ng/dL**; approximately 45% of men with azoospermia are seen to have levels below this threshold.
2. 30%–44% of testosterone is bound to SHBG, 54%–68% loosely bound to albumin, and 0.5%–3.0% is unbound; only the free and loosely bound participate in cellular activity.
3. Total testosterone exhibits a circadian rhythm, **peaks in early morning and trough levels in late afternoon**, therefore assays are typically performed in the morning.

4. In hypoandrogenism, LH will be elevated if primary cause is testicular Leydig cell dysfunction, and LH is decreased in pituitary dysfunction.
5. FSH is used in combination with testis size to predict if azoospermia is a result of obstruction or spermatogenic dysfunction; normal FSH values (< 7.6) and larger testis size (length > 4.6 cm) could be a predictor of obstruction. However, patients with maturation arrest of sperm may also have normal testicular size and a normal FSH; thus a normal FSH should not rule out an issue of sperm production.
6. Initial laboratory screen should be performed in the morning and should include **total testosterone and FSH** in men presenting with impaired libido, ED, subfertile semen parameters or azoospermia, atrophic testes, or evidence of hormonal abnormality on physical exam. If these values are abnormal, prolactin, LH, and estradiol should also be checked.
7. **Prolactin** levels should be obtained if low testosterone is found or if the patient has gynecomastia, severe headaches, or visual disturbances. Prolactin-secreting pituitary tumors produce high levels of circulating prolactin, and these lesions tend to reduce LH and FSH levels.

GENOMIC ASSESSMENT

1. Fluorescent in situ hybridization (FISH) uses fluorescent probes that bind to DNA allowing for identification of specific regions or entire chromosomes.
2. **Genetic testing including karyotype is critical for males with azoospermia and severe oligospermia (less than 5 million sperm/mL)** as well as patients with poor IVF outcomes and/or recurrent pregnancy loss.
3. **A region in the long arm of the Y chromosome is critical to the formation of sperm in men, known as the azoospermia factor. Microdeletions in three regions are associated with azoospermia and oligospermia: AZFa, AZFb, and AZFc.** Deletions of AZFa and AZFb have a much poorer prognosis for testicular sperm retrieval by surgery than patients with AZFc deletions, which has an approximately 50% sperm retrieval rate during microsurgical testicular sperm extraction (microTESE). No sperm have ever been retrieved in men with a complete AZFa and/or AZFb microdeletion.

4. Men with vasal agenesis or idiopathic obstructive azoospermia should also undergo **cystic fibrosis transmembrane conductance regulator (CFTR) mutation carrier testing** (including assessment of the 5T allele). For men who harbor a *CFTR* mutation, genetic evaluation of the female partner should be recommended.

IMAGING DURING INFERTILITY EVALUATION

1. **Transrectal ultrasound (TRUS):** This is indicated in men with azoospermia and acidic, very low-volume ejaculate (< 1.5 mL) and palpable vas deferens to rule out **EDO.** EDO may be identified by seminal vesicle dilatation (greater than 1.5 cm in diameter with or without a midline prostatic cyst). Often EDO caused by stones, scar, prostatic cysts, or a persistent utricle can be diagnosed by TRUS. **Seminal vesiculography**, **chromotubation** (antegrade injection of diluted indigo carmine monitored by flexible cystoscopy), and **ejaculatory duct manometry** are three dynamic tests that can improve the accuracy of the EDO diagnosis; however, they are more invasive. **Seminal vesicle aspiration** is also used to confirm the presence of sperm in patients with suspected obstruction.
2. **Vasography:** Intraoperative, transscrotal vasography is currently used to detect abdominal vas deferens, seminal vesicle, and ejaculatory duct patency prior to definitive surgery for epididymal or vasal obstruction. It should only be performed simultaneously with microsurgical vasectomy reversal.
3. **Scrotal ultrasound:** This should not be routinely performed in the initial evaluation of the infertile man. However, this may be indicated when the testes are not easily palpable because of coexistent hydrocele, to confirm the origin and character (solid versus cystic) of intrascrotal masses, and for confirming a clinically suspicious varicocele (however, physical exam should remain the gold standard for identifying and grading a clinical varicocele). Physicians should not pursue surgical treatment of subclinical varicoceles (< 4 mm) that are not palpable on examination, since it does not result in improved seminal outcomes.
4. **Renal ultrasound:** This should be recommended for patients with vasal agenesis (unilateral and bilateral) to assess for renal abnormalities. In men with unilateral absence of the vas deferens,

26%–75% will have ipsilateral renal anomalies including agenesis. In men with bilateral vas agenesis, the prevalence is approximately 10%.

Classification of Abnormalities

GENETIC SYNDROMES

1. **Klinefelter syndrome (KS; 47 XXY) is the most commonly identified genetic cause of infertility.** Men with KS have primary testicular failure, nonobstructive azoospermia (NOA), low testosterone, and high FSH and LH. 95% of affected adults have azoospermia, small testes, and elevated gonadotropin levels. **Half of men with this syndrome have sufficient sperm during surgical sperm retrieval for IVF.**
2. **Cystic fibrosis is autosomal recessive, characterized by an abnormal chloride transporter, and results in congenital bilateral absence of the vas deferens (CBAVD).**
3. **Primary ciliary dyskinesia (PCD) is autosomal recessive, which results in impairment in motile cilia; Kartagener syndrome is likely the most well-known PCD.**
4. **Kallmann syndrome, absence of GnRH production, is characterized by anosmia, poorly developed secondary characteristics, atrophic testicles, sub/infertility, hypogonadotropic hypogonadism. Supplementation with gonadotropins achieves a return of spermatogenesis in 95%.**

TESTICULAR CAUSES

1. Testicular causes can be divided into pathology in the production in the seminiferous epithelium, synthesis of testosterone by Leydig cells, or obstruction in the transporting system.
2. Dysfunction in seminiferous epithelium is defined as a decrease in sperm production. Pathologic conditions that disrupt blood-testis barriers can lead to antibody formation, which can reduce fertilizing potential.
3. Steroidogenic dysfunction is caused by Leydig cell dysfunction. Men with low serum testosterone should be optimized by medications to boost endogenous testosterone production, such as aromatase inhibitors, selective estrogen receptor modulators (SERMs), or hCG, with reevaluation of semen parameters

3 months later to assess for improvement. There is currently no accepted therapy for azoospermia with low testosterone and high LH, and treatment is surgical sperm extraction. Nonetheless, one can try medications to improve endogenous testosterone production and see if any of these interventions stimulate increased testosterone synthesis.

PITUITARY DYSFUNCTION

1. LH directs Leydig cell steroidogenesis. FSH controls spermatogenesis in Sertoli cells, though spermatogenesis is also influenced by intratesticular testosterone levels as well.
2. Hypogonadotropic hypogonadism: Kallmann syndrome results in decreased pituitary hormonal secretion with mutation in GNRHR and KAL1 gene. **Treatment includes replacement of LH with hCG and replacement of FSH with recombinant FSH (rFSH) or human menopausal gonadotropin (hMG).**
3. Incomplete forms with hypoandrogenism associated with LH concentrations above those with Kallmann can be treated with SERMs (clomiphene or tamoxifen) or with aromatase inhibitors.
4. Tumors in the sella turcica can compress the anterior pituitary and result in LH and FSH suppression; **if prolactin levels are significantly elevated, cranial MRI should be obtained.** Dopamine agonists such as bromocriptine and cabergoline can be prescribed if not a candidate for surgery.

EXTRATESTICULAR ENDOCRINE DYSFUNCTION

1. **AR insensitivity is associated with increased testosterone, estradiol, and LH with variable FSH levels.**

DEVELOPMENTAL DISORDERS

1. Hypospadias and epispadias may result in deposition of semen too distal in vaginal vault.
2. Unilateral absence of the vas may signal renal agenesis because renal development is coupled with Wolffian ductal development.
3. **Congenital bilateral absence of the vas results in low-volume, acidic, obstructive azoospermia,** identified in 1%–2% of infertile males and 4%–17% of azoospermic patients. CFTR gene mutations are seen in 80% of men with CBAVD and 20% of congenital unilateral absence of the vas deferens (CUAVD).

VARICOCELES

1. More common on the left. However, a solitary right varicocele with abrupt onset should be investigated for renal pathology.
2. They are found in approximately 15% of the population, 35% of men with primary infertility, and 75%–81% of men with secondary infertility.
3. It is thought that reproductive dysfunction caused by varicoceles is due to an increase in intratesticular temperature due to interruption in the countercurrent heat exchange. Surgical correction can improve semen parameters.

CRYPTORCHIDISM

1. Associated with future infertility via several potential mechanisms, congenital testicular and Wolffian duct anomalies, hormonal alterations, heat-induced damage, higher risk of infertility with higher testicular location and bilateral cryptorchidism.

EJACULATORY DYSFUNCTION

1. **Evaluation for ejaculatory ductal obstruction is needed if seminal volume < 1.0 mL. It affects 1%–5% of infertile men.**
2. Antegrade ejaculation requires bladder neck to close and external sphincter to close to create a high-pressure compartment that empties when it is opened again.
3. **Sympathomimetic agents such as synephrine, pseudoephedrine, ephedrine or phenylpropanolamine can be used to treat retrograde ejaculation.**
4. **Anejaculation is lack of seminal emission and projectile ejaculation usually caused by neurologic conditions or long-standing diabetes;** therapy includes stimulation with penile vibratory devices, electroejaculation, and surgical sperm extraction.

SUBSTANCE ABUSE

1. Alcohol, cocaine, marijuana, methamphetamines, opioids, tobacco and exogenous testosterone have been associated with infertility.
2. Following exogenous testosterone discontinuation, normal spermatogenesis returns in about 4–6 months. These patients are typically treated with medications to boost endogenous testosterone production to prevent the recurrence of hypogonadal symptoms.

SURGERY

1. Testicular injury during pediatric hernia repair is estimated at 1%–2% while bilateral repair can cause bilateral vas obstruction in 40%.

Evaluation of the Infertile Male

ALL PARAMETERS NORMAL

1. When two semen analyses are normal and the history and physical examination are unrevealing in the male, further evaluation of the female partner is recommended.
2. If the evaluation of the female partner is also found to be normal, and the couple still has not conceived, then sperm function tests noted earlier may be useful. Most couples with unexplained infertility will go on to be treated with **IUI or IVF.**

AZOOSPERMIA

1. When no sperm are found on semen analysis, the specimen should be centrifuged and further examined to confirm the finding. In addition, **collection error** and/or retrograde ejaculation must be ruled out as causes of azoospermia. If **retrograde ejaculation** is identified by the finding of sperm in the postejaculate urinalysis (more than 10 to 15 sperm per high-power field [HPF]), treatment can be initiated with sympathomimetic agents to promote antegrade ejaculation. Alternatively, sperm can be retrieved from the bladder, processed, and used for IUI and/or IVF.
2. The results of the fructose test and gonadotropin levels determine what additional evaluation and treatment is necessary.
   a. The LH, FSH, and testosterone levels can differentiate **primary testicular failure** from secondary testicular failure caused by either pituitary or hypothalamic dysfunction.
   b. A serum **FSH more than three times normal** along with atrophic testicles on physical examination constitutes a diagnosis of NOA and indicates severe testicular failure. **However, it does not mean that no sperm are in the testis because one-half of men can have low numbers of testicular sperm on more extensive evaluation.** Sperm production in men with NOA is heterogenous and these patients should

be offered microTESE. Sperm found in these men can be used in conjunction with IVF/ICSI.

3. After ruling out a major endocrine abnormality, the major differential diagnosis is **ductal obstruction** or **testicular failure;** consider female-factor infertility.
   a. Negative semen fructose test: Three possibilities exist in the azoospermic patient with normal hormone studies and a negative fructose test. These include CBAVD and seminal vesicle atrophy, bilateral EDO and, rarely, **seminal vesicle dysfunction** similar to bladder myopathy. The treatment of CBAVD is direct sperm aspiration from the epididymal remnant or testicle. The sperm are then processed and used in combination with IVF and ICSI. EDO is managed by transurethral resection of the ejaculatory ducts (TURED) or by unroofing midline cysts.
   b. Positive fructose test: A positive fructose test usually rules out complete obstruction of the ejaculatory ducts and severe dysfunction of the seminal vesicles but does not assess the patency of the ductal system from the level of the testis to the ejaculatory ducts. Therefore a positive fructose test in azoospermia does not differentiate between proximal ductal obstruction and testicular failure.
   c. Testicular biopsy: A testicular biopsy is important in the azoospermic patient with normal hormones and normal-sized testes with fructose in the ejaculate. The microscopic examination of the biopsy will indicate whether spermatogenesis is progressing normally. With the advent of IVF and ICSI, sperm found on testicular biopsy should also be cryopreserved for future use (Fig. 22.2).

MULTIPLE ABNORMAL PARAMETERS ON THE SEMEN ANALYSIS

1. Diffuse abnormalities of all or many of the seminal parameters are the most common pathologic pattern identified (55%). Determination of the LH, FSH, and testosterone levels rule out an endocrine abnormality.
2. Stress, infections, and other environmental factors such as hot tubs or bath, drugs, and toxin exposures may produce a transient abnormality of all seminal parameters. Therefore when other factors are not identified by the history or physical

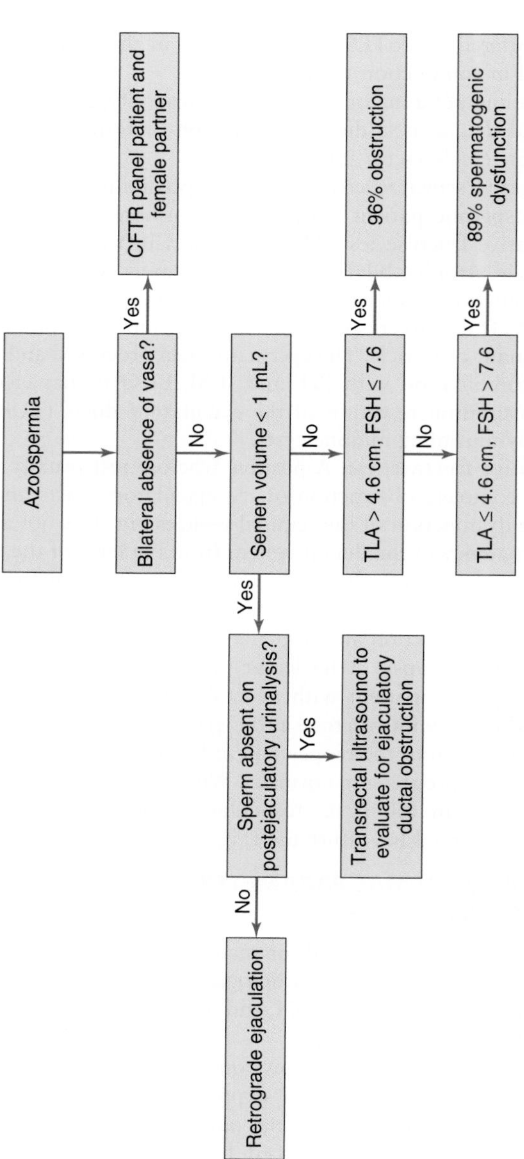

FIGURE 22.2 Algorithm for evaluation of azoospermia. *CFTR,* Cystic fibrosis transmembrane conductance regulator; *FSH,* follicle-stimulating hormone; *TLA,* testicle length in an adult.

examination, it may be prudent to follow patients for 3 to 6 months to assess self-correction. If spontaneous correction has not occurred, nonspecific therapy can be instituted as discussed later. Couples can also be offered ART (IUI, IVF).

3. Varicoceles: Historically varicocelectomy was reserved for the treatment of infertile men but there is an emerging concept for early repair of varicoceles to prevent future infertility and Leydig cell dysfunction.
   a. A **varicocele** is defined as **dilated, varicose internal spermatic veins** producing fullness, dilatation, and **poor drainage of the pampiniform plexus.** A varicocele is found in **15%** of males in the general population and in **35% to 40% of men presenting with infertility** problems and results in abnormal semen parameters.
   b. Varicoceles are **classified according to size as either large (grade III), medium (grade II), or small (grade I).** Large varicoceles can be seen as a "bag of worms" under the scrotal skin. Medium varicoceles are readily detected by palpation, especially on standing. Small varicoceles can only be identified by feeling an impulse in the scrotum with the Valsalva maneuver or by feeling a difference in the size and fullness of the spermatic cord when the patient moves from the standing to the supine position. The majority (90%) of varicoceles occurs on the left side, and the remainder is bilateral. Isolated right varicoceles suggest intraabdominal or retroperitoneal pathology and may merit abdominal and pelvic imaging.
   c. The exact mechanism through which the varicocele exerts a detrimental effect on fertility is unclear; the leading theory is that it leads to **increased intrascrotal temperature** through retrograde venous blood flow. It characteristically decreases normal sperm morphology with an increase in immature and tapered sperm forms (**stress pattern**). Decreased sperm motility and varying degrees of oligospermia also may exist.
   d. Varicocele treatment involves surgical ligation or transvenous angiographic identification and embolization of involved internal spermatic veins. Surgical approaches can be **laparoscopic, inguinal, or subinguinal** with ligation of the internal spermatic and collateral veins, though most male

fertility experts agree that subinguinal microsurgical varicocelectomy is the gold standard. For venous occlusion via embolization, a variety of techniques is used, including sclerosing solutions, balloons, and stainless steel coils.

e. Results of varicocele ligation from published series indicate that **semen analysis improvement occurs in 70%** of cases, with an associated **40% pregnancy rate.** With baseline sperm counts greater than 10 million sperm/mL, pregnancy rates are significantly higher than when the initial counts are lower. Generally, varicocele recurrence rates are lower with surgical (5%) versus angiographic (20%) treatments.

f. For men with clinical varicoceles and NOA, couples should be informed of the absence of definitive evidence supporting varicocele repair prior to ART. Varicocele repair defers treatment with ART for at least 6 months. However, there have been several small studies, without control groups, which have reported the return of adequate motile sperm in the ejaculate sufficient to avoid surgical sperm retrieval. This is also the hypothesis that varicocele repair may improve the testicular microenvironment and lead to a better outcome of surgical sperm retrieval.

ISOLATED ABNORMAL PARAMETER ON SEMEN ANALYSIS

1. Abnormal semen volume
   a. Large ejaculate volume: A volume greater than 5.5 mL may result in dilution of the spermatozoa and poor cervical placement of seminal fluid during intercourse. Mechanical concentration of the spermatozoa and IUI may overcome this issue.
   b. Absent or low ejaculate volume (Fig. 22.3): Once a collection abnormality has been ruled out, it is essential to consider **retrograde ejaculation, infection of the accessory sex glands, or endocrine dysfunction (low testosterone).** The presence of retrograde ejaculation is confirmed by the finding of large quantities of spermatozoa in the postejaculatory urine sample (greater than 15 sperm per HPF). Sympathomimetic drugs with alpha-adrenergic activity can reverse this issue in one-third of patients, and generally in those without scar tissue at the bladder neck from prior surgery.

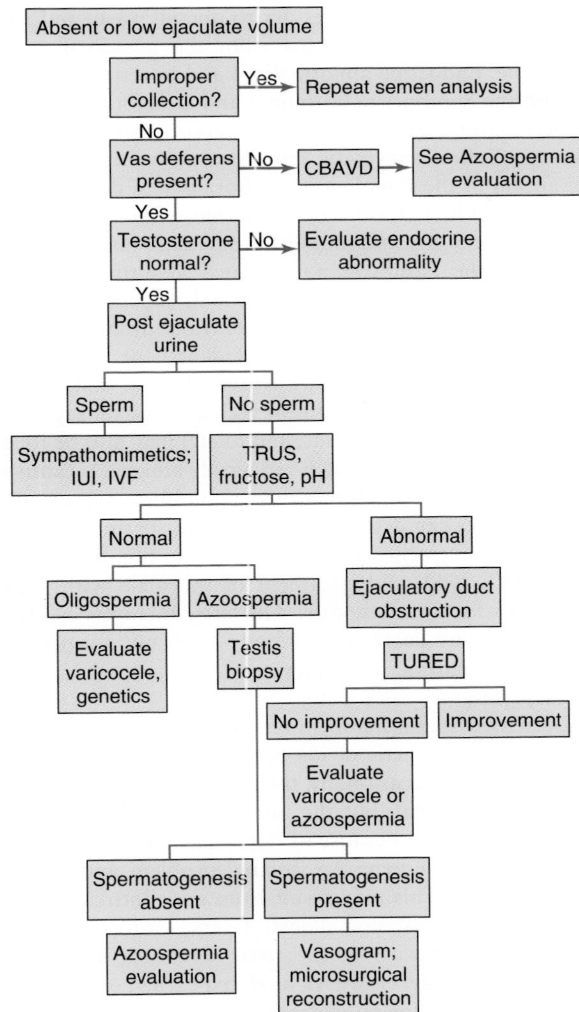

FIGURE 22.3 Algorithm for patients with absent or low-volume (less than 1.5 mL) ejaculate. *CBAVD*, Congenital bilateral absence of the vas deferens; *IUI*, intrauterine insemination; *IVF*, in vitro fertilization; *TRUS*, transrectal ultrasound; *TURED*, transurethral resection of the ejaculatory ducts.

In others, it may be necessary to obtain, wash, and inseminate (IUI) sperm collected from the postejaculate urine sample. Endocrine abnormalities and infections are treated with the appropriate hormones and antibiotics.

2. Hyperviscosity: Problems with hyperviscous semen are rare and may reflect enzymatic imbalance in semen. Mechanical disruption of the sample in the laboratory to decrease viscosity, followed by IUI, is useful in this situation.
3. Decreased motility and forward progression (asthenospermia)
   a. This is the most common isolated abnormality found in semen and can be due to endocrine dysfunction, infection of accessory glands, varicocele, epididymal dysfunction, genetics, reactive oxygen species (oxidants), or environmental exposures. Specific therapy is available for some of these problems. Empirical treatment with antioxidant supplements (vitamins A, C, and E, zinc, and folate) may also be tried.
   b. Sperm motility may also be adversely affected by **antisperm antibodies** that agglutinate or immobilize sperm. Special sperm tests can determine levels of antisperm antibodies in semen. Treatments are available for antibodies, including IUI, IVF, ICSI, and treatment of the male with systemic steroids for 6 to 9 months. The latter therapy has been associated with decreased antibody levels but not necessarily increased natural pregnancy rates.
4. Oligospermia
   a. Decreased sperm numbers may be secondary to endocrine dysfunction, genetic or idiopathic conditions, or unilateral obstruction. Occasionally, the absolute number of sperm is relatively normal, but the number of sperm per milliliter may appear low because of large ejaculate volume.
5. Abnormal morphology: An isolated problem with morphology is unusual. This may result from gonadotoxic exposures (e.g., tobacco), systemic illness, fevers, varicocele, or idiopathic causes. Reversing the toxic exposure may improve sperm morphology. However, as stated earlier, one should not pursue treatment for an isolated morphology defect as it has no impact with natural pregnancy rates or those during IUI. If an isolated morphology defect exists and the couple is pursuing IVF (for other reasons), the embryologists will frequently employ ICSI as opposed to conventional IVF.

Treatment Options

EMPIRICAL TREATMENT OF IDIOPATHIC MALE-FACTOR INFERTILITY

1. Second only to those with varicoceles, **idiopathic male infertility** is the next largest group of infertility patients. Essentially, idiopathic infertility refers to men who have an abnormal semen parameter or parameters on the semen analyses with a normal history, physical examination, and screening hormone analysis. The etiology of the abnormal semen quality is unclear and probably reflects our incomplete knowledge of the genetics of spermatogenesis and sperm maturation. Many of these cases will likely be seen to have genetic etiologies in the future.
2. Nonpharmacologic treatments. Various nonpharmacologic treatments have been suggested, but their efficacy has not been rigorously demonstrated. These include:
   a. Vitamins and diet: Changes in dietary habits and vitamin supplements have been associated with improved semen quality and fertility. Antioxidant therapy has been shown to increase motility of in vitro isolated sperm, but a similar treatment of men with unexplained severe asthenospermia did not reliably improve motility in a large, randomized study. This therapy may be beneficial for smokers to reduce the oxidative effects on sperm.
   b. Prostatic massage.
   c. Antibiotics for occult infection.
   d. Varicocelectomy for the occult or **subclinical varicocele:** Three randomized, controlled clinical trials demonstrated no benefit to varicocelectomy for nonpalpable, ultrasound-detected lesions.

MEDICAL TREATMENT FOR MALE INFERTILITY

Endocrinopathies are the primary etiology in $< 3\%$ of cases of male infertility; can be divided into cases of hormonal deficiency or hormonal excess.

1. Hypogonadotropic hypogonadism: (1) Gonadotropic agents to replace LH/FSH, agents include hCG, hMG, and rFSH and (2) SERMs (i.e., clomiphene citrate) that bind to hypothalamic and pituitary estrogen receptor sites. Aromatase inhibitors (i.e., anastrozole) can also be used to improve endogenous

testosterone production. A combination of these agents can also be used. These patients should never be treated with conventional testosterone replacement.

2. **Hypergonadotropic hypogonadism:** Results from testicular failure; aromatase inhibitors, gonadotropins, and antiestrogen agents have all been investigated and should still be attempted in this patient population to improve endogenous testosterone production. Some of these patients will still have a benefit.
3. **SERMs, AIs, and gonadotropic agents should not be used as empiric treatment for men with idiopathic male infertility.**
4. **Androgen excess:** Usually from taking exogenous testosterone or anabolic steroids; most patients will have spontaneous recovery of spermatogenesis with cessation of androgens and starting on medications to induce endogenous testosterone production, with the intention to avoid the development of hypogonadal symptoms. Some with persistent azoospermia will require hCG and/or hMG.
5. **Estrogen excess: T:E ratio should be > 10:1;** aromatase inhibitors used to diminish E2 production and increase serum testosterone levels.
6. **Prolactin excess:** High levels of prolactin inhibit secretion of GnRH; medical therapy consists of dopamine agonists (bromocriptine, cabergoline, pergolide, quinagolide), radiation therapy, or transphenoidal surgical resection of prolactinoma.
7. **Retrograde ejaculation:** Should be suspected in patients with low semen volume or absence of antegrade ejaculate; **postejaculate urinalysis** should be examined. Once diagnosis is made, treatment with alpha-adrenergic agents (ephedrine, pseudoephedrine, phenylpropanolamine) or TCA (imipramine) may result in bladder neck closure and antegrade ejaculation.

SURGICAL MANAGEMENT OF MALE INFERTILITY

Surgical management in male infertility can be categorized into (1) diagnostic procedures, (2) procedures that optimize spermatogenesis, (3) procedures that improve sperm delivery, and (4) sperm retrieval (Fig. 22.4).

1. Testis biopsy is indicated in azoospermic men with normal size testis and consistency; palpable vas, normal FSH can be diagnostic and determine obstructive from NOA. However, this

	Advantages	Disadvantages
MESA (microsurgical epididymal sperm aspiration)	Microsurgical procedure allows lower complication rate Epididymal sperm has better motility than testicular sperm Large number of sperm can be harvested for cryopreservation of multiple vials in a single procedure	Requires anesthesia and microsurgical skills Not indicated for nonobstructive azoospermia
PESA (percutaneous epididymal sperm aspiration)	No microsurgical skill required Local anesthesia Epididymal sperm has better motility than testicular sperm	Complications include hematoma, pain, and vascular injury to testes and obstruction of the epididymis Variable success in obtaining sperm Small quantity of sperm obtained than the MESA Not indicated in nonobstructive azoospermia
TESA (testicular sperm aspiration)	No microsurgical skill required Local anesthesia Can be used for obstructive azoospermia	Immature or immotile testicular sperm Small quantity of sperm obtained Poor results in nonobstructive azoospermia Complications include hematoma, pain, and vascular injury to testes and epididymis
TESE (testicular sperm extraction)	Low complication rate if performed microsurgically Preferred technique for nonobstructive azoospermia	Requires anesthesia DNA microsurgical skills

FIGURE 22.4 Surgical techniques for sperm retrieval.

should be performed with the plan to convert to a microTESE if the patient has NOA. Sperm may also be cryopreserved at the time of biopsy for future IVF/ICSI. Alternatively, this can also be performed at the time of egg retrieval with fresh sperm being used for a synchronized IVF cycle.

2. For men with NOA undergoing sperm retrieval, microdissection testicular sperm extraction (microTESE) should be performed.
3. For men with azoospermia due to obstruction, sperm may be extracted from the epididymis via percutaneous epididymal sperm aspiration (PESA) or testicle via testicular sperm aspiration (TESA) or testicular sperm extraction (TESE).
4. For men with aspermia, surgical sperm extraction (PESA/TESA/TESE) or induced ejaculation via sympathomimetics, vibratory stimulation, or electroejaculation may be performed depending on the patient's condition and clinical experience.
5. **Vasovasostomy: 2%–6% of vasectomized men will seek reversal;** iatrogenic injury usually from hernia repair occur in 6% of azoospermic men. Before reconstruction, history of adequate spermatogenesis should be documented (prior children). Reconstruction is preferable to sperm retrieval if time since vasectomy is < 12 years and no female fertility risk factors are present. Couples interested in conception status post (s/p) vasectomy should be counseled about both surgical reconstruction and/or simultaneous surgical sperm retrieval with cryopreservation.
6. **TURED: EDO is suspected in azoospermic or severely oligo/athenospermic men with at least one palpable vas, low semen volume, acid semen pH, negative/equivocal or low semen fructose levels.** Estimated 1%–5% of infertile men have EDO. Transrectal sonography can show a midline cystic lesion or dilated ejaculatory ducts and seminal vesicles.
7. **Electroejaculation:** Indicated for men with neurologic impairment in sympathetic outflow and who do not respond to vibratory stimulation. If patient has a high above T6 thoracic lesion or a history of autonomic dysreflexia, pretreatment with sublingual nifedipine 15 minutes before procedure is required.

ASSISTED REPRODUCTIVE TECHNOLOGY

No apparent difference exists in pregnancy rates between fresh versus cryopreserved sperm in patients with obstructive azoospermia. However, in patients with NOA, there is the concern that if rare sperm are found, they may not survive the freeze/thaw process and the sperm usability rate is higher in patients undergoing microTESE with a coordinated, synchronized egg retrieval. This also contributes to a higher pregnancy and live birth rate in these men.

1. ART can improve conception rates by bypassing many or all the barriers associated with normal fertilization. The simplest techniques involve sperm processing and insemination of the female; more sophisticated ones involve manipulation of the sperm and ova extracorporeally. Fertilization with these procedures can occur in vitro or in vivo.
2. Semen processing is used as an isolated procedure or in conjunction with oocyte processing. **Sperm washing, swim-ups, sedimentation, and gradient centrifugations** are common ways to remove seminal plasma and leukocytes and to select for and concentrate highly motile sperm. With these procedures, fewer sperm than normal are needed because they are placed higher within the female reproductive tract than an ejaculate during intercourse.
3. **IUI** is a common treatment for couples presenting with male-factor infertility. **In this technique, a small catheter is used to inject processed sperm through the cervix and into the uterine cavity.** By bypassing the cervical mucus, more motile sperm can progress to the fallopian tubes where normal fertilization occurs. Indications for IUI include male infertility caused by mechanical or anatomical problems (e.g., ED, hypospadias), low semen quality, and cervical mucus problems. Effectiveness decreases if the total motile count in the ejaculated sample is < 5 million motile sperm. For some patients, IUI outcomes can be improved with ovulation induction medications.
4. **IVF** was developed to manage fallopian tube obstruction and the first live birth was in 1978. Female partners undergo ovarian hyperstimulation to induce the maturation of multiple oocytes that are then harvested just prior to ovulation. Processed semen and recovered oocytes are mixed in vitro. If fertilization occurs, embryos are placed back into the uterus transcervically. **ICSI has made it possible to use cryopreserved testicular sperm, which allows for sperm and ova to be retrieved on different days.**
5. In gamete intrafallopian transfer (**GIFT**), sperm and oocytes are placed into the fallopian tubes prior to fertilization. This is done in lieu of uterine placement with the hope that higher pregnancy rates will be achieved with more physiologic placement of gametes. Because GIFT does not improve the fertilizing capacity of sperm, it has no benefit over IVF in male-factor

infertility. Given the recent success of IVF and ICSI, tubal transfers constitute fewer than 2% of ART cases.

6. Micromanipulation: Sperm and oocyte micromanipulation by **ICSI has become the mainstay of addressing the poor fertilizing capacity of sperm often seen in male infertility.** By injecting a single sperm directly into an oocyte, multiple barriers of fertilization are bypassed and success rates (when compared to standard IVF) are greatly improved. Pregnancy rates of 40% to 50% have been obtained using this technique even in the most severe cases of male infertility. In addition, not only ejaculated sperm but sperm retrieved from the male reproductive tract are capable of pregnancy with ICSI. **Vasal, epididymal, and even testicular sperm, from both obstructed and unobstructed men, are now routinely used with IVF and ICSI.**
7. **IVF with ICSI** should not be performed without **karyotype analysis on both partners.** Despite its great success, concerns remain with ICSI.
   a. **Multiple gestations may occur in up to 30% of pregnancies compared to 1% to 2% of naturally conceived pregnancies.** Multiple gestations are associated with lower birth weights, higher overall complication rates, and increased learning disabilities relative to singletons. In addition, the **delivery costs** associated with managing multiple, often premature, gestations are at least **10 to 20 times higher** than that associated with the singleton deliveries. Among respectable ART programs, the trend is to transfer as few embryos back as possible to reduce multiple gestations.
   b. **ICSI bypasses many mechanisms of natural selection such that many men who would not be able to conceive under normal circumstances are now able to father children.** Although overall rates of **major birth defects** (3.3%) associated with IVF and ICSI may be similar to intercourse, there is concern about elevated risks of specific malformations, including **hypospadias,** with this technology. In addition, concerns exist regarding possible **developmental issues.** There is a significant increase in sex chromosomal abnormalities among ICSI offspring (**0.8% versus 0.2% naturally**) that is likely attributable to the chromosomal status

of the fathers rather than to the technique itself. As previously mentioned, from 5% to 8% of men with severe oligospermia have deletions in the AZF region of the Y chromosome. It has been shown conclusively that these genetic deletions are passed to the male offspring produced by these fathers through IVF/ICSI.

c. More recently, concerns have arisen regarding whether **rare imprinting diseases such as Beckwith-Wiedemann syndrome and Angelman syndrome** are increased in children conceived with ICSI. For these reasons, genetic counseling is recommended for all couples considering IVF-ICSI.

8. Preimplantation genetic diagnosis (**PGT-A/M**) is now possible by sampling a single cell from the developing embryo in vitro and performing FISH, single cell polymerase chain reaction (PCR), or comparative genomic hybridization (CGH) to **examine for aneuploidy, chromosomal translocations, or specific diseases caused by point mutations**. Current indications for PGD include lethal disease prevention and screening in advanced maternal age couples, patients with certain autosomal-dominant disorders, or with couples sharing positive carrier screens.

CONCLUSION

Our knowledge of testis development, testis stem cells, and sperm production are rapidly revolving. As the chromosomal and molecular mechanisms that underlie sperm production are further elucidated, fewer male patients with infertility will have undefined etiologies. Concurrently, fast-paced ARTs now allow us to bypass many natural selection barriers that had been present throughout evolution. As a consequence, the study of human reproduction is more important than ever to allow us to understand how our evolution is being altered by technology. Despite these advances in technology, classical treatments for male infertility still remain cost effective. Indeed, a properly conducted male-factor infertility evaluation has immense value on several levels: (1) it can identify treatable diseases that underlie the infertility; (2) it can identify those individuals who might be at risk for future diseases such as prostate and testis cancer; and (3) it can cure, and not simply bypass, the infertility.

CLINICAL PEARLS

1. Semen quality and male fertility are reasonable mirrors of overall health of an individual. Likewise, when semen quality is impaired, efforts should be made during the infertility evaluation to find out why.
2. Classic medical treatments for male infertility, such as repair of blockages and varicoceles, continue to be cost effective when compared to assisted reproduction.
3. Dramatically low or zero sperm counts that are genetic in origin do not generally respond to classical medical and surgical therapies for male infertility. Such cases are excellent candidates for assisted reproduction.

Additional content, including Self-Assessment Questions and Suggested Readings, may be accessed at www.ExpertConsult.com.

Disorders of the Adrenal Gland

Marshall Strother, MD, and Alexander Kutikov, MD

Urologists care for patients with adrenal disorders principally from the surgical perspective. This chapter provides an overview of adrenal pathophysiology and addresses tactics used in urologic clinical practice to assess and manage surgical adrenal disease.

Adrenal Anatomy

OVERVIEW

1. The adrenal glands each weigh approximately 4 to 5 g and measure 5 × 3 × 1 cm.
2. They are positioned in the retroperitoneum within Gerota's fascia anterior and superomedial to each kidney.
3. The right adrenal, described as triangular, lies posterior and lateral to the inferior vena cava (IVC) and contacts the liver anteriorly.
4. The smaller left gland tends to be semilunar and is intimately related to the upper pole of the left kidney. Anterior to the left adrenal lies the tail of the pancreas and the splenic artery.
5. The diaphragm borders both adrenals posteriorly.

VASCULATURE

Blood flow through the adrenals is substantial, given the endocrine function of the glands. Understanding adrenal vasculature is critical for safe retroperitoneal surgery. The venous drainage of the right gland differs from that of the left, and the surgeon must be aware of this fact.

Arterial Supply

1. No one dominant artery supplies either adrenal.

2. Small vessels enter the glands from three main sources:
   a. Inferior phrenic artery: superior adrenal arteries, majority of blood supply.
   b. Aorta at the level of the superior mesenteric artery (SMA): middle adrenal arteries.
   c. Renal artery: inferior adrenal arteries.
3. Arteries rapidly branch, and as many as 60 separate vessels may penetrate the adrenal capsule in a stellate fashion.

Venous Drainage

1. Right adrenal vein
   a. Short vessel which drains directly into the posterior aspect of the IVC.
   b. If torn during dissection, can result in life-threatening bleeding and has been called "the vein of death."
   c. In some patients, joins with a right hepatic vein prior to entering the vena cava.
   d. Accessory right adrenal vein(s) occasionally may be present.
2. Left adrenal vein
   a. The left adrenal vein is substantially longer than the right.
   b. Drains directly into the left renal vein.
   c. Usually joins with the inferior phrenic vein at some point in its course.
   d. As on the right, accessory veins may be present.

Innervation

1. Sympathetic
   a. Cortex: postganglionic fibers from splanchnic ganglia
   b. Medulla: preganglionic sympathetic fibers from the sympathetic trunk
2. Parasympathetic: poorly defined. May arise from the vagus nerve.

HISTOLOGIC STRUCTURE

The adrenal gland is surrounded by a fibrous capsule and is composed of a yellowish cortex and a red to gray medulla.

1. Cortex—the adult cortex is composed of three distinct concentric regions and comprises 80% of total adrenal weight (see "Adrenal Physiology").

2. Medulla—lies in the center of the gland beneath the zona reticularis. Rich in chromaffin cells—named so because they precipitate chromium salts—the medulla produces catecholamines such as epinephrine, norepinephrine, and dopamine.

EMBRYOLOGY

1. The cortex stems from the intermediate mesoderm of the urogenital ridge.
2. The medulla originates from the neural crest cells of the neuroectoderm.
3. At birth, the adrenal gland is twice the weight of the adult adrenal gland. The gland rapidly begins to involute following delivery, losing tissue from a region known as the "fetal cortex," which is completely resorbed by 12 months age.
4. Adrenal development is mostly independent of renal development. In the absence of a normally positioned ipsilateral kidney, the adrenal gland takes on a more discoid shape but functions normally and is found in the normal position in the retroperitoneum.
5. Ectopic adrenal tissue, known as "adrenal rests," can be found anywhere along the path of gonadal descent. This tissue is found in 50% of neonates, but only 1% of adults. In cases of congenital adrenal hyperplasia, this tissue hypertrophies and can be mistaken for malignancy.

Adrenal Physiology

ADRENAL CORTEX PHYSIOLOGY

Each of the three zones of the cortex contains different enzymes along the three major synthetic pathways, resulting in three different classes of steroid hormones produced in each zone (Fig. 23.1).

1. **Zona glomerulosa** produces aldosterone, the major mineralocorticoid in humans. It can produce up to 150 mg daily. Secretion of aldosterone is directly influenced by the body's angiotensin II and potassium levels. Atrial natriuretic peptide (ANP) is the main inhibitor of aldosterone secretion. It is important to note that while adrenocorticotrophic hormone (ACTH) can weakly stimulate aldosterone secretion, the hypothalamic-pituitary-adrenal axis plays little role in aldosterone secretion overall. Thus, the zona

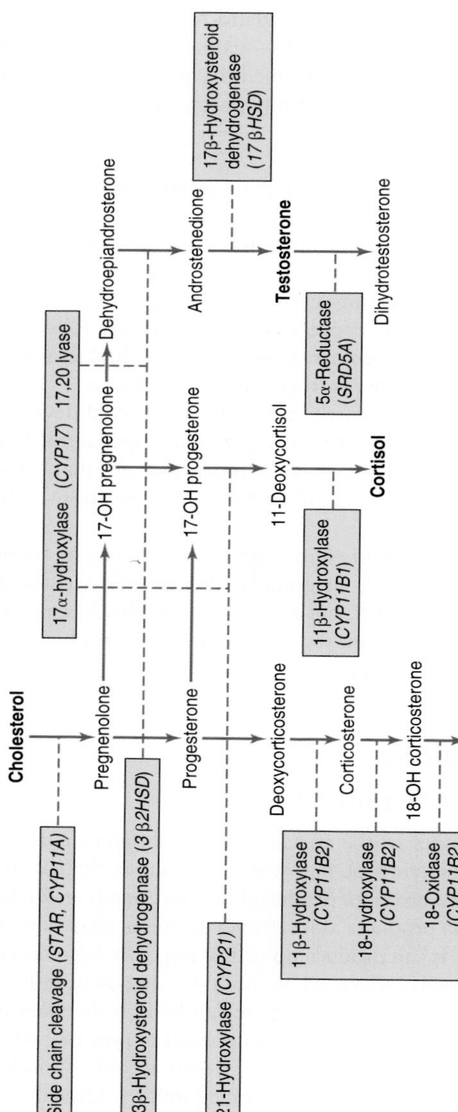

FIGURE 23.1 **Cholesterol-steroid biosynthesis pathway. Enzymes are listed in boxes and genes in parentheses.** (From Hyun G, Kolon TF. A practical approach to intersex in the newborn period. *Urol Clin North Am*. 2004;31:435-443.)

glomerulosa is the only region of the adrenal cortex that does not atrophy following loss of pituitary function.

2. **Zona fasciculata** is the site of glucocorticoid production and excretes up to 30 mg of cortisol (aka hydrocortisone when given exogenously) each day. Unless pathology is present, cortisol secretion is under tight control by pituitary ACTH through the hypothalamic-pituitary-adrenal axis.
3. **Zona reticularis,** the innermost zone of the adrenal cortex, is the source of adrenal androgens. The major sex steroid hormone of the adrenal is dehydroepiandrosterone (DHEA) followed by DHEA-S and androstenedione (> 20 mg/day). These act as weak androgens and appear to be under the control of ACTH. In normal physiologic states, these hormones have little influence; however, they become important when secreted in excess (e.g., congenital adrenal hyperplasia) and in states of androgen deprivation.

ADRENAL MEDULLA PHYSIOLOGY

Chromaffin cells located in the adrenal medulla secrete norepinephrine, epinephrine, and dopamine in response to stimulation by preganglionic sympathetic nerve fibers.

1. Liver rapidly metabolizes catecholamines that are released by the medulla. This breakdown is catalyzed by:
   a. Catechol-O-methyltransferase (COMT).
   b. Monoamine oxidase (MAO).
2. Catecholamine metabolites and small amounts of norepinephrine are excreted in the urine. The major metabolites include:
   a. Metanephrine.
   b. Normetanephrine.
   c. Vanillylmandelic acid (VMA).

Adrenal Disorders

INCREASED ADRENAL FUNCTION

Conn syndrome, cortisol excess, and pheochromocytoma.

1. **Primary hyperaldosteronism** (aka Conn syndrome)
   a. Differentiated from secondary hyperaldosteronism by characteristically low renin levels. In cases of secondary

hyperaldosteronism (usually due to renal artery stenosis or congestive heart failure [CHF]), renin levels are high.

b. Signs and symptoms stem from physiologic action of aldosterone to promote renal sodium reabsorption by opening sodium channels in cells of the renal cortical collecting system lumen.
   1) Hypertension
      i. Results from intravascular volume expansion.
      ii. Mean BP of 180/110 mm Hg in patients with aldosterone-secreting adenomas and 160/100 mm Hg in those with idiopathic bilateral adrenal hyperplasia.
      iii. Normotensive patients are extremely rare.
   2) Hypokalemia
      i. Not present in all patients—63%–91% of patients are normokalemic at presentation.
      ii. Balanced by the renal potassium-sparing effects of hypokalemia itself. Can be exacerbated by sodium loading.
      iii. Can result in polyuria, polydipsia, and muscle weakness.
   3) Metabolic alkalosis is caused by potassium-induced H^+ wasting.
   4) Edema is generally not present, despite the overall hypervolemic state. This is due to what has been called the "aldosterone-escape phenomenon." Despite high mineralocorticoid levels, urinary fluid loss quickly equilibrates with intake, resulting in only mild volume expansion.
   5) Other metabolic abnormalities include mild hypernatremia (~145 mEq/L) and hypomagnesemia.
   6) Increased cardiac risks—patients with hyperaldosteronism have higher rates of cardiovascular events independent of hypertension and potassium levels.

c. Causes of Conn syndrome
   1) Adrenal adenoma: cause of up to 70% of cases of primary hyperaldosteronism (see "Adrenal Neoplasia").
   2) Adrenal carcinoma: less than 1% of primary hyperaldosteronism. 2.5%–5% of adrenocortical carcinoma (ACC) (see "Adrenal Neoplasia").
   3) Bilateral adrenal hyperplasia: less severe phenotype than adenomas
      i. Idiopathic
         A. Responsible for 30%–40% of Conn syndrome.

B. Poor response to surgery. Treated with aldosterone receptor blockade.

ii. Familial hyperaldosteronism (types I–III)

A. All forms show autosomal dominant inheritance and result in bilateral adrenal hyperplasia.

B. Type I (aka glucocorticoid-suppressible hyperaldosteronism) results from fusion of 11β-hydroxylase promoter to aldosterone synthase gene, resulting in ACTH stimulating aldosterone secretion.

C. Type II is indistinguishable from idiopathic hyperplasia except by its inheritance pattern.

D. Type III has a severe phenotype. Consider testing in Conn syndrome presenting in patients less than 20 years old.

d. Evaluation of patients with hyperaldosteronism as it relates to urologic practice is addressed later in this chapter (see "Evaluation of Adrenal Pathology in Urologic Practice")

2. **Cortisol excess**

a. Terminology

1) Cushing syndrome: excessive systemic glucocorticoid exposure causing associated signs and symptoms. Note: there are no widely accepted strict diagnostic criteria for this syndrome in cases where laboratory testing and clinical exam are ambiguous.

2) Subclinical Cushing syndrome: deprecated term denoting increased serum cortisol levels without the signs/symptoms of Cushing syndrome.

3) "Autonomous cortisol secretion" (ACS): term recommended by the 2016 European Society of Endocrinology (ESE) guidelines panel to replace "subclinical Cushing syndrome." It is defined as a serum cortisol during a low-dose dexamethasone suppression test (LDDST) of > 5.0 mcg/dL without signs/symptoms of Cushing syndrome. LDDST cortisol of 1.8–5.0 mcg/dL is termed "possible autonomous cortisol secretion" (PACS) (see "Testing for Cortisol Excess"). Use of these terms is not yet universally accepted.

4) Hypercortisolism and cortisol excess: general terms denoting higher-than-normal levels of cortisol. No strictly defined criteria.

5) Cushing disease: Cushing syndrome caused by an ACTH-secreting pituitary tumor.

b. Signs and symptoms
   1) More specific signs/symptoms: moon facies, buffalo hump, proximal muscle weakness, easy bruisability, and abdominal striae.
   2) Less specific signs/symptoms: central obesity, depression, diabetes, hypertension, osteoporosis.
   3) Symptoms of particular interest to urologists
      i. Urolithiasis—50% of patients with Cushing syndrome will form stones
      ii. Hypogonadotropic hypogonadism is also common

c. Causes of cortisol excess syndrome: only a minority arise from pathology of the adrenal gland itself.
   1) Primary (ACTH-independent) adrenal hypercortisolism is a rare cause of Cushing syndrome.
      i. **Adrenal adenoma** and **adrenal carcinoma** cause approximately the same number of cases of Cushing syndrome per year (10% and 8% of all cases of Cushing syndrome per year respectively) (see "Adrenal Neoplasia").
      ii. Bilateral **micronodular hyperplasia** is a rare cause of primary adrenal hypercortisolism. The pigmented variant is called **primary pigmented nodular adrenocortical disease.** Associated with Carney complex.
      iii. Bilateral ACTH-independent **macronodular hyperplasia**—adrenals replaced by nodules (up to 4 cm). Adrenals each weigh over 60 g and up to 500 g each. Responsible for < 1% of cases of hypercortisolism. Associated with McCune-Albright syndrome.
      iv. Management of micronodular and micronodular hyperplasia is bilateral adrenalectomy, although partial adrenalectomy and unilateral adrenalectomy have been described. Medical hormonal manipulation may be used as a bridge to surgery or when surgery is impossible.
   2) Nonadrenal causes of cortisol excess—exogenous glucocorticoids and ACTH-dependent processes
      i. Iatrogenic steroid administration is a very common cause of Cushing syndrome.

ii. **ACTH-producing pituitary tumors** are responsible for up to 70% of cases of endogenous cortisol excess and 80% of ACTH-dependent cases. Cushing *syndrome* resulting from primary pituitary pathology is called "Cushing *disease*." Adrenal glands are hyperplastic (6–12 g) but less so than in cases of ectopic ACTH secretion.

iii. **Ectopic ACTH** is responsible for up to 15% of cases of endogenous Cushing syndrome. Half are caused by paraneoplastic action of small-cell lung cancer. Other malignancies such as carcinoid and pancreatic and thyroid tumors can also be culprits. Adrenal glands become extremely hyperplastic (12–30 g).

iv. **Ectopic corticotropin-releasing hormone (CRH)** is extremely rare.

d. Comprehensive patient evaluation for hypercortisolism is complex and is beyond the scope of this text. Diagnostic strategies as they relate to urologic practice, however, are discussed later in this chapter (see "Evaluation of Adrenal Pathology in Urologic Practice").

3. **Adrenal sex steroid excess**—can be caused by metabolic defects (see "Abnormal Adrenal Function") or rarely by adrenal neoplasms (see "Adrenal Neoplasia").
4. **Pheochromocytoma** is a tumor of the adrenal medulla that generates, stores, and secretes catecholamines.
   a. Signs and symptoms are a result of epinephrine, norepinephrine, and dopamine release into the bloodstream by neoplastic chromaffin cells.
      1) Classic symptom triad of headache, palpitations, and diaphoresis.
      2) Paroxysmal hypertension present in only 30%–50%, whereas other patients behave identical to those with essential hypertension. 20% of patients are entirely asymptomatic.
      3) Orthostatic hypotension (result of hypovolemia), papilledema, weight loss, leukocytosis, polycythemia, hyperglycemia, and cardiovascular complications have all been associated with pheochromocytoma.
      4) Patients with pheochromocytoma as part of a genetic syndrome are often asymptomatic and account for 25% of all patients with pheochromocytomas.

b. Clinical characteristics—classically described as "the rule of 10s," although this "rule" has been repeatedly challenged.
   1) 10% extra-adrenal (actually ~25%).
      i. Known as paragangliomas (though some authors reserve this term for extra-adrenal pheochromocytoma of the head and neck only).
      ii. Most common extra-adrenal site is the organ of Zuckerkandl (chromaffin bodies at aortic bifurcation).
      iii. Can also occur in neck, abdomen, and pelvis including the bladder.
      iv. More common with familial disease.
      v. Up to tenfold higher risk for recurrence if tumor is extra-adrenal.
   2) 10% familial (actually ~30%)—associated with RET (multiple endocrine neoplasia type II), VHL (von Hippel-Lindau), NF1 (neurofibromatosis type I), and SDH mutations. Screening for genetic disorders in patients presenting with pheochromocytoma is recommended for patients younger than 50 years old and patients with a suggestive clinical or family history.
   3) 10% malignant (actually 5% for adrenal pheochromocytoma and as high as 30% for extra-adrenal pheochromocytoma)—pathologic documentation of malignancy is problematic as even benign lesions exhibit capsular penetration and vascular invasion. Histologic features are also nonspecific. Malignancy, therefore, is defined as presence of metastasis or invasion of surrounding tissues.
      i. More common in women.
      ii. More common in extraadrenal disease.
      iii. Five-year survival 36%–60%.
      iv. See "Management of Metastatic Disease."
   4) 10% bilateral—more common with familial disease. Interesting to note that solitary right-sided tumors are ~40% more common than left-sided tumors for unclear reasons and have a threefold higher risk of recurrence.
   5) 10% pediatric—common in familial cases.

c. Diagnosis—see "Evaluation of Adrenal Pathology in Urologic Practice."

d. Treatment—sporadic pheochromocytoma should be resected. Treatment strategies for familial cases are more controversial as bilateral disease and recurrence rates are high, yet mortality and morbidity of bilateral adrenalectomy are also significant. Partial adrenalectomy has gained popularity in recent years. A multidisciplinary management approach is advised in these patients.
   1) Preoperative catecholamine blockade is paramount for symptomatic patients, as life-threatening catecholamine surges may occur perioperatively. Prior to routine use of prophylactic blockade, surgical mortality was as high as 50%. Patients who are asymptomatic and normotensive preoperatively do not necessarily require blockade.
      i. Alpha-blockade (or calcium channel blockade) should be initiated 10–14 days preoperatively.
         A. Phenoxybenzamine 10 mg PO twice daily is started and titrated by daily increases of 10–20 mg to a systolic blood pressure (SBP) of 120/80 mm Hg in a seated position. Mild postural hypotension (SBP > 90 mm Hg in standing position) is tolerated and is a sign of appropriate dosing.
         B. In children, 0.2 mg/kg (max 10 mg) four times daily dosing should be used with incremental increases by 0.2 mg/kg.
         C. Some investigators have shown that calcium channel blockade is just as effective and may be safer than alpha-blockade for preoperative management of pheochromocytoma.
         D. Doxazosin alpha-blockade and foregoing blockade altogether have been described for asymptomatic patients.
      ii. Beta-blockade can be lethal if initiated prior to appropriate alpha-blockade. It is only used to treat tachycardia, which may result from alpha-blockade and alpha-blockade-induced arrhythmias. Beta-blockade must be administered with great care as CHF, bradycardia, myocardial depression, asystole, and death have all been documented in patients with pheochromocytoma.

iii. α-Methyl-para-tyrosine (metyrosine) is sometimes added to alpha-blockade if alpha-blockade inadequately controls blood pressure or based on institutional preference. Administration results in depletion of stored catecholamine, as the agent inhibits tyrosine hydroxylase, the rate-limiting enzyme in biosynthesis of catecholamines. Causes significant central nervous system side effects.

iv. Preoperative optimization of volume status—after alpha-blockade is initiated, the patient should be encouraged to increase salt intake to increase intravascular volume.

A. Admission at least 24 hours prior to surgery is advisable, so that intravenous (IV) hydration can be administered and appropriate volume status secured.

B. The last dose of phenoxybenzamine and/or metyrosine is usually given on the night before surgery. Phenoxybenzamine and metyrosine should not be given on the day of surgery.

v. Intraoperative management—intraoperative hypertension is generally managed with a nitroprusside drip.

vi. Postoperative management—following surgery in patients who required significant blockade, a short intensive care unit (ICU) stay is recommended for BP and blood sugar monitoring as rebound hyperinsulinemia may occur. Aggressive IV fluids and glucose administration are the postoperative routine.

2) Management of metastatic disease

i. Catecholamine blockade for symptomatic relief.

ii. High-dose radioactive ^{131}Iodine metaiodobenzylguanidine (^{131}I-MIBG) if lesions visible on MIBG scan.

iii. Chemotherapy with cyclophosphamide, vincristine, and dacarbazine (CVD) if invisible or after ^{131}I-MIBG failure.

iv. Many consider metastatectomy standard of care despite limited evidence.

3) Prognosis
   i. Familial, right-sided, and extra-adrenal tumors are more likely to recur.
   ii. Follow-up should be indefinite, because tumors, whether malignant or benign, can recur many years following resection.

DECREASED ADRENAL FUNCTION

Addison disease (primary adrenal insufficiency), a nonsurgical entity. Etiologies include:

1. Autoimmune/idiopathic.
2. Infectious—tuberculosis, cytomegalovirus (CMV) adrenalitis in human immunodeficiency virus (HIV) patients, fungal infections, syphilis.
3. Infarction/hemorrhage—meningococcemia (Waterhouse-Friderichsen syndrome), pseudomonal and other infections, coagulopathy, trauma.
4. Metastasis—although metastases to the adrenals are common, adrenal insufficiency resulting from metastases is extremely rare.
5. Exogenous glucocorticoid administration—results in suppression of native adrenal function, which may diminish the body's ability to respond to stress. The necessity of perioperative stress dose steroids is controversial.
6. Surgical resection of a cortisol-secreting tumor due to suppression of the contralateral gland's function by the hypercortisolemic state or bilateral adrenalectomy. Patients undergoing synchronous or metachronous bilateral renal procedures are at risk for unintended damage to both glands.

ABNORMAL ADRENAL FUNCTION

Congenital adrenal hyperplasia is addressed in Chapter 27, Disorders of Sexual Development of this text.

ADRENAL NEOPLASIA

1. **Benign adenoma**—benign tumor of the adrenal cortex.
   a. Prevalence of up to 6% in large autopsy series.
   b. 90% of all adrenal incidentalomas. 93% are metabolically inactive.

c. Rich in intracellular lipid, resulting in characteristic imaging features.
d. Management: no treatment, surveillance, or resection depending on characteristics. See "Evaluation of Adrenal Pathology in Urologic Practice."
e. **Perioperative considerations**
   1) Adenomas causing primary hyperaldosteronism
      i. Treatment with preoperative spironolactone has been suggested. Long-term spironolactone or its counterpart eplerenone, which has lesser binding affinity to androgen and progesterone receptors, is used to treat poor surgical candidates.
      ii. Aldosterone-to-renin ratio (ARR) should be measured postoperatively. Patients should be counseled on a high sodium diet and monitored for hyperkalemia in the postoperative period.
      iii. 94% of patients with have normal potassium and ARR after surgery for Conn syndrome. Only 37%–52% will require no antihypertensive medications postoperatively, likely reflecting persistence of other factors contributing to hypertension in these patients.
   2) Adenomas causing hypercortisolism
      i. Monitor for postoperative Addisonian crisis and consider postoperative glucocorticoid supplementation, since cortisol hypersecretion by functional adenoma results in atrophy of the contralateral gland.

2. **Adrenal carcinoma**—rare cancer with a poor prognosis.
   a. Clinical features
      1) Annual incidence is 0.5–2 in 1,000,000.
      2) Occurs in patients 40–50 years of age (most common) and children younger than 5 years of age.
      3) Linked to MEN1, Beckwith-Wiedemann, and Li-Fraumeni syndromes as well as Lynch syndrome, Carney complex, neurofibromatosis type 1, familial adenomatous polyposis, and McCune-Albright syndrome.
      4) Left-sided tumors are more common.
      5) 60% of tumors are functional.
         i. ~40% Cushing syndrome.
            A. Cortisol production per unit volume of tumor is low.

B. Hypercortisolism results from larger masses.

ii. ~25%–50% Cushing with virilization—this combination is suggestive of carcinoma, as it is almost never seen with adrenal adenomas.

iii. 20%–30% virilization alone (most common presentation in children).

A. Serum testosterone, DHEA, DHEA-S elevated.

B. 17-ketosteroids are elevated.

iv. Feminization (~6%) and hyperaldosteronism (2.5%) are rare.

6) Up to 20% of tumors can have vena caval extension.

7) 92% of adrenal carcinomas are greater than 6 cm at diagnosis. Median size at presentation is 11 cm.

b. Diagnosis—See "Evaluation of Adrenal Pathology in Urologic Practice."

c. Treatment

1) Surgical resection is the only treatment that impacts survival.

i. Aggressive resection with en bloc resection of organs subject to local invasion is recommended. Lymph node dissection is optional.

ii. Laparoscopy is possible, but some data suggest worse outcomes and increased rates of tumor spillage.

iii. Cytoreductive adrenalectomy with debulking metastatectomy is generally recommended for metastatic disease if at least 90% of tumor burden can be removed.

iv. Resection of local or distant recurrences should be considered, especially with low-grade primary disease and long disease-free intervals.

v. Adjuvant chemotherapy and radiation should be considered.

vi. Hormonally active adrenal carcinomas are subject to the same perioperative considerations as benign adenomas.

2) Chemotherapy

i. Mitotane, a drug which poisons mitochondria of the adrenal cortical cells, in combination with etoposide, doxorubicin, and cisplatin (M-EDP) is currently considered first line, though outcomes remain poor.

3) Hormonal therapy (e.g., with ketoconazole, metyrapone, aminoglutethimide, etomidate, or mifepristone) can be used to palliate hormonal symptoms.

d. Prognosis.
   1) Children have superior prognosis to adults.
   2) Stage is the most significant prognostic indicator.
      i. Stage I
         A. Tumor ≤ 5 cm, no local invasion, negative nodes.
         B. 5-year survival is up to 33%–66%.
      ii. Stage II
         A. Tumor > 5 cm, no local invasion, negative nodes.
         B. 5-year survival is up to 20%–58%.
      iii. Stage III
         A. Local invasion into periadrenal fat or positive nodes without local invasion.
         B. 5-year survival is 18%–24%.
      iv. Stage IV
         A. Metastatic disease or locally invasive tumor with positive nodes.
         B. 5-year survival is < 5%.
         C. Over 40% of patients present with stage IV disease.

3. **Neuroblastoma**—addressed in Chapter 26.
4. **Pheochromocytoma**—See "Increased Adrenal Function."
5. **Oncocytoma**—extremely rare. Fifty cases reported in the literature. Unlike renal oncocytomas, a high percentage of adrenal oncocytomas prove malignant. Diagnosis is made on final pathology after resection.
6. **Ganglioneuroma**—rare benign tumor which can grow very large and encase vessels without impinging on the vessel lumen. Diagnosis is made on final pathology after resection.
7. **Myelolipoma**—rare, benign, nonfunctional cortical tumor consisting of fat and hematopoietic elements.
   a. Diagnosis easily made on imaging. Presence of macroscopic fat (< −30 Hounsfield unit [HU]) is pathognomonic; however, care should be made not to confuse with extraadrenal lesions such as teratoma, angiomyolipoma, or liposarcoma.
   b. The need for metabolic workup is controversial. Myelolipomas are not hormonally active; however, concurrent functional adenomas can be present and can be missed on

imaging in the presence of a myelolipoma, so some advocate for routine metabolic testing, especially in the setting of signs/symptoms.

c. Growth rates vary widely, and tumors can regress. No standard observation protocol exists but ultrasound or cross-sectional imaging every 2–3 years is reasonable.
d. Treatment is rarely indicated. Resection can be considered for symptomatic disease or very large tumors (usually > 10 cm), which confer a small risk of rupture and hemorrhage.

8. **Cysts**—rare adrenal lesions seen in only ~0.2% of autopsies; associated with 6% chance of malignancy.
   a. Endothelial cysts are most common (~40%).
      1) Benign.
      2) Calcifications are common and do not suggest malignancy.
   b. Pseudocysts are second most common adrenal cystic lesion.
      1) Lack epithelial lining.
      2) Arise from encapsulation of foci of previous adrenal hemorrhage.
      3) Can grow very large and cause symptoms. They are otherwise benign.
   c. Cystic lymphangiomas are benign.
   d. Echinococcal cysts can be found in the adrenal but are almost always found concurrently in other organs as well.
   e. Epithelial cysts are the most common cystic lesion in the kidney but very rare in the adrenal gland.
   f. Management should include metabolic workup. There is no consensus regarding the management of metabolically inactive lesions; however, surveillance and resection are both generally reasonable, with larger lesions (>4–5 cm) being favored for resection.
9. Metastasis.
   a. In patients with prior malignancy, over 50% of newly discovered adrenal lesions represent metastases.
   b. Most common primary is the lung followed by kidney.
   c. Fine needle aspiration is helpful in differentiating primary adrenal mass from metastatic disease.
   d. The decision to perform adrenalectomy in the setting of a solitary adrenal metastasis should be made in a multidisciplinary setting and depends on the primary tumor type and other clinical factors.

Evaluation of Adrenal Pathology in Urologic Practice

Urologists routinely face patients who are referred with an adrenal mass incidentally discovered on imaging (incidentaloma).

IMAGING OF ADRENAL MASSES

Imaging characteristics, size, and interval growth of tumor are used to assess risk of malignancy. Imaging characteristics also afford ability to differentiate between various benign pathologic entities.

1. Imaging characteristics
   a. Ultrasound is rarely used to evaluate adrenals as normal glands and small nodules are difficult to visualize, especially on left.
   b. Cross-sectional imaging with computed tomography (CT) or magnetic resonance imaging (MRI) affords anatomical detail and quantification of intracellular lipid content.
      1) Macroscopic fat (< −30 HU) is pathognomonic for myelolipoma.
      2) Microscopic fat is diagnostic of adrenal adenoma:
         i. < 10 HU on noncontrast CT:
            A. 98% specific for adenoma.
            B. 70% of adenomas exhibit this finding. The remainder of adenomas are called are “lipid-poor.”
            C. Metastases and low-density pheochromocytomas are the few adrenal lesions that may also measure < 10 HU, but these are usually easy to suspect based on clinical history and metabolic workup. They never measure < 0 HU. PET may be useful if these are suspected.
            D. Loss of signal on out-of-phase MRI sequences also demonstrates intracellular lipid and is similarly specific for adrenal adenomas, but it is less sensitive.
   c. A lesion measuring > 10 HU on noncontrast CT or lacking signal dropout on MRI requires 15-minute CT triphasic washout study:
      1) If lesions exhibit > 60% absolute percent washout or > 40% relative percent washout, this is largely diagnostic of adenoma.

   2) Lack of washout is consistent with pheochromocytoma, metastasis, and potentially adrenocortical carcinoma.
 d. Pheochromocytoma-specific imaging—FDG-PET (or more recently ^{68}Ga-DOTATATE PET/CT) is indicated in patients with metabolic testing concerning for pheochromocytoma to rule out extraadrenal or metastatic disease. MIBG isotope scanning should be used instead in patients with MEN-2 germline mutations or in the rare circumstance when there is an excess of norepinephrine and normetanephrine but not epinephrine or metanephrine.

2. Size and growth
 a. Adrenal lesions < 4 cm can be observed, since only 4%–5% are carcinoma. Masses > 6 cm (other than myelolipoma) should be resected, even if their other imaging characteristics are suggestive of benign adenoma, since 25% of masses > 6 cm are malignant, although there is growing interest in observation of these lesions. Masses 4–6 cm can be observed in the setting of otherwise reassuring imaging features; however, resection is recommended in the setting of other concerning features and should be particularly considered in young and otherwise healthy patients.
 b. Interval growth—guidelines state that surgical resection should be prompted by a 20% increase in tumor diameter or a 5 mm increase in diameter, whichever is larger.
   1) Up to 25% of benign adenomas will have > 1 cm increase in size.
   2) Resection of lesions for interval growth very rarely uncovers malignancy, especially if growth is sluggish.
   3) Average growth rate of tumors eventually discovered to be carcinoma were 1.9 cm/year.

3. Follow-up
 a. Metabolically inactive lesions < 4 cm with imaging features consistent with benign adenoma require no further imaging.
 b. Lesions that are not resected and are either greater than 4 cm in diameter or show other features not consistent with benign adenoma (in addition to HU > 10) should undergo reimaging in 6, 12, and 24 months, though more frequent imaging may be considered if suspicion of malignancy is high. (Lesions greater than 4 cm in diameter with such imaging features should generally undergo resection.) (See Fig. 23.2.)

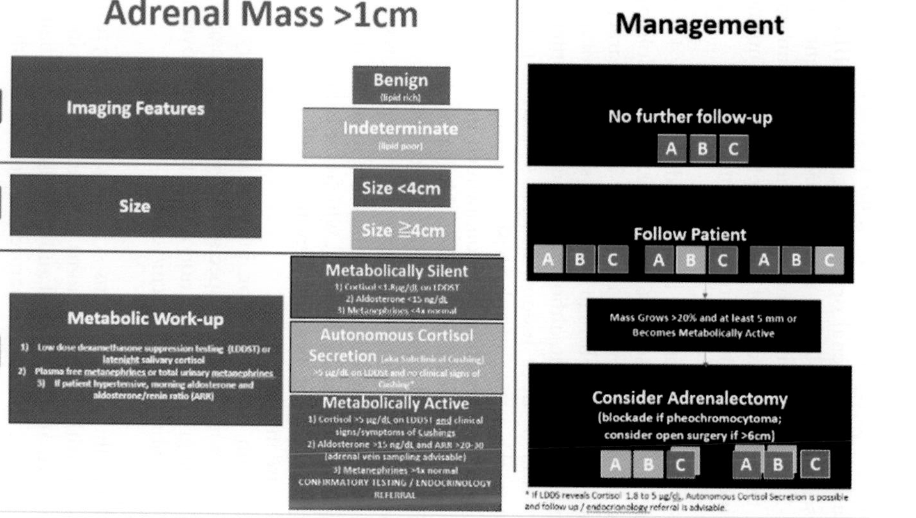

FIGURE 23.2 Management algorithm for newly diagnosed incidental adrenal mass. Masses known to be myelolipomas are exceptions. Masses found in the setting of a known extraadrenal malignancy may be considered for biopsy. (From Kutikov A, Crispen P, Uzzo R. Pathophysiology, Evaluation, and Medical Management of Adrenal Disorders. In: Partin AW, Dmochowski RR, Kavoussi LR, Peters CA, eds. *Campbell-Walsh-Wein Urology*. 12th ed. Elsevier; 2020. Figure 65-33)

BIOPSY OF ADRENAL MASSES

1. Risk of bleeding, hypertension, track seeding, and disruption of surgical planes.
2. Only indicated to assess for adrenal metastasis in the setting of a patient with another known malignancy and only if results will change management.
3. Pheochromocytoma must be biochemically ruled out prior to biopsy due to risk of biopsy provoking hypertensive crisis.
4. Biopsy should not be used if adrenal carcinoma is suspected. Biopsy is unable to differentiate adenoma from carcinoma, and adrenal carcinoma is prone to track seeding.
5. Larger needles (at least 19G) should be used to provide more accurate results.

ASSESSMENT OF FUNCTION OF ADRENAL MASSES

1. Over 10% of incidentalomas harbor metabolic function.
   a. 5.3% Cushing syndrome
   b. 5.1% pheochromocytoma
   c. 1% aldosteronoma
2. Metabolic workup—all adrenal masses > 1 cm in size must be assessed for metabolic function. (See Table 23.1.)
   a. **Testing for Conn syndrome**
      1) Testing not indicated in patients without hypertension.
      2) Morning (between 8 and 10 AM) aldosterone to renin ratio (ARR) and morning aldosterone level are obtained as a screening test. Cutoff values of 20 and 15 ng/dL, respectively, have sensitivity/specificity > 90%.
      3) Hypokalemia should be repeated, since low potassium level may lead to false-positive results.
      4) Patients, who are usually otherwise instructed to adhere to a low sodium diet, should be instructed to liberalize their sodium intake prior to testing.
      5) Chewing tobacco and licorice should be avoided.
      6) Potassium-sparing diuretics and mineralocorticoid blockers must be stopped for at least 4 weeks prior to testing.

TABLE 23.1 Summary of Hormonal Testing for Adrenal Lesions

	Test	Performance	Interpretation	Precautions and Preparation	Confirmatory Testing
Aldosterone	Morning aldosterone-to-renin ratio with serum aldosterone.	Draw plasma renin activity and aldosterone level between 8 AM and 10 AM.	**Serum aldosterone level > 15** ng/dL and **ARR > 20** and have sensitivity and specificity > 90%.	• Institute normal sodium diet • Replete hypokalemia • Avoid chewing tobacco and licorice • Stop K-sparing diuretics and aldosterone inhibitors • Ok to continue anti-HTN medication in screening setting	Always required. Fludrocortisone suppression, sodium loading, captopril suppression, and/or adrenal vein sampling. Refer to endocrine.
Cortisol	Low-dose dexamethasone suppression testing (LDDST)	• 1 mg dexamethasone taken between 11 PM and 12 AM • Cortisol level drawn between 8 AM and 9 AM • Optional dexamethasone level at time of cortisol level	• **Cortisol > 5** mcg/dL 95% specific but 18% false negative • **Cortisol > 1.8** mcg/dL 90% sensitive, 80% specific • Dexamethasone levels should be > 0.22 mcg/dL	• Stop OCPs • Consider stopping other medications which may interact with steroid metabolism	• Confirmation only required if equivocal • Patients testing positive should be screened for hypertension, diabetes, and vertebral fractures • Morning ACTH level required for further workup of etiology

	Late-night salivary cortisol	Saliva sample taken between 11 PM and 12 AM	**Cortisol > 145 ng/dL** has > 90% sensitivitsy and specificity	Inaccurate results may be caused by: • altered circadian rhythm • acute or chronic illness • tobacco products used on the day of testing	
Catecholamines	Plasma-free meta-nephrines	Blood draw	The following values are highly specific: • **Normetanephrine > 2.2 nmol/L** (400 ng/L) • **Metanephrine > 1.2 nmol/L** (236 ng/L)	Hold the following medications: • Alpha-1 antagonists (esp phenoxybenzamine) • Tricyclic antidepressants • Caffeine (24 hours) • Acetaminophen (5 days)	Confirmation only required if equivocal
	24-Hour urinary fractionated meta-nephrines	24-Hour urine collection. Test: • Metanephrine • Normetanephrine • Total metanephrine • Creatinine	Any of the following values have sensitivity of 97% and specificity of 91%: • **Metanephrine > 1531 nmol/day** • **Normetanephrine > 4011 nmol/day** • **Total metanephrine > 1563 nmol/day**	Hold: • Tricyclic antidepressants • Phenoxybenzamine Measure total creatinine to ensure complete collection	

7) Most antihypertensive agents can be continued for initial testing.
   i. Beta-blockers—can lead to false-positive results (need to be stopped for confirmatory testing).
   ii. ACE-inhibitors—minority of patients can exhibit false-negative results.
   iii. Calcium channel blockers do not affect testing.
8) Confirmatory testing with fludrocortisone suppression, sodium loading, or captopril suppression tests is required. These generally require referral to endocrinology.
9) Adrenal vein sampling (AVS) to prove laterality of aldosterone hypersecretion prior to surgery is controversial. It was previously considered mandatory; however, it is probably not necessary in patients < 40 years old with a clear unilateral adenoma and a normal contralateral gland. One randomized trial suggested that AVS is never beneficial, and there are numerous alternative studies available which have sought to replace it; however, it is still often recommended.
10) Adrenal tumors confirmed to be causing primary hyperaldosteronism should undergo resection. See Adrenal Neoplasia.

b. **Testing for cortisol excess**—two valid initial tests
   1) Low-dose dexamethasone suppression test—most often utilized test for screening
      i. Patient takes 1 mg of dexamethasone between 11 PM and 12 AM. Cortisol level drawn the next morning between 8 AM and 9 AM. Cortisol > 5 mcg/dL is 95% specific but yields 18% false negatives; > 1.8 mcg/dL is 90% sensitive but only 80% specific. If the 1.8 mcg threshold is used, the test should be repeated in 3–12 months.
      ii. A dexamethasone level may be drawn with the AM serum cortisol level to confirm the medication was taken properly. Dexamethasone levels should be > 0.22 mcg/dL; however, this test is costly and has limited availability, so it is not required.
      iii. Oral contraceptives can yield false-positive results in up to 50% of cases due to increasing cortisol binding globulin levels. Numerous other medications can

cause inaccurate results due to interaction with steroid metabolism.

2) Late-night salivary cortisol testing—cortisol > 145 ng/dL measured in saliva sample taken between 11 PM and midnight has > 90% sensitivity and specificity. False positives may be caused by:
   i. Interference with normal circadian rhythm: altered sleep patterns, depression
   ii. Acute or chronic illness
   iii. Tobacco products used on the day of testing
3) A 24-hour urinary cortisol—now felt to not be adequately sensitive for initial screening purposes. Results only meaningful in patients with normal renal function.
4) Combining multiple of these testing modalities may be useful in ambiguous cases.
5) Morning basal ACTH levels should be drawn and confirmed to be low prior to resection of an adrenal mass suspected of hypersecretion of cortisol to rule out an ACTH-dependent process.
6) All patients diagnosed with "autonomous cortisol secretion" (see "Increased Adrenal Function") should undergo screening for hypertension, diabetes, and asymptomatic vertebral fractures (with plain x-ray or with reevaluation of CT demonstrating the adenoma if available).
7) Adrenal adenomas causing cortisol excess without overt Cushing syndrome do not require resection. These are at < 1% risk of progressing to overt Cushing syndrome but generally undergo some further monitoring.
8) Adenomas causing cortisol excess with overt Cushing syndrome should undergo resection.

c. **Testing for adrenal sex steroid excess**
   1) Routine screening of patients with adrenal masses for androgen/estrogen secretion is not recommended, unless adrenocortical carcinoma is highly suspected.
   2) Sex steroids may be used as tumor markers to detect recurrence or monitor response of adrenal carcinoma to therapy.
   3) Testing should include serum DHEA-S and testosterone. Men and postmenopausal women should undergo testing for 17β-estradiol. Full evaluation with serum 17-OH

progesterone, androstenedione, 17-OH pregnenolone, 11-deoxycorticosterone, progesterone, and estradiol is optional and should be more strongly considered with higher levels of suspicion for adrenal carcinoma.

d. Testing for pheochromocytoma—two valid initial tests
   1) Plasma-free metanephrines
      i. Plasma-free metanephrines are slightly less specific; however, they can be measured on the same blood draw as cortisol, aldosterone, and renin levels.
      ii. Alpha blockers, tricyclic antidepressants, caffeine (within 24 hours), and acetaminophen (within 5 days) interfere with results.
      iii. Ideally the patient should be fasting on the day of the study and supine for 20 minutes prior to the blood draw. β-blockade should be stopped beforehand to prevent false positives. These requirements for ideal testing are generally only indicated only for confirmatory testing.
      iv. Serum levels > 2.2 nmol/L (400 ng/L) for normetanephrine and/or > 1.2 nmol/L (236 ng/L) for metanephrine are highly specific. Lesser elevations above the upper limit of normal should prompt repeat testing with endocrinology.
   2) 24-hour urinary fractionated metanephrines
      i. Collect all urine in a 24-hour period, discarding the first morning void and including the first morning void from the following day.
      ii. Measure creatinine to ensure adequate collection.
      iii. Tricyclic antidepressants and phenoxybenzamine must be stopped.
      iv. Metanephrine > 1531 nmol/day, normetanephrine > 4001 nmol/day, or total metanephrine > 1563 nmol/day; sensitivity of 97% and specificity of 91%.

e. **Repeat functional testing** of nonfunctional adenomas is indicated only in the presence of new clinical signs of Cushing or Conn syndrome, according to recent guidelines. In the past, annual repeat testing was recommended for 3 to 4 years; however, only ~2% of initially metabolically silent adrenal masses gain function on follow-up.

SUMMARY OF SURGICAL INDICATIONS

See also Figure 23.2.

1. Functional adrenal mass, except ACS without overt Cushing syndrome.
2. Increased risk of malignancy
   a. Mass > 4 cm AND washout characteristics not consistent with benign adenoma.
   b. Mass > 4 cm OR washout characteristics not consistent with benign adenoma in young and/or noncomorbid patient.
   c. Mass > 6 cm.
   d. Mass that is rapidly increasing in size (> 20% and > 5 mm in diameter).
3. Bilateral adrenalectomy for ACTH-independent macronodular adrenal hyperplasia, primary pigmented nodular adrenocortical disease, select patients with ectopic ACTH syndrome, and failed neurosurgical treatment of Cushing disease.
4. Select patients with isolated adrenal metastasis.

CLINICAL PEARLS

- All adrenal masses > 1 cm require a metabolic workup.
- Adrenal CT washout study is superior to MRI in characterizing indeterminate adrenal masses.
- Adrenal biopsy cannot differentiate between adrenal adenoma and adrenal carcinoma.
- Possibility of pheochromocytoma must be ruled out before biopsy or surgery.

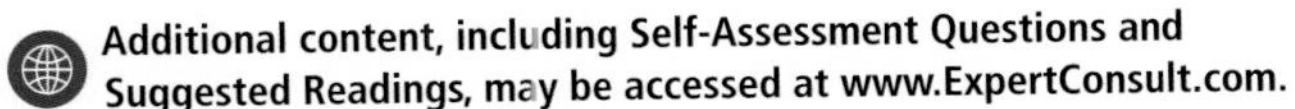

Additional content, including Self-Assessment Questions and
Suggested Readings, may be accessed at www.ExpertConsult.com.

Retroperitoneal Tumors and Retroperitoneal Fibrosis

Daniel Roberson, MD, and Daniel J. Lee, MD

Retroperitoneal Anatomy

Many pathologies treated by urologists exist in the retroperitoneal space, and thus it is imperative that all urologists develop and maintain a strong knowledge base of retroperitoneal anatomy (Table 24.1). The borders of the retroperitoneal cavity are as follows: the posterior parietal peritoneum of the peritoneal cavity anteriorly, the diaphragmatic reflection superiorly, the inlet to the true pelvis inferiorly, the musculature and associated connective tissues of the body wall posteriorly with extension to flank musculature laterally.

Nearly every organ system passes through the retroperitoneum. Notable for urologists, the upper urinary tract including the kidneys and proximal to middle portions of the ureters are contained in the retroperitoneum as are both adrenal glands. Found in the retroperitoneum are major vascular structures of the body including the aorta and inferior vena cava (IVC) from the diaphragm down to common iliac divisions with all critical branches in between, including lumbar vessels and anterior branches to the contents of the peritoneal cavity. Associated with these vessels are lymphatic networks. Large nerve plexuses of the sensory, motor, and autonomic nervous systems, including the celiac, hypogastric, and sacral plexuses, are located in the retroperitoneum. Portions of the gastrointestinal tract, including the pancreas, the second and third portions of the duodenum, and the ascending and descending colon lie within the retroperitoneum. The splenic hilum is within the retroperitoneum as splenic vasculature passes into the peritoneal cavity. Connective tissues including fat occupy a significant portion of retroperitoneal space.

TABLE 24.1 Differential Diagnoses

Retroperitoneal Fibrosis	Retroperitoneal Hemorrhage	Retroperitoneal Tumor
Aortic aneurysm Carcinoid Infectious process (histoplasmosis, actinomycosis, tuberculosis) Inflammatory bowel disease Lymphoma Metastatic disease (colon, breast, lung, genitourinary, thyroid) Pancreatitis Retroperitoneal sarcoma Retroperitoneal hemorrhage	Great vessel rupture Hematologic origin (anticoagulation therapy, blood dyscrasias) Iatrogenic (percutaneous or vascular procedure) Pancreatic hemorrhage Renal hemorrhage (angiomyolipoma)	Direct extension of local tumor (renal, adrenal) Hamartoma Lipoma Leiomyoma Metastatic disease (colon, breast, lung, genitourinary, thyroid) Sarcoma (liposarcoma, leiomyosarcoma) Schwannoma

Anatomic relationships between the aforementioned structures are important to understand as urologic surgeons perform evaluation of retroperitoneal pathology and plan surgical approach and resection borders. Loss of usual fat planes of the right and left colonic mesentery on preoperative imaging raises concern for their involvement in tumor growth. Neoplastic growth into or iatrogenic injury of the psoas muscles can cause motor weakness with lower extremity hip flexion and knee extension. Similarly, anterior and medial thigh paresthesia can result from growth into or damage of the genitofemoral nerve. Malignant processes or surgical procedures in the left retroperitoneum raise concern for involvement of the aorta, spleen, and pancreatic tail, while on the right there is similar concern of involvement of the IVC and duodenum. Somewhat unique to surgery of the retroperitoneum is the frequent need for a multidisciplinary approach involving different surgical teams.

Benign Diseases of the Retroperitoneum

RETROPERITONEAL FIBROSIS

The idiopathic form of retroperitoneal fibrosis accounts for about two-thirds of retroperitoneal fibrosis cases with the remaining third of cases being secondary to other factors (Table 24.2). Idiopathic retroperitoneal fibrosis is a diagnosis of exclusion; thus a thorough evaluation must be completed before the diagnosis can be made. **It is paramount to exclude a primary or metastatic malignancy as the cause of retroperitoneal fibrosis.**

Idiopathic retroperitoneal fibrosis is an uncommon entity and epidemiologic data is sparse. Mean age at presentation is between 50 and 60 years old. Men have a two to three times higher incidence than women. No familial clustering has been observed. Pathogenesis was originally thought to be related to chronic periaortitis due to an exaggerated local reaction to atherosclerotic plaques, though now it is believed to be more of a manifestation of systemic autoimmune disease. It is often found in patients with immunoglobulin G4 (IgG4)–related diseases. Classically, idiopathic retroperitoneal fibrosis appears as a dense mass in the center of the retroperitoneum, usually at the L4 to L5 vertebral

TABLE 24.2 Causes of Retroperitoneal Fibrosis

Drugs	Malignancies	Infections
Methysergide	Primary retroperitoneal tumors	Chronic UTI
Beta-blockers	Metastatic retroperitoneal tumors	Tuberculosis
Ergot alkaloids	Carcinoid retroperitoneal tumors	Gonorrhea
Haloperidol	Chemicals	Syphilis
Reserpine	Asbestos	Inflammatory processes
Phenacetin	Talcum powder	Endometriosis
Methyldopa	Avitene	Sarcoidosis
LSD	Iatrogenic	Collagen vascular disease
Amphetamines	Radiation	
Traumatic		
Hemorrhage		
Urinary extravasation Postsurgical		

LSD, Lysergic acid diethylamide; *UTI*, urinary tract infection.

level. It can envelope the great vessels and involve nearly any structure in the retroperitoneum. Presentation of retroperitoneal fibrosis varies widely with symptoms oftentimes being vague having an insidious onset. The most common presenting complaints are back pain and abdominal pain, though weight loss, vomiting, and fatigue are common. It is not uncommon for patients to present in renal failure due to ureteral obstruction.

No standardized diagnostic criteria exist for retroperitoneal fibrosis. Historically, on intravenous (IV) pyelography, the triad of proximal hydroureteronephrosis, medial ureteral deviation, and extrinsic compression of the ureters was noted. Magnetic resonance imaging (MRI) and computed tomography (CT) scan are both valuable in the evaluation of retroperitoneal fibrosis. It is important to perform cross-sectional imaging with IV contrast to look for lymphadenopathy and other findings that would raise suspicion for malignancy. In cases of patients with decreased glomerular filtration rate (GFR), an MRI with contrast can be used to achieve adequate imaging evaluation. Fluorodeoxyglucose positron emission tomography (FDG-PET) **scans have more recently been shown to reliably distinguish between malignant and benign retroperitoneal fibrotic plaques as well as predict a patient's response to steroids.** This has the potential to reduce the need for biopsy and aid in individualization of care. Laboratory tests are nonspecific for the diagnosis of retroperitoneal fibrosis, though erythrocyte sedimentation rates, C-reactive protein levels, and gamma globulin levels are often elevated.

In patients presenting with acute renal failure and bilateral obstruction, decompression of the urinary tract and restoration of metabolic homeostasis are a must prior to definitive treatment of the retroperitoneal fibrosis. This can be done with ureteral stenting or placement of percutaneous nephrostomy tubes. Following upper tract decompression ruling out malignancy is the next step. **Should any ambiguity of malignancy remain following a complete workup, a biopsy should be performed.**

Initial treatment for retroperitoneal fibrosis can be either medical or surgical, though medical therapy is often pursued first. Glucocorticoids and various immunosuppressive agents are the mainstay of medical therapy. No standardized steroid dosing schedule exists. A studied regimen with noted effectiveness is as follows: 60 mg of oral prednisolone taken every other day for 2 months, over the next 2 months the dose was tapered to 40 mg for 2 weeks, 30 mg for 2 weeks, 20 mg for 2 weeks, and 10 mg for 2 weeks with administration still being every other day, and finally a maintenance dose of 5 mg daily for a total treatment period of 2 years. It is important that steroid therapy is not abandoned early as regression of fibrotic plaques can be seen up to 20 months after treatment. Immunosuppressants alone and in combination with steroids also play a role in the medical treatment of retroperitoneal fibrosis. Success has been seen with rituximab used alone and in combination with steroids for both idiopathic and secondary retroperitoneal fibrosis. Additionally, there are reports of success with tamoxifen, azathioprine, cyclophosphamide, penicillamine, and mycophenolate mofetil.

Surgical treatment is in the form of operative retroperitoneal exploration and ureterolysis. Surgery can be performed should medical therapy not be effective or upfront depending on patient preference and overall clinical picture. Preoperative ureteral stent placement greatly aids in ureteral identification and dissection. At the time of surgical exploration, deep biopsies should be performed to rule out any undiagnosed malignancy. Once the ureters are completely freed of the fibrotic plaque, they can be intraperitonealized or wrapped with omentum to ensure success and durability of the operation. **Regardless of whether the disease process is unilateral or bilateral, a bilateral ureterolysis should be performed.** Postoperative steroid therapy is often used in an attempt to prevent recurrence. Regardless of treatment paradigm, it is important that patients maintain long-term follow-up as relapses may occur.

RETROPERITONEAL HEMORRHAGE

Spontaneous retroperitoneal hemorrhage is rare and can occur in a wide variety of age groups depending on the etiology that can be highly varied (Table 24.3). When the bleeding is renal in origin, it has been classically referred to as Wunderlich syndrome. This is frequently the initial presentation of a renal angiomyolipoma, which is, in fact, the most common cause of spontaneous retroperitoneal hemorrhage. Patients may present in hypovolemic shock or complain of back, flank, abdominal, hip, or upper thigh pain. Physical examination may be significant for flank ecchymosis,

TABLE 24.3 Causes of Spontaneous Retroperitoneal Hemorrhage

Retroperitoneal Tumors	
Benign	**Malignant**
Angiomyolipoma	Renal cell carcinoma
Lipoma	Sarcoma
Adenoma	Wilms tumor
Fibroma	Granulosa cell tumors
Hamartoma	
Papilloma	
Hemorrhagic renal cyst	
Vascular	**Hematologic**
Panarteritis nodosa	Anticoagulation therapy
Renal artery arteriosclerosis	Hemophilia
Renal artery aneurysm rupture	Blood dyscrasia
Aortic aneurysm rupture	

hypotension, or gross hematuria. Cross-sectional imaging is most useful in uncovering the extent of bleed and the possibility of a malignant origin.

Patients should first be resuscitated and stabilized, anticoagulant medications should be discontinued, and any potential coagulopathies treated and reversed. Patients can be monitored with serial imaging to evaluate for resolution of the hematoma and bleeding. If conservative therapy fails and the patient becomes unstable, angiography with selective embolization of active bleeding vessels can be performed. **Retroperitoneal exploration should be approached with caution as it often results in massive blood loss and, when bleeding is renal in origin, nephrectomy.**

PELVIS LIPOMATOSIS

Pelvic lipomatosis is a benign condition in which an excessive deposition of mature unencapsulated fat is in the pelvic retroperitoneum. The etiology of pelvic lipomatosis is unknown though obesity is a common association. It occurs predominantly in men in the age range of 20–50 years old, with Black men having the highest incidence.

Half of patients with pelvic lipomatosis will present with voiding dysfunction. Constipation is also a common presenting complaint. Hypertension is common as well as azotemia due to extrinsic compression of the ureters. Cystitis glandularis, cystitis cystica, and cystitis follicularis have been observed in association with pelvic lipomatosis in as high as 75% of patients in some series. **Pelvic lipomatosis classically shows "pear-shaped" or "teardrop-shaped" bladder on imaging.** The upper urinary tracts can range from normal to severely dilated, and the distal ureters are typically deviated medially. CT scan is valuable in diagnosis given its ability to detect fat.

Conservative management includes weight reduction and monitoring for renal deterioration with lab work and imaging. Progressive hydronephrosis or azotemia should prompt urinary tract decompression. Ureteral stenting, nephrostomy tube placement, ureteral reimplantation into the bladder dome, and urinary diversion have all been employed in this setting. Debulking of pelvic fatty tissue has also been reported though it is technically challenging and comes with a high risk of serious complications.

MYELOLIPOMA

Myelolipomas are benign growths composed of mature fat and bone marrow elements. They most commonly occur in the adrenal gland but may be seen in other extramedullary locations throughout the retroperitoneum. These lesions are generally seen in patients older than 40 years and are typically smaller than 5 cm. They are often discovered incidentally. **They may be surgically removed if the patient is symptomatic; however, good evidence supports observation regardless of the size of the lesion.**

LEIOMYOMA

Leiomyomas are benign tumors of smooth muscle origin. They are most commonly found in the female reproductive organs, but they can be seen in the retroperitoneum and the bladder. Leiomyomas are difficult to distinguish from malignant lesions based on imaging alone and are generally surgically excised for this reason. Leiomyomas can be distinguished from malignant leiomyosarcoma histologically because of their positivity for desmin.

CLINICAL PEARLS

Benign Disease of the Retroperitoneum

1. Once malignancy has been ruled out, the treatment of retroperitoneal fibrosis typically revolves around relief of ureteral obstruction through ureteral stenting, percutaneous nephrostomy tube placement, or ureterolysis.
2. Retroperitoneal hemorrhage is most commonly renal in origin. No matter the site, this can represent life-threatening bleeding and requires astute attention to resuscitation and source control.
3. Leiomyomas often grow very large in size and are difficult to distinguish radiographically from malignant lesions. They are generally surgically excised for this reason.

Malignant Pathology of the Retroperitoneum

EPIDEMIOLOGY AND ETIOLOGY

Primary retroperitoneal sarcomas are rare tumors accounting for 0.1% to 0.2% of all malignancies and 10% to 15% of all soft tissue sarcomas. The incidence is approximately 2.7 cases per 10^6 persons per year. They most commonly present within the 50–60 years old age range, though age at presentation is highly variable. Both sexes seem to be affected equally and there is no documented racial or ethnic predilection.

Information with regard to risk factors for retroperitoneal sarcomas is sparse, but prior radiation, trauma, and environmental exposure to dioxin and asbestos have all been documented. Germline mutations such as Li-Fraumeni syndrome also put individuals at risk for the development of sarcomas. Approximately 0.1% of patients who have received radiation therapy will develop a sarcoma at or near the treatment site. Sarcomas are thought to develop from mesenchymal stem cells residing in muscle, fat, and connective tissues. Retroperitoneal sarcomas arise primarily from soft tissues of fibrous and adipose origin. Abnormalities on chromosome 12 resulting in amplification of certain gene products involved in p53 inactivation have also been cited in the carcinogenesis of retroperitoneal sarcomas.

PATHOLOGY

Liposarcomas are the most common primary retroperitoneal tumor and approximately 20% of all liposarcomas are retroperitoneal in origin. They are most commonly seen during the fifth to sixth decade of life and can grow to be quite large. Grossly, liposarcomas have a "fish flesh" appearance and tend to be encapsulated. Well-differentiated liposarcomas are more common than dedifferentiated liposarcomas and are classified as low grade with less potential to metastasize. Higher-grade liposarcomas tend to bear little resemblance histologically to fat-filled structures and often are locally invasive, have a high potential to metastasize, and recur after local excision. It is thought that high-grade, dedifferentiated liposarcomas arise from well-differentiated liposarcomas.

Leiomyosarcomas are less common, though remain the second most common subtype of retroperitoneal sarcoma. They are believed to be more common in women and are found most commonly in the sixth decade of life. Low-grade lesions can be distinguished from leiomyomas by the increased number of mitoses seen with high-power microscopy (more than five mitoses per high-power field). **There is no definitive evidence that these sarcomas arise from malignant degeneration of leiomyomas.** In the retroperitoneum it is theorized that they originate from the IVC, its tributary veins, or any small vessel. Therefore they often present with lower extremity swelling/edema.

Following liposarcomas and leiomyosarcomas, undifferentiated/unclassified soft tissue sarcomas are the third most common histologic type of retroperitoneal sarcoma. These tumors were previously included within the older category of malignant fibrous histiocytoma (MFH). Among the pediatric population, the most common subtypes are extraskeletal Ewing sarcoma/primitive neuroectodermal tumor (PNET), alveolar rhabdomyosarcoma, and fibrosarcoma.

DIAGNOSIS

Because of their relatively slow growth and concealed location, retroperitoneal sarcomas are generally quite large at the time of diagnosis. Symptoms are often due to tumor mass effect or local invasion. The vast majority of patients will present with abdominal pain or an abdominal mass (60% to 80%). Patients will often also complain of accompanying nausea, vomiting, early satiety, and weight loss (20% to 30%). Lower extremity edema, stemming from extrinsic compression of the IVC, is also a common finding on initial physical examination (20% of patients) as is a protuberant abdomen. Urinary symptoms tend to be infrequent.

On physical examination, a protuberant abdomen is often easily identifiable. Palpable lymphadenopathy is uncommon, found in approximately 5% of presenting patients. If a tumor arises primarily from retroperitoneal vessels, presentation correlates with the vessel involved (e.g., lower extremity edema in the case of the iliac vessels, Budd-Chiari syndromic findings with involvement of the perihepatic IVC).

Cross-sectional imaging with either CT or MRI is essential in the workup of patients suspected of having a retroperitoneal mass. The size of the mass, its relationship to other important anatomic structures, the presence of lymphadenopathy, and visceral metastases can all be assessed with these modalities. CT is also excellent for the detection of bony invasion. If there is a question of vascular involvement after initial imaging, it is often advisable to obtain magnetic resonance angiography to more precisely delineate the relationship of important vascular structures to the retroperitoneal mass.

If imaging does not provide a diagnosis with reasonable certainty, CT or ultrasound-guided biopsy may be used to obtain a tissue diagnosis. Because of the infrequency of these lesions and the low sensitivity and specificity of diagnostic biopsy of these lesions in inexperienced hands, it is recommended that biopsies be performed at a center experienced in dealing with masses of this nature. In specific cases, open biopsy can be performed. Independent of the operative approach, care must be taken during biopsy to avoid tumor spillage.

STAGING

Tumor grade plays an integral role in the staging of primary retroperitoneal tumors. Tumor grading is determined by the overall appearance of differentiation of cells, the number of atypical mitoses, and the presence of necrosis. Tumors are graded from well differentiated (low grade) to poorly differentiated (high grade) in a three-tier system (G1 to G3). The tumor-node-metastasis (TNM) system is combined with tumor grading (GTNM system) for the complete clinical staging of these tumors (Tables 24.4 and 24.5).

Clinical staging should include a thorough physical examination, bone scan, and CT of the chest, abdomen, and pelvis. It is beneficial to obtain information on bilateral renal function prior to exploration in case nephrectomy is warranted intraoperatively.

TABLE 24.4 American Joint Commission on Cancer (AJCC) Grade-Tumor-Node-Metastasis (GTNM) Classification of Soft Tissue Sarcomas, Eighth Edition (2017)

Tumor Grade
GX—Grade cannot be assessed
G1—Total differentiation,[a] mitotic count,[b] and necrosis score[c] of 2 or 3
G2—Total differentiation, mitotic count, and necrosis score of 4 or 5
G3—Total differentiation, mitotic count, and necrosis score of 6, 7, or 8

Primary Tumor
TX—Primary tumor cannot be assessed
T0—No evidence of primary tumor
T1—Tumor 5 cm or less in greatest dimension
T2—Tumor more than 5 cm and less than or equal to 10 cm in greatest dimension
T3—Tumor more than 10 cm and less than or equal to 15 cm in greatest dimension
T4—Tumor more than 15 cm in greatest dimension

Regional Lymph Node Involvement
N0—No regional lymph node metastasis of unknown lymph node status
N1—Regional lymph node metastasis

Distant Metastasis
M0—No distant metastasis
M1—Distant metastasis

[a]Differentiation: *1* = cancer cells look similar to normal cells; *2* = cancer cells look moderately different to normal cells; *3* = cells look abnormal and very different to normal cells.
[b]Mitotic count: *1* = there are less than 10 cells dividing; *2* = there are more than 10 cells, but less than 20 cells dividing; *3* = there are more than 20 cells dividing.
[c]Necrosis: *0* = there is no dying tissue; *1* = less than half of the cancer is dying tissue; *2* = more than half of the cancer is dying tissue.

SURGERY

Extirpative surgery is the most effective form of therapy for patients with primary retroperitoneal tumors. **Complete resection, with negative margins, has proven to be the most important predictor of favorable outcomes in this patient population.** It is essential to be aware of the extent of the disease preoperatively and

TABLE 24.5 American Joint Commission on Cancer (AJCC) Staging System for Soft Tissue Sarcomas, Eighth Edition (2017)

IA			
T1	N0	M0	G1
IB			
T2, T3, T4	N0	M0	G1
II			
T1	N0	M0	G2, G3
IIIA			
T2	N0	M0	G2, G3
IIIB			
T3, T4	N0	M0	G2, G3
IV			
Any T	N1	M0	Any G
Any T	Any N	M1	Any G

From Amin MB, Edge SB, Greene FL, et al., eds. *AJCC Cancer Staging Manual.* 8th ed. Switzerland: Springer; 2017.

the organs that potentially may need to be sacrificed to optimize the chances of obtaining a negative margin.

The surgical approach is generally through a large midline, chevron, or thoracoabdominal incision. Regardless of approach, it is of paramount importance to gain wide exposure to the retroperitoneum to assess the ability to safely resect tumor. En bloc removal of all tumor and affected organs is essential for good patient outcomes, and it is very common to require removal of at least one adjacent organ in order to obtain negative margins. Major vascular structures, kidneys, portions of the diaphragm, liver, stomach, gallbladder, spleen, pancreas, and bowel can all be involved. **The most frequently resected organ is the ipsilateral kidney, followed by a portion of the colon, adrenal gland, pancreas, and spleen.** Surgical morbidity and mortality in contemporary series range from 6% to 25% and 2% to 7%, respectively. Hemorrhage, intraabdominal abscess, and enterocutaneous fistula formation are commonly described complications.

OUTCOMES

Classically, the overall survival for patients with primary retroperitoneal sarcomas has been poor. Survival at 2, 5, and 10 years has been cited at 56%, 34%, and 18%, respectively, for all outcomes. In patients without metastatic disease, 2- and 5-year survivals can be as high as 70% and 50% to 60%, respectively.

Patients receiving a complete surgical resection with negative margins achieve superior survival compared to patients in whom complete surgical resection is incomplete. Five-year survival for patients with complete surgical resection averages 54% compared to 17% for those with incomplete resections. Unfortunately, tumor recurrence, even after complete surgical resection, is the rule rather than the exception. **Tumor recurrence can be as high as 70% at 5 years and up to 90% at 10 years.** In the absence of metastatic disease, surgery is the mainstay of treatment for recurrent local disease. Studies support that a significant number of patients can experience prolonged disease-free survival when all recurrent tumor can be resected.

Tumor grade has a significant impact on patient survival. Low-grade lesions demonstrate an approximately 50% survival advantage compared to intermediate- and high-grade lesions. This survival advantage is maintained regardless of margin status. Due to the rarity of retroperitoneal sarcomas and the need for complex, multidisciplinary surgical and medical care, treatment at a high-volume center has been shown to have a significant beneficial impact on overall survival. **When feasible, patients with retroperitoneal sarcoma should be referred to a high-volume center.**

Given that the vast majority of failures occur in the abdomen, with an additional 20% to 30% of recurrences in the lungs, a surveillance regimen including physical examination, combined with CT of the chest, abdomen, and pelvis appears to be the most reasonable approach. The current guidelines from the National Comprehensive Cancer Network for the surveillance of retroperitoneal sarcomas include physical examination with chest, abdomen, and pelvis CT at strict intervals. For low-grade disease, this is carried out every 3 to 6 months for 2 to 3 years then annually thereafter. For well-differentiated liposarcoma, omission of chest imaging can be considered. For high-grade disease, the schedule is every 3 to 4 months for 3 years, then every 6 months for 2 years, and annually thereafter. Chest imaging should always be obtained for high-grade sarcoma and for leiomyosarcoma.

RADIATION AND CHEMOTHERAPY

Much of the data supporting the use of radiation therapy and chemotherapy for treatment of sarcoma come from the extremity sarcoma literature; however, there is growing evidence on the use of applications for retroperitoneal diseases. The use and timing of radiotherapy in patients with retroperitoneal sarcoma is controversial.

Retrospective studies on the benefit of adjuvant radiotherapy have yielded mixed results, but a decrease in local recurrences has been cited in some studies. Postoperative radiation has been associated with significant gastrointestinal toxicities. Intraoperative radiotherapy has been used in a small amount of patients at specialized centers. Intraoperative radiotherapy allows for the ability to directly target the resection bed while sparing nearby radiosensitive tissue. Historically, it was thought that neoadjuvant radiation therapy may be beneficial as a lower dose is required and toxicity may be lower because the mass effect of the tumor often displaces organs out of the treatment field and the lack of surgical adhesions decreases the risk of bowel toxicity. This being said, the only phase III randomized controlled trial comparing outcomes from preoperative radiotherapy and surgery with surgery alone for patients with resectable, primary retroperitoneal sarcoma showed that patients who had preoperative radiotherapy had a significantly higher rate of complications and a shorter median time to abdominal recurrence-free survival. **Therefore the role of neoadjuvant radiation therapy prior to surgical resection of retroperitoneal sarcoma remains highly controversial and appears to be less favorable given contemporary literature.**

The exact role and benefit of chemotherapy in the treatment of retroperitoneal sarcoma is also controversial. Modest benefits have been noted using adjuvant doxorubicin chemotherapy in patients with extremity sarcomas, but these benefits are difficult to extrapolate to patients with retroperitoneal sarcomas. **For patients with advanced or metastatic disease, doxorubicin is the principal chemotherapeutic agent.** A response rate of 20% to 25% has been noted, but complete or sustained responses are rare. A 4% overall survival advantage has been seen in patients with high-grade lesions. Combination agents have been employed but have not demonstrated superior responses compared to single-agent treatment and have shown significantly increased rates of toxicity.

CLINICAL PEARLS

Malignant Pathology of the Retroperitoneum

1. Due to their relatively slow growth and concealed location, retroperitoneal sarcomas are generally quite large at the time of diagnosis. Symptoms are typically due to tumor mass effect or local invasion, with the most common presenting symptom being abdominal pain or an abdominal mass.
2. Surgical resection is the most effective form of treatment for primary retroperitoneal tumors. Complete resection, with negative margins, is the most important predictor of outcome.
3. Radiation therapy may be administered pre-, intra-, or postoperatively, though preoperative radiotherapy is more recently not supported by high-quality data in the treatment of localized disease in a patient who is a surgical candidate. Chemotherapy has a limited role in the treatment of retroperitoneal sarcomas, but doxorubicin represents the most commonly used agent.

Additional content, including Self-Assessment Questions and Suggested Readings, may be accessed at www.ExpertConsult.com.

Embryology and Differences of Sex Development

Katherine M. Fischer, MD, and Thomas F. Kolon, MD, MS

Human sex development occurs in an organized, sequential manner beginning with the chromosomal sex which is established at fertilization. The chromosomal sex directs the development of the undifferentiated gonads into testes or ovaries, giving rise to the gonadal sex, and finally the phenotypic sex results from differentiation of the internal ducts and external genitalia under the influence of local and systemic hormones as well as transcription factors. Discordance between any of these three processes (chromosomal, gonadal and phenotypic sexual differentiation) results in a Difference of Sex Development (DSD).

DSD replaced the prior term intersex disorder after a 2006 panel of professionals, parents, and individuals affected by DSD put out a consensus statement on management of these conditions as well as introduced new nomenclature. The term DSD replaced previous terms such as hermaphrodite, pseudohermaphrodite, ambiguity, and intersex with a karyotype-based subclassification. The intention was to acknowledge progress in the understanding of molecular and genetic bases for the diagnoses, but also to remove, to the extent possible, gender implications and potentially pejorative terminology. Use of a specific diagnosis, if known, is ultimately preferred over reference to only the karyotype. Some still prefer the term intersex. This chapter will use the term DSD throughout for consistency but acknowledge that this term may not be universally embraced. In addition, for the sake of historicity, congenital adrenal hyperplasia (CAH) will be discussed under the 46XX heading with the understanding that it is better served as a separate entity and not included in DSD.

This chapter begins with a brief overview of normal sexual development to provide a context in which to understand DSD and then covers common etiologies as well as the evaluation and management of these patients. The differential diagnosis for patients presenting with ambiguous genitalia is quite large and can seem overwhelming at times. It is helpful to work through the differential diagnosis pathway in a careful and methodical manner based upon exam and laboratory findings as many possible diagnoses can be eliminated in this manner and in most cases a precise cause of DSD can be elucidated (Fig. 25.1).

Normal Sexual Development

In order to understand how various DSDs can arise, it is helpful to have a general understanding of normal in utero sexual development. Sexual differentiation is a complex process regulated by more than 50 different genes located on both the sex (X and Y) chromosomes as well as autosomes. These genes encode a variety of transcription factors, gonadal steroid and peptide hormones as well as tissue receptors (Fig. 25.2).

During the first 6 weeks of development the gonadal ridge, germ cells, internal ducts, and external genitalia are bipotential in all embryos and then based upon genetic influences the gonadal ridge differentiates into either ovaries or testes and germ cells into oocytes or spermatocytes. *SRY* (sex-determining region Y gene) is located on the short arm of the Y chromosome and has been termed testis determining factor as it induces a genetic cascade that directs the development of the bipotential gonads toward testes although additional upstream (*SF1, WT1*) and downstream (*DAX1, SOX9, Wnt4, AMH,* homeobox) genes are involved in this process as well. The precise time when this happens is unknown but differentiation of Sertoli cells occurs by 6 to 7 weeks gestation.

The newly differentiated Sertoli cells produce anti-müllerian hormone (AMH) which is a glycoprotein encoded on the short arm of chromosome 19. AMH is critical to the regression of müllerian ductal structures and formation of wolffian (male) internal ductal structures instead. Leydig cells differentiate slightly later, around 8 to 9 weeks gestation, and produce testosterone (T), the other hormone necessary for male sexual differentiation. Testosterone exerts both systemic and local effects to direct male sexual development and in some peripheral tissues, including the

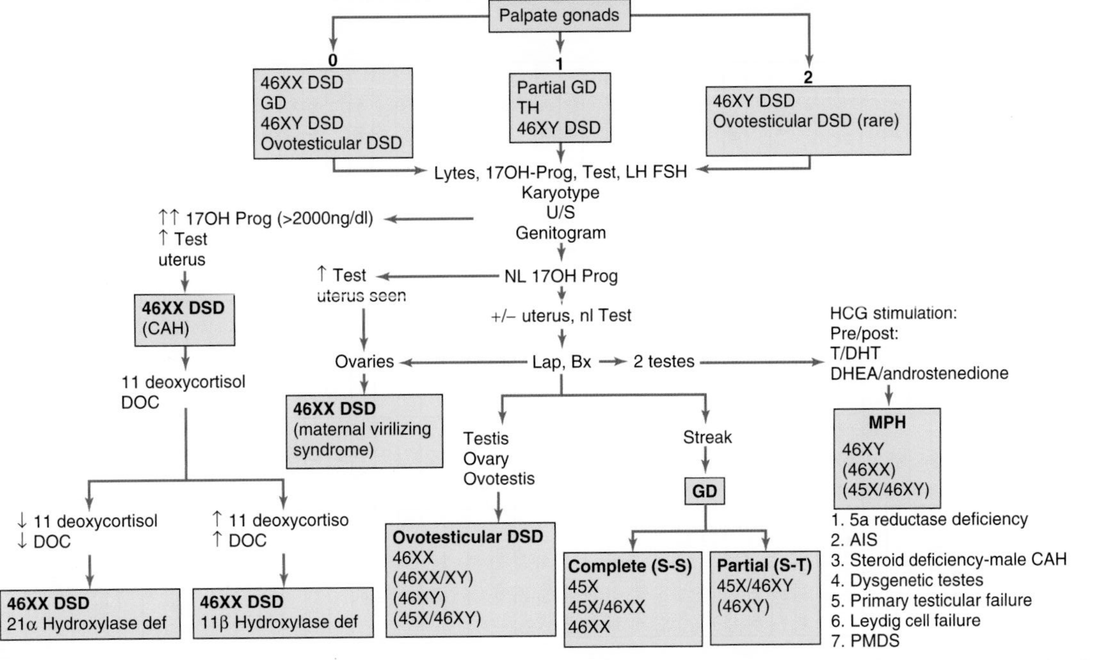

FIGURE 25.1 Decision pathway for evaluation of congenital adrenal hyperplasia *(CAH)* and Differences of Sex Development *(DSD)*. *DHEA*, Dehydroepiandrosterone; *GD*, gonadal dysgenesis; *PMDS*, persistent müllerian duct syndrome; *S*, streak gonad; *T*, testis.

Genetic Etiology of DSD				
Syndrome	**Karyotype**	**Genital Phenotype**	**Gene**	**Locus**
21-Hydroxylase deficiency	XX	virilized	CYP21B	6p21.3
11-Hydroxylase deficiency	XX	virilized	CYP11 (B1,B2)	8q21-22
3BHSD deficiency	XX XY	ambiguous	HSD3B2	1p13.1
17a-Hydroxylase or 17,20 lyase deficiency	XX XY	ambiguous	CYP17	10q24-25
17BHSD deficiency	XY	ambiguous	17BHSD3	9q22
Lipoid adrenal hyperplasia	XX XY	female, ovarian failure (XX)	StAR	8p11.2
Leydig cell failure	XY	ambiguous	hCG/LH receptor	2p21
Androgen insensitivity	XY	ambiguous (female-AIS 7)	AR	Xq11-12
5a-Reductase deficiency	XY	ambiguous, pubertal virilization	SRD5A2	2p23
Persistent müllerian duct	XY	male	AMH AMH II receptor	19q13.3 12q13
Gonadal dysgenesis:				
complete	XX	female,	FSH receptor	2p16-21
	45X, 45X/46XX	sexual infantilism	X monosomy	paternal X loss
	XY		SRY	Yp53.3
			DSS (DAX-1)	Xp 21-22
			SOX9	17q24.3-25.1
			WT-1	11p13
Partial	45X/46XY	ambiguous	unknown	unknown
	XY			
XY Dysgenesis	XY	ambiguous	SRY	Yp53.3
	45X/46XY		DSS (DAX-1)	Xp 21-22
			XH-2	Xq13.3
			WT-1	11p13
			SOX9	17q24.3-25.1
			SF-1	9q33
Ovotesticular DSD	XX	ambiguous	SRY	Yp53.3
	XX/XY		testis cascade	unknown
	XY		downstream genes	
Klinefelter	47XXY	variable androgen	XY	sex chromosome
	46XY/47XXY	deficiency		nondisjunction
XX Testicular DSD	XX	ambiguous to normal	SRY	Y translocation to X

FIGURE 25.2 Genetic characteristics of Differences of Sex Development *(DSD)*.

urogenital sinus, testosterone is converted to dihydrotestosterone (DHT) by 5α-reductase. DHT binds androgen receptors with a greater affinity and stability than testosterone making DHT the active androgen in tissues that possess 5α-reductase.

Without *SRY*, ovaries begin to develop as opposed to testes. Unlike in males, no gene has been identified that directs ovarian development in the way that *SRY* directs testicular development. However, it is no longer believed that female differentiation is merely a "default" pathway. It does appear to be necessary to have two copies of at least one locus on the X chromosome for normal ovarian development, explaining the development of streak gonads in 45X Turner syndrome patients. Estrogen synthesis begins in the female embryo just after 8 weeks. Unlike testosterone, estrogen is not necessary for female differentiation; however, it can interfere with male differentiation.

Until 8 weeks gestation, the urogenital tract is identical in males and females with both wolffian and müllerian duct systems present. In the male fetus, production of AMH by Sertoli cells acts to suppress the müllerian ducts and production of testosterone by Leydig cells promotes the development of the wolffian ducts instead. The wolffian ducts give rise to the internal male reproductive structures which include the epididymis, vas deferens, seminal vesicles, and ejaculatory ducts. Both of these hormonal affects are local which accounts for the variability of internal duct structures seen in patients with ovotesticular DSDs. In the absence of AMH and testosterone, the wolffian ducts regress in females and the müllerian ducts persist and develop into the female internal reproductive tract including the fallopian tubes, uterus, and proximal two-thirds of the vagina.

Unlike the local effects of testosterone and AMH on the internal reproductive tract, testosterone acts systemically to result in masculinization of the external genitalia, with conversion to DHT playing an important role in this process as well. Starting at 10 weeks, testosterone and DHT induce thickening and elongation of the genital tubercle to become the penis and fusion of the urethral folds from posterior to anterior. The urogenital swellings migrate posterior to the genital tubercle and fuse to become the scrotum. By 12 to 13 weeks the male external genitalia are complete though penile growth, and testicular descent into the scrotum occurs in the third trimester under the influence systemic of androgens. In the female fetus, without circulating testosterone, the genital tubercle develops only slightly to form the clitoris, the lateral genital swellings become labia majora, and the urethra folds become the labia minora.

DSD Categories

46XX DSD

As previously stated, CAH will be discussed under this 46XX heading, but most acknowledge (especially patients and families) that CAH is a separate entity and not included in DSD. 46XX DSD is the most common cause of ambiguous genitalia in the newborn and results from masculinization of the female fetus secondary to exposure to androgens during development. This can be from endogenous overproduction of adrenal androgens and precursors secondary to defects in the steroid biosynthesis pathway or as a result of exposure to exogenous maternal androgens. This group of patients has normal ovaries and müllerian duct structures and typically presents with masculinization of the external genitalia and urogenital sinus at birth to a variable extent.

CAH accounts for the majority of 46XX DSD cases. Inactivation or loss of function mutations affecting multiple enzymes and genes in the steroid synthesis pathway can cause CAH, including steroidogenic acute regulatory (*StAR*), 3β-hydroxysteroid dehydrogenase (3β-HSD), 17β-hydroxysteroid dehydrogenase (17β-HSD), 17-hydroxylase, 17,20 lyase, 21-hydroxylase, and 11-hydroxylase deficiencies. CAH is most often a result of deficiency in 21-hydroxlyase or 11-hydroxylase, which are the two terminal enzymes in glucocorticoid synthesis. This causes a compensatory increase in adrenocorticotrophic hormone (ACTH) secretion leading to increased production of adrenal steroids proximal to the defect including testosterone (Fig. 25.3).

While all of these defects cause impaired cortisol secretion, only 21-hydroxylase (*CYP21*), 11-hydroxylase (*CYP11B1*) and to a much lesser degree 3β-HSD (*HSD3B2*) deficiencies cause overproduction of adrenal androgens leading to masculinization of 46XX fetuses. Males affected by these conditions may present later with precocious puberty or in infancy with salt wasting but typically do not have genital ambiguity noted at birth. In contrast, 3β-HSD, 17β-HSD, 17-hydroxylase, 17,20 lyase and *StAR*

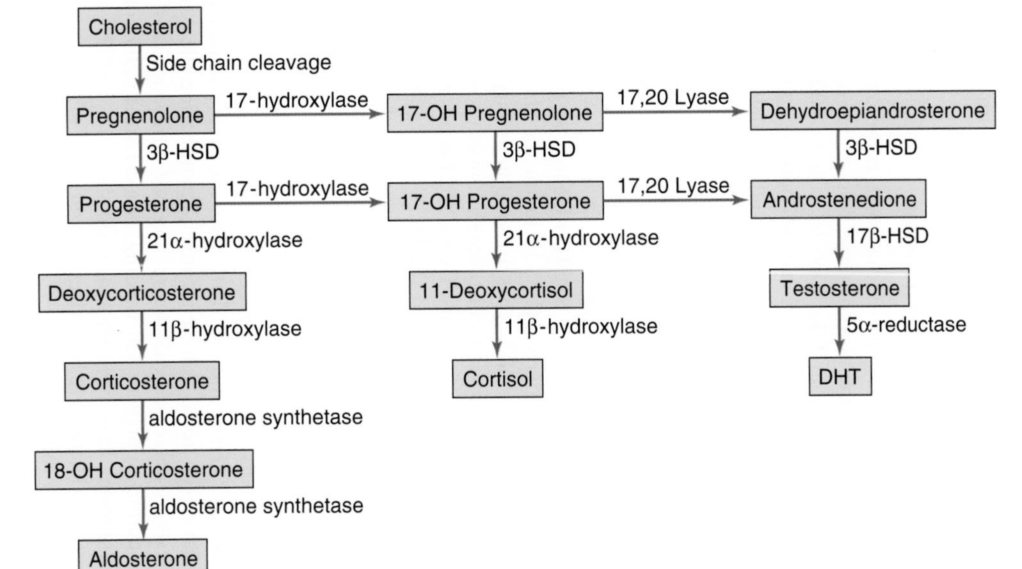

FIGURE 25.3 The steroid biosynthetic pathways with responsible enzymes.

deficiencies block androgen production resulting in 46XY DSD (male undervirilization) with normal genitalia in affected females at birth and genital ambiguity to varying degrees in males. The defects associated with CAH are all inherited in an autosomal recessive pattern.

21α-Hydroxylase (CYP21) Deficiency

Deficiency of 21α-hydroxylase is the most common cause of ambiguous genitalia in the newborn and responsible for 95% of CAH cases occurring from 1 in 5000 to 1 in 15,000 births in the United States and Europe. Affected individuals can be divided into three categories based upon their clinical manifestations: (1) salt wasters (patients with virilization and aldosterone deficiency), (2) simple virilizers (patients with virilization but no salt wasting), and (3) nonclassic patients (patients without evidence of virilization or salt wasting). The majority of patients present with one of the two classic forms with approximately 75% having salt wasting and 25% simple virilizing.

The 21α-hydroxylase gene (*CYP21*) is located within the major human leukocyte antigen (HLA) locus on the short arm of chromosome 6 (6p21.3). HLA types are co-dominantly inherited and can be used as a marker to distinguish homozygous, heterozygous, and unaffected individuals. Two *CYP21* genes are located on chromosome 6 between HLA-B and HLA-DR: a functional 10 exon *CYP21B* gene and a *CYP21A* pseudogene that is nonfunctional due to the presence of multiple stop codons. Recombination between *CYP21B* and the homologous but inactive *CYP21A* accounts for approximately 95% of 21α-hydroxylase deficiency (21OHD) mutations resulting in a variable decrease in 21α-hydroxylase activity. These conversions usually involve the transfer of inherent *CYP21A* mutations. Patients with simple virializing 21OHD have been noted to have a conversion mutation (Ile-Asn) causing severely decreased enzyme activity but sufficient aldosterone production to prevent salt wasting. Nonclassical CAH conversion mutations have been shown to display 20% to 50% of normal activity. There have been over 200 different *CYP21* mutations reported to cause 21OHD.

Females with the classic salt-wasting or simple virilizing forms present with masculinization of the eternal genitalia including enlargement of the clitoris and varying degrees of labial fusion with the vagina and urethra opening into a common urogenital sinus. The enlargement of the clitoris can be so dramatic that it appears to be a hypospadiac penis or rarely a fully masculinized urethra can exist with a meatus at the tip of what appears to be a normal glans. Virilization is often more severe in patients with salt wasting but this is not always the case.

In both male and female patients with salt-wasting CAH, symptoms occur within the first few weeks of life with failure to gain weight and weight loss, dehydration and in severe cases adrenal crisis. In untreated patients there will be progression of masculinization with pubic and axillary hair growth, deepening of the voice and premature epiphyseal plate closure leading to decreased skeletal growth. This continued masculinization occurs in both males and females leading to a precocious puberty in affected males who may have had normal phenotypic appearance at birth. Twenty-five to 30% of affected males will also have testicular adrenal rest tissue, which has been associated with infertility, and is caused by hypertrophy of adrenal rests in response to excess ACTH stimulation.

The diagnosis of 21OHD can be made by elevated levels of plasma 17-hydroxyprogesterone as well as pelvic ultrasound (US) demonstrating müllerian structures. Neonatal screening programs for CAH, which are now present in all 50 states and over 40 countries, have helped increase prompt diagnosis, particularly in males and patients with nonclassic forms. HLA typing of amniotic fluid cells in mothers with a previously affected offspring has been used to identify a fetus with a *CYP21* deficiency. This has led to prenatal treatment of CAH in some cases with good results of decreasing the masculinization. This remains controversial though because of potential risk of treating a fetus who may not need the therapy. Treatment typically needs to be initiated prior to confirmation of the diagnosis and only one in eight fetuses of parents with a previous child with CAH will be affected and benefit.

11β-Hydroxylase (CYP11B1) Deficiency

11β-hydroxylase deficiency (11OHD) accounts for about 5% of CAH cases and can occur with both classic and mild forms. This defect results from mutations in *CYP11B1* gene located on chromosome 8. In 11OHD, lack of cortisol results in increased production of 11-deoxycortisol, deoxycorticosterone (DOC), and androgen by the adrenal gland. Hypertension, which occurs in about two-thirds of patients, is presumed to be a consequence of excess DOC, with resultant salt and water retention. Excess androgen secretion in utero masculinizes the external genitalia of the female fetus with phenotypes ranging from significant masculinization present at birth, similar to classic 21-hydroxylase deficiency to late onset forms with mild virilization in adolescent patients. After birth, untreated males and females progressively masculinize and experience rapid somatic growth and skeletal maturation, similar to 21-hydroxylase deficiency CAH patients.

Two distinct enzymes, *CYP11B1* and *CYP11B2*, are encoded by two tandem and homologous genes at 8q21–22. *CYP11B1* encodes 11β-hydroxylase, which converts DOC to corticosterone and 11-deoxycortisol to cortisol. This gene's protein is expressed in the adrenal zona fasciculata and is primarily under the influence of corticotropin. Alternatively, *CYP11B2* encodes for aldosterone synthetase, which converts corticosterone to 18-hydroxycorticosterone and 18-hydroxycorticosterone to aldosterone. It is expressed in the zona glomerulosa and is under the influence of angiotensin II and potassium. Although *CYP11B1* and *CYP11B2* are extremely homologous, both genes are functional. Thus gene conversions are not the cause of impaired enzyme activity, as was described for 21OHD. Similar to *CYP21*, alterations with less enzyme activity usually result in more severe phenotypes, but heterogeneity can occur.

The diagnosis of 11OHD can be confirmed with increased plasma levels of 11-deoxycortisol and DOC. This disorder can be detected prenatally, and the masculinization of the fetus can be decreased following in utero dexamethasone treatment, as previously described for 21OHD. Other defects in androgen synthesis resulting in CAH such as 3β-HSD deficiency, *CYP17* deficiency, and StAR deficiency are covered under disorders of 46XY DSD as they tend to cause feminization as opposed to masculinization of the external genitalia.

46XY DSD

46XY DSD is a heterogenous group of conditions affecting 46XY individuals who have differentiated testes but varying degrees of feminization of either the internal and/or external genitalia. These conditions result from defects in androgen production, androgen activity or impaired production or activity of AMH. Depending upon the specific defect, the degree of masculinization of the external genitalia and internal ducts is highly variable. This can range from a normal female phenotype (complete androgen insensitivity syndrome [CAIS]) to a normal male with unilateral undescended testis.

LEYDIG CELL APLASIA/HYPOPLASIA

Leydig cell aplasia/hypoplasia is an autosomal recessive condition resulting from the failure of Leydig cell differentiation secondary to abnormalities in the luteinizing hormone (LH) receptor. This results in elevated LH levels but markedly decreased testosterone levels as there is no Leydig cell response to LH stimulation. Follicle stimulating hormone (FSH) levels will be unaffected and human chorionic gonadotropin (hCG) stimulation will not be able induce a rise in testosterone. There will be normal internal wolffian duct structures because Sertoli cell secretion of AMH is unaffected, but the testicles will be undescended and the external genitalia will have a phenotypically female appearance as these processes are both normally testosterone driven. Incomplete forms of this syndrome can occur with the mildest form being a phenotypically normal male with primary hypogonadism. The diagnosis of Leydig cell aplasia is typically made as a result of sexual infantilism or failure of secondary sexual characteristics to develop at puberty or after gonads are palpated in the groin or labia on examination.

ANDROGEN BIOSYNTHESIS DEFECTS

StAR Deficiency

The first step in gonadal and adrenal steroid synthesis is the conversion of cholesterol to pregnenolone which is mediated by p450scc, the *CYP11A* gene product. Congenital lipoid adrenal hyperplasia was originally thought to be secondary to defects in *CYP11A*; however, it was later discovered that these defects would be incompatible with fetal survival and that lipoid CAH is a result of mutations in the *StAR* gene. *StAR* is a protein that stimulates cholesterol transport from the outer to inner mitochondrial membrane where this first step in steroid synthesis catalyzed by p450scc occurs.

Over 40 *StAR* mutations causing congenital lipoid adrenal hyperplasia have been discovered, most commonly occurring in patients of Asian descent. These patients are often born after an uncomplicated pregnancy and present a few days to weeks after birth with severe adrenal insufficiency and require both glucocorticoid and mineralocorticoid replacement for survival. 46XY males will be born with female or ambiguous external genitalia, often rudimentary wolffian duct structures, and both the adrenal glands and testes will be massively engorged with lipid deposits. 46XX females will have a normal female phenotypic appearance and will undergo normal pubertal changes but invariably develop polycystic ovaries and have lipid-laden adrenal glands similar to males. Abdominal imaging will demonstrate large, lipid-laden adrenal glands in these patients.

3β-Hydroxysteroid Dehydrogenase Deficiency

3β-HSD deficiency results in impaired adrenal production of aldosterone and cortisol and impaired gonadal testosterone and estradiol formation. In complete forms, severe adrenal insufficiency will be seen in the first week of life and salt wasting can be present depending upon the severity of the defect. Males will exhibit variable degrees of 46XY DSD whereas females will generally have mild clitoromegaly and masculinization of the external genitalia. This counterintuitive masculinization occurs from the conversion of steroid precursors to testosterone by extragonadal fetal 3β-HSD (found in the placenta and peripheral tissues). Diagnosis is made with increased serum levels of 17-hydroxypregnenolone and dehydroepiandrosterone (DHEA).

17α-Hydroxylase and 17,20 Lyase (CYP17) Deficiency

The *CYP17* gene is located on chromosome 10q24.3 and the cytochrome p450 c17 protein catalyzes 17α-hydroxylase and 17,20 lyase (desmolase) activities. Therefore, abnormalities in *CYP17* cause findings consistent with both 17α-hydroxylase and 17,20 lyase deficiencies including decreased cortisol and sex hormone production. Females will generally present at puberty with sexual infantilism due to lack of ovarian estrogen production. Males may have a range of phenotypic development from normal female external genitalia to ambiguous male genitalia with hypospadias. Overproduction of DOC and corticosterone leads to hypertension, hypokalemic alkalosis, and carbohydrate intolerance.

Though 17α-hydroxylase and 17,20 lyase are linked by the *CYP17* gene, patients with only 17,20 lyase deficiency have been reported. These individuals have normal secretion of aldosterone, cortisol, and ACTH and typically do not display hypertension. 46XY patients with isolated 17,20 lyase deficiency typically have ambiguous as opposed to female genitalia.

17β-Hydroxysteroid Dehydrogenase Deficiency

There are at least five known isoenzymes of 17β-HSD. The type 3 17β-HSD catalyzes the reduction of androstenedione to testosterone and is expressed only in the testis. Different isoenzymes catalyze the reduction of estrone to estradiol and androstenedione to testosterone. As expected, these patients have elevated plasma androstenedione (up to 10 times normal) levels, low plasma testosterone, elevated LH, and normal-to-high FSH levels. In these patients more than 90% of plasma testosterone is produced from extragonadal conversion of androstenedione to testosterone whereas less than 1% of testosterone is produced this way in normal males. Some patients may have normal DHT levels suggesting conversion from androstenedione.

These patients are usually 46XY males with ambiguous or female external genitalia and normal internal wolffian duct structures and undescended testes. They are often raised as girls but may undergo significant virilization at puberty and adopt a male gender role, similar to that seen in 5α reductase deficiency. At puberty, the expression of other 17βHSD isoenzymes in the peripheral tissues partially compensates for testicular 17βHSD-3 deficiency; however, the phenotype is variable. Some patients develop gynecomastia at puberty, depending on their testosterone to estradiol ratio. Diagnosis is often not made during the neonatal period if genitalia appear female and a karyotype has not been performed for any reason. It may be made when a testis is found during hernia repair. Labs would show the abnormalities described previously and diagnosis is confirmed with hCG stimulation test resulting in increased androstenedione to testosterone ratio as opposed to androgen insensitivity where increased testosterone would be seen.

Cytochrome P450 Oxidoreductase Deficiency

Cytochrome P450 oxidoreductase (POR) is a co-factor for all microsomal P450 enzymes which include 17-hydroxylase, 17,20-lyase, 21-hydroxylase, and aromatase. POR deficiency has been added to the list of 46XX and 46XY DSDs after the discovery of patients with apparent combined 17-hydroxylase and 21-hydroxylase deficiencies.

5α-Reductase Deficiency

5α-Reductase deficiency is an autosomal recessive condition resulting from alterations in the 5α reductase-2 gene. 5α-reductase catalyzes the conversion of testosterone to DHT, which is necessary for normal masculinization of the external genitalia. These patients often have a clitoris-like phallus with severely bifid scrotum and perineoscrotal hypospadias; however, some patients may present with less severe external genitalia ambiguity and rarely isolated microphallus. These patients typically have normal wolffian structures with cryptorchidism and a rudimentary prostate since 5α-reductase is also highly expressed in the prostate. At puberty, these patients will show signs of virilization with increased muscle mass, deepening of the voice, penile growth, and hyperpigmentation of the scrotum and rarely even migration of the testis into the scrotum. They do not experience gynecomastia or male pattern balding, facial hair is decreased, and their prostates remain infantile. Although these patients are usually oligospermic or azoospermic, fertility via intrauterine insemination has been reported.

Diagnosis is made by laboratory studies showing elevated plasma testosterone but low serum DHT. After hCG stimulation the testosterone to DHT ratio will increase to greater than 20:1. The virilization at puberty is believed to occur secondary to markedly higher levels of testosterone binding the androgen receptor or increased activity of the 5α-reductase type 1 isoform.

Androgen Insensitivity Syndromes

Disorders of androgen receptor function are the most common definable cause of 46XY DSD and the undervirilized male. These patients have a 46XY karyotype and present with a broad phenotypic spectrum ranging from normal female external genitalia to normal phenotypic males with infertility.

CAIS is an X-linked disorder affecting 1 in 20,000 live male births. The androgen receptor (AR) gene is found on long arm of chromosome X. 46XY males therefore only have one copy of this gene and mutations in it are present in 95% of CAIS cases. When testosterone or DHT binds the androgen receptor, the receptor is activated resulting in downstream mRNA synthesis and protein production. Abnormalities in the androgen receptor that account for androgen insensitivity syndrome (AIS) include decreased quantity of apparently normal receptors, qualitatively abnormal receptor (such as unstable binding), absence of receptor binding, or defective action after binding such as defective upregulation.

Patients with CAIS will have a normal female phenotype with the exception of decreased axillary and pubic hair and a short, blind-ending vagina (Fig. 25.4). They have bilateral testes, which are often undescended, and lack internal müllerian structures since the testis produce AMH. In some cases, these patients can have well-developed wolffian duct structures but classically do not since testosterone binding is needed to stabilize their development. CAIS is most often diagnosed when patients present with amenorrhea or when a testis is found at the time of inguinal hernia repair, as up to 50% of these patients will have inguinal hernias (Fig. 25.5). Laboratory findings will show a normal male androgen profile and karyotype will confirm 46XY. Pelvic US will confirm the absence of müllerian structures (uterus). Histologically the testes in these patients will have incomplete or absent spermatogenesis with normal or hyperplastic Leydig cells. Endocrine evaluation in the neonatal period demonstrates normal male levels of testosterone, DHT, and gonadotropins. At puberty, gonadotropin levels rise, leading to increased levels of plasma estradiol and also peripheral aromatization of testosterone, which result in development of female secondary sex characteristics, including some breast development.

Partial androgen insensitivity syndrome (PAIS) is also an X-linked disorder and presents with incomplete masculinization with variable ambiguity of the external genitalia. The classic phenotype is perineoscrotal hypospadias with cryptorchidism, rudimentary wolffian structures, gynecomastia and infertility; however, wide variability is possible even within the same family. The diagnosis of PAIS can be difficult given the variation in findings. It should be suspected with 46XY karyotype, ambiguous genitalia,

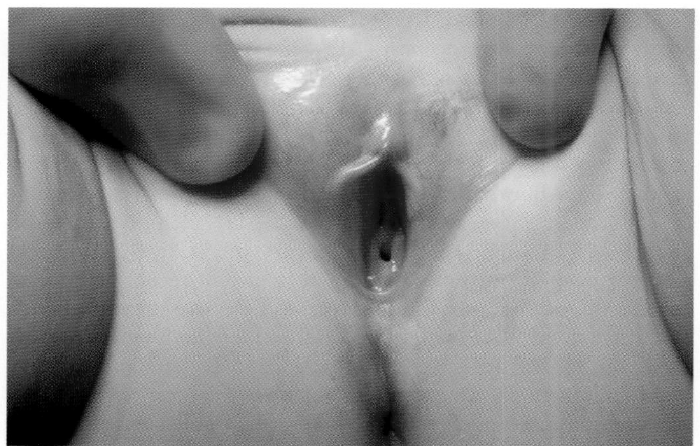

FIGURE 25.4 Normal introitus and female external genitalia appearance in 46XY patient with complete androgen insensitivity syndrome (CAIS).

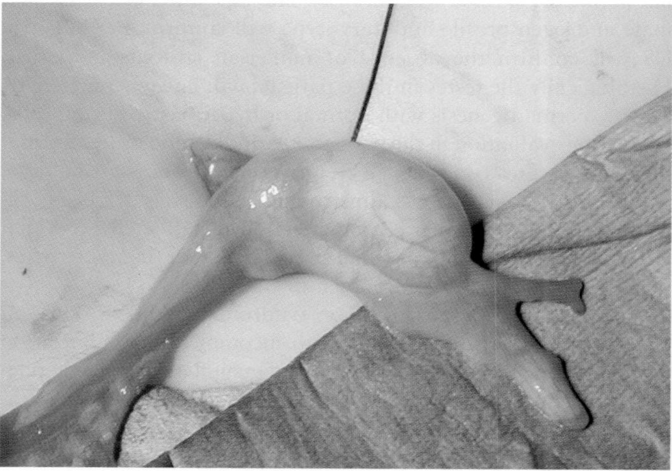

FIGURE 25.5 Abdominal testis identified at the time of inguinal hernia repair in 46XY patient with complete androgen insensitivity syndrome (CAIS).

and absent müllerian structures on pelvic US. Laboratory studies should show a normal male level of androgens and gonadotropins with a normal testosterone to DHT ratio. The androgen receptor gene can be characterized in serum DNA by polymerase chain reaction (PCR) and can confirm the diagnosis as well as whether partial verses complete insensitivity is present.

A variety of mutations of the androgen receptor have been found in patients presenting with male factor infertility with no other identifiable cause. This has led to the classification of a mild AIS with a normal male phenotype or sometimes mild hypospadias but azoospermia or severe oligospermia. On laboratory analysis these patients will have normal to elevated testosterone and LH levels. These findings have suggested that infertility in otherwise normal males may be the result of a mild form of PAIS.

Persistent Müllerian Duct Syndrome (Hernia Uteri Inguinale)

Persistent müllerian duct syndrome (PMDS) is an autosomal recessive disorder that arises from a lack of müllerian inhibiting substance (MIS) (AMH) activity on the ducts leading to persistence of these structures in an otherwise phenotypically normal male. Affected patients often have unilateral or bilateral undescended testis as well as bilateral fallopian tubes, a uterus, and proximal vagina that drains into a prostatic utricle (Fig. 25.6). The majority of patients with PMDS will have intraabdominal testes in a position analogous to ovaries and up to 10% have transverse testicular ectopia with both testes located in the same hernia sac along with the fallopian tubes and uterus. Penile development is normal.

PMDS can be caused by a defect either in the AMH gene or in the receptor. The AMH gene is found on chromosome 19p13 and the receptor is located on chromosome 12q13. Alterations in the AMH gene appear to occur mostly in Arab and Mediterranean countries in families with consanguinity. Patients with type I PMDS will have low or undetectable levels of serum MIS, whereas those with type II PMDS secondary to a defective AMH receptor will have high normal or elevated serum MIS levels. The diagnosis of PMDS is often made at the time of hernia repair or orchiopexy when müllerian structures will be found in the groin along with a normal testis. Historically treatment with hysterectomy was

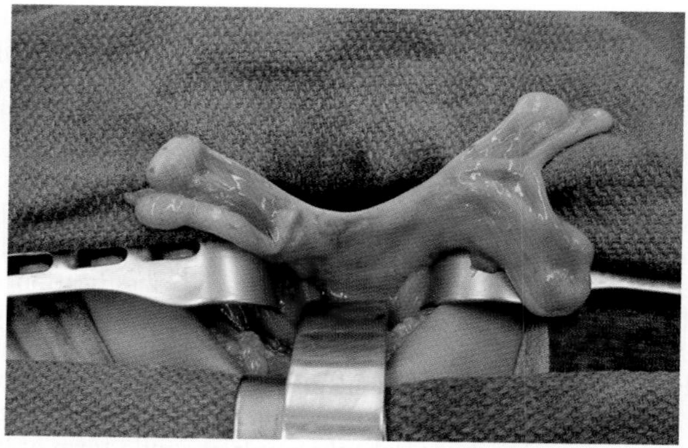

FIGURE 25.6 Retained müllerian structures in 46XY patient with persistent müllerian duct syndrome (PMDS).

recommended but it is now recognized that the vas deferens is closely related to the lateral edge of the müllerian structures and may be injured during attempts to remove them so that leaving the structures in place may be preferable. In addition, skip areas of vassal atresia may occur. This risk of injury to the vas deferens must be weighed against the risk of malignancy in the retained müllerian remnants which is reported to be 3%–8%.

Vanishing Testis Syndrome

Vanishing testis syndrome or congenital anorchia describes a spectrum of anomalies occurring in 46XY patients that result from cessation of testicular function and absence of testes before birth with clear evidence that there was testicular function at some point during development. The etiology of these disorders is not always clear and testicular loss may be related to regression secondary to genetic mutation, a teratogen, or bilateral torsion events. The phenotype present will depend upon when loss of testicular function occurs with more female phenotypes occurring with earlier loss. Loss of testes prior to 8 weeks gestation results in 46XY patients with female external and internal genitalia with agonadism or streak gonads. Loss at 8 to 10 weeks leads to ambiguous genitalia and variable ductal development. Loss of testis function after the critical male differentiation period

(12–14 weeks) results in normal male phenotype externally and internally but anorchia requiring androgen replacement.

46XX Testicular DSD

About 1 in 20,000 phenotypic males have a 46XX karyotype with testicular differentiation despite lacking a Y chromosome. Eighty to 90% of 46XX males result from an anomalous Y to X translocation involving the *SRY* gene during meiosis. The amount of DNA material involved in the exchange varies, but, in general, the greater the amount of Y DNA present, the more masculinized the phenotype. Patients with undetectable *SRY* are more likely to have genital ambiguity. In those patients who are *SRY* negative, sex reversal may occur from downstream mutations of either autosomal of X chromosomal genes that permit testicular differentiation despite the absence of *SRY* or undetected mosaicism.

The majority of 46XX males will have normal male external genitalia development with 10% presenting with ambiguity or hypospadias. All of these patients are infertile with similar findings to Klinefelter syndrome including hypogonadism, gynecomastia, azoospermia, and hyalinization of the seminiferous tubules with low testosterone and elevated FSH and LH at puberty. However, unlike Klinefelter syndrome, these patients have normal skeletal proportions and are shorter. Treatment includes androgen replacement in some cases and also reduction mammoplasty if needed. These patients classically lack germ cell elements, so fertility is not possible even with assisted techniques.

GONADAL DYSGENESIS

This category includes a wide spectrum of anomalies that range from complete absence of gonadal development to delayed gonadal failure. Patients with dysgenetic gonads exhibit ambiguous development of the internal genital ducts, urogenital sinus, and external genitalia.

Complete Gonadal Dysgenesis

Complete gonadal dysgenesis (CGD) can affect both genetic males (46XY CGD) and females (46XX CGD) due to chromosomal abnormalities that result in failure of gonadal development. Unlike patients with Turner syndrome, 46XX CGD patients have normal stature and normal external and internal female genitalia and müllerian strictures; however, they have bilateral streak gonads and sexual infantilism and most commonly present with amenorrhea and lack of puberty. 46XX CGD is most often a sporadic occurrence but familial clusters have also been reported consistent with autosomal recessive inheritance.

Turner syndrome occurs in 1 in 2500 live female births and refers to female patients with only one normally functional X chromosome, as well as short stature, gonadal dysgenesis (GD), a lack of secondary sexual characteristics, and a variety of other somatic abnormalities. The karyotype is classically 45X but mosaic 45X/46XX or less commonly 45X/46XY are also possible. A 45X constitution may be due to nondisjunction or chromosome loss during gametogenesis in either parent resulting in a sperm or ovum without a sex chromosome. Mosaicism is thought to occur in 30%–40% of these patients. It is critical to detect the presence of any occult Y chromosome material as this predisposes patients to possible masculinization and also gonadoblastoma, which may occur in 30%–35%. Given reports of gonadoblastoma occurring as early as 5 months of age, prophylactic excision of streak gonads in Y mosaic Turner syndrome patients is generally recommended.

The typical Turner syndrome stigmata Include short stature, shield chest, wide spaced nipples, cardiac anomalies (coarctation of the aorta), and webbed neck. It is believed that in Turner syndrome, follicular cells that normally surround the germ cells and protect them are inadequate leading to rapid attrition of oocytes via apoptosis with few or no oocytes remaining by birth, resulting in streak gonads. Similar to 46XX CGD patients, they will have sexual infantilism and amenorrhea, but because of the associated features, this condition is more commonly detected prior to puberty. Though bilateral streak gonads are the rule, there have been descriptions of primary follicles in the genital ridges of some 45X individual correlating to rare occurrences of menarche. Rare conceptions have been documented despite karyotyping revealing only 45X cell lines.

46XY CGD, also called XY sex reversal or Swyer syndrome, occurs when there is failure of testicular development despite the presence of a Y chromosome. Because testes do not develop, there is no testosterone or MIS production either resulting in phenotypically female external genitalia and normal müllerian duct structures (fallopian tubes, uterus, and vagina). These patients will display sexual infantilism and amenorrhea at puberty, and this is often how they initially present given normal female phenotype present at birth. It is a heterogenous condition that can result from mutations or deletions in any of the genes involved in the testis differentiation cascade including *SRY* and others such as *WT1*, *DAX1*, or *SOX9*, or duplications of the *DSS* locus on the X chromosome.

Histologic analysis of dysgenetic gonads of XY males has revealed that those with normal *SRY* had some element of rete testis and tubular function, whereas those with *SRY* mutations had completely undifferentiated gonads similar to those of 45X individuals. Thus, *SRY* may have a direct role in testicular formation in addition to its indirect role in initiating the male differentiation cascade. Duplication of the *DSS* (dosage-sensitive sex reversal) locus has been associated with 46XY GD and other anomalies. It has been mapped to the Xp21 region, which contains the *DAX1* gene. Mutations in *DAX1* can cause X-linked congenital adrenal hypoplasia and hypogonadotropic hypogonadism. It is hypothesized that the duplicated gene escapes normal X inactivation, therefore disrupting testis formation despite the presence of *SRY*. Similar to other forms of GD, these patients are at increased risk of germ cell tumors, most commonly gonadoblastoma, which occur in up to 35% by 30 years of age.

Noonan syndrome patients (often referred to as *male Turner syndrome*) display Turner-like stigmata including short stature, webbed neck, and right heart disease. They have a normal 46XY sex chromosome constitution often with cryptorchidism of hypoplastic testes. Puberty is delayed and androgen deficiency can be seen. However, fertility may occur in the absence of cryptorchidism. Most cases are sporadic, but familial clusters are consistent with an autosomal dominant inheritance.

Partial Gonadal Dysgenesis

Partial gonadal dysgenesis (PGD) includes disorders with variable degrees of bilateral testicular dysgenesis and usually a 46XY karyotype. They occur secondary to impaired testicular development despite the presence of *SRY*. This results in a variable degree of ambiguous genitalia with undescended testes depending upon the ability of the testis to produce testosterone. Internally, there is also variability from normal wolffian structures to persistence of rudimentary müllerian structures based upon the local secretion of MIS by the dysgenetic testes. These patients are also at increased risk of gonadoblastoma.

Mixed gonadal dysgenesis (MGD) is characterized by a unilateral streak gonad and contralateral dysgenetic testis most commonly with karyotype 45X/46XY. The intraabdominal streak gonad is typically associated with ipsilateral rudimentary müllerian structures secondary to a lack of local paracrine MIS activity. The dysgenetic testis can be undescended or in a normal scrotal position and varying degrees of ambiguous genitalia are present. MGD is the second most common cause of ambiguous genitalia presenting in the newborn period (after CAH) so must be kept in the differential diagnosis.

The risk for developing gonadoblastoma or dysgerminoma in MGD is 15% to 35% and can occur in both the dysgenetic testis and streak gonad. The risk of tumor has been reported to be highest (approximately 50%) with streak gonads and ambiguous genitalia versus closer to 10% in those with scrotal testis and mild undervirilization. Patients with MGD are also at increased risk of Wilms tumor and a large number of patients with Denys-Drash syndrome have MGD.

Male patients with Denys-Drash syndrome have ambiguous genitalia with streak or dysgenetic gonads, progressive neuropathy, and Wilms tumor. Analysis of these patients revealed heterozygous mutations of the Wilms tumor suppressor gene (WT1) at 11p13. Most *WT1* mutations in Denys-Drash syndrome occur de novo and act as dominant negative mutations.

The WAGR syndrome (Wilms tumor, Aniridia, Genitourinary [GU] abnormalities, developmental delay) is also associated with *WT1* alterations (heterozygous deletions). The GU anomalies in the WAGR syndrome are usually less severe than in Denys-Drash syndrome.

The *SOX9* gene (17q24.3-25.1) has been associated with campomelic dysplasia, an often lethal skeletal malformation, and 46XY GD. Affected 46XY males have phenotypic variability from normal males to normal females, depending on the function of the gonads. The *SOX9* protein is expressed in the developing gonad, rete testis, seminiferous tubules, and skeletal tissue.

OVOTESTICULAR DSD

Ovotesticular DSD occurs when an individual is born with both ovarian and testicular tissue present. Ovotestis is the most common gonad present and cases of ovotesticular DSD can be classified into three groups based upon the gonads present: (1) lateral with one testis and one ovary, (2) bilateral with two ovotestes, and (3) unilateral with an ovotestis and either an ovary or testis contralaterally. The development of the internal duct structures is determined based upon the local hormonal effects of the ipsilateral gonad and the external genitalia are ambiguous with hypospadias, cryptorchidism, and incomplete fusion of the labioscrotal folds. The ovarian portion of ovotestis may be normal whereas the testicular portion is typically dysgenetic. Rare ovulation and pregnancy has been reported for female 46XX ovotesticular DSDs but no clear male fertility documented.

The most common karyotype is 46XX, followed by 46XX/46XY mosaicism and 46XY. Most 46XX ovotesticular DSD patients are *SRY* negative and the genes responsible have not yet been identified. Although sex chromosome mosaicism arises from mitotic or meiotic errors, 46XX/46XY chimerism is usually a result of double fertilization (an X sperm and a Y sperm) or, less commonly, fusion of two normally fertilized ova. Thus, chimeric patients have two distinct cell populations. The least common form of ovotesticular DSD, 46XY, may result from a cryptic 46XX cell line or gonadal mosaicism with a mutated sex determination gene. While ovotesticular DSD is rare, accounting for 3%–10% of DSD worldwide, it seems to be more common in South Africa representing approximately 50% of DSD in this population.

OTHER DSD

Mayer-Rokitansky-Küster-Hauser Syndrome

Mayer-Rokitansky-Küster-Hauser (MRKH) syndrome is a rare disorder involving congenital absence of the uterus and vagina that occurs in 1 in 4000 to 5000 female births. These individuals have a 46XY karyotype with normal external genitalia and secondary sexual characteristics. Though the external genitalia appear normal, they have only a shallow vaginal pouch and uterine remnants. Normal ovaries with normal function as well as normal fallopian tubes are present. The genetic basis for this DSD is largely unknown but there has been some suggestion of the involvement of *WNT4*. These patients will most often present with primary amenorrhea although infertility or dyspareunia may also bring them to attention. Importantly, upper urinary tract anomalies including renal agenesis, pelvic, or horseshoe kidney are present in approximately one-third of MRKH patients.

Evaluation and Management of Ambiguous Genitalia at Birth

It is important to recognize that ambiguous genitalia in the neonate represents a medical emergency and requires prompt and thorough evaluation to rule out life-threatening causes (i.e., CAH). Additionally when a prenatal diagnosis is not suspected, this can represent a psychosocial emergency for the family requiring sensitivity and support from the medical team. Evaluation and management of these patients is best accomplished via a pediatric multidisciplinary team approach including a urologist, endocrinologist, geneticist, and psychiatrist or psychologist. The goal should be to make a precise diagnosis and initiate medical therapy if warranted, and always with the help of the parents, to agree upon a proper gender of rearing based upon the diagnosis, child's individual anatomy, functional potential of the genitalia, and reproductive potential.

HISTORY AND PHYSICAL EXAMINATION

A thorough patient and family history should be obtained, including prematurity, any abnormalities on prenatal US, whether a fetal karyotype was performed, and if there was any discordance of this with prenatal US findings. The mother should also be questioned regarding ingestion of any exogenous hormones such as those used for assisted reproductive techniques and maternal use of steroids or contraceptives during the pregnancy. Family history of sudden infant death, urologic abnormalities, infertility, amenorrhea, hirsutism, and consanguinity may also be helpful. Any masculinization or cushingoid appearance of the mother is important to note as well.

On physical examination, any dysmorphic features such as a short, broad neck or widely spaced nipples should be noted. A genital exam should be performed in a warm room with the patient supine in the frog leg position. Phallic size should be documented included width and stretched length. This can be easily accomplished by grasping the glans with a gauze pad, pressing down on the penopubic angle with a cotton tip applicator and stretching the penis against the applicator to measure the dorsal length. The position of the urethral meatus and degree of phallus curvature should also be recorded (Fig. 25.7). The number of perineal openings—three (urethra, vagina, anus) or two (urethra or urogenital sinus, anus)—is important to note as well. Rectal exam to palpate for a uterus can be helpful.

The finding of palpable versus absent gonads on exam is of critical importance to narrowing the differential diagnosis (Fig. 25.1). The inguinal exam for palpable gonads should be performed with warmed hands beginning at the anterior superior iliac crest and sweeping the groin from lateral to medial with the nondominant hand. Once a gonad is palpated, it should be grasped with the dominant hand while the other hand continues to sweep toward the scrotum in an attempt to bring the gonad down. The size, location, and texture of both gonads should be noted if palpable.

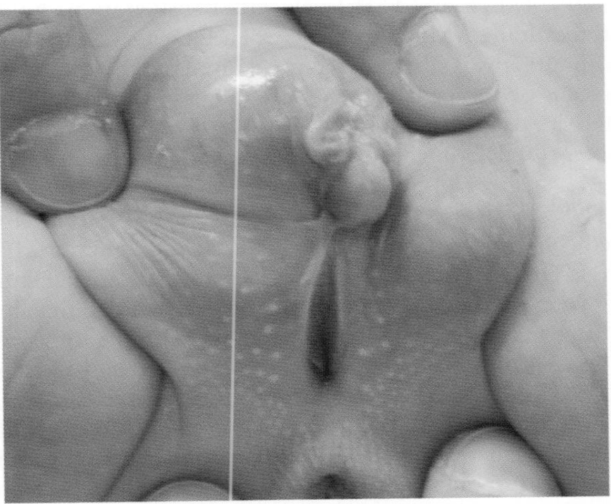

FIGURE 25.7 46XY patient with severe hypospadias and bilateral cryptorchidism secondary to 46XY testicular dysgenesis.

The undescended testis can be found anywhere along the normal path of descent including the inguinal canal to the scrotum or ectopically in the superficial inguinal pouch or occasionally femoral, perineal, or contralateral scrotal regions. The development and pigmentation of the labioscrotal folds can also be helpful.

Unless associated with a patent process vaginalis, ovaries and streak gonads do not descend and ovotestes do so rarely. Therefore, any palpable gonad is likely a testis and can help narrow the differential. If gonads are nonpalpable bilaterally any DSD diagnosis is possible with 46XX CAH being most common. If one gonad is palpable, 46XX DSD, CGD is ruled out. If both gonads are palpable, 46XY DSD and less commonly ovotesticular DSD are the likely diagnoses. Importantly, the patient with bilateral or unilateral nonpalpable gonads and hypospadias should be regarded as having DSD until proven otherwise even when the genitalia are not ambiguous.

LABORATORY STUDIES

All patients should have a karyotype, with FISH for Y chromosome as indicated, serum electrolytes, 17OH-progesterone (17OHP), T, LH, and FSH levels, and consideration should be given to adding AMH and DHT when indicated as well. These tests should always be ordered after discussion with and at the discretion of the pediatric endocrinologist. Markedly elevated 17OHP levels indicate 21OHD. If 17OHP values are not suggestive of 21OHD, a high-dose ACTH test can identify rare forms of CAH, such as 11OHD. Markedly elevated 11-deoxycortisol and DOC levels are seen in 11OHD. If the 17OHP level is elevated, 11-deoxycortisol and DOC levels differentiate 21OHD from 11OHD. If the 17OHP level is normal, a T:DHT ratio along with androgen precursors, such as androstendione, before and after hCG stimulation will help elucidate the 46,XY DSD etiology. The hCG stimulation test is not needed in the first 60 to 90 days of life when there is a natural gonadotropin surge with a resultant increase in T level. After this age, an hCG test would be needed to further examine androgen imbalance as above. Either a failure to respond to hCG or low level of AMH, in combination with elevated LH and FSH levels during the mini-puberty of infancy, is indicative of functional anorchia in 46XY DSD.

IMAGING

Pelvic US is useful in assessing for the presence or absence of müllerian structures. A genitogram obtained with fluoroscopy and contrast injection through a catheter or catheters can be helpful in evaluating a urogenital sinus and understanding the level of confluence of the urethra and vagina. MRI with gadolinium may also be used to provide greater anatomic detail for complex anomalies. This can require general anesthesia in some children, but a "feed and swaddle" technique has been successful in allowing MRI of the newborn to be obtained without the need for anesthesia. Diagnostic laparoscopy is often used to evaluate for the presence and relationship of wolffian and müllerian ductal structures as well as allow for visualization of the gonads with bilateral deep longitudinal gonadal biopsies for histologic evaluation prior to making a decision as to how to manage the gonads going forward.

Treatment Options and Indications

Much current research is aimed at understanding the influence of androgens on the fetal and newborn brain and its relationship to gender identity. Diagnosis and management of these children is very individualized and should always involve a team approach, which includes the pediatric urologist, endocrinologist, geneticist, psychologist, and the child's parents. The general management considerations for CAH and DSD are discussed later.

46XX-CAH

Early diagnosis and treatment of newborns with CAH is essential to prevent potentially life-threatening electrolyte abnormalities. Initial treatment is aimed at correcting dehydration and salt losses with fluid therapy and mineralocorticoid replacement. Once the diagnosis is confirmed, glucocorticoid replacement with hydrocortisone is then added. In all CAH patients, steroid replacement is the cornerstone of medical management as this both replaces the needed steroids and suppresses the increased ACTH secretion that causes a buildup of precursors and androgens which give rise to the manifestations of virilization and hypertension. Glucocorticoid and mineralocorticoid therapy replacement is typically lifelong with stress dosing needed at times of illness or surgery.

Surgical decisions are made by the parents with information and counseling by the local multidisciplinary team along with peer and advocate support groups. Surgery remains common in the management of infants with CAH, including clitoriplasty, vaginoplasty and labiaplasty. The practice of early surgical intervention has recently been questioned especially with increasing consideration for the irreversible nature of some procedures. Conversely, the consequences of raising children with highly ambiguous genitalia is mostly unknown, as are the results of deferring surgery until the pediatric patients are old enough to make the decision themselves. Surgery has three main aims: reducing the size of the enlarged masculinized clitoris, reconstructing the female labia, and increasing the opening and possibly length of the vagina. These procedures have gone through many changes during the history of surgery. Surgical technique continues to be revised to optimize the girl's external appearance and functional size while maintaining adequate sensation.

Reduction clitoroplasty may be employed for infants with severe clitoromegaly. The central portions of the corporal bodies are excised, and the surgeon preserves the dorsal neurovascular bundles by incising Buck fascia laterally at the 3 o'clock and 9 o'clock positions. The remaining proximal and distal portions of the bodies are then reapproximated and placed in the investing fascia. This optimizes future erectile function and sensation. A glansplasty for an extremely large glans is rarely indicated. A vulvoplasty is carried out by extending the incision for the clitoroplasty on either side of the midline strip of introital tissue down to the level of the vaginal orifice as labia minora. Redundant labial scrotal skin is brought down as preputial flaps to form the labia majora.

The position of the vagina should be accurately determined preoperatively by the genitogram as part of the workup for DSD. There are four main types of vaginal repair: a simple "cutback" of the perineum, a "flap" vaginoplasty, a "pull-through" vaginoplasty, or a more extensive rotation of skin flaps or segmental bowel interposition. Usually a low vaginoplasty can be performed at the same time as the clitoroplasty. When the vagina opens very low, a simple cutback with a vertical midline incision may be all that is needed to open the introitus. Usually, however, a posterior-based U-shaped flap is necessary for a tension-free anastomosis, reducing the risks of postoperative vaginal stenosis. Exposure of the high vagina requires either a perineal approach, a posterior vaginoplasty, or an anterior sagittal transanorectal vaginoplasty. When the vagina is extremely high and small, replacement with a bowel segment will be necessary, usually with the sigmoid colon.

46XY DSD

Decreased masculinization (hypospadias with cryptorchidism or more ambiguous development) is seen in most patients with XY DSD. In untreated patients with 5α-reductase deficiency, significant virilization occurs at puberty as testosterone levels increase into the adult male range, whereas DHT remains disproportionately low. Treatment is currently unclear for this enzyme deficiency when diagnosed in infancy. Male gender assignment has been recommended because the natural history of this deficiency is virilization at puberty with subsequent change to male gender. However, this decision requires surgical hypospadias repair and orchiopexy with male hormonal replacement.

Rarely do patients with dysgenetic testes have fully masculinized external genitalia. The surgical issues are dependent on the degree of virilization in each individual case. This will also influence the decision process of gender assignment. If a 46XY infant with testicular dysgenesis is raised as male, he will need a hypospadias repair, orchiopexy, or possibly orchiectomy. Müllerian ducts have usually not fully regressed and may be fully or partially removed at the time of other repairs to facilitate orchiopexies. Extensive dissection behind the bladder neck and up to the area where the müllerian structures insert into the urethra is usually contraindicated to avoid damage to the sphincter mechanism risking incontinence. Both open and laparoscopic excisions have been reported. Arguments for removal of the müllerian structures include the possibility of cyclic hematuria postpuberty or the formation of stones or chronic urinary tract infections if the continuity with the urethra is maintained and stasis occurs in a dilated müllerian remnant. Arguments against removal maintain that complications from the structures are uncommon and their removal risks injury to the vas deferens, the bladder neck, and the urethral sphincter.

Dysgenetic testes may appear normal grossly but microscopically are disorganized and poorly formed; thus, a biopsy of the gonad is recommended in most children undergoing DSD evaluation. Currently, the recommendation is to remove an undescended dysgenetic testis because of the risk of malignancy though orchiopexy and follow-up is also acceptable. In 45X/46XY patients, if the biopsy is normal and the testis is scrotal or can be placed in the scrotum, it should not be removed, but a risk of malignancy correlates with the extent of testicular decent as discussed previously and careful surveillance is needed. Tumors have also been reported in scrotal dysgenetic testes. A scrotal testis needs to be followed very closely for this reason. The possibility does exist of a male gender in these patients who would require a hypospadias repair yet would have removal of severely dysgenetic testis requiring replacement hormones. It would seem obvious that treatment in these cases needs to be individualized. The child's parents should discuss with the pediatric urologist, endocrinologist, geneticist, and psychiatrist the issues of T imprinting in utero, the need for hormones prepuberty and postpuberty, the degree of masculinization, the function of the testis, and the extent of surgery that is required.

Affected boys with errors in testosterone production are undermasculinized with varied degrees of hypospadias, cryptorchidism, bifid scrotum, or a blind vaginal pouch. For the patient reared as a boy, testosterone therapy may be indicated to augment penile size and to aid in the hypospadias repair. Some enzyme deficiencies require glucocorticoid and mineralocorticoid replacement (CAH as discussed earlier), and all of these patients need testosterone replacement at puberty for masculinization. Gonadectomy is recommended in 46XY patients raised as girls to address the risk of tumor formation in the future.

Traditionally, a child with CAIS would be raised as a girl. Most of these children are not diagnosed until a workup is performed when amenorrhea occurs at puberty. Occasionally, it is discovered at the time of inguinal hernia repair or when a prenatal karyotype does not match the external phenotype of the newborn child. If the child is to be raised female, an orchiectomy is recommended for future cancer risk. The testes are at risk for cancer development and the incidence of malignant tumors is estimated to be 5% to 10%. Seminoma is the most common tumor seen, but nonseminomatous germ cell tumors and other malignancies have also been reported. Tumor risks appear to be greater in older patients and in those with partial rather than complete androgen insensitivity; tumor formation appears to occur after puberty. Intratubular germ cell neoplasia has been identified in prepubertal boys with partial AIS but not complete AIS. Vaginal dilation or vaginal augmentation may or may not be needed. This usually is reserved until after puberty and a number of techniques are available. In patients with partial AIS, orchiectomy is recommended soon after diagnosis to avoid further virilization in patients who will be raised in the female gender. Male gender assignment is usually successful in AIS patients with a predominantly male phenotype; however, predicting the adequacy of masculinization in adulthood may not be possible based on the maternal family history or characterization of the AR genetic defect. Some children respond well to high-dose androgen therapy, but its durability is not yet clear.

The timing of gonadectomy is controversial (prepuberty versus postpuberty), and endocrine, oncologic, and psychological issues must be taken into account. The incidence of malignancy associated with CAIS is about 0.8% and usually occurs after puberty, though there has been a case report of a malignant abdominal yolk sac tumor in a 17-month-old child, uncommon carcinoma in situ (CIS), and several reports of benign abdominal masses. The incidence of tumor formation in PAIS is much higher, and early gonadectomy is recommended unless the testis can be brought into the scrotum and adequately monitored. In an infant with complete AIS, some advocate that the testes should be left in place until after puberty to take advantage of the endogenous hormonal function, and in this way, natural female pubertal changes can occur by testosterone conversion to estrogen, which can then be augmented by exogenous estrogen. These purported advantages, though, have not been documented in a scientific study.

After puberty is completed, the testes would be removed and replacement estrogen continued. Other risks to be discussed include: inguinal testes are easily injured; psychologic issues, including explaining to a mature postpubertal patient of the need to remove her testes; the risk of testis cancer increases if the patient is lost to follow-up care; and early orchiectomy requires full replacement hormones for pubertal changes.

GONADAL DYSGENESIS

Management of the gonads in patients with gonadal dysgenesis DSD is an important consideration. There is increased risk of gonadoblastoma and dysgerminoma in dysgenetic gonads if any Y chromosome material is present, so removal in these cases is typically recommended. Streak gonads do not descend, but they may be palpable as a small remnant of tissue in an inguinal hernia sac. If a dysgenetic testis is in the inguinal position, it can be removed using an incision in the groin as for a traditional orchiopexy or hernia repair. If the gonad is in the abdomen as is more often the case, then the treatment options include open abdominal exploration and removal of the gonads or laparoscopic gonadectomy, which usually preferred.

If these patients are raised male and the testicles can be brought to the scrotum, a careful decision should be made between orchiopexy verses prophylactic gonadectomy. Traditionally about two-thirds of MGD and PGD patients have been raised as female and typically the degree of masculinization of the genitalia can serve as a guide in this decision. In cases of incomplete GD, the testis may be able to produce some meaningful testosterone to decrease the amount of supplementation needed for normal phenotypic male appearance; however, if the dysgenetic testes are not removed, they need to be carefully monitored for the development of malignancy.

Growth hormone supplementation is usually recommended early in childhood, and estrogen or testosterone therapy is begun after puberty to optimize the patient's height and maintain appropriate secondary sexual characteristics. Although rare cases of spontaneous pregnancy have been reported, infertility usually occurs. Pregnancy may be possible using donor eggs and assisted reproductive techniques.

OVOTESTICULAR DSD

Generally, a female sex has been assigned to most patients because of the presence of a vagina, uterus, and ovarian tissue and the possibility of fertility in some of these patients if raised female. Less commonly, the patient has a 46XY karyotype with adequate penile development and without a uterus present, so a male sex assignment might be more appropriate. The decision of sex of rearing should always be deferred until the child has had an adequate evaluation of the GU system. Usually, the internal organs need to be visualized and the gonads biopsied. This can be done through an open abdominal exploration or laparoscopically.

If raised female, the child should have dysgenetic testicular tissue removed because of the risk of malignancy. For patients who have a separate ovary, this is straightforward; however, with an ovotestis, a cleavage plane between the testicular and ovarian portions may or may not be present allowing for the selective removal of the testicular tissue. Successful removal of all testicular tissue can be confirmed with a postoperative hCG stimulation test. If vaginoplasty is needed this can be performed early or deferred until puberty. When normal ovarian tissue is preserved, sufficient ovarian function may be present at puberty, though sometimes hormonal supplementation is needed.

If the child is raised male, he should have any hypospadias or cryptorchidism repaired as an infant. Testosterone supplementation may be needed if the amount of testicular tissue present is inadequate to begin or continue puberty. Careful surveillance for testicular tumor is needed if testicular tissue is preserved and gonadectomy after puberty may be beneficial given the high risk for malignancy and low likelihood of male fertility.

A persistent müllerian duct, such as a uterus and fallopian tubes, has usually not fully regressed and connects to the urethra near the bladder at the verumontanum. If there is a decision to rear the child as a boy, the structures may be left in place as removal may injure the vas deferens which usually runs alongside the uterus. As previously discussed, retained female structures have the potential for urinary tract infections, stones, or even cyclic hematuria at puberty.

Gender

Gender choice in the patient with DSD can be a difficult decision for both parents and physicians. There are two differing views regarding timing of gender assignment. Choice of genital reconstructive surgery shortly after birth has the goal of avoiding any internal conflicts for the patient or external familial or societal conflicts as the child develops. Opponents argue that the decision of gender assignment should be made by the affected individual once they are old enough to participate in decision-making after puberty. They argue that neither physicians nor the patient's family can predict gender identity, so a decision should be deferred, and no surgical reconstruction undertaken in early childhood. Regardless of the timing of the decision, it should be guided by three equally important factors: the functional and anatomic abilities of the genitalia (phallus or vaginal size, fertility potential), the cause of the DSD, and the family's values and desires. It is important to remember that the optimal gender confers reproductive potential (if possible), good sexual function, minimal medical procedures, an overall gender appropriate appearance, a stable gender identity, and psychosocial well-being.

One factor in the decision-making process that is becoming clearer is the large body of evidence to support the notion that the prenatal and postnatal hormonal milieu has an important role in predicting gender and sexual identity. For instance, genetically female rats given testosterone shortly after birth do not exhibit typical female behavior during adulthood. One study showed that among CAH girls with excessive prenatal androgen exposure, many have tomboyish personalities and are more likely to have bisexual or homosexual interests than women without CAH. Among women affected by CAH from 21-OH deficiencies, there appears to be outcome differences between the more severe salt-losing form and simple virilizing forms. Women with simple masculinizing CAH (when the deficiency is partial) reported greater satisfaction and fewer concerns with regard to their psychosexual outcomes compared to women with the more severe salt-losing form.

In general, newborns with ambiguous genitalia from CAH have normal ovaries and uterus and should be raised as females. In cases of bilateral testicular dysgenesis where a vagina and uterus are present, female assignment may be desirable. Likewise, in cases of CAIS, a female orientation is correct. For most other instances of partial resistance, it is desirable to opt for male rearing. Male rearing is also appropriate when a deficit in 5α-reductase is identified because further virilization occurs during puberty. In cases where ovarian function may be preserved, female assignment is preferable for these cases of ovotesticular DSD. When a decision for female rearing is made in 46XY DSD, removal of testicular tissue is generally recommended. If raised as males, these patients require careful follow-up because of the increased risk of gonadal tumors.

Follow-Up

Treatment of the child with ambiguous genitalia should not end with the first postoperative visit. A boy should be evaluated 6 to 12 months after orchiopexy for testes size, location, and viability. The parents should be made aware of the issues regarding increased malignancy risk and infertility. Starting at puberty, the boy should be taught how to perform monthly testicular self-exams and offered a semen analysis check at age 18. Orchiopexy is not protective against testis cancer development, but it does allow easier palpation for subsequent physical exams. Although intraabdominal testes comprise only 10% to 15% of all undescended testes, they account for almost 50% of those testes that develop cancer. The most common tumor in an undescended testis is a seminoma. Up to 35% of dysgenetic testes may develop cancer, most commonly a benign tumor called gonadoblastoma. Although this tumor does not spread, it can develop into a malignant form called a dysgerminoma. Patients with a 45X/45XY mosaic karyotype also have an increased risk of CIS. Some surgeons have recommended US and biopsy of a testis at puberty. US is then performed yearly until age 20 when a repeat biopsy is performed. Absence of CIS at age 20 years suggests that the risk of CIS is minimal.

The patient with hypospadias repaired as a child should remain in follow-up with his physician to identify and correct any long-term complications of the surgery. It is also important to document adequate control of voiding and the force of urinary stream. There appears to be no increase in infertility from a purely urethral point of view rather than that previously described for cryptorchidism.

Cosmetic and functional results improve yearly with advances in optical magnification, instrumentation and sutures, and tissue handling. Continuous research in this area allows the surgeon to refine the technique and provide the patient with the best repair possible. Girls who have undergone a feminizing genitoplasty require long-term follow-up for issues of menstruation, intercourse, and sensation as previously described. With proper care, DSD individuals should be able to lead well-adjusted lives and ultimately obtain sexual satisfaction. Simple yet comprehensive discussions with all physicians involved and the parents must take into account parental anxieties and social, cultural, and religious views regarding gender choice.

New molecular biology techniques have allowed genetic analysis to be commonplace for patient evaluation. As new genes have been described, a complex yet specific pathway of sex determination and development has evolved that allows us to formulate clinical algorithms for both prenatal and postnatal diagnosis and treatment. The future holds great promise for the further definition of the genes involved in urogenital development and function.

Congenital Anomalies

Jason P. Van Batavia, MD, and Karl Godlewski, MD

Upper Urinary Tract

ABNORMALITIES OF THE KIDNEY

1. **Simple ectopia**

   The incidence of renal ectopia is approximately 1 per 900 (pelvic: 1 per 3000, solitary: 1 per 22,000; bilateral: 10%) with a left-sided predominance. Associated findings include decreased size, persistent fetal lobulations, anterior or horizontal renal pelvis, anomalous vasculature, contralateral agenesis, hydronephrosis (56%), and vesicoureteral reflux (VUR, 30%). In females, 20%–60% have müllerian anomalies. In males, 10%–20% have associated genital defects including undescended testes, hypospadias, or urethral duplication. The adrenal gland is in a normal location.

   A workup for simple ectopia typically includes ultrasound (US; to monitor for dilatation and growth of kidneys) and possibly a voiding cystourethrography (considered routine in the past, now more selective and only in those with urinary tract infection [UTI]). These patients may also be at an increased risk for stone formation.

2. **Thoracic ectopia**

   Thoracic ectopia comprises less than 5% of ectopic kidneys (overall incidence 1:13,000). It remains uncertain whether the origin is a delayed closure of diaphragmatic anlage, versus accelerated renal ascent. The kidney is located in the posterior mediastinum (Foramen of Bochdalek) and is not within the pleural cavity. The adrenal gland is located in its normal location. A diagnosis is typically made on a plain chest radiograph. No treatment is required.

3. **Crossed ectopia and fusion (Bauer)** (Fig. 26.1)
Crossed ectopia is defined as a kidney located on the side opposite that which its respective ureter inserts into the bladder. Over 90% of all crossed ectopic kidneys are fused. The incidence is 1 per 1000 to 1 per 2000, with a 2:1 male predominance and 3:1 left-crossed predominance. The fusion originates from an abnormal migration of ureteral bud or rotation of caudal end of fetus at the time of bud formation. Associated findings include multiple or anomalous vessels arising from the ipsilateral side of the aorta, ureteropelvic junction (UPJ) obstruction (29%), and VUR (15%). Approximately 20%–50% of those with solitary crossed kidney have associated genital, skeletal, and hindgut anomalies. A diagnosis can be made with US, renal scan, or magnetic resonance urography (MRU).
4. **Horseshoe kidney**
Horseshoe kidney is the most common fusion anomaly with an incidence of 1 in 400 live births and a 2:1 male predominance. It is caused by a fusion of the lower poles before or during rotation (4 to 6 weeks gestation). Ascent is impeded by the inferior mesenteric artery (IMA). The isthmus usually consists of bulky, parenchymal tissue with its own blood supply. The kidney units fail to rotate and so calyces face posteriorly and the renal pelvis is anterior. Blood supply is variable and only 30% have just one renal artery to each kidney. Patients can suffer from associated

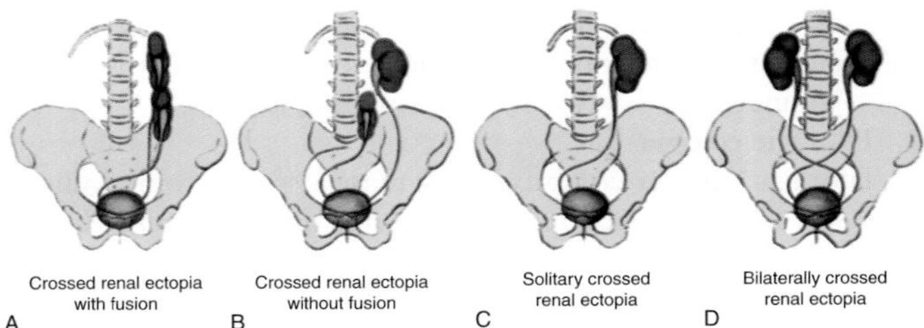

FIGURE 26.1 **(A–D) Four types of crossed renal ectopia.** (From Shapiro E, Bauer SB, Chow JS. Anomalies of the upper urinary tract. In: Partin AW, Dmochowski RR, Kavoussi LR, Peters C, Wein AJ, eds. *Campbell-Walsh-Wein Urology*. 12th ed. Philadelphia: Elsevier; 2020.)

anomalies of the skeletal, cardiovascular, and central nervous systems. Other associated anomalies include hypospadias and cryptorchidism (4%), bicornuate uterus (7%), duplex ureters (10%), UPJ obstruction (previously thought to occur in up to 33%), and nephrolithiasis (17%). As many as 20% of trisomy 18 and up to 60% of Turner syndrome patients have a horseshoe kidney. Excluding other anomalies, survival is not affected. Hydronephrosis is commonly seen but rarely represents true obstruction (Fig. 26.2).

5. **Bilateral renal agenesis**
   The incidence of bilateral renal agenesis is 1 per 4800 births or 1 per 400 newborn autopsies (75% are male) and the diagnosis is typically lethal. It originates from either failure of ureteral bud development from the Wolffian duct or absence of the nephrogenic ridge. Renal agenesis is associated with absent renal arteries (25%), complete ureteral atresia in (> 90%), bladder atresia or severely hypoplastic bladder (50%), and flattened, but normal, adrenal glands. It is also associated with *Potter syndrome* characterized by intrauterine growth retardation (IUGR), Potter facies (prominent epicanthal folds, flat nasal bridge), oligohydramnios, pulmonary hypoplasia, bowed limbs, and gastrointestinal (GI) anomalies (60%). Bilateral renal agenesis may result from inactivation of *PAX2/8, Gata3, Lim1* or *Grem1* genes.
6. **Unilateral renal agenesis**
   The incidence of unilateral renal agenesis (URA) is 1 per 1100 births. It occurs more often in males than in females (1.8:1) and the left kidney is more often absent. Embryologically, the condition is a result of ureteral bud failure. Associated findings include an absent ureter with hemitrigone (60%), contralateral UPJ or ureterovesical junction (UVJ) obstruction (11% and 7%, respectively), VUR (30%), adrenal agenesis (10%), and genital anomalies (20%–40% in both sexes). Females can suffer from multiple müllerian anomalies including unicornuate uterus, bicornuate uterus with rudimentary horn on affected side, uterovaginal atresia (Mayer-Rokitansky-Küster-Hauser syndrome), uterus didelphys, and proximal vaginal agenesis. In males, the Wolffian

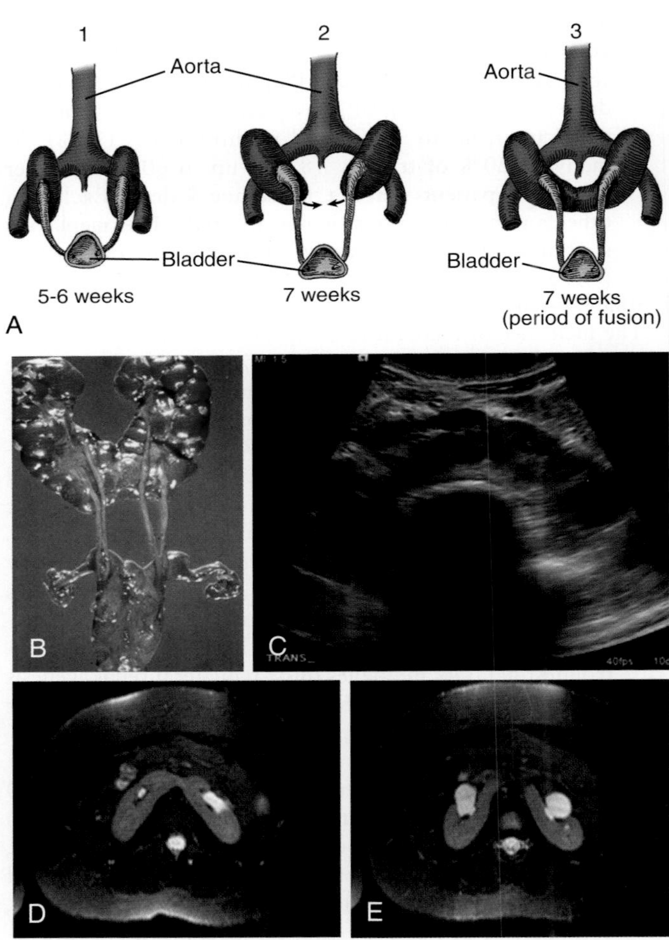

FIGURE 26.2 (A) Embryogenesis of horseshoe kidney. The lower poles of the two kidneys touch and fuse as they cross the iliac arteries *(1, 2)*. Ascent is stopped when the fused kidneys reach the junction of the aorta and inferior mesenteric artery *(3)*. (B) Postmortem specimen showing horseshoe kidney with bilateral duplicated ureters. (C) Ultrasonogram of horseshoe kidney at the level of the isthmus. (D) Magnetic resonance urogram (MRU) shows axial T2 fat-saturated image at the level of the isthmus. (E) Axial T2 fat-saturated image demonstrates extrarenal pelvis.

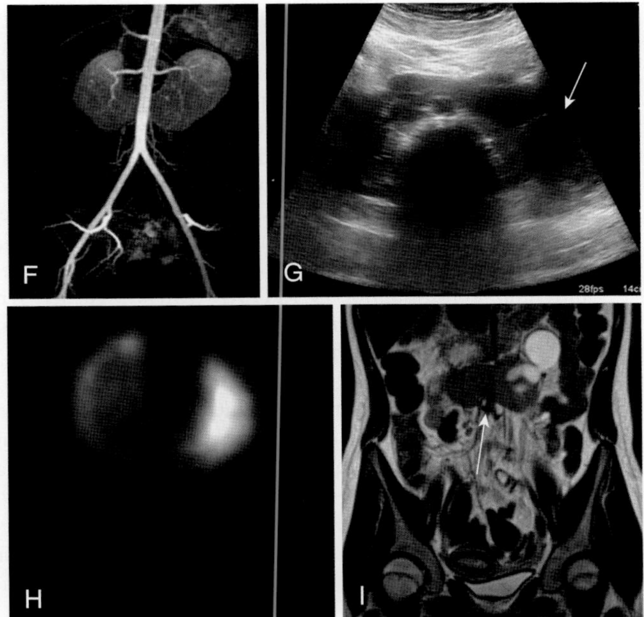

FIGURE 26.2, Cont'd (F) Angiographic sequence shows variable blood supply to the kidney. (G) Transverse ultrasonogram of 14-year-old girl with left flank pain found to have marked left hydronephrosis in a horseshoe kidney *(arrow)*. (H) Mercaptoacetyltriglycine (MAG3) scan demonstrates left uretero-pelvic junction obstruction (UPJO). (I) Coronal T2 images of MRU show the isthmus *(arrow)* and severe left hydronephrosis. (A, From Benjamin JA, Schullian DM. Observation on fused kidneys with horseshoe configuration: the contribution of Leonardo Botallo [1564]. *J Hist Med Allied Sci*. 1950;5:315-326; B, From Weiss MA, Mills SE. *Atlas of Genitourinary Tract Disorders*. Philadelphia: JB Lippincott; 1988. [Reprinted in: Shapiro E, Bauer SB, Chow JS. Anomalies of the upper urinary tract. In: Partin AW, Dmochowski RR, Kavoussi LR, Peters C, Wein AJ, eds. *Campbell-Walsh-Wein Urology*. 12th ed. Philadelphia: Elsevier; 2020.])

structures distal to the epididymal head are absent in 50%, including the body and tail of epididymis, vas, and seminal vesicles. Cardiac (15%), GI (9%), neurologic (3%), and hematologic (6%) anomalies can also be present. Maternal insulin-dependent diabetes mellitus is associated with a threefold increased risk of URA. If the single kidney is normal, no special precautions are required, and survival is not affected. Management is focused on the genital, cardiac, GI, and skeletal abnormalities. In 2008, the American Academy of Pediatrics Council on Sports Medicine and Fitness published a statement—"injury to solitary kidney is rare and each individual athlete needs individual assessment for particular sport." They suggested that wearing protective padding may reduce risk of injury. Other conditions associated with renal agenesis include vertebral defects, anal atresia, cardiac defects, tracheo-esophageal fistula, renal anomalies, and limb abnormalities (VACTERL) (30%), Turner syndrome, Poland syndrome, Fraser syndrome, Branchio-oto-renal (BOR) syndrome, and DiGeorge anomaly.

7. **Supernumerary kidney** (Fig. 26.3)
   The incidence of supernumerary kidney is unknown. Males and females are affected equally with a left-sided predominance. It originates from combined defects of the ureteral bud and metanephros. It is an accessory organ with its own distinct blood supply, collecting system, and encapsulated parenchyma. Associated findings include hydronephrosis (50%), common ureter (40%), duplex ureter (40%), and ectopic ureter.

CYSTIC ABNORMALITIES OF THE KIDNEYS

1. **Autosomal-dominant polycystic kidney disease (ADPKD)**
   ADPKD is the most common inheritable renal cystic disease with an incidence of 1 in 400–1000 live births. ADPKD accounts for 7% to 15% of all end-stage renal disease (ESRD) patients. There are two major genetic forms with different phenotypes. The first, PKD1 (located on chromosome 16), is more common (85%), rapidly progressive, and presents in the fourth or fifth decade of life. The second, PKD2 (located on chromosome 4), is relatively less common (15%), progresses more slowly, and presents in eighth decade of life. ADPKD typically presents with abdominal/flank pain, hematuria, and progressive renal insufficiency (Table 26.1).

   ADPKD is associated with liver cysts (33%), berry aneurysms (circle of Willis; 10% to 40%), as well as cysts of the seminal vesicle (40%), pancreas (5%), spleen, and lungs. Colonic diverticulosis, aortic aneurysms, and mitral valve

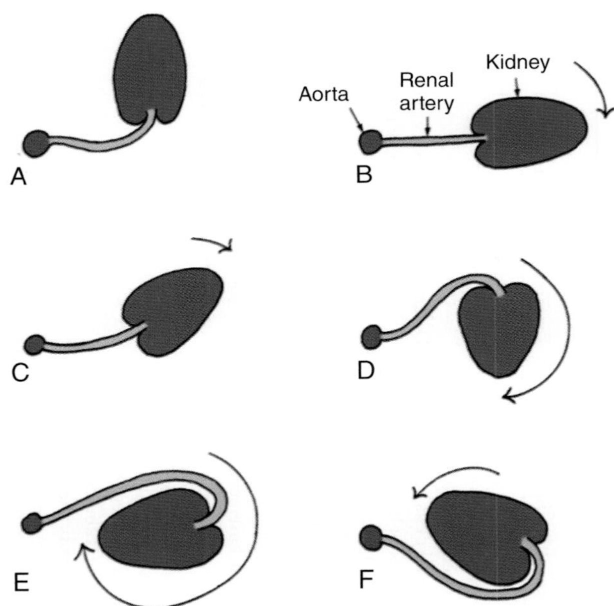

FIGURE 26.3 Rotation of the kidney during its ascent from the pelvis. The left kidney with its renal artery and the aorta are viewed in transverse section to show normal and abnormal rotation during its ascent to the adult site. (A) Primitive embryonic position; hilus faces ventrally (anterior). (B) Normal adult position; hilum faces medially. (C) Incomplete rotation. (D) Hyperrotation; hilus faces dorsad (posterior). (E) Hyperrotation; hilus faces laterad. (F) Reverse rotation; hilus faces laterad. (A, From Shapiro E, Bauer SB, Chow JS. Anomalies of the upper urinary tract. In: Partin AW, Dmochowski RR, Kavoussi LR, Peters C, Wein AJ, eds. *Campbell-Walsh-Wein Urology*. 12th ed. Philadelphia: Elsevier; 2020; B, From Skandalakis JE, Gray SW. *Embryology for Surgeons: The Embryological Basis for the Treatment of Congenital Defects*. Philadelphia: WB Saunders; 1972.)

prolapse are also more common in patients with ADPKD. There is no increased risk of renal cell carcinoma.

Complications of ADPKD include renal failure, hypertension, myocardial infarction, and intracranial hemorrhage (9%).

There is no cure, and therapy is predicated on delaying the onset of ESRD and preventing complications. It is imperative to control blood pressure (BP), to decrease cardiac disease

TABLE 26.1 Characteristics of Major Inheritable and Noninheritable Cystic Kidney Diseases

Inheritable

Disease Entity	Chromosomal Defect	Renal Findings	Extrarenal Manifestations
Autosomal-recessive polycystic kidney disease (ARPKD)	Chromosome 6	In newborn, usually large, homogeneous, echogenic kidneys	Congenital hepatic fibrosis; biliary dysgenesis
Autosomal-dominant polycystic kidney disease (ADPKD)	*PKD1:* chromosome 16 *PKD2:* chromosome 4 *PKD3;* not mapped	Renal cysts scattered throughout parenchyma; large kidneys	Diverticulitis; liver, spleen, pancreatic cysts; mitral valve prolapse; intracranial (berry) aneurysms
Juvenile nephronophthisis/medullary cystic disease complex Juvenile nephronophthisis (autosomal recessive)	Chromosome 2; not mapped	Cysts of corticomedullary junction; develop after onset of renal failure; always thickened tubular basement membrane	Retinitis pigmentosa (16%; also known as Senior-Loken syndrome); rarely skeletal abnormalities, hepatic fibrosis, Bardet-Biedl syndrome, ocular motor apraxia, and other neurologic defects
Medullary cystic disease (autosomal dominant)		Cysts of corticomedullary junction; develop before onset of renal failure; tubular basement membrane may NOT be thickened	None

Tuberous sclerosis (autosomal dominant)	*TSC1:* chromosome 9 *TSC2:* chromosome 16	Cysts and angiomyolipomas throughout kidney; cysts even present in utero; 3% incidence of RCC	Adenoma sebaceum; epilepsy; mental retardation; cranial tumors
von Hippel-Lindau disease (autosomal dominant)	Chromosome 3	Cysts, adenomas, and clear cell RCC (35%–38% of cases)	Cerebellar hemangioblastomas; retinal angiomas; pheochromocytomas; cysts of pancreas and epididymis

Noninheritable

Disease Entity	Renal Findings	Extrarenal Manifestations
Multicystic dysplastic kidney	Renal maldevelopment with diffuse cysts and remnants of early metanephros; minimal, if any, nephron development; most frequent renal cystic disease in newborns	Unusual
Benign multilocular cyst	Benign cystic neoplasm of the kidney; remainder of kidney has normal nephrons that may be compromised by growing mass; present more often in males when less than 4 years of age and females when greater than 30 years of age	None

Continued

TABLE 26.1 Characteristics of Major Inheritable and Noninheritable Cystic Kidney Diseases—cont'd

Noninheritable		
Disease Entity	Renal Findings	Extrarenal Manifestations
Simple cysts	Single or multiple cysts; normal nephrons throughout kidney; very common in normal kidneys with increasing age	None
Medullary sponge kidney	Ectatic collecting ducts; nephrons usually normal	None
Acquired renal cystic disease	Diffuse cysts; adenomas; occasionally RCC; increases with duration of ESRD	None

ESRD, End-stage renal disease; *RCC*, renal cell carcinoma.
From Pope JC IV. Renal dysgenesis and cystic disease of the kidney. In: Wein AJ, Kavoussi LR, Novick AC, et al, eds. *Campbell-Walsh Urology*. 10th ed. Philadelphia: Saunders; 2012.

and prevent deterioration of renal function. Patients may encounter issues with pain typically due to renal capsular stretching by cysts. Screening for asymptomatic berry aneurysms is only recommended if there is a family history of aneurysms or subarachnoid hemorrhage, upcoming major elective surgery, or high-risk occupation (i.e., pilot).

2. **Autosomal-recessive (infantile) polycystic kidney disease**

   Autosomal-recessive polycystic kidney disease (ARPKD) is caused by mutations of the *PKHD1* gene on chromosome 6 leading to fusiform dilation of collecting ducts and tubules, resulting in numerous small subcapsular cysts. The infantile type is rare (1 per 10,000 to 50,000 live births) and usually presents with bilateral flank masses in infancy, but can present in childhood with renal or hepatic insufficiency. Historically, mortality for the infantile type is 50% in first few days of life.

   Imaging shows large (12 to 16 times normal) kidneys with a characteristic, streaked appearance on intravenous urogram (IVU) ("sunburst" pattern). In newborns, renal US reveals bilaterally enlarged hyperechogenic kidneys with numerous microcysts.

   Associated findings include congenital hepatic (periportal) fibrosis (in all cases) and dilation of bile ducts. The degree of hepatic insufficiency varies inversely with the severity of renal disease and directly with the age of presentation. Although respiratory support, BP control, and dialysis can improve survival, all patients will ultimately develop cirrhosis.

3. **Medullary sponge kidney (precalyceal canalicular ectasia)**

   Medullary sponge kidney is an adult disease pathologically characterized by dilated distal collecting ducts with numerous cysts in the medullary pyramids. It can be diagnosed on computed tomography (CT) or an IVU showing collections of contrast adjacent to the calyces ("bristles on a brush" also called "blushing") often with calcifications in the medulla. Clinically, patients often remain asymptomatic. When patients do develop issues, the most common are nephrolithiasis (50%–60%), infection (20%–33%), distal renal tubular acidosis (30%–40%), and hematuria (10%–18%). Medical management of stone disease (calcium oxalate and calcium phosphate) and infections is often required. Approximately 33% of patients have hypercalciuria.

4. **Medullary cystic kidney disease (MCKD) and juvenile nephronophthisis (NPH)**

   This group of disorders has various genetic patterns characterized pathologically by bilateral small kidneys, an attenuated basement membrane, atrophic tubules, corticomedullary cysts, and interstitial fibrosis (hallmark). MCKD is inherited in an autosomal-dominant fashion and leads to ESRD by the third of fourth decade of life. Juvenile NPH is inherited in an autosomal-recessive fashion and is rapidly progressive with most patients developing ESRD at a mean age of 13 and almost always by age 25. Medical management of renal failure can delay the need for transplant; however, most patients will need sodium replacement. Both MCKD and juvenile NPH result in polydipsia and polyuria in the majority (80%) of patients. MCKD patients develop hypertension while those with juvenile NPH can develop retinitis pigmentosa (16%).

5. **Multicystic dysplastic kidney (MCDK)**

   MCDK is the most common cystic disease of the newborn (1 in 1000 to 4000 live births) and results in multiple renal cysts of various sizes without identifiable renal parenchyma. Many theories exist on its origin including (1) severe obstruction from atresia of the ureter or renal pelvis, (2) abnormal signaling between the ureteric bud and metanephric mesenchyme resulting in development arrest and failure, (3) ischemia from inadequate development of vasculature as the kidney migrates. Contralateral renal abnormalities are common—VUR (18%–43%) and ureteropelvic junction obstruction (UPJO, 3%–12%). Voiding cystourethrogram (VCUG) is not routinely recommended for all infants with MCDK; however, should be considered in those with contralateral renal abnormalities on US or those with a history of UTI.

   The natural history is benign and 40% will involute spontaneously. There is no increased risk of malignancy or hypertension. US is the most diagnostic study and typically shows cysts of varying sizes without visible communication and no hydronephrosis. If US is nondiagnostic then renal scintigraphy (dimercaptosuccinic acid [DMSA] or mercaptoacetyltriglycine [MAG3]) can confirm the diagnosis with no flow or function present (must have no function to be true MCDK). Most will decrease in size over time and can be followed conservatively. Reports of hypertension are rare and malignant transformation is no higher than a normal renal unit. Surgical intervention (nephrectomy) is only warranted if enlarging over time.

COLLECTING SYSTEM ABNORMALITIES

1. **Calyceal diverticulum**

   A calyceal diverticulum is a cystic cavity within the kidney lined with urothelium that communicates with a calyx (type 1) or renal pelvis (type 2) via a narrow infundibulum. The incidence of these diverticula is 4.5 per 1000. The embryological origin is thought to be failure of third- and fourth-order branches of the ureteral bud to degenerate, which form the diverticulum cavity. Most are asymptomatic, but approximately one-third of patients will form stones, and some may have recurrent infections because of urinary stasis. The diagnosis is made with CT or magnetic resonance imaging (MRI) with delayed-phase imaging (diverticulum will only have contrast on delayed imaging since the lining urothelium does not have nephrons and will only backfill). Treatment is only indicated if symptomatic or large and includes removal of stones, drainage of purulence, and marsupialization to the renal surface with closure of the collecting system and cauterization of the epithelium. Calyceal diverticula with stones can be treated laparoscopically, endoscopically, or percutaneously depending on location and stone burden.

2. **Hydrocalycosis**

   Hydrocalycosis is a rare dilation of a major calyx resulting from either vascular compression, cicatrization, or achalasia of the infundibulum (i.e., Fraley syndrome). It may present with flank pain, hematuria, or UTI but rarely requires any intervention.

3. **Megacalycosis**

   Megacalycosis is a congenital enlargement of calyces without dilation of the renal pelvis. It is easily mistaken for obstruction—however, the dilation is nonobstructive. The dilation results from a malformation of the renal papillae. It is commonly associated with increased number of calyces (12–20). The condition affects males more than females (6:1) and bilateral disease is almost exclusively seen in males while unilateral segmental disease is more often seen in females. Megacalycosis may be associated with stones or infection, but by itself causes no deterioration of renal function.

4. **Infundibulopelvic stenosis**
   This is a rare, typically bilateral, condition that leads to dilated calyces proximal to diminutive infundibulum and renal pelvis. Most will have progressive renal failure. It is commonly associated with VUR and less frequently with dysplasia and lower urinary tract anomalies (posterior urethral valves [PUVs]). Treatment options include infundibuloplasties or multiple calicocalicostomies draining into lower pole ureterocalicostomy.
5. **Ureteropelvic junction obstruction**
   UPJO is the most common cause of abdominal masses in children (hydronephrosis). There is a 2:1 male to female predominance in children and left-sided predominance in all ages. There are several possible etiologies for UPJO including segmental ureteral muscular attenuation or malorientation, true stenosis, angulation, and extrinsic compression (Figs. 26.4 and 26.5). Crossing lower pole vessels are present in approximately 20% to 30% of cases. Rarely, lower pole UPJO can occur in duplex ureters. A secondary UPJO can occur from severe VUR causing a markedly tortuous dilated and kinked ureter. In these cases, staged surgical intervention is preferred as correction of the VUR may result in better upper tract drainage.
   Associated findings include VUR (5% to 10%), contralateral agenesis (5%), contralateral UPJO (10%), and rarely dysplasia or MCDK. Many infants with UPJO will be identified in utero with routine prenatal screening US. If not detected prenatally, symptoms include episodic flank pain and/or palpable mass, hematuria, infection, nausea, and vomiting. In older children, GI distress and poorly localized upper abdominal pain may be the only symptoms.

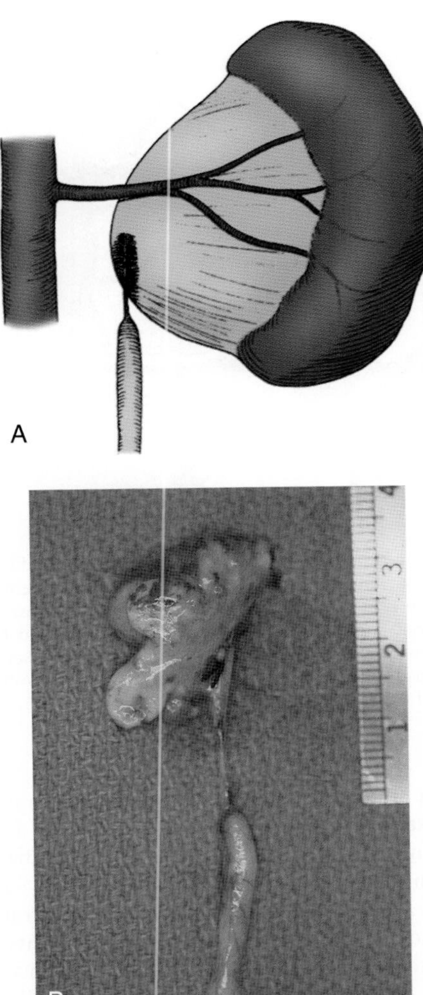

FIGURE 26.4 (A) Intrinsic narrowing of upper ureter contributing to ureteropelvic junction obstruction (UPJO). (B) Surgical specimen of nonfunctioning kidney with significant proximal ureteral narrowing. (From Carr MC, Casale P. Anomalies and surgery of the ureter in children. In: Wein AJ, Kavoussi LR, Novick AC, Partin AW, Peters C, eds. *Campbell-Walsh Urology*. 10th ed. Philadelphia: Saunders; 2012.)

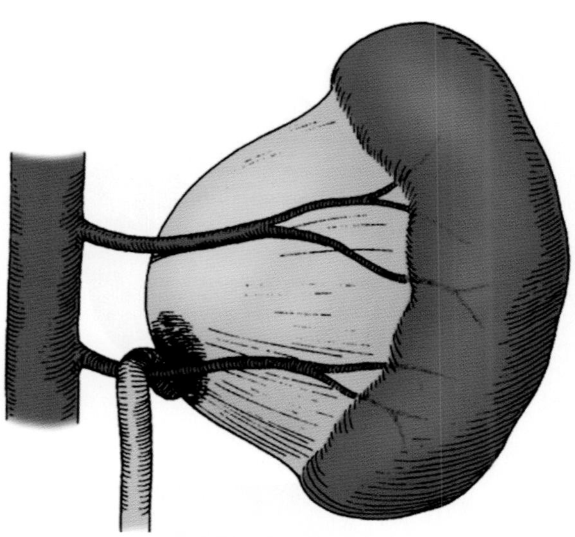

FIGURE 26.5 A lower pole crossing vessel contributes to significant kinking at the ureteropelvic junction (UPJ) and resultant intermittent obstruction. Often, when the ureter is mobilized, no evidence of intrinsic narrowing is found. Insertional anomaly and peripelvic fibrosis may also be present as secondary obstructive factors. (From Carr MC, Casale P. Anomalies and surgery of the ureter in children. In: Wein AJ, Kavoussi LR, Novick AC, Partin AW, Peters C, eds. *Campbell-Walsh Urology*. 10th ed. Philadelphia: Saunders; 2012.)

Radiologic findings include hydronephrosis, an enlarged anteroposterior (AP) renal pelvis diameter on US (multiple interconnected hypoechoic areas with identifiable cortical rim), and delayed excretion of radiotracer (> 20 minutes) on the affected side despite Lasix administration during renal scan (i.e., MAG3/Lasix). Most infants diagnosed antenatally can be followed with surveillance (combination of US and renal scan). Up to 66% will not require treatment and will improve on repeat imaging. Those that have worsening dilation on US, worsening drainage curves, decreasing or poor function, breakthrough infections, or intractable pain warrant prompt surgical consultation and intervention. Many techniques exist for surgical repair including dismembered (Anderson-Hynes) pyeloplasty, spiral flap, vertical flap, and Foley Y-V pyeloplasty (Fig. 26.6). These can be done via open, laparoscopic, or robotic-assisted techniques.

Generally, success rates after surgery are 90%–100% with few complications. Failures can be managed by either repeat pyeloplasty, endoscopic incision, or ureterocalicostomy. Follow-up varies but may consist of US at 1 month, renal scan at 3 months, and US at 1 year postoperatively in most cases. In order to limit radiation exposure, repeat renal scans are not always obtained if US examinations are reassuring.

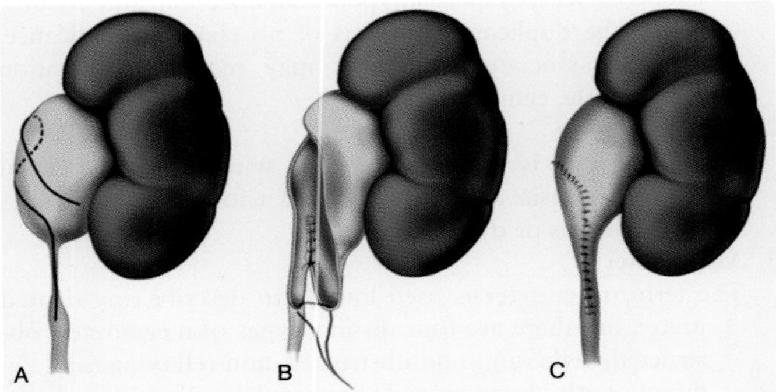

FIGURE 26.6 (A) A spiral flap may be indicated for relatively long areas of proximal ureteral obstruction when the ureteropelvic junction (UPJ) is already in a dependent position. The spiral flap is outlined with the base situated obliquely on the dependent aspect of the renal pelvis. The base of the flap is positioned anatomically lateral to the UPJ, between the ureteral insertion and the renal parenchyma. The flap is spiraled posteriorly to anteriorly or vice versa. The anatomically medial line of incision is carried down completely through the obstructed proximal ureteral segment into normal-caliber ureter. The site of the apex for the flap is determined by the length of flap required to bridge the obstruction. The longer the segment of proximal ureteral obstruction, the farther away is the apex because this will make the flap longer. However, to preserve vascular integrity of the flap, the ratio of flap length to width should not exceed 3:1. (B) Once the flap is developed, the apex is rotated down to the most inferior aspect of the ureterotomy. (C) The anastomosis is then completed, usually over an internal stent, again using fine absorbable sutures. (From Partin AW, Dmochowski RR, Kavoussi LR, Peters C, Wein AJ, eds. *Campbell-Walsh-Wein Urology*. 12th ed. Philadelphia: Elsevier; 2020.)

URETERAL ANOMALIES

1. **Duplication of ureter**
   Ureteral duplication occurs in 1 per 125 autopsies, with a female predominance. Up to 85% of cases are unilateral and the condition is inherited in an autosomal-dominant fashion with incomplete penetrance. Most cases seem to arise from two ureteral buds meeting the metanephros. Another embryological explanation is a bud that bifurcates immediately after arising from Wolffian (mesonephric) duct but before meeting the metanephros. Ureteral duplication is associated with reflux (42%), renal scarring and dilation (29%), ectopic insertion (3%), large kidneys with excess calyces, dysplasia/hypoplasia, infection, and ureteroceles. The duplication itself is of no clinical significance, but the associated anomalies may require intervention (ureterocele, ectopia, etc.).
2. **Ureteral atresia**
   Ureteral atresia is usually associated with a MCDK. Distal segment atresia is often associated with contralateral hydronephrosis or dysplasia (50%).
3. **Megaureter**
   The term megaureter is used loosely to describe any dilated ureter, but there are four distinct types of megaureter: obstructed, refluxing, non-obstructed non-refluxing, and refluxing with obstruction. There is a 3:1 male to female ratio and a 3:1 left-sided predominance. Megaureter is responsible for 10%–25% of all antenatally detected upper tract dilation.

   In a primary obstructing megaureter there is general agreement that obstruction occurs from an abnormal aperistaltic terminal segment of ureter at or near the UVJ. A non-refluxing, non obstructed megaureter results from widened ureteral bud forming a ureter dilated down to the orifice, which is in the normal position. A refluxing megaureter usually has a laterally ectopic orifice and may be associated with a dysplastic kidney.

   US typically shows moderate to severe hydronephrosis and proportionately greater ureteral dilation versus renal dilation. A VCUG can diagnose the reflux type. A MAG3/Lasix renal scan can help distinguish obstructed from unobstructed megaureters. Recently, MR urogram has been used to delineate drainage, split renal function, and anatomy (i.e., insertion point of ureters).

There has been an increasing trend towards conservative management of megaureters as the majority will be asymptomatic and resolve with time. Some studies have shown that the degree of ureteral dilation (> or < 10 mm) may be prognostic in terms of risk for complications or surgical interventions. Continued surveillance of persistent dilation is warranted as studies have shown worsening of previous stable dilation at or during puberty. Surgical correction is indicated when patients have recurrent UTIs, progressive dilation, or loss of renal function. If prompt decompression is needed in a neonate, cutaneous ureterostomy or nephrostomy tube placement is preferred. Tapering of the ureter is commonly needed for refluxing megaureters prior to reimplantation in a non-refluxing fashion.

4. **Vesicoureteral reflux**

The incidence of VUR is approximately 1–2 per 100 in the general population (in childhood), but VUR is 8 to 40 times more frequent in affected families. It can be found in 70% of infants and 30% of children diagnosed with a UTI. It may occur in as many as 17% of children without a UTI undergoing VCUG for other indications.

Primary VUR is thought to occur when the ureteral bud arises ectopically leading to a laterally placed orifice and short submucosal tunnel. Alternatively, VUR may result from delayed or incomplete development of the intrinsic smooth muscle of the distal ureteral segment. Secondary VUR occurs when excessive voiding and storage pressures overwhelm a marginally competent UVJ. Bladder bowel dysfunction (BBD) can also play a major role in the development or exacerbation of VUR.

Primary VUR is graded I to V by the International Reflux Study system depending on the degree of dilation (Fig. 26.7). VUR can transmit bacteria from the bladder to the upper tracts leading to pyelonephritis and renal scarring. Higher grades of VUR can predispose to increased renal scarring (Table 26.2). VCUG is the gold standard for diagnosing VUR.

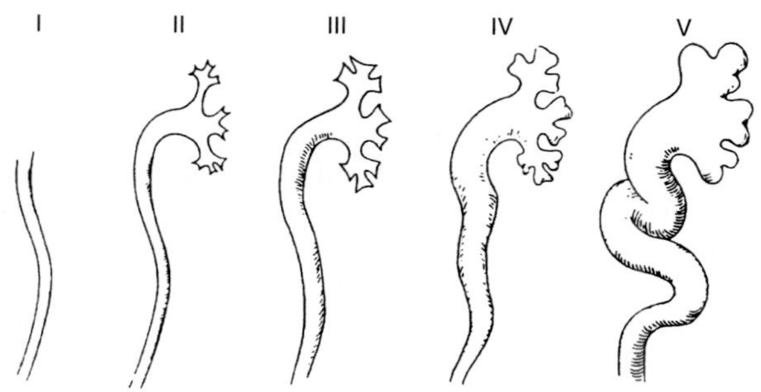

FIGURE 26.7 **International Reflux Study classification of vesicoureteral reflux (VUR).** (From Atala A, Keating MA. Vesicoureteral reflux and megaureter. In: Partin AW, Dmochowski RR, Kavoussi LR, Peters C, Wein AJ, eds. *Campbell-Walsh-Wein Urology*. 12th ed. Philadelphia: Elsevier; 2020.)

TABLE 26.2 Congenital Renal Scarring

Grade of Vesicoureteral Reflux	Number of Patients Normal	Slight Damage	Severe Damage
1–3	13 (100%)	–	–
4	8 (53%)	5 (34%)	2 (13%)
5	2 (15%)	5 (38%)	6 (46%)

Modified from Marra G, Barbieri G, Dell'Agnola CA, et al. Congenital renal damage associated with primary vesicoureteric reflux. *Arch Dis Child Fetal Neonatal Ed.* 1994;70:F147. (Table 122-4 from Wein AJ, Kavoussi LR, Novick AC, et al, eds. *Campbell-Walsh Urology*. 10th ed. Philadelphia: Saunders; 2012:3280.)

In recent years, contrast-enhanced voiding urethrosonogram (ceVUS) has been utilized as it eliminates radiation exposure to the child. Since the overarching goal in VUR management and treatment is to prevent functional loss and renal scarring (with subsequent hypertension and renal failure), some advocate for utilizing renal scintigraphy or DMSA to screen and follow children with VUR as it is the gold standard for capturing renal scarring.

The initial management of children with reflux is typically conservative. Depending on sex, circumcision status, and VUR

TABLE 26.3 Treatment of the Child with VUR and UTI Over One Year of Age

	CAP	Observation
No BBD, recurrent febrile UTI, renal cortical abnormalities	option	option
BBD, recurrent febrile UTI, OR renal cortical abnormalities	recommended	not recommended

Option: Surgical intervention for VUR, including both open and endoscopic methods, may be used. Prospective randomized, controlled trials have shown a reduction in the occurrence of febrile urinary tract infections in patients who have undergone open surgical correction of VUR as compared to those receiving continuous antibiotic prophylaxis.

grade, children with VUR may be placed on prophylactic antibiotics (amoxicillin if < 2 months of age and trimethoprim-sulfamethoxazole or nitrofurantoin if > 2 months of age). Children with VUR are closely monitored with periodic US, periodic VCUG or ceVUS (usually at 18–24 months if no interval UTIs) based on their age, sex, and clinical history (Table 26.3).

Spontaneous resolution of reflux is common, particularly in low-grade reflux (grades 1–3), but resolution also depends on the initial grade and the initial age at presentation. These two variables are inversely proportional to one another. Low-volume VUR (grades 1–3) resolves at a rate of 17% per patient-year, whereas grade 4 VUR resolves at a rate of 4% per patient-year. Timing of VUR initiation on VCUG may also be associated with resolution, with VUR occurring during the filling phase being less likely to spontaneously resolve compared with VUR that occurs later in the voiding phase. Reimplantation of the refluxing unit either by an open intravesical approach (i.e., Cohen cross-trigonal or Glenn-Anderson techniques), open extravesical approach (i.e., Lich-Gregoir technique), or robotic extravesical detrusorrhaphy approaches is the standard surgical management. Surgical success rates are excellent. Duplicated ureters are reimplanted together in their common distal muscular sheath. Some centers advocate for subureteric injection of bulking agents, although the longevity of these methods is unclear. Breakthrough infections, failure to comply with the antibiotic prophylaxis regimen, persistent reflux into puberty in females, progressive scarring, and worsening renal function are all considerations that favor surgical intervention, but ultimately there are no absolute indications for surgical correction of reflux.

5. **Ectopic ureter**

   An ectopic ureter is defined as any ureter, duplex or single, that does not insert into the trigone of the bladder. The incidence of ectopic ureters is 1 per 1900 live births with a 3:1 female predominance. Ectopic ureter is often duplex in females (80%) and a single ureter in males.

   The embryological cause is thought to be a failure of the ureteral bud to separate from the mesonephric duct, most likely due to its ectopic origin on the duct. Possible locations for ectopic ureters are shown in Fig. 26.8. In females these locations include anywhere between the bladder neck to perineum including the vagina, uterus, and rectum. In males the ectopic ureter always inserts proximal to the external sphincter, including Wolffian structures such as the vas deferens, seminal vesicles, or ejaculatory duct.

   Associated findings include renal dysplasia, ureteral obstruction, and incontinence. The degree of renal dysplasia correlates with the degree of ectopy. Incontinence is variable and presents when the ectopic orifice is located distal to the sphincter in females or if there is a failure of bladder neck development. Bilateral ectopic ureters, in which the orifices are distal to the bladder neck, lead to a poorly developed bladder and incontinence because of outlet incompetence and failure of bladder cycling.

   Multiple surgical strategies exist including heminephroureterectomy (for poorly functioning units) and salvage procedures such as ureteroureterostomy or common sheath reimplantation. MR urogram is an excellent imaging tool to help define anatomy for surgical planning (in young infants $< \sim$ 4–5 months, a feed and swaddle MR can be obtained without sedation/anesthesia).

6. **Ureterocele**

   A ureterocele is a cystic dilation of the distal aspect of the ureter that is located in the bladder. The incidence is

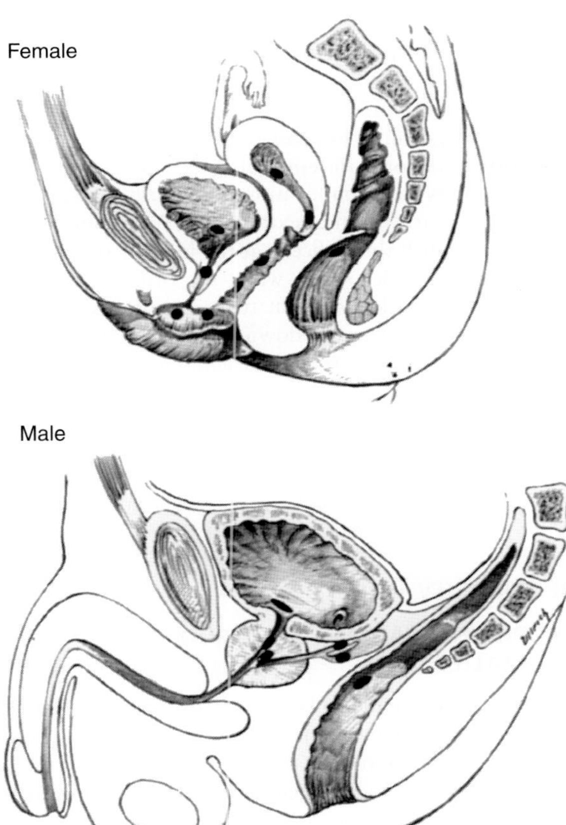

FIGURE 26.8 Sites of ectopic ureteral orifices in females and males. (From Schlussel R, Retik AB. Ectopic ureter, ureterocele, and other anomalies of the ureter. In: Walsh PC, Vaughn ED, Retik AB, et al, eds. *Campbell's Urology*. 8th ed. Philadelphia: Saunders; 2002:2014.)

1 per 500 to 4000 live births; bilateral ureteroceles are present in 10% to 15% of cases and there is a 4:1 female predominance. A ureterocele is thought to develop from a failure of the distal ureteral membrane (Chwalla's membrane) to rupture causing distal ureteral dilation. The

ureter is duplicated in most children (80%), with the ureterocele almost always draining the upper pole ureter. Associated anomalies include contralateral ureteral duplication (50%), renal segmental dysplasia, renal fusion, renal ectopia, reflux, bladder outlet obstruction, and rarely, incontinence (only in females).

Classification is based on location of the orifice and is typically defined as intravesical or extravesical. An ectopic ureterocele is one in which the orifice is at the bladder neck or urethra. A cecoureterocele occurs when the orifice of the affected ureter is in the bladder but the ureterocele cavity extends beyond the bladder neck down the urethra; it may be associated with poor bladder neck development and incontinence.

Management is varied depending on the severity. In newborns, puncture of the ureterocele relieves obstruction but may cause secondary reflux in 10%–15% of patients. Excision of the ureterocele with upper pole heminephroureterectomy may also be considered.

Lower Urinary Tract

EXSTROPHY/EPISPADIAS—SPECTRUM OF ANOMALIES

The embryological origin of bladder exstrophy is hypothesized as failure of the cloacal membrane to migrate toward the perineum around 4 weeks gestation, thus preventing ingrowth of the lateral mesoderm and coalescence of genital tubercles. Exstrophy is rare with an incidence of 2.15 per 100,000 live births. Bladder exstrophy, cloacal exstrophy and epispadias are variants of the exstrophy-epispadias complex. The most reproducible finding among these variants is some degree of separation of symphysis pubis.

Epispadias (30%) occurs in about 1 in 100,000 live births. It may be penopubic with incontinence in males (55%), penile (20%) with or without incontinence, balanitic (5%), or it may occur in females with incontinence (20%). It consists of a dorsal meatus with a distal mucosal groove, flattened glans, or bifid clitoris in females. In males, there is a variable degree of dorsal chordee with shortening of the corporal bodies in severe forms (penopubic). Nearly all cases of epispadias require complete disassembly with or without complete separation of the distal urethra from the glans (Mitchell technique).

Classic bladder exstrophy (60%) occurs in 1 per 50,000 births with 3:1 male predominance. In classic bladder exstrophy the bladder and the urethra are open dorsally, and the penis is short or the clitoris is bifid.

Cloacal exstrophy (10%) results from the condition of failure of the urorectal septum to descend. It occurs approximately in 1 per 200,000 births, about equally in males and females.

In classic bladder exstrophy, undescended testes and inguinal hernias are common because of a shortened inguinal canal and frequent failure of the infraumbilical rectus musculature to develop. The upper urinary tract is usually normal or may be duplex. In cloacal exstrophy, there is a vesicointestinal fissure opening into the center of the exstrophied bladder, a short blind-ending distal colon, an absent or duplicated appendix, and often an omphalocele. Two-thirds of females have an absent or duplex and stenotic vagina; nearly all have a tethered spinal cord with 50% having a myelomeningocele. The OEIS complex consists of omphalocele, cloacal exstrophy, imperforate anus, and spinal defects. The penis or clitoris is bifid or may be absent.

Classic bladder exstrophy may be managed either with a staged surgical approach or with a primary single-stage repair. In the multistage repair the initial procedure typically includes bladder closure, penile lengthening (freeing the corpora from attachment to the pubic bone), and tubularization of the bladder neck. In cloacal exstrophy, the omphalocele and vesicoenteric fissure must be dealt with by lateral closure of the bowel, end colostomy, and omphalocele repair. The bladder halves are also approximated in the first stage. The second stage is epispadias repair, in most cases at approximately 1 to 2 years of age. The goal of the third stage in those with a functional, sufficiently large bladder is to achieve continence via bladder neck reconstruction (60% success). Those patients who fail are considered candidates for augmentation with or without a catheterizable channel.

Alternatively, the single-stage exstrophy repair includes complete penile disassembly, bladder closure, bladder neck reconstruction, and epispadias repair all within one operation, often during the newborn period. In the single-stage repair, the urethral meatus is often left in a hypospadiac location. Despite the name, many of these children require additional procedures to achieve urinary continence.

All patients require careful follow-up throughout adolescence, puberty, and adulthood with surveillance of the upper tracts, monitoring of acid-base balance, renal function tests, sexual function, and supportive counseling. Transitional urology is an emerging field dedicated to care of these complex patients as they enter adulthood.

URACHUS

The urachus is an embryological remnant of the allantois that typically obliterates. Anomalies are detected postnatally using a combination of US, CT, or VCUG. Urachal anomalies include a patent urachus, urachal sinus, urachal cyst, or vesicourachal diverticulum. Most urachal anomalies can be observed and will resolve spontaneously. If patients develop infections, abscess, or have continuous drainage, treatment consists of excision either via open or laparoscopic technique ± antibiotics. Rarely, the urachal segment may undergo malignant transformation (adenocarcinoma), however this occurs almost exclusively in adults. When removing a urachal anomaly that connects to the bladder, a bladder cuff is often removed.

POSTERIOR URETHRAL VALVES

The incidence of PUVs is 1 per 5000 to 8000 boys. The most commonly used classification system was first described by Hugh Hampton Young in 1919. **Type 1 valves** are the most common (95%) and are thought to be due to a hypertrophied inferior urethral crest formed by the insertion of the distal ends of the Wolffian ducts into the anterior-lateral walls of the cloaca. The leaflets arise from the verumontanum and fuse anteriorly just proximal to the external urethral sphincter. **Type II valves** are non-obstructing normal folds in the prostatic urethra and not currently recognized as true valves. **Type III valves** represent an annular ring similar to a congenital urethral stricture formed by persistence of the urogenital membrane. More recent literature suggests that all PUVs are type III and become type I after insertion of a urethral drainage tube.

PUVs are associated with VUR in 50% of patients. VUR typically resolves within about 2 years in approximately 25%–40% of cases. Persistent unilateral reflux is usually associated with a nonfunctioning kidney, most commonly the left one. Severe renal dysplasia is common in those with severe obstruction.

Concentrating defects lead many to develop polyuria. Acute renal failure and acidosis in the newborn are obstructive phenomena; chronic renal insufficiency may occur into adolescence and adulthood from dysplasia.

Valve bladder syndrome describes a vicious cycle of progressive bladder dysfunction caused by detrusor hypertrophy, high-pressure voiding and eventual bladder decompensation leading to deterioration of renal function and worsening dilation.

There should be high suspicion for PUVs when antenatal US shows findings of a distended thick-walled bladder, bilateral ureterectasis and pelviectasis with or without oligohydramnios. The definitive radiologic study for diagnosis postnatally is a VCUG and should be completed in any infant with the aforementioned antenatal findings. Clinically, PUVs should be suspected in a male newborn with a palpable bladder, urinary ascites, and minimal/no urine output. Occasionally the diagnosis can be missed at birth and diagnosed later on after a UTI or complaints of poor stream in an infant or older child. Ultrasonography and renal scan are employed to assess the extent of upper tract damage and postoperative recovery.

In any newborn or infant suspected of having PUVs, initial management consists of bladder drainage with a small feeding tube (5 or 6 Fr) per the urethra; VCUG may be done when infant is stable with this catheter in place. The healthy infant or older child should undergo transurethral incision of valves. A sick infant should undergo treatment when creatinine stabilizes and sepsis resolves. A cutaneous vesicostomy can be utilized in very–low-birth-weight infants whose urethra cannot accommodate an endoscope or in those that have high residual urine volumes with worsening renal function despite endoscopic valve ablation. Circumcision should be recommended in infants with PUVs as their overall risk of UTI is 50%–60%. Circumcision decreases this risk by 83%–92%, to a level similar to unaffected males. Nonfunctioning kidneys with refluxing ureters are typically preserved as they act as a "pop off valve" for the high-pressure system. Additionally, native ureters may be used as tissue for augmentation of the bladder if needed at the time of renal transplant. Ureteral reimplantation is almost never indicated and is often fraught with failure. Antibiotic prophylaxis is maintained as long as reflux persists or upper tract emptying is slow.

In the long term, approximately 20%–50% of all children with PUVs develop ESRD and require renal transplantation. Children whose creatinine levels stabilize below 0.8 mg/dL at 1 year of life have better outcomes than those with creatinine levels above 1.2 mg/dL. Continence is eventually achieved in virtually all who undergo valve incision.

MEGALOURETHRA

This rare lesion is usually associated with prune belly syndrome. Megalourethra occurs in two distinct types: scaphoid and fusiform. The scaphoid type results from a deficiency of corpus spongiosum allowing ballooning of the urethra during voiding. This type can be repaired with hypospadias techniques. The fusiform type involves a deficiency of corpora cavernosa and corpus spongiosum, resulting in an elongated flaccid penis with redundant skin. This form is seen usually in stillborn infants with other cloacal anomalies and is difficult to correct because of the lack of adequate corporal tissue.

MISCELLANEOUS

1. An anterior urethral valve is much less common than PUV and is caused by an anterior urethral diverticulum. The diverticulum can be excised with careful attention to prevent the distal flap from obstructing.
2. *Enlarged utriculus masculinus* is a dilated müllerian remnant that is typically asymptomatic. A prostatic utricle is associated with hypospadias and disorders of sexual development (DSD). The utricle can be surgically excised retrovesically or transvesically if urinary stasis leads to UTI or the utricle interferes with bladder emptying. Utricles rarely require surgical intervention.
3. Aphallia and diphallia are exceedingly rare conditions. These occur with failure of fusion of the genital tubercles or failure of differentiation of phallic mesenchyme.

External Genital Malformations

HYPOSPADIAS

The classic triad for hypospadias is incomplete dorsally hooded foreskin, an ectopically located urethral meatus, and ventral penile curvature. Hypospadias occurs in 1 per 150–300 live male births and there is a 9%–15% incidence in first-degree relatives (brother/father). The exact mechanism is debated but is thought to result from failure of the mesodermal urethral folds to converge in the midline between 8 and 16 weeks gestation.

Boys with hypospadias may also have a blunted human chorionic gonadotropin response to gonadotropin-releasing hormone and low androgen-receptor levels (few cases). Undescended testes occur in 7% of boys with hypospadias and that number rises to 10% in those with more severe proximal variants. Up to one-third of boys with hypospadias and undescended testes have a DSD diagnosis, usually genetic mosaicism. As per the updated American Urological Association (AUA) guidelines these boys should be evaluated for DSD, especially with increasing severity of hypospadias. Other associated conditions include inguinal hernia (9%) and upper tract anomalies (46% when associated with imperforate anus, 33% with meningomyelocele, 12% to 50% when one other system anomaly is present, 5% with isolated hypospadias). Appropriate classification (Fig. 26.9) should include assessing the degree of chordee (penile curvature) as well as the location of the urethral meatus after degloving. Ultimately, most hypospadias

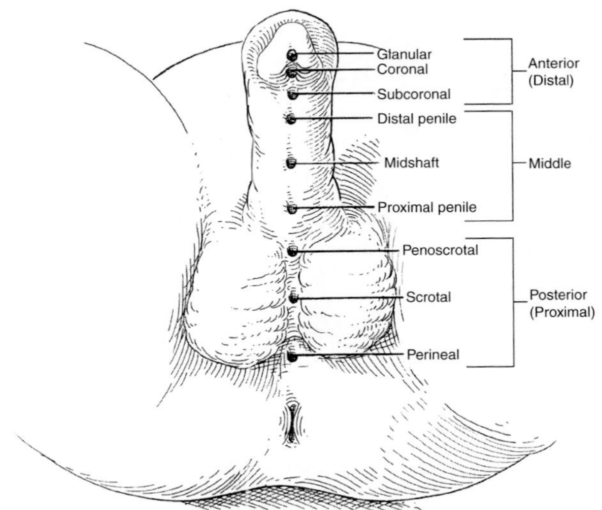

FIGURE 26.9 Anatomically descriptive levels of hypospadias within the three major categories, based on the level of the meatus following orthoplasty. (From Retik AB, Borer JG. Hypospadias. In: Partin AW, Dmochowski RR, Kavoussi LR, Peters C, Wein AJ, eds. *Campbell-Walsh-Wein Urology*. 12th ed. Philadelphia: Elsevier; 2020.)

(70%–85%) is classified as distal, with 10%–25% being proximal. GMS score (glans, meatus, penile shaft [curvature]) objectively stratifies hypospadias severity by incorporating examination findings in the operating room with quality of the glans and urethral plate, location of meatus, and degree of penile curvature.

As there are over 300 described techniques in the literature, surgical technique is often based on surgeon preference as well as meatal location, quality of urethral plate, availability of adjacent tissue, and degree of chordee. A single-stage repair between 6 and 18 months of age is preferred for distal hypospadias without severe chordee. Meatal advancement and glanuloplasty (MAGPI) can be utilized for glanular hypospadias (Fig. 26.10). Coronal or distal penile hypospadias is commonly repaired with a tubularized incised plate (TIP) or Thiersch-Duplay urethroplasty (Fig. 26.11).

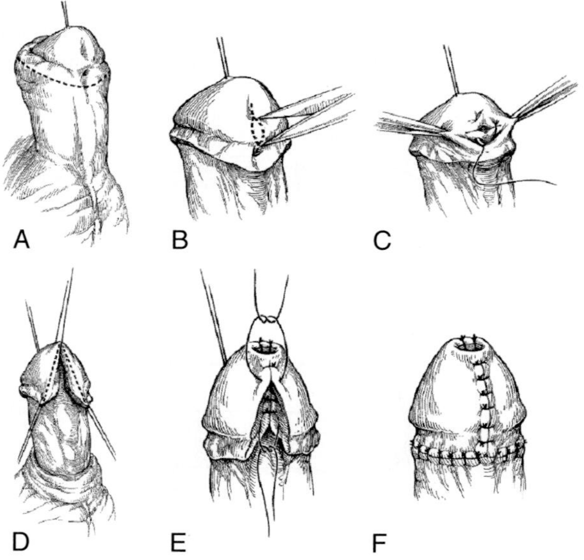

FIGURE 26.10 Meatal advancement and glanuloplasty (MAGPI). (A) Circumferential subcoronal incision is marked. (B) Longitudinal incision and (C) transverse approximation (Heineke-Mikulicz procedure) of transverse granular "bridge" in urethral plate. (D) Ventral edge of meatus is pulled distally, and medial glan "trimming" incisions are marked. (E) Deep suture approximation of the glan. (F) Superficial approximation of the glans and skin. (From Duckett JW. Hypospadias. In: Walsh PC, Retik AB, Vaughan ED Jr, et al, eds. *Campbell's Urology*. 7th ed. Philadelphia: Saunders; 1998.)

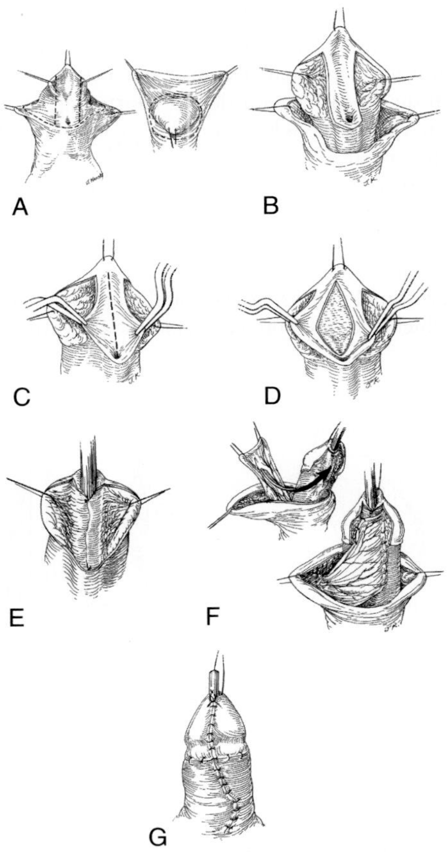

FIGURE 26.11 Tubularized incised plate (TIP) urethroplasty in distal, primary hypospadias repair. (A) Stay sutures are placed, and proposed urethral plate demarcating and circumferential incisions are marked. (B) Parallel longitudinal and circumferential incisions have been made. (C) Proposed longitudinal line of incision in the midline of the urethral plate. (D) Urethral plate has been incised. (E) Urethral plate tubularized over a 6-F Silastic catheter taking care not to close the distal extent (meatus) of the incised urethral plate too tightly. (F) Subcutaneous (dartos) tissue flap is harvested from lateral or dorsal penile shaft and repositioned over the neourethra as a second layer of coverage. (G) Glans penis has been approximated in two layers, redundant skin excised, and indwelling bladder catheter secured. (From Retik AB, Borer JG. Primary and reoperative hypospadias repair with the Snodgrass technique. *World J Urol*. 1998;16:186-191.)

Penile shaft or more proximal hypospadias may be managed by inner preputial transverse island flap (Figs. 26.12 and 26.13).

When chordee is present it can be corrected via either plication or grafting. Plication is a dorsal shortening technique used to straighten the penis when chordee is mild (0–30 degrees). Grafting is a ventral lengthening technique used for more severe chordee (> 30 degrees). Commonly utilized grafts include dermal patch (from groin), tunica vaginalis, and small intestine submucosa (SIS). Grafting to correct chordee typically necessitates a staged procedure.

Severe proximal hypospadias usually requires a staged approach in which the first stage corrects the curvature and lays in

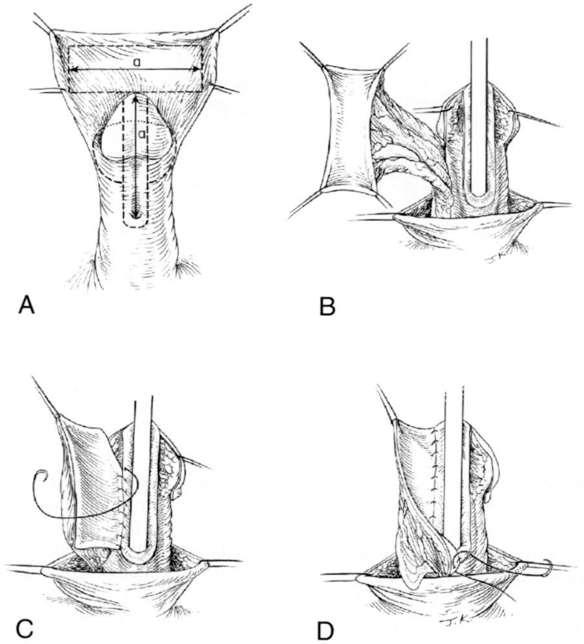

FIGURE 26.12 Onlay island flap repair. (A) Proposed incisions for urethral plate and preputial skin onlay. (B) Pedicled preputial skin onlay with stay. (C) Initial full-thickness suture approximation of onlay flap and urethral plate. (D) Approximation at proximal extent.

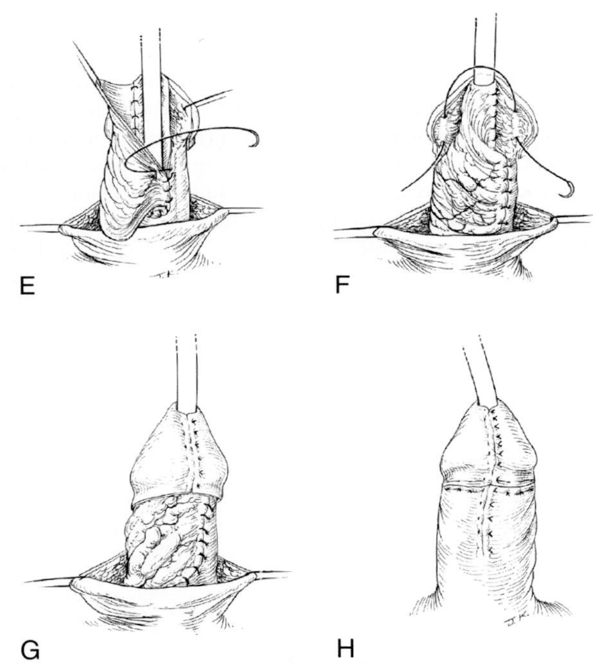

FIGURE 26.12, cont'd (E) Completion of anastomosis with running subcuticular technique. (F) Inferolateral border of onlay pedicle has been advanced as a second-layer coverage of proximal and longitudinal suture lines. (G) Approximated glans. (H) Completed repair. (From Atala A, Retik AB. Hypospadias. In: Libertino JA, ed. *Reconstructive Urologic Surgery*. 3rd ed. St. Louis: Mosby; 1998.)

skin onto the ventrum for future urethroplasty and the second stage relocates the urethral meatus to an orthotopic location on the glans or to the coronal margin via urethroplasty. A multilayer closure without overlapping suture lines is critical to preventing postoperative complications.

Occasionally, a simple degloving of the penis and mobilizing the urethra may treat chordee without urethral involvement.

Urinary diversion via urethral stent is used to allow the urethroplasty to heal. Some distal repairs without formal urethroplasty do not require urethral stents. Antibiotics may be administered either during stent removal or for as long as the urethral stent remains in place depending on surgeon preference.

Overall, long-term follow-up suggests complications are more common in proximal repairs (23%–68%) than distal repairs (10%–15%). Urethrocutaneous fistula is the most common complication (10%) and typically requires surgical repair as it rarely spontaneously resolves. Fistulae can result from distal obstruction (i.e., meatal stenosis) or high-pressure voiding. UTI occurs in less than 10% of cases and can be treated with oral antibiotics. Urethral strictures are rare and usually occur at the meatus or the proximal end of the repair. These are treated by Y-V meatoplasty,

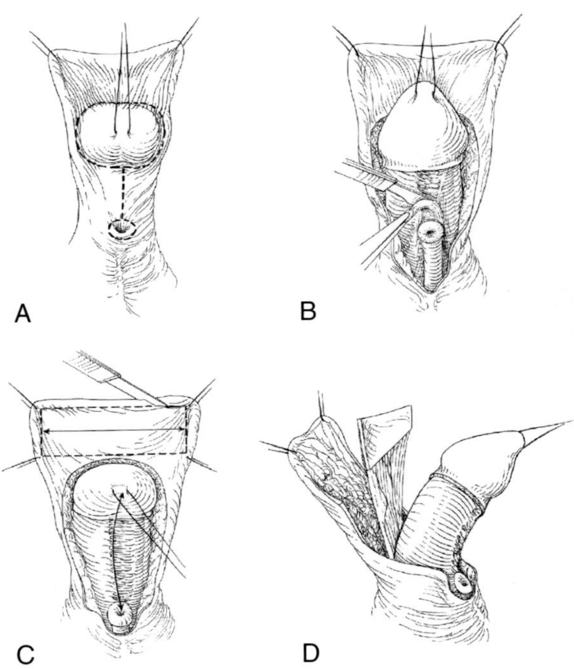

FIGURE 26.13 Transverse preputial island flap repair. (A) Proposed initial incisions for proximal shaft/penoscrotal hypospadias. (B) Release of tethering urethral plate and "dropping" of meatus proximally. (C) Incision of preputial skin of appropriate dimensions for length of defect and width for desired luminal diameter. (D) Harvested transverse preputial island flap.

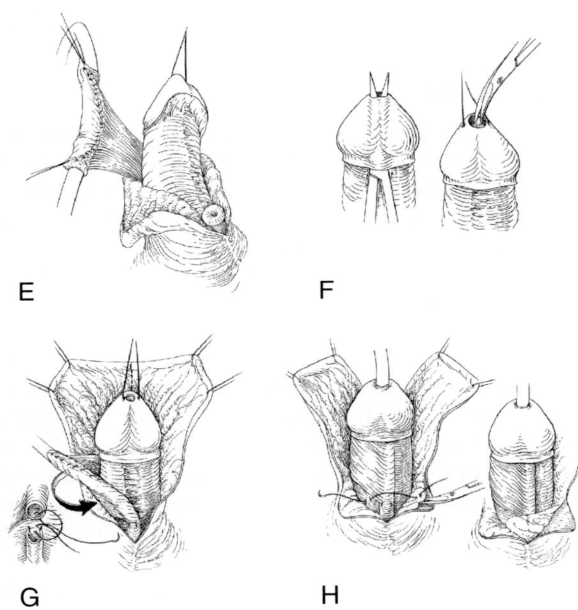

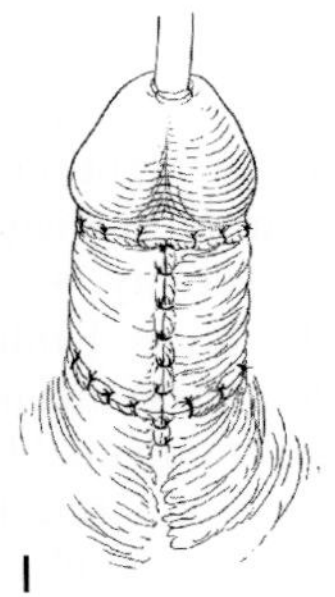

FIGURE 26.13, cont'd (E) Running subcuticular suture tubularization has been performed over a Silastic catheter to be followed by a second-layer running Lembert suture. (F) Generous glans channel is fashioned for neourethral passage. A core of glans tissue is excised to achieve sufficient caliber. (G) Native urethral meatus is fixed to corpora cavernosa prior to performing proximal anastomosis with the neourethra. (H) Subcutaneous (dartos) tissue coverage of anastomosis. (I) Finished surgery with skin suture lines. (From Atala A, Retik AB. Hypospadias. In: Libertino JA, ed. *Reconstructive Urologic Surgery*. 3rd ed. St. Louis: Mosby; 1998.)

excision with revision urethroplasty. Strictures can also lead to the development of a urethral diverticulum, which should be suspected in patients presenting with a weakened stream, postvoid dribbling or ballooning of the penile shaft. When carefully done, the procedures outlined can provide a functional and cosmetically "normal" penis and meatus even in the most severe hypospadias cases.

CRYPTORCHIDISM

The incidence of cryptorchidism is 1% to 4% in full-term males and 15%–45% in premature and low-birth-weight infants. The etiology is largely unknown, but many theories are based on various genetic, environmental, and hormonal risk factors that predispose a boy to develop cryptorchidism. Gestational testicular descent is regulated by two hormones—insulin-like 3 (INSL3) and testosterone.

Cryptorchidism is associated with a patent processus vaginalis in 90% of cases. The fertility rate is likely no different in those with treated unilateral cryptorchidism compared to controls (90% versus 93%); however, infertility may be as high as 50% in bilateral cryptorchidism. The risk of testicular cancer is increased two- to five-fold over the general population in these patients. A careful examination can discriminate retractile from undescended testis in most cases. Approximately 80% of cryptorchid testes are palpable and up to 90% are unilateral. A testis that can be manipulated into the scrotum with a gentle stretch of the cremaster and does not retract into the canal is retractile and requires no surgery. Retractile testes should be observed through puberty as 10%–16% will ascend (acquired cryptorchidism) and require intervention. A nonpalpable testis warrants exploration of the groin or diagnostic laparoscopy. Both US and MRI have poor sensitivity, 45% and 65%, respectively, in detecting nonpalpable testes. Findings also do not change the need for surgery; therefore these imaging studies are not recommended. In cases of bilateral nonpalpable testes, a karyotype and hormonal testing (follicle-stimulating hormone [FSH], luteinizing hormone [LH], inhibin, anti-Mullerian hormone, testosterone) can be helpful although will not preclude a confirmatory diagnostic laparoscopy.

Typically, inguinal exploration after 6 months of age for a palpable cryptorchid testis is the preferred surgical management (spontaneous testicular descent can occur in up to 67% of undescended testicles by 3 months of age thought secondary to the testosterone surge, i.e., "mini-puberty" that occurs in males around 2 months of life). If the canal is empty, the peritoneum is opened; either a testis or blind ending vas deferens and gonadal vessels are found overlying the psoas above the internal inguinal ring. A vanishing testis (blind-ending vessels) is thought to be due to an in utero vascular accident. In cases where the gonadal vessels are intrinsically too short, a laparoscopic two-staged Fowler-Stephens orchidopexy can be used to bring down an intraabdominal testis. In the first stage, the gonadal vessels are ligated (usually with clips) and 3–6 months later, once collateral blood supply via the cremasteric and vasal arteries has become more robust, a second-stage laparoscopic orchidopexy is performed. The traditional open, primary orchidopexy carries a success rate of > 90% while a staged Fowler-Stephens repair is successful approximately 70% of the time.

HERNIA/COMMUNICATING HYDROCELE

The incidence of infant/childhood inguinal hernia is 1% to 5% of full-term infants. This increases to 30% in infants who are born before 32 weeks and in infants weighing less than 1 kg. There is a right-sided predominance, which is attributed to delayed right testicular descent. There is a higher incidence of contralateral hernia in preterm infants that should be evaluated at the time surgery. In infants, hernias are caused by a failure of the processus vaginalis to obliterate after testicular descent.

Neonatal scrotal hydroceles are present in 5% of infants and will usually be reabsorbed by 12 months of age. No surgery is required. A communicating hydrocele is suspected if parents or practitioners note fluctuations in the volume of fluid surrounding the testicle. Unlike a true hernia, which is repaired promptly in infants because of the risk of incarceration, a true communicating hydrocele may be fixed electively after 6 months of age.

APPENDAGES

Testicular and epididymal appendages are present at the upper pole of the testis or epididymis. They represent müllerian or wolffian duct remnants and are only bothersome when torsion of the appendage occurs. Torsion of the appendix can sometimes be differentiated from testicular torsion by point tenderness and swelling at the upper pole of the testis. Examiners may note a "blue dot" sign where the infarcted tissue is apparent beneath the scrotal skin. Boys with torsion of the appendix testis may have a visible cremaster reflex. Diagnosis is usually made with scrotal US with Doppler. When diagnosis is in doubt scrotal exploration is recommended. If the diagnosis is certain, treatment is conservative with nonsteroidal antiinflammatory drugs (NSAIDs) and scrotal support as the pain will usually resolve in 3 to 5 days.

Cloacal Dysgenesis/Persistent Cloaca

CLOACA ANOMALY

Cloaca anomaly represents failure of the urorectal septum to descend, resulting in a single perineal opening or a sinus into which the rectum, vagina, and urethra enter. The upper urinary tract should be evaluated with ultrasonography as there can be associated hydronephrosis (due to hydrocolpos), dysplasia, fusion anomalies, ectopia, UPJO, and ureteral duplication. Echocardiography to rule out cardiac anomalies and lumbosacral spine US or MRI to assess for spinal cord anomalies and tethering should also be ordered. Genitosonography, VCUG if possible, and cystovaginoscopy are necessary to assess the anatomy. Diverting colostomy is usually performed early in infancy and urologic assessment can be performed under the same anesthetic.

Reconstruction via a midline posterior approach is carried out between 4 and 12 months of age. This reconstruction includes a tapering and pull through of the rectum, as well as total or partial mobilization of the vagina and urethra, with longitudinal separation of the urogenital sinus for cloacas that are shorter than 3 cm. Longer cloacas may need abdominal and perineal mobilization of the bladder, vagina, and rectum. Clitoroplasty, labioplasty, and vaginoplasty can then follow mobilization. Spinal anomalies and neurogenic bladders are common.

VAGINAL ATRESIA AND VAGINAL AGENESIS (MAYER-ROKITANSKY-KÜSTER-HAUSER SYNDROME)

1. **Vaginal atresia**
   Vaginal atresia occurs when the urogenital sinus fails to contribute to the distal portion of vagina. This differs from vaginal agenesis and testicular feminization because

müllerian structures remain unaffected; therefore the uterus, cervix, and upper portion of the vagina are normal. Hormonal assays can be used to distinguish primary vaginal atresia from a short vagina in girls with testicular feminization. Females with primary vaginal atresia have normal LH, FSH, and low testosterone levels. This condition often presents at puberty with amenorrhea. Surgical management involves a transverse incision at the level of the hymenal ring, through the fibrous area of absent lower vagina, until the upper vagina is reached. A vaginal pull through can then be performed with perineal skin flaps or simple vaginal mobilization.

2. **Vaginal agenesis**

Vaginal agenesis (müllerian aplasia), also known as Mayer-Rokitansky-Küster-Hauser (MRKH) syndrome occurs in 1 in 5000 live female births. This results in the congenital absence of the proximal portion of vagina in an otherwise phenotypically normal 46XX female. It is caused by a failure of sinovaginal bulbs to develop and form the vaginal plate. Vaginal agenesis is associated with variable absence or hypoplasia of cervix, uterus, and fallopian tubes. There are two forms of MRKH syndrome—the typical form (type A) where there are symmetrical uterine remnants and normal fallopian tubes and the atypical form (type B) where there are asymmetrical uterine buds or abnormal fallopian tubes. Other associated abnormalities in type B include renal anomalies (URA or ectopia in 75%) and skeletal and vertebral anomalies (10%–20%). It may present in the newborn period with hydrocolpos but commonly presents with primary amenorrhea or hematocolpos at puberty.

US is the study of choice for the evaluation of these genital and associated renal anomalies. VCUG is used to evaluate for reflux and cystovaginoscopy helps to delineate the introital anatomy. Those with complete uterovaginal agenesis are managed with nonoperative approaches (Frank technique of perineal pressure) or vaginal replacement surgery, described techniques include skin neovagina (McIndoe split-thickness skin graft], muscle flap neovagina, or intestinal neovagina.

CLINICAL PEARLS

1. Most congenital disorders and their associated anomalies are predictable if the embryology is known.
2. Understanding the nuances of ureteral duplication and ureteral ectopia helps predict the associated clinical manifestations of each anomaly of the upper urinary tract.
3. Despite lasting commitment to hypospadias repair and numerous approaches to correction, reconstruction of hypospadias and associated chordee remains challenging.

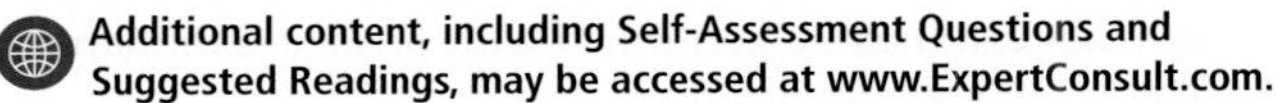

Additional content, including Self-Assessment Questions and Suggested Readings, may be accessed at www.ExpertConsult.com.

Pediatric Oncology

Christopher J. Long, MD, and Thomas F. Kolon, MD, MS

Wilms Tumor

GENERAL

First described by Rance in 1814 and characterized by Wilms in 1899, there are approximately 450 to 500 new cases per year of Wilms tumor (WT) in North America. WT is the most common pediatric renal tumor. WT represents 80% of all genitourinary (GU) cancers in children younger than 15 years of age. The median age of presentation is 3.5 years, and 90% occur before 7 years. WT is typically sporadic although 10% of patients will have an associated syndrome. 5%–10% of tumors will be bilateral, multifocal at presentation. The at-risk syndromes are divided into those with a risk of somatic overgrowth and those without. Common overgrowth syndromes include Beckwith-Wiedemann syndrome and isolated hemihypertrophy and are linked to chromosome *11p15*. Non-overgrowth syndromes include WAGR (Wilms tumor, aniridia, genital anomalies, developmental delay) and Denys-Drash, which are associated with the WT1 gene on chromosome *11p13*. Patients with at-risk syndromes are enrolled in early surveillance protocols with screening ultrasound every 3 to 4 months. Bilateral WT is more likely in patients with a predisposition syndrome.

DIAGNOSIS

Most patients will present with symptoms of a palpable abdominal mass, abdominal pain, or hematuria. In contrast to neuroblastoma, the mass typically does not cross the midline of the abdomen. Hematuria can be present in up to 25% of patients and can indicate tumor extension into the renal pelvis. Hypertension accompanies 25% to 60% of cases.

The differential diagnosis is vast and can be age driven. Other malignant abdominal tumors can masquerade as a renal mass, such as a hepatoblastoma or sarcoma. Renal-specific tumors include renal cell carcinoma and rhabdoid tumors, both of which are more likely to occur in the second decade of childhood yet remain quite rare in pediatric patients. Neuroblastoma is common and is more likely to present at a younger age. Benign abdominal masses include renal abscess, multicystic dysplastic kidney, hydronephrosis, multilocular cystic nephroma (CN), polycystic kidney, angiomyolipoma, and congenital mesoblastic nephroma (CMN). CMN typically occurs in newborns or infants. Other potential lesions include mesenteric cysts, choledochal cysts, intestinal duplication cysts, and splenomegaly.

Imaging typically begins with a renal bladder ultrasound (RBUS). If a malignant lesion is suspected, cross-sectional imaging with IV contrast should be performed, either a magnetic resonance imaging (MRI) (preferred) or computed tomography (CT) scan of the abdomen. This helps to identify tumor rupture or hemorrhage, multifocal or bilateral disease, renal vein/inferior vena cava (IVC) thrombus, and nodal involvement. A CT of the thorax should be performed to rule out metastatic disease, as this is the most common site of distant metastasis.

PATHOLOGY

Gross pathologic features include a lesion that is sharply demarcated with a pseudocapsule. Most lesions are solitary, though they can be bilateral and/or multifocal. WT are frequently large and can have hemorrhage or necrosis. Extension into the renal pelvis is rare while venous (renal vein or IVC) invasion occurs in 20% of patients.

The specific pathology varies across a wide spectrum and plays a key role in prognosis. The classic WT is triphasic, containing elements of metanephric blastema, epithelium (glomerulotubular), and stroma (myxoid, occasionally differentiated into striated muscle, cartilage, or fat). The makeup of the tumor consists of one to three of these elements to varying degrees. Epithelial differentiation is more favorable and more likely to be present in stage I tumors. Blastemal elements tend to have a better response to chemotherapy while epithelial and stromal elements respond relatively poorly. Patients with a blastemal predominant tumor have a higher risk of recurrence after chemotherapy. Unfavorable histology (UH) is present in up to

10% of lesions and includes the presence of anaplasia. Anaplasia occurs more frequently in older patients and is highly resistant to chemotherapy, regardless of tumor stage. It confers a particularly poor prognosis and diffuse anaplasia is worse than a focal distribution.

Nephrogenic rests are a precursor of WT and consist of persistent primitive metanephric elements beyond 36 weeks of gestation. They exhibit a variable natural history of maturation, involution, and sclerosis. A later in embryogenesis form consists of primarily blastemal and tubular components. An earlier embryogenesis form consists of primarily stromal elements. Multiple nephrogenic rests in a kidney confer a high risk of WT development in the contralateral kidney and warrant close surveillance. Rests are present in 100% of bilateral WT compared to only 35% of unilateral WT, though only approximately 1% of rests will progress to WT.

Additional Renal Tumors

Cystic nephroma (CN) and cystic, partially differentiated nephroblastoma (CPDN) are benign neoplasms with malignant potential (considered by many experts to be part of the spectrum of nephroblastoma). Tumors occur in both adults and children, are often associated with *DICER1* mutations, and are generally asymptomatic but may cause hematuria. CNs are all cystic, without solid component, with septa made of pure stromal tissue and lack any blastemal elements. CPDN is also cystic, but septae contain blastemal elements (or nephrogenic rests). It is important to note that nephroblastomas, clear cell sarcomas, and mesoblastic nephromas may also be predominantly cystic.

CMN occurs in early infancy and is often detected prenatally. It is associated with polyhydramnios, resembles leiomyoma grossly, and histologically exhibits sheets of spindle-shape uniform cells that appear to be fibroblasts. There is no capsule but when completely excised, it follows a benign course; it may be a hamartoma. The spindle-cell variant may behave with a more malignant potential. Treatment is typically nephrectomy given the large size at presentation.

Clear cell sarcoma of the kidney is seen in up to 3% of pediatric renal tumors. These patients receive chemotherapy and radiation therapy due to a high concern for relapse, even for low stage disease. In contrast to WT, this tumor does carry a risk for brain and bone metastasis.

Rhabdoid tumor of the kidney is relatively rare (2% of pediatric renal masses) but is the most aggressive and lethal renal mass. Patients are typically young (< 16 months of age) and present at an advanced stage. The tumor can metastasize to the brain and is poorly responsive to chemotherapy. Unfortunately, these factors lead to its high mortality rate.

STAGING

Historically, histopathology and tumor stage are the most important predictors of survival in WT patients (Table 27.1). At diagnosis the surgeon determines whether the tumor is resectable. If the tumor is thought to be unresectable, this is categorized as stage III disease and preoperative chemotherapy is performed.

TABLE 27.1 Wilms Tumor Staging of the Children's Oncology Group

Stage	Description
I	• Tumor limited to the kidney and completely excised • The renal capsule is intact, and the tumor was not ruptured prior to removal • There is no residual tumor
II	• Tumor extends beyond the kidney but is completely excised • There is regional extension of tumor (i.e., penetration of the renal capsule, invasion of the renal sinus) • Extrarenal vessels may contain tumor thrombus or be infiltrated by tumor
III	• Residual nonhematogenous tumor confined to the abdomen • Lymph node involvement • Peritoneal implants • Any tumor spillage either before or during surgery • Tumor extension beyond surgical margin either grossly or microscopically, or tumor not completely removed
IV	Hematogenous metastases (lung, liver, bone, brain) or lymph node metastases outside the abdominopelvic region are present
V	Bilateral renal involvement at diagnosis

Beyond tumor staging and node status, biologic markers are key predictors for treatment stratification and success. Loss of heterozygosity at chromosomes *16q* and/or *1p* is present in up to 20% of WT and is noted to have a higher risk of tumor recurrence. Gain of 1q is noted in up to 25% of patients with familial WT and confers a poor prognosis as well. These markers have been an important adjunct to tumor stage and histology to identify more aggressive tumors.

TREATMENT

Clinical trials are performed by several groups across the world and their efforts have drastically improved the therapeutic outcomes for patients with WT. The National Wilms Tumor Study Group (NWTSG), Children's Oncology Group (COG), International Society of Pediatric Oncology (SIOP), and United Kingdom Children's Cancer Group (UKCCSG) have created paradigms that are followed closely for these patients.

COG recommends primary surgery prior to chemotherapy and does not recommend biopsy if the tumor is deemed resectable. Radical nephrectomy with lymph node sampling is the standard protocol and all efforts should be focused on preventing tumor spillage. SIOP protocols differ in that preoperative chemotherapy is given to all patients prior to surgical resection, the justification for this being a decrease in intraoperative tumor spillage and a migration toward more lower stage tumors. UKCCSG also utilize preoperative chemotherapy but they also incorporate pretreatment biopsy. Their reasoning is the potential to avoid WT treatment for those lesions that clinically appear suspicious, as biopsy data did not identify WT in up to 12% of patients.

Current chemotherapy regimens are as follows: regimen EE-4A, vincristine, and dactinomycin for 18 weeks after nephrectomy; regimen DD-4A, vincristine, dactinomycin, doxorubicin for 24 weeks after nephrectomy or after biopsy and subsequent nephrectomy; regimen I, vincristine, doxorubicin, cyclophosphamide, and etoposide for 24 weeks after nephrectomy; regimen M, vincristine, dactinomycin, doxorubicin, cyclophosphamide, and etoposide with radiation therapy. Regimen I is used when anaplasia is identified in the tumor.

There are some specific management highlights that warrant mention. Tumors with blastemal elements are at higher risk for recurrence and stage III patients, meaning those with tumor positive nodes or tumor spillage, do benefit from radiation treatment after nephrectomy. Very low risk WT is a subset of patients that are less than 2 years of age with a stage I FH tumor that is < 550 g with negative lymph nodes. Surgery alone is indicated in these patients.

Partial nephrectomy (PN) is allowed per COG protocols for patients with bilateral disease, WT in a solitary kidney, or patients with unilateral WT with a predisposing syndrome. Patients with bilateral disease should also undergo upfront chemotherapy prior to surgical intervention. PN is performed after neoadjuvant chemotherapy is administered. Upfront chemotherapy is given for 6 weeks, at which point imaging is repeated to gauge response. If a good response is noted, another 6 weeks of chemotherapy is administered prior to surgical resection, though biopsy or surgical resection is recommended if there is a poor response. Concern does exist for a higher risk of tumor spillage, positive surgical margins, and postprocedure complications, but the literature to date has proven PN a safe and efficacious approach in select patients. PN is recommended if possible, although radical nephrectomy for the larger tumor and PN of the contralateral tumor is also an option instead of bilateral nephrectomy. If anaplasia is present in the specimen, recurrence is likely and nephrectomy is recommended.

Treatment of tumor relapse is based on the histology (presence of anaplasia) and the chemotherapy treatment to date. COG protocols divide patients into standard, high, and very high risk. Patients without anaplasia and who were treated with two-agent therapy are considered standard risk and have a high survival rate (70%–80%). These patients are given radiation therapy if they have not already received it. Patients that were treated with three agents initially are considered high risk and have a lower survival rate (40%–50%); patients with anaplasia and/or blastemal elements are considered very high risk and have a survival rate closer to 10%. These patients are given a combination of chemotherapy, surgical resection is considered if feasible, radiation therapy, and hematopoietic stem cell transplantation.

Treatment evolution has resulted in drastic improvements in cancer control and longer lifespans for patients. Although cancer control is paramount, secondary health problems after chemotherapy and radiation therapy are significant for these patients and have become a concern as these patients age, with the incidence of long-term morbidity increasing with time. Patients have a higher mortality risk compared to their peers that persists for their lifetime after completion of treatment. Cardiac toxicity is another long-term concern, with congestive heart failure significantly increased for patients who received chemotherapy. Infertility is common in patients, particularly if radiation is administered. Sperm banking is performed for older patients prior to treatment initiation, but the majority of these patients are prepubertal and this is not an option for them. Current protocols include testicular biopsy and cryopreservation in hopes of future fertility from these precursor cells. Secondary malignancy rates increase with further follow-up and this effect is amplified if radiation therapy is administered. Due to the increased survival for these patients, an increased focus has been placed on these concerns, especially as they enter adulthood and are at risk for early onset of chronic disease.

SURGICAL MANAGEMENT OF WILMS TUMOR

Surgical resection is the mainstay of WT management. For patients with a unilateral mass, nephrectomy with hilar lymph node dissection is the first step in management. Exploration is carried out as soon as the child is medically stable and the previously mentioned studies are completed. Historical teaching included exploration of the contralateral kidney with biopsy as needed, though this is no longer needed with modern imaging techniques. Resectability depends largely on the degree of attachment to surrounding organs or major vascular invasion into the vena cava. Heroic extirpation involving major resection of these organs or cardiopulmonary bypass to remove high caval or atrial tumors is not warranted. Unresectable lesions should be treated first with neoadjuvant chemotherapy, after which there is a higher chance of successful resection with negative margins. Pretreatment of large tumors reduces the rate of intraoperative rupture and may shift to a more favorable histology.

Transverse abdominal incision provides adequate exposure in most cases, from the tip of the 12th rib on the involved side to the ipsilateral rectus abdominis (the rectus can be spared in many cases). The colon is completely reflected, and complete mobilization of kidney is required for adequate visualization. Beginning the dissection along the posterior abdominal wall inferiorly and the great vessels medially, with early ureteral ligation, allows early exposure and ligation of renal vessels prior to mobilization of the mass.

Biopsy of the tumor or localized operative spill upstages the tumor and prompts abdominal radiation due to an increased incidence of abdominal recurrence. The adrenal is taken if the tumor involves the upper pole. Gross assessment of lymph nodes has a 40% false-positive and 0% false-negative rate, and thus routine dissection of hilar and periaortic nodes is warranted as it does improve staging. The absence of lymph node biopsy is associated with an increased relative risk of recurrence, which was largest in children with presumed stage I disease because of under staging. Remaining tumor in nodes or other organs should be marked with surgical clips to facilitate direction of radiation therapy.

Neuroblastoma

Traditionally neuroblastoma has been grouped with WT due to an overlap in the age of presentation, but contemporary management has been mainly by pediatric general surgery, so our discussion will be abbreviated. Neuroblastoma represents 8% to 10% of all childhood malignancies and is the most common malignant tumor of infancy. Following brain tumors, it is the most common malignant solid tumor of childhood. One-third of cases are diagnosed in the first year of life and an additional one-fourth between 1 and 2 years of age.

Tumor cells arise from primitive, pluripotent sympathetic cells derived from the neural crest. Neuroblastoma can arise anywhere along the sympathetic chain from the head to pelvis; more than half arise in the abdomen and two-thirds of these in the adrenal. Lesions are lobular, tend to be infiltrative, and are often associated with a classically described stippled calcification on imaging. Histologically, neuroblastoma is one of the "small, round blue-cell tumors" of childhood. There is a malignancy gradient from neuroblastoma (most malignant) to ganglioneuroblastoma (intermediate) to ganglioneuroma (benign). As many as 70% of patients have metastasis at presentation (liver is most common in younger children, bone in older children). Classically these patients are described as being "sick" at diagnosis, commonly with unexplained fever, malaise, anorexia, weight loss, and irritability. This contrasts with WT patients, who are less likely to have metastatic disease at presentation. Pareneoplastic syndromes are also common at presentation with secretion of catecholamines and vasoactive intestinal peptide resulting in hypertension and diarrhea, respectively.

Bone marrow aspirate is indicated in all suspected cases and 50% to 70% will be positive. Most patients will be anemic due to bone marrow metastasis. Ninety-five percent of patients have elevation of urinary catecholamines (vanillylmandelic acid and/or homovanillic acid). Appropriate radiographic imaging will depend on the site. An abdominal x-ray can identify a calcified mass (the classic stippled appearance). Cross-sectional imaging with a CT or MRI will differentiate a neuroblastoma from a WT due to the presence of intratumor calcification and vascular encasement, which is common in neuroblastoma (Table 27.2). A meta-iodobenzylguanidine

TABLE 27.2 International Neuroblastoma Staging System

Stage	Description
1	• Localized tumor confined to the area of origin with complete gross excision, with or without microscopic residual disease • Identifiable ipsilateral and contralateral lymph nodes negative microscopically
2A	• Localized tumor with incomplete gross excision • Ipsilateral, nonadherent lymph nodes negative microscopically
2B	• Localized tumor with complete or incomplete gross excision • Ipsilateral, nonadherent lymph nodes positive • Contralateral enlarged nodes must be negative for tumor
3	• Unresectable unilateral tumor crossing the midline, with or without regional lymph node involvement • Localized unilateral tumor with contralateral regional node involvement • Midline tumor with bilateral extension by infiltration (unresectable) or by node involvement
4	Dissemination of tumor to distant lymph nodes, bone, bone marrow, liver, skin, and/or other organs (except as defined in stage 4S)
4S	Localized primary tumor as defined for stage 1 or 2 with dissemination limited to liver, skin, and/or bone marrow

(MIBG) scan will be taken up by tumors cells and can help identify both primary and metastatic disease.

Children under 1 year of age have favorable survival outcomes, as do patients with lower stage disease. Children at higher risk include those over 1 year of age, and those with higher stage, amplification of *N-MYC* gene, unfavorable histology, and DNA ploidy. N-MYC amplification is more commonly found in patients with higher stage disease and is an independent predictor for a poor prognosis.

Surgery is reserved for initial biopsy and complete resection if the tumor is small enough and amenable to removal. Otherwise, surgery is performed after chemotherapy is administered. Based on International Neuroblastoma Staging System (INSS) criteria, the operative protocol begins by assessing resectability of primary or metastatic tumor, which is determined by the tumor location, relationship to major vessels, ability to control the blood supply, and overall prognosis of patient. Nonadherent, intracavitary lymph nodes should be sampled. Routine biopsy of the liver in situations involving an abdominal neuroblastoma without evidence of metastatic disease has been advocated.

Chemotherapy consists of carboplatin, cyclophosphamide, doxorubicin, and etoposide. Treatment of intermediate-risk disease, which includes children with metastatic disease to regional lymph nodes and infants with INSS stage 4 tumors, involves chemotherapy for 12 to 24 weeks of the same chemotherapy as described previously. In addition, radiation therapy is utilized to enhance disease-free survival, specifically in patients with Stage III or IV disease (excluding IV-S). Treatment of high-risk disease, specifically patients with disseminated disease, requires intensive treatment with multiagent therapy of various combinations, although overall survival has remained disappointingly low (below 15%). All patients with stage I disease can be cured and the vast majority of stage II disease has excellent outcomes. Patients with IV-S disease, which occurs in infants, overall do quite well, with most having spontaneous tumor involution.

Genitourinary Rhabdomyosarcoma

Rhabdomyosarcoma (RMS) arises from primitive totipotential embryonal mesenchyme, specifically striated muscle. GU tract involvement occurs with the second greatest frequency after head and neck tumors. Sites include bladder, prostate, vagina, and cervix or paratesticular tissue. GU sites comprise approximately 20% of all RMSs. The incidence of GU RMS is 0.5 to 0.7 cases per 1 million in children younger than 15 years. Most tumors arise sporadically, although patients with Li-Fraumeni syndrome, basal cell nevus syndrome, Costello syndrome, Noonan syndrome, and multiple endocrine neoplasm type 2A (MEN 2A) have been associated with a higher risk of RMS development.

PATHOLOGY

Tumor subtypes differ based on extent of differentiation from mesenchymal progenitor. Tumor classification by Intergroup Rhabdomyosarcoma Study (IRSG)/COG include embryonal RMS (ERMS), alveolar RMS (ARMS), and anaplastic or undifferentiated. Embryonal subtypes are considered a more favorable variant and occur more frequently. Genetic translocation plays an important role for prognosis, particularly for ARMS. The *PAX3* (chromosome 2) or *PAX7* (chromosome 1) fusion with *FOX01* (chromosome 13) translocation occurs in up to 80% of ARMS tumors. Of the 20% of patients without a translocation, the prognosis of ARMS and ERMS tumors is equal. Undifferentiated tumors have a very poor prognosis. Botryoid tumors, which occur in the vagina, typically have an excellent prognosis.

PRESENTATION

Signs and symptoms are dependent on organ of involvement and size of the primary tumor at initial assessment. Bladder and/or prostate lesions typically present with obstructive symptoms including urinary retention, stranguria, incontinence, or infection. Trigonal involvement leads to hydronephrosis and progressive obstruction. Hematuria and constipation are also seen. Vaginal tumors can present with a visible mass and vaginal discharge. Paratesticular RMS presents as a painless scrotal mass.

EVALUATION

Imaging typically begins with an ultrasound. Suspicious lesions should prompt a CT or MRI to evaluate the tumor, nodal involvement, and for any evidence of metastatic disease. CT thorax should be performed in all patients. Bone scan is reserved for patients with node positive disease and those with a positive CT thorax. Biopsy of the primary lesion occurs after staging and most of these tumors are amenable to endoscopic biopsy, though the location may require percutaneous or rarely open biopsy. If a bladder lesion cannot be biopsied endoscopically, an open approach with pelvic and paraaortic lymph node biopsy is indicated, though this is a rare event. The goals of therapy are organ preservation and complete tumor resection should only be performed if the primary organ be left intact. The exception to this paradigm is for a paratesticular RMS, in which case radical orchiectomy is performed.

STAGING

Pretreatment RMS staging is dependent on the size and location of the primary tumor, the status of draining lymph nodes, and the presence or absence of metastatic disease (Table 27.3). The bladder and prostate are unfavorable sites, while paratesticular, vaginal, vulvar, cervical, and uterine tumors are favorable sites. Additional factors in prognosis include patient age, tumor histology, and the tumor fusion gene status. The ultimate outcome predictor for these patients incorporates the pretreatment stage, the surgical resection outcome, and the histologic subtype, as opposed to surgical staging alone (Table 27.3–27.5).

TABLE 27.3 IRS TNM Clinical Staging

Stage	Stage 1: favorable site, nonmetastatic Stage 2: unfavorable site, small tumor, negative nodes, nonmetastatic Stage 3: unfavorable site, larger or positive nodes, nonmetastatic Stage 4: any site, metastatic
Tumor	T1: confined to site of origin T2: fixation to surrounding tissue
Site	Favorable: paratesticular, vagina, vulva, cervix, uterus Unfavorable: bladder, prostate
Regional lymph nodes	N0: regional lymph nodes not clinically involved N1: regional lymph nodes clinically involved
Metastasis	M0: no distant metastasis M1: metastasis present

TABLE 27.4 Postoperative Clinical Group Assignments

Clinical Group	Tumor Status
1	Localized disease, completely resected
2	• Grossly resected tumor with microscopic residual disease • Regional disease with involved nodes, completely resected with no microscopic residual • Regional disease with involved nodes, grossly resected, but with evidence of microscopic residual and/or histologic involvement of the most distal regional node (from primary site) in the dissection
3	Incomplete resection or biopsy with gross residual mass
4	Distant metastasis

TABLE 27.5 Rhabdomyosarcoma Risk Stratification

Histology	Clinical Group	Stage	Age	Risk Group
Embryonal	I, II, III	1	All	Low
Embryonal	I, II	2, 3	All	Low
Embryonal	III	2,3	All	Intermediate
Embryonal	IV	4	< 10 years	Intermediate
Embryonal	IV	4	> 10 years	High
Alveolar	I, II, III	1, 2, 3	All	Intermediate
Alveolar	IV	4	All	High

TREATMENT

RMS treatment is multimodal in nature, incorporating chemotherapy and radiation therapy in addition to surgical resection. As mentioned earlier, outside of paratesticular tumors, complete primary tumor resection should only be attempted if the tumor can be completely excised with an organ-sparing approach. Primary resection can be more successful after a chemotherapy treatment course depending upon the tumor response. The chemotherapeutic regimen of choice includes vincristine, D-actinomycin, and cyclophosphamide (VAC). RMS tumors are responsive to radiation therapy and studies have shown a higher risk of local recurrence if radiation is not administered.

There are several primary tumor site-specific treatment patterns. Bladder and prostate RMS are higher risk sites, and chemotherapy is initiated after biopsy and radiation therapy is initiated due to improved survival rates. Vaginal and other gynecologic RMS tumors have an excellent survival and combined chemotherapy and radiation therapy is the treatment of choice. Brachytherapy or endovaginal radiation therapy is an option for this group, though long-term concerns of vaginal stenosis, atrophy, and dyspareunia must be considered for these patients.

Once treatment has completed, follow-up imaging can identify the presence of a residual mass and endoscopy combined with biopsy can confirm pathology. Biopsy will often reveal the presence of rhabdomyoblasts representing dormant, treated tumor cells rather than oncologically active tumor cells. No further intervention of rhabdomyoblasts is required, other than close surveillance. Our protocol after treatment is repeat surveillance biopsies confirming the presence of rhabdomyoblasts or normal cells for 4 years after therapy (5 years from diagnosis).

Radical cystectomy is relatively rare now given the tendency toward bladder preservation. If we proceed with cystectomy, we surveil the subsequent continent bladder diversion for 2 years to ensure no tumor recurrence. We begin with a bilateral cutaneous ureterostomy at the time of cystectomy (though an ileal loop diversion is reasonable) and Indiana pouch at the time of continent diversion.

Testis Tumors

Testis tumors are uncommon in children, accounting for approximately 1% to 2% of all pediatric solid tumors. Incidence in children is 1 per 100,000. There is a bimodal peak incidence, first within the first 2 years of life and again in the postpubertal ages. Children have more benign tumors and fewer germinal testis tumors than do adults. Puberty is an important transition period, after which children with testicular tumors have a similar risk profile as adults.

CLASSIFICATION

We will outline the tumor types according to the bimodal distribution mentioned earlier (Table 27.6). In prepubertal children germinal tumors constitute approximately 77%, compared with 95% of testis tumors in adults. The two most common tumors are yolk sac tumor and teratoma.

Yolk sac carcinoma (YST) comprises up to 60% of all testis tumors in children and is the most common malignant tumor in this age group. YST is unique in that it rarely spreads to retroperitoneal nodes (4%), instead spreading to the lungs (20%) via hematogenous route. Alpha-fetoprotein (AFP) is elevated 90% of time, and if elevated is pathognomonic of yolk sac tumor presence. Of note AFP is physiologically elevated during the first year of life (typical nadir occurs between 6 and 8 months of age). Presentation is typically within the first 2 years of life and can occur in the newborn period.

Teratoma constitutes approximately 40% of tumors in prepubertal boys and is the most common benign testis tumor in this

TABLE 27.6 Classification of Prepubertal Testis Tumors

Prepubertal Testicular Tumors	Adolescent/Adult Testicular Tumors

Germ cell tumors
• Yolk sac tumor
• Teratoma
• Seminoma
Gonadal stromal tumors
• Leydig cell tumor
• Sertoli cell tumor
• Juvenile granulosa cell tumors
Gonadoblastoma
Lymphoma and leukemia
Paratesticular rhabdomyosarcoma
Benign lesions
• Mature teratoma
• Epidermoid cyst
• Simple cyst
	Germ cell tumors
	• Seminoma
	• Non-seminomatous germ cell tumor
	  • Choriocarcinoma
	  • Embryonal carcinoma
	  • Yolk sac tumor
	  • Teratoma
	  • Mixed germ cell tumor

age group, referred to as mature teratoma. It includes all three embryologic germ cell layers to varying degrees. Tumor markers should be normal. This contrasts with postpubertal males, in whom there is risk for metastatic disease and, and the mass is termed immature teratoma. Seminoma is extremely rare before puberty and should be considered a postpubertal tumor.

Gonadal stromal tumors (nongerm cell) typically present between 4 and 5 years of age. Interstitial cell (Leydig cell) tumors represent approximately 18% of all testis tumors, can present with virilizing (precocious puberty) or virilizing with gynecomastia (rarely malignant). These must be differentiated from Leydig cell hyperplasia (nodules that develop in testes of boys with poorly controlled congenital adrenal hyperplasia). Leydig tumors are unresponsive to adrenocorticotropic hormone (ACTH) and dexamethasone and gonadotropin stimulation. Sertoli cell tumors are approximately 8% of all prepubertal testis tumors; they are usually present as a painless mass and are rarely malignant. They are rarely metabolically active, with about 10% presenting with gynecomastia. Juvenile granulosa cell tumor presents in neonates and is distinguished preoperatively from yolk sac tumor if AFP is negative.

Paratesticular RMS constitutes approximately 4% of testis tumors in children and can arise from the epididymis, spermatic cord, or the testicular tunics. These tumors are not metabolically active and tumor markers are not elevated.

Gonadoblastoma contains both germline and stromal cell tumor types but only occurs in patients with a history of Difference of Sex Development (DSD or intersex), specifically those with a mosaic karyotype containing a Y component (i.e., mosaic Turner syndrome). These tumors are at increased risk for malignant degeneration into dysgerminoma or seminoma.

Reticuloendothelial malignancy, primarily lymphomas and leukemias, may present with testicular tumor(s) in 2% to 3% of patients. If the initial presenting symptoms include bilateral testicular masses, an examination for systemic disease is warranted.

DIAGNOSIS

Patients will typically present with a painless testicular or scrotal mass. Some will complain of pain or have concerns for scrotal skin changes. Others can present with an incidental mass noted on scrotal imaging completed for alternative reasons. The exam should also include palpation of the cord as well as regional lymph nodes. One should be able to differentiate a testicular from a paratesticular mass. The patient should be examined for signs of precocious puberty. Patients can present with signs of metastatic disease, such as weight loss, chest pain, abdominal pain, and/or shortness of breath.

Scrotal ultrasound should be done in most patients with a testicular mass. The sensitivity for detecting a mass nears 100%. A teratoma can contain both cystic and solid components. A YST can be well circumscribed but is typically well vascularized and can have areas of necrosis and/or hemorrhage. A multifocal hypoechoic pattern is characteristic of leukemia or lymphoma. A small (<1 cm), solitary mass that has well-defined borders and no necrosis or hemorrhage suggests a benign lesion. An epidermoid cyst is a benign lesion and classically described as having an onion skin appearance on ultrasound.

Malignant lesions require additional workup. A chest CT is performed to rule out metastasis. MRI of the abdomen and pelvis is a mainstay of retroperitoneal evaluation if a mass is suspicious for a malignancy. CT scan can also be considered but MRI avoids radiation for the child.

Serum tumor markers should be performed in all patients, even those with a suspected benign lesion. AFP, human chorionic gonadotropin-β (β-HCG), and lactate dehydrogenase (LDH) aid in the diagnosis and treatment course. In cases of Leydig cell tumor, serum testosterone and urinary 17-ketosteroids are evaluated. Chorionic gonadotropins, follicle-stimulating hormone (FSH), and luteinizing hormone (LH) are normal or low. Height, weight, bone age, and pubertal changes are advanced. Sertoli cell tumors exhibit normal or elevated estrogens and androgens in urine and serum; 17-ketosteroids are normal, as are gonadotropins.

MANAGEMENT

As in adults, radical inguinal orchiectomy is standard unless preoperative evaluation suggests benign tumor, in which case an inguinal approach is taken but partial orchiectomy is performed after control of the inguinal cord. Surgical excision of the primary tumor should be expedited, with tumor markers performed prior to or just before making an incision. Staging is similar to that of adult testis tumors (Table 27.7). Early control of the cord should be performed to prevent tumor spillage. If a partial orchiectomy is planned, preoperative counseling should include the possible need for orchiectomy. Intraoperative US can be used to localize small tumors. An intraoperative frozen pathologic analysis should rule out a malignant process.

For those patients with organ-confined YST, AFP will fall rapidly to normal. If the CT scan is negative, close surveillance is the treatment of choice and no chemotherapy or radiation therapy is administered. Monitoring should include monthly AFP and chest x-ray for the first year, then bimonthly during the second year. CT scan of the chest and abdomen may also be obtained every 3 months for the first year and every 6 months for the second year (varies by institution). In contrast to adult germ cell tumor (GCT) management, retroperitoneal lymph node resection (RPLND) has little to no role in the management of YST due to its hematogenous spread. Patients who have adenopathy and persistently

TABLE 27.7 Children's Oncology Group Staging System for Testicular Germ Cell Tumors

Stage	Extent of Disease
I	• Limited to testis (testes), completely resected by high inguinal orchiectomy • No clinical, radiographic, or histologic evidence of disease beyond the testis • Tumor markers normal after appropriate half-life decline (AFP, 5 days; ß-hCG, 16 hours) • Patients with normal or unknown tumor markers at diagnosis must have a negative ipsilateral retroperitoneal node sampling to confirm stage I disease if imagining identified nodes > 2 cm
II	• Microscopic disease in scrotum or high in spermatic cord (≤ 5 cm from proximal end) • Tumor markers remain elevated after appropriate half-life interval • Tumor rupture or scrotal biopsy before orchiectomy
III	• Retroperitoneal lymph node involvement • Nodes > 4 cm are considered metastasis • Biopsy of nodes 2–4 cm to confirm diagnosis
IV	Distant metastases

elevated AFP after orchiectomy will undergo chemotherapy and cure rates approach 100% in these patients.

Mature teratoma in the prepubescent male is cured with a partial orchiectomy as metastases from a mature teratoma have never been reported in children. Epidermoid cysts can also be cured with testis-sparing surgery. Reticuloendothelial tumors are managed by biopsy and systemic therapy.

Gonadal stromal tumors (Leydig, Sertoli) are thought to be benign in almost all cases and are preferentially treated with a partial orchiectomy but may warrant orchiectomy depending on the size. Tumors have ultrasound appearance of an intraparenchymal, homogenous, hypoechoic lesion. Enucleation of the tumor is a possible alternative to radical orchiectomy, depending on its size. Regression of virilizing signs is unpredictable and endocrine referral is mandatory. Patients can have advanced bone age in response to excessive virilization.

Patients with paratesticular RMS are treated with radical orchiectomy and high ligation of the cord. This is typically curative in patients with normal abdominal imaging. RPLND is recommended for patients ≥ 10 years of age, regardless of the abdominal CT imaging as this does increase their overall and disease-free survival rates.

Postpubertal GCT are managed the same as in adult patients, so we will refer the reader to this specific chapter 17 (Adult Genitourinary Cancer: Renal and Testicular) of the book for further discussion.

Postpubertal males should be counseled to undergo sperm cryopreservation before initiation of chemotherapy, RPLND, or radiation therapy due to the concerns for treatment effects. Prepubertal males are eligible for testicular tissue cryopreservation at select centers. Although current technology has not achieved fertilization, it does yield the best chance for achieving this in the future for these patients.

PROGNOSIS

Compared to postpubertal tumors, pediatric masses are more likely to be benign and to have a better prognosis even if malignant. Children younger than 2 years with yolk sac tumors have approximately a 98% chance of survival. The prognosis is worse in older children and those with metastatic disease. Patients with paratesticular RMS typically have a favorable diagnosis, though those presenting at an age ≥ 10 years and a primary tumor ≥ 5 cm have a worse prognosis.

CLINICAL PEARLS

1. **Wilms tumor**—Children often present with large tumors that typically result in nephrectomy. Chemotherapy can dramatically shrink Wilms tumor and, as a result, nephron sparing surgery has emerged as a treatment option for these patients, particularly those with bilateral masses. Neoadjuvant chemotherapy is warranted in patients with bilateral tumors. Surgical resection includes resection of the tumor intact with lymph node dissection to fully stage the tumor. The presence of anaplasia is a poor prognostication.
2. **Neuroblastoma**—Neuroblastoma remains the most common extracranial solid cancer in childhood that displays marked heterogeneity, from low- to high-risk tumors. Those with high-risk disease can be difficult to treat, with even the most intensive multimodal therapies achieving only 30% cure rates.
3. **Genitourinary (GU) rhabdomyosarcoma**—The evolution in the management of GU rhabdomyosarcoma has shifted from primarily radical exenteration to organ-sparing procedures. The histologic diagnosis is made with biopsy, followed by chemotherapy, and then assessing radiographically for a decrease in tumor size. Surgical resection can then provide accurate staging of the patient, with some situations lending themselves to endoscopic resection of the tumor to attempt to spare organs. In younger children, avoiding radiation therapy, particularly to the pelvis, can be beneficial to prevent both short-term and long-term morbidity.
4. **Testis tumors**—In general pediatric testes tumors are more likely to be benign and those that are malignant typically have a better prognosis. Pediatric testis tumors with an elevation of alpha fetoprotein (AFP) generally denote yolk sac carcinoma and require orchiectomy. Other prepubertal testes that are not associated with elevation of AFP may be amenable to partial orchiectomy or enucleation if a discreet lesion is noted. Once a patient demonstrates pubertal changes and is found to have a potential testicular teratoma, radical orchiectomy is indicated as opposed to performing a testis-sparing procedure.

Pediatric Urolithiasis

John K. Weaver, MD, and Arun K. Srinivasan, MD

Pediatric Nephrolithiasis

PRESENTATION

There has been a significant increase in the prevalence of nephrolithiasis from 5% (1988–1994) to 9% (2007–2010).[1,2] A disproportionate increase has been reported in children with the greatest change seen in female adolescents. Incidence among girls aged 15 to 19 increased from 75 per 100,000 in 1997 to 120 per 100,000 in 2012.[3] As a result, it is more critical than ever for practitioners to develop the necessary skills to diagnose and treat pediatric patients who present with nephrolithiasis.

Pediatric patients often do not present with the classic localized flank pain that physicians are accustomed to seeing in adults. Children are often unable to reliably localize their pain. Nonspecific abdominal pain is often their initial presenting complaint. It is critical for physician to possess a high degree of suspicion for stones in patients presenting with abdominal pain, particularly if the patient has a prior history of kidney stones.

All patients with a potential kidney stone should undergo a thorough history and physical exam. Patients who have a stone will often describe a history of nausea and vomiting in conjunction with their pain. Some patients will endorse gross hematuria which can help guide the clinician to the appropriate diagnosis. The hematuria results from the stone irritating the urothelium. If the stone has migrated into the distal ureter, the patient may complain of frequency, irritation, and dysuria with voiding.

Occasionally patients will complain of fevers and chills during an acute stone episode. This occurs if the stone has resulted in obstruction of the flow of urine. If urinary flow is obstructed, the static urine is susceptible to becoming infected. Patients with infection in the setting of a urinary obstruction can develop sepsis very quickly. It is critical for a practitioner to quickly identify these patients, as they will require the emergent placement of a ureteral stent or nephrostomy tube in order to bypass the obstruction and drain the infection.

A urologic history should be obtained from all stone patients. This is critical, as subsequent potential treatment options are dependent on a patient's current urologic condition. Additionally, any patients at risk of urinary stasis are prone to both stone formation and infection.

A family history of nephrolithiasis should be obtained. Inherited metabolic or genetic conditions that place patients at risk for nephrolithiasis include cystinuria, primary hyperoxaluria, *CY24A1* gene mutations, or Dent disease. A complete dietary history should also be obtained including daily fluid intake, salt intake, vitamin and mineral supplementation, as well as inquiring if the patient is on a special diet, such as a ketogenic diet. Certain medications can also place patients at an increased risk for stones. These include, but are not limited to, corticosteroids, diuretics (furosemide, acetazolamide), protease inhibitors (indinavir), antibiotics, and antiepileptics (topiramate).[4]

A complete abdominal and genitourinary exam should be performed on all children presenting with a potential stone. Patients may endorse costovertebral or lower quadrant tenderness on the affected side.

LABORATORY EVALUATION

A urinalysis is a critical component of the nephrolithiasis workup. There will often be red blood cells present for reasons previously discussed. Finding bacteria in a urine specimen suggests the presence of a urinary tract infection (UTI). The threshold for the classic definition of bacteriuria is 5+, which is roughly equivalent to 100,000 colony-forming units (CFUs)/mL.[5] Pyuria, defined as urine WBC > 10 or positive leukocyte esterase, indicates the presence of inflammation.[6]

Nitrites will be positive if an organism that reduces nitrate is present within the urine. Not all urinary pathogens are nitrate reducers; for example, *Pseudomonas* and gram-positive organisms are not, but a positive test is highly specific for bacterial infection.

The pH of a urine specimen can also be helpful in identifying the most likely type of stone that is present. Calcium phosphate and struvite stones will form in alkaline conditions, while calcium oxalate, cystine, and uric acid stones generally form in acidic urine.

Crystals may be seen in the microscopic analysis of urinary sediment and can both indicate the potential presence and the composition of a stone. Calcium oxalate crystals tend to have a refractile square "envelope" shape. Cystine crystals are generally hexagonal in shape and the triple phosphate crystals from struvite stones have a "coffin-lid" appearance.[5]

A complete metabolic panel should also be obtained when evaluating a patient for a potential stone episode. A patient may be found to have an elevated creatinine as a result of dehydration from the associated nausea and vomiting. Electrolytes may also be significantly abnormal depending on how long the patient has been symptomatic. See Figs. 28.1 and 28.2 for nonemergent and emergent clinical care pathways for kidney stones.

Urinary Metabolic Abnormalities

CALCIUM

Urinary metabolic abnormalities should be checked in all pediatric stone patients. These results can be helpful in terms of identifying the etiology of the stone and determining the best treatment course. Approximately 30%–50% of children with kidney stones are found to have hypercalciuria. Idiopathic hypercalciuria is defined as hypercalciuria that occurs in the absence of hypercalcemia in patients in whom no other cause can be identified.[7,8] It appears to be transmitted in an autosomal dominant fashion with incomplete penetrance.[9,10]

A 24-hour urine collection can be performed to determine a patient's daily calcium excretion. While a 24-hour urine collection is the gold standard, it is not always practical in children, particularly in very young children who are not toilet trained. In these patients a urine calcium/creatinine ratio can be used to estimate daily calcium excretion. The majority of normocalcemic hypercalciuric patients are idiopathic, but this is a diagnosis of exclusion and known causes for normocalcemic hypercalciuric should first be ruled out. These include prematurity, diuretic exposure (furosemide, acetazolamide), anticonvulsants (topiramate), ketogenic diet, Dent disease, Bartter syndrome, distal renal

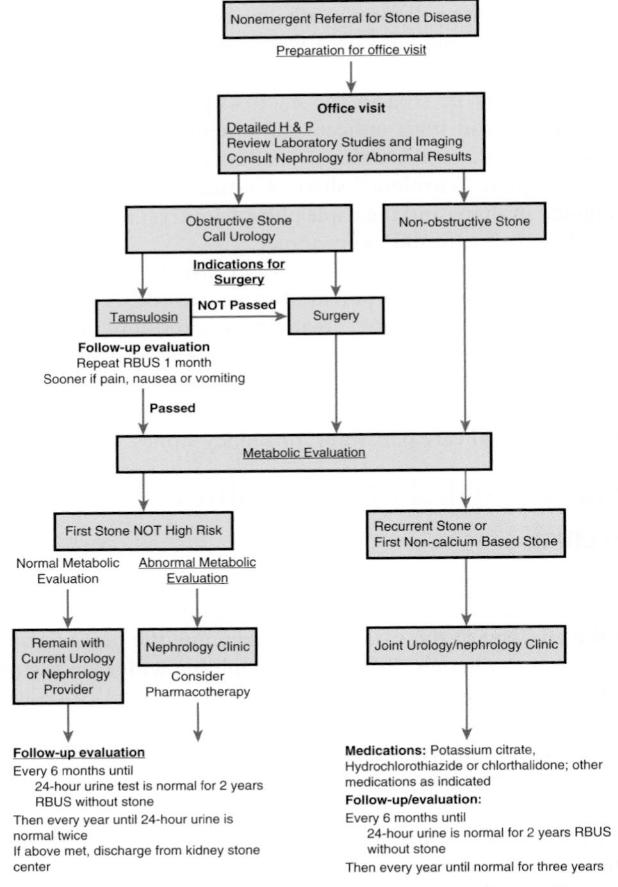

FIGURE 28.1 **The standard care pathway for patients presenting with a nonemergent kidney stone at the Children's Hospital of Philadelphia. *RBUS,* Renal bladder Ultrasound.** (From Tasian GE, Copelovitch L, Plachter N, et al. Outpatient clinical pathway for the evaluation/treatment of child with nephrolithiasis. Children's Hospital of Philadelphia Center for Healthcare Quality and Analytics. https://www.chop.edu/clinical-pathway/nephrolithiasis-outpatient-specialty-care-clinical-pathway; 2019.)

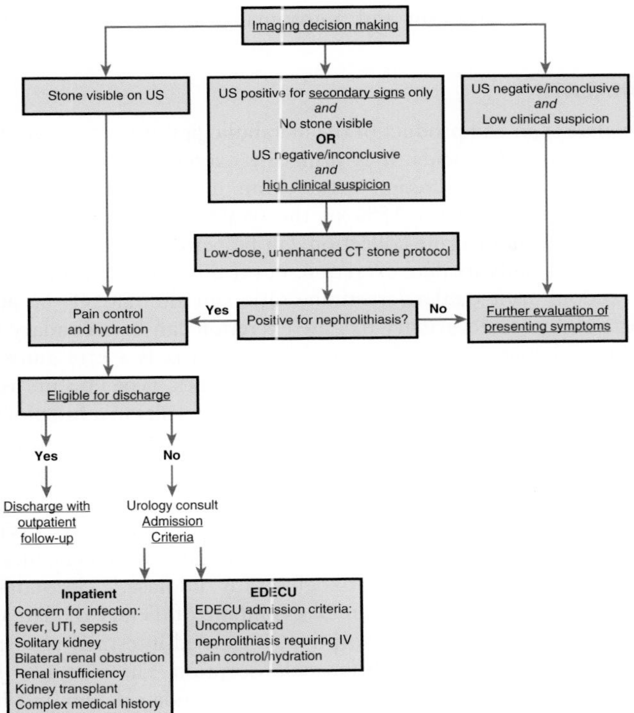

FIGURE 28.2 The clinical care pathway for patients presenting to the emergency room with a kidney stone at the Children's Hospital of Philadelphia. *CT*, Computed tomography; *US*, ultrasound; *UTI*, urinary tract infection. (From Zonfrillo M, Lavelle J, Piro J, Kim S, Darge K. ED pathway for evaluation and treatment of children with suspected nephrolithiasis. Children's Hospital of Philadelphia Center for Healthcare Quality and Analytics. https://www.chop.edu/clinical-pathway/nephrolithiasis-suspected-emergent-care-clinical-pathway; 2018.)

tubular acidosis (dRTA), hereditary hypophosphatemic rickets with hypercalciuria, familial hypomagnesemia with hypercalciuria and nephrocalcinosis, and possibly medullary sponge kidney.

Potential causes of hypercalcemic hypercalciuria include hyperparathyroidism, biallelic CYP24A1 mutations, hypervitaminosis D, prolonged immobilization, sarcoidosis, malignancy, and corticosteroid excess. Hypocalcemic hypercalciuria can be secondary to hypoparathyroidism and autosomal dominant hypocalcemic hypercalciuria.

OXALATE

Oxalate is an end product of the metabolic pathways for glyoxylate and ascorbic acids. It is primarily excreted by the kidneys. Urinary oxalate excretion arises from metabolic homeostasis. Diet contributes 10%–15% of the oxalate that is excreted in urine. A 24-hour urine collection can be performed to determine a patient's daily oxalate excretion, but if this is not feasible, then a random urine oxalate/creatinine ratio can alternatively be performed. Increased urinary oxalate excretion can be secondary to primary hyperoxaluria. Primary hyperoxaluria is a rare autosomal recessive disorder consisting of three types. Type I occurs as a result of a mutation in the AGXT gene that results in a functional defect of the hepatic peroxisomal enzyme alanine-glyoxylate aminotransferase. Type II which is milder than type I is caused by a mutation in the *GRHPR* gene which results in deficient glyoxylate reductase-hydroxypyruvate reductase enzyme activity.[11] Type III results from a mutation in the HOGA1 gene which encodes a mitochondrial 4-hydroxy-2-oxoglutarate aldolase.[12] Secondary hyperoxaluria results from an excess intake of dietary oxalate or an increase in intestinal absorption. Increased intestinal absorption occurs in patients with fat malabsorption. The excess fat in the gastrointestinal tract of these patients binds calcium and by doing so does not allow calcium to bind oxalate. Unbound oxalate is then free to be absorbed in excess.

CITRATE

When intracellular acidosis is present in the proximal tubules, citrate is reabsorbed in order to counteract the acidosis. This results in hypocitraturia. Hypocitraturia can be seen in the setting of a ketogenic diet, acetazolamide, topiramate, dRTA, and chronic diarrhea, but most cases are idiopathic. Additionally, a diet high in animal protein and low in vegetable fiber and potassium promotes lower citrate excretion.[13]

CYSTINE

Cystinuria is an autosomal recessive disorder that results from mutations in the SLC3A1 or SLC7A9 genes. It is characterized by a lack of reabsorption of cystine as well as the dibasic amino acids lysine, ornithine, and arginine. Patients typically present with renal colic and stones in the second and third decade of life; however, they may present as early as infancy with staghorn calculi. The poor solubility of the excess cystine in the urine of these patients places them at risk of recurrent nephrolithiasis and even renal failure.[14]

URIC ACID

Uric acid excretion is greater in children than in adults; however, despite the higher uric acid excretion observed in children, uric acid nephrolithiasis is rare in children. Hyperuricosuria in the setting of low urinary pH is the greatest risk factor for uric acid stone formation. Hyperuricosuria associated with significant hyperuricemia is usually associated with inherited disorders of purine metabolism, lymphoproliferative disorders or polycythemia. Other causes of hyperuricosuria include excessive purine intake (animal protein), hemolysis, and medications (probenecid, salicylates, and cyanotic congenital heart disease).[14]

IMAGING

Ultrasonography has been found to be a safe and effective initial imaging modality for pediatric patients presenting with possible nephrolithiasis. Studies have found that although ultrasound (US) is less sensitive and specific than computed tomography (CT), US accurately identifies clinically significant kidney stones in children. US has > 70% sensitivity and > 95% specificity for detecting urinary tract stones, including stones located in the mid-ureter, which are generally poorly visualized on US.[15,16]

On US, a kidney stone will show up as a hyperechoic focus in the renal papillae, calyces, or renal pelvis and will potentially exhibit twinkle artifact (Fig. 28.3). Twinkle artifact is a multicolor signal that overlies stones when exposed to Doppler. Historically posterior acoustic shadow was important for diagnosis, but modern harmonic and spatial compounding US technology does not generate shadows as readily.

Nonenhanced CT is exceptionally accurate for diagnosing kidney stones with nearly 100% sensitivity and specificity. Nonetheless, because CT scans deliver ionizing radiation, which is associated with an increased risk for malignancy later in life,

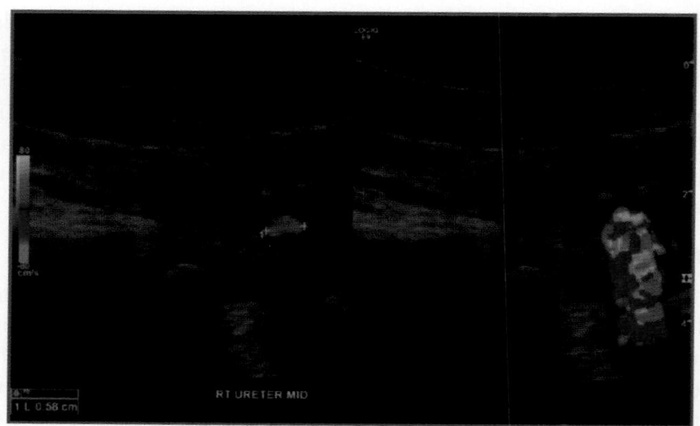

FIGURE 28.3 Ultrasonographic appearance of ureteral stone. A stone appears as an echogenic focus on gray-scale with confirmatory "twinkle artifact" on color Doppler.

efforts have been made to minimize their use in children. A technical paper by the American Urological Association also supports using US as the initial imaging study for children with suspected nephrolithiasis. They recommend obtaining a noncontrast CT scan only for children with a nondiagnostic US in whom the clinical suspicion for stones remains high.

Low-dose CT protocols have been developed with the goal of reducing radiation dose with adequate image quality, but even those should only be used when US is equivocal.[17] The attributable risk for cancer from a single CT scan is small (0.2%–0.3% above baseline), but this risk increases with each additional CT scan.[18] Of note, halving the dose of radiation for children weighing 50 kg or less has been shown to not affect the diagnostic accuracy of a CT for renal stones.[19] Studies have even showed CT scans with as much as a threefold decrease in radiation dose are still very effective at identifying renal stones in children.[20]

Patients with a history of nephrolithiasis are at a high risk of recurrence and therefore a high risk of needing additional imaging in the future. The risk of cumulative radiation exposure is particularly concerning for children because of their long life expectancy and the greater sensitivity of developing tissues to the effects of radiation.

TREATMENT

When a patient presents with an incidental finding of an asymptomatic, non-obstructing renal calculi they may not require any treatment in the acute setting. The American Urological Association (AUA) published a guideline for this clinical situation in which they state: "In pediatric patients with asymptomatic and non-obstructing renal stones, clinicians may utilize active surveillance with periodic ultrasonography." However, when patients present with a symptomatic, obstructing renal calculi, treatment is warranted in the form of either observation with pain control, medical expulsive therapy (MET), or surgical intervention. MET is the use of medication, primarily alpha-blockers, to facilitate passage of a ureteral stone. The AUA guidelines, with respect to MET, state: "In pediatric patients with uncomplicated ureteral stones less than or equal to 10 mm, clinicians should offer observation with or without MET using alpha-blockers." A multi-institutional retrospective cohort study demonstrated that tamsulosin was associated with higher stone passage (56%) compared with those treated with analgesics alone (44%).[21] These results were pooled in a systemic review and meta-analysis, which demonstrated that MET with an alpha-blocker was associated with increased odds of stone passage compared with placebo or analgesic alone (OR 2.21, 95% CI, 1.4–3.49).[22] The use of alpha-blockers in children remains off-label, but they are well tolerated, with $< 1\%$ of treated children withdrawing from studies due to adverse effects.[22]

Up to 60% of children with kidney or ureteral stones will require surgery.[21,23,24] There are three types of surgeries that a patient with nephrolithiasis can be offered. They include shockwave lithotripsy (SWL), ureteroscopy (URS), and percutaneous nephrolithotomy (PCNL).

When deciding whether or not to offer a patient SWL, multiple factors must be taken into account. These include, but are not limited to, stone size, location, stone composition, and body habitus of the patient. Body habitus may become an issue when patients reach adolescence, but generally, body habitus is less of a factor in children as compared to adults as the skin to stone distance in children is usually shorter.[25]

With respect to SWL the AUA currently recommends: "Clinicians should offer URS or SWL for pediatric patients with ureteral stones who are unlikely to pass the stones or who failed observation and/or MET, based on patient-specific anatomy and body habitus, and for patients with a total renal stone burden of less than or equal to 2 centimeters clinicians may offer SWL or URS as first-line therapy." For patients with a renal stone burden over 2 cm the AUA states both PCNL and SWL are acceptable treatment options, but if SWL is utilized, they recommend clinicians place an internalized ureteral stent or nephrostomy tube.

Stones in the lower pole are notoriously difficult to treat with SWL. A recent systematic review and meta-analysis comparing SWL, URS, and PCNL in adults for lower pole stones less than 2 cm in size favored PCNL over SWL and URS over SWL, particularly in stones 10 to 20 mm in size.[26] The Hounsfield units (HU) of a patient's stones should be noted prior to proceeding with SWL if the patient has had a preoperative CT scan. Stone attenuation less than 1000 HU was associated with treatment success in children.[27,28]

Per the AUA, antimicrobial prophylaxis for patients undergoing SWL is unlikely to provide any benefits except in patients at increased risk for infection. Administration of a laxative, such as polyethylene glycol 3350, the night before the procedure to decrease the stool load can also assist with intraoperative localization. However, this is not used in our practice to avoid dehydration and electrolyte imbalance postoperatively.

Complications associated with SWL include hematuria (up to 44%); subcapsular or perirenal hematoma; steinstrasse; and injury to adjacent structures such as colon, vasculature, lung, spleen, and pancreas.[29] Additionally, Krambeck et al. reported an increased risk for hypertension and diabetes mellitus related to bilateral treatment, number of administered shocks, and treatment intensity.[30]

In the past, URS placed patients at unacceptably high risk for complications such as ureteral perforation, ureteral ischemia, and ureteral stricture formation; however, with the miniaturization of ureteroscopes over time, URS is now a much safer and more widely utilized procedure. The utilization of URS has been rising while the utilization of SWL has been declining. This trend was shown by Seklehner et al. in two papers.[31,32] Both of their studies analyzed Medicare data to find trends in stone treatment in adult patients. They found that for ureteral calculi, URS was initially performed in 62.9% of patients in 2001, increasing to 70.2% by 2010 at the cost of a declining use of SWL (34.9%–29.3%) ($P < .001$), and for renal calculi, the utilization of URS increased over time from 8.4% in 2001 to 20.6% of cases by 2010 ($P < .0001$). A similar study has not yet been performed for pediatric patients. The smaller kidneys of children provide less room for the surgeon to maneuver a ureteroscope and have sharper angles (Fig. 28.4).

URS is mainly performed for patients with a total stone burden under 2 cm. A recent systemic review reported the results of 14 studies of children and found the average stone clearance was 87.5%, and 10% of patients experienced complications less than or equal to Clavien III.[33] Complications associated with URS include ureteral perforation, postoperative UTIs, ureteral stricture formation, and ureteral obstruction from stone fragment pass or from residual mucosal edema postoperatively.

PCNL is a very effective treatment option for stone burdens over 2 cm. In the earliest study, Woodside et al. rendered seven patients stone free without complications. Since that time, pediatric PCNL has become widely adopted and the miniaturization of instruments has facilitated this process. PCNL is considered first-line therapy for renal stones greater than 20 mm in children, with stone clearances of approximately 90%.[34] The AUA guidelines recommend a CT scan for preoperative planning prior to performing PCNL.[34] A CT allows a urologist to accurately determine stone size and location as well as identify any aberrant renal anatomy such as malrotation. A preoperative urine culture should be obtained 2 to 3 weeks prior and treated if positive. Antibiotic prophylaxis is recommended for all patients undergoing PCNL and the AUA's antimicrobials of choice are first- or second-generation cephalosporins or an aminoglycoside plus metronidazole or clindamycin for 24 hours. Risks of the procedure include bleeding requiring transfusion, delayed renal hemorrhage requiring angioembolization, sepsis, pneumothorax, hemothorax, urothorax, incomplete stone clearance, and injuries to adjacent organs. Approximately 15% to 39% of children will experience some form of complication. Most of the complications are minor, but greater or equal to Clavien III complications occur in 1% to 16%.[35]

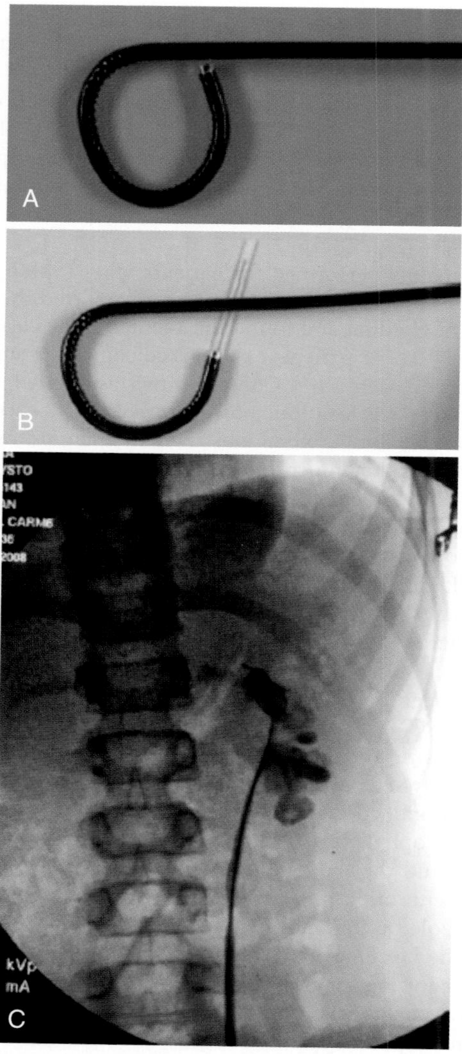

FIGURE 28.4 (A) Flexible ureteroscope displaying its 270-degree deflection at its distal tip. (B) The degree of tip deflection becomes restricted when a laser fiber is passed through the scope (C). Significant deflection is required for the ureteroscope to handle the sharp angles that lead to a lower pole calyx.

STONE PREVENTION

Increasing fluid intake is often one the most effective ways to prevent stone formation. It acts by reducing the concentration of lithogenic factors within the urine. In adults the general recommendation is greater than 2 to 2.5 L of fluid per day; children should take in at least equal to their calculated maintenance rates.[36] Many specific fluids have been tested with regard to their effect on stone formation. For instance, orange juice, lemonade, and black currant juice can increase urinary pH and citrate excretion and decrease stone formation in patients with acidic urine. Additionally, diuretics such caffeine and alcohol increase urine volume and by extension decrease stone formation. Grapefruit juice has been shown to increase the risk for calcium-based stones. The impact of soft drinks on stone formation is controversial.[37,38]

Increased salt intake promotes calciuria by sodium competing with calcium for reabsorption in the renal tubules. Thus, a low-salt diet is recommended for patients with hypercalciuria or calcium-containing stones.[38] It may also be beneficial for cystine stone formers.

The general recommendation with respect to calcium intake in the setting of kidney stones is to not restrict calcium. A moderate intake of daily calcium is recommended.[39] This is because calcium binds oxalate within the gastrointestinal tract thereby preventing oxalate absorption. If high levels of oxalate are absorbed, patients are placed at increased risk for calcium oxalate stone formation. As described previously, patients with fat malabsorption develop a pseudo–low calcium diet because excess fat within their gastrointestinal tract binds to calcium leaving excess oxalate unbound and free to be absorbed. This is again why patients with fat malabsorption are at increased risk for calcium oxalate stone formation.

Animal proteins, but not vegetable and dairy protein sources, increase the risk of calcium oxalate stone formation. Animal proteins possess sulfur-containing amino acids which are metabolized to sulfuric acid. This excess acid load results in hypocitraturia, decreased urine pH, and increased urinary calcium. Additionally, high dietary animal protein results in an increased purine load and increased uric acid production. This can result in uricosuria and acidic urine. Children at risk for stone formation should still eat their full daily allowance of protein, but they should not eat excessive amounts.

Foods high in oxalate include nuts, spinach, soybeans, beets, tofu, okra, and chocolate. Calcium oxalate stone formers are advised to avoid these foods; however, only approximately 15% of urinary oxalate excretion is from the diet. Oxalate is a by-product of ascorbic acid metabolism, so patients with a history of oxalate stones should refrain from taking vitamin C supplements.[40]

Citrate is protective against calcium oxalate stone formation. Fruits and vegetables are usually high in citrate. Additionally, foods high in potassium have been found to indirectly result in elevated citrate levels.[41] Magnesium binds oxalates in the gastrointestinal tract and prevents its absorption. Magnesium supplementation has been shown to decrease stone formation and may be helpful in children with secondary hyperoxaluria.[39,40]

MEDICATIONS

Thiazide diuretics are known to decrease hypercalciuria. They are critical in the treatment of patients with a history of hypercalciuria who have not responded to a low-sodium diet. Alkylating agents such as potassium citrate or potassium magnesium citrate reduce the recurrence of calcium oxalate stones in patients with low or normal citrate levels.[14,42] These medications are associated with only mild gastrointestinal side effects. They can also be beneficial in patients with uric acid stones, cystinuria, and hyperoxaluria.

Patients with cystinuria are generally managed with dietary modifications, and alkalinization of the urine. However, if these interventions are not proving effective, thiol-containing agents can be given to these patients. The two most common medications are D-penicillamine and alpha-mercaptopropionylglycine. Cystine is composed of two cysteine molecules that are connected via a disulfide bond. These medications work by reducing this bond and forming the more soluble cysteine by-products. These medications should be used with caution, however, as they are both associated with significant side effects including febrile reactions, gastrointestinal discomfort, liver dysfunction, impaired taste, bone marrow suppression, trace metal deficiencies, membranous glomerulopathy, and myasthenia gravis.

Allopurinol is indicated in patients with hyperuricemia in conjunction with hyperuricosuria such as phosphoribosyl pyrophosphate synthetase superactivity (PRPSS) or hypoxanthine guanine pohospho ribosyl transferase (HGPRT) deficiency. It may also be used for treating hyperuricosuric calcium oxalate urolithiasis if there is no concomitant evidence of hypercalciuria, hyperoxaluria or hypocitraturia.[43]

FOLLOW-UP

Approximately 50% of patients who develop kidney stone disease during childhood will develop a recurrent stone within 3 to 5 years.[44-46] Additionally, children with an identifiable metabolic abnormality have an up to fivefold increased risk for recurrence compared with children with no identifiable metabolic disorder.[47] Consequently, all children should undergo a comprehensive metabolic evaluation. Analysis should begin with an infrared spectroscopy or radiograph diffraction analysis of a passed stone. This study will be diagnostic if a cysteine or struvite stone is present. Following a stone episode, all patients should perform a 24-hour urine collection that is then analyzed for calcium, oxalate, uric acid, sodium, citrate, creatinine, volume pH, and cysteine (cyanide-nitroprusside screening test). Results are evaluated with respect to weight, body surface area, or creatinine to be properly interpreted in children. Urine creatinine excretion (normal 15–25 mg/kg/day for adults) is useful in assessing the adequacy of the urine collection. Supersaturations for calcium oxalate, calcium phosphate, and uric acid can be calculated from computer models based on the results of the urine collection. Obtaining a 24-hour urine collection from young patients, particularly those who are not yet toilet trained, may not be possible, but analysis of a random spot urine sample measuring the ratio of calcium, uric acid, citrate and oxalate to creatinine ratio can be performed in these patients.

Pediatric stone patients should all be followed with regular imaging postoperatively. US is sufficient to screen for stone recurrence without putting the patient at risk for radiation.

REFERENCES

1. Scales Jr CD, Smith AC, Hanley JM, et al. Prevalence of kidney stones in the United States. *Eur Urol*. 2012;62(1):160-165.
2. Stamatelou KK, Francis ME, Jones CA, et al. Time trends in reported prevalence of kidney stones in the United States: 1976-1994. *Kidney Int*. 2003;63(5):1817-1823.

3. Tasian GE, Ross ME, Song I, et al. Annual incidence of nephrolithiasis among children and adults in South Carolina from 1997 to 2012. *Clin J Am Soc Nephrol*. 2016;11(3):488-496.
4. Tasian GE, Jemielita T, Goldfarb DS, et al. Oral antibiotic exposure and kidney stone disease. *J Am Soc Nephrol*. 2018;29:1731.
5. Simerville JA, Maxted WC, Pahira JJ. Urinalysis: a comprehensive review. *Am Fam Physician*. 2005;71:1153-1162.
6. Gordon LB, Waxman MJ, Ragsdale L, Mermel LA. Overtreatment of presumed urinary tract infection in older women presenting to the emergency department. *J Am Geriatr Soc*. 2013;61:788-792.
7. Milliner DS, Murphy ME. Urolithiasis in pediatric patients. *Mayo Clin Proc*. 1993;68(3):241-248.
8. Stapleton FB, McKay CP, Noe HN. Urolithiasis in children, the role of hypercalciuria. *Pediatr Ann*. 1987;16(12):980-981, 984-992.
9. Kruse K, Kracht U, Kruse U. Reference values for urinary calcium excretion and screening for hypercalciuria in children and adolescents. *Eur J Pediatr*. 1984;143(1):25-31.
10. Coe FL, Parks JH, Moore ES. Familial idiopathic hypercalciuria. *N Engl J Med*. 1979;300(7):337-340.
11. Hoppe B, Beck BB, Milliner DS. The primary hyperoxaluria. *Kidney Int*. 2009;75(12):1264-1271.
12. Belostotsky R, Sebound E, Idelson GH, et al. Mutations in DHDPSL are responsible for primary hyperoxaluria type III. *Am J Hum Genet*. 2010;87(3):392-399.
13. Hess B, Michel R, Takkinen R, et al. Risk factors for low urinary citrate in calcium nephrolithiasis: low vegetable fibre intake and low urine volume to be added to the list. *Nephrol Dial Transplant*. 1994;9(6):642-649.
14. Ettinger B, Pak CY, Citron IT, et al. Potassium-magnesium citrate is an effective prophylaxis against recurrent calcium oxalate nephrolithiasis. *J Urol*. 1997;158(6):2069-2073.
15. Johnson EK, Faerber GJ, Roberts WW, et al. Are stone protocol computed tomography scans mandatory for children with suspected urinary calculi? *Urology*. 2011;78(3):662-666.
16. Passerotti C, Chow JS, Silva A, et al. Ultrasound versus computerized tomography for evaluating urolithiasis. *J Urol*. 2009;182(suppl 4):1829-1834.
17. Kwon JK, Chang IH, Moon YT, et al. Usefulness of low-dose nonenhanced computed tomography with iterative reconstruction for evaluation of urolithiasis: diagnostic performance and agreement between the urologist and the radiologist. *Urology*. 2015;85:531.
18. Kuhns LR, Oliver WJ, Christodoulou E, et al. The predicted increased cancer risk associated with a single computed tomography examination for calculus detection in pediatric patients compared with the natural cancer incidence. *Pediatr Emerg Care*. 2011;27(4):345.
19. Karmazyn B, Frush DP, Applegate KE, et al. CT with a computer-simulated dose reduction technique for detection of pediatric nephroureterolithiasis: comparison of standard and reduced radiation doses. *Am J Roentgenol*. 2009;192:143.
20. Spielmann AL, Heneghan JP, Lee IJ, et al. Decreasing the radiation dose for renal stone CT: a feasibility study of single and multidetector CT. *Am J Roentgenol*. 2002;178:1058.

21. Tasian GE, Cost NG, Granberg CF, et al. Tamsulosin and spontaneous passage of ureteral stones in children: a multi-institutional cohort study. *J Urol.* 2014;192(2):506-511.
22. Velazquez N, Zapata D, Wang HH, et al. Medical expulsive therapy for pediatric urolithiasis: systematic review and meta-analysis. *J Pediatr Urol.* 2015;11(6):321-327.
23. Routh JC, Graham DA, Nelson CP. Epidemiological trends in pediatric urolithiasis at United States freestanding pediatric hospitals. *J Urol.* 2010;184(3): 1100-1104.
24. Dangle P, Ayyash OT, Shaikh H III, et al. Predicting spontaneous stone passage in prepubertal children: a single institution cohort. *J Endourol.* 2016;30(9): 945-949.
25. Kurien A, Symons S, Manohar T, et al. Extracorporeal shock wave lithotripsy in children: equivalent clearance rates to adults is achieved with fewer and lower energy shock waves. *BJU Int.* 2009;103:81.
26. Donaldson JF, Lardas M, Scrimgeour D, et al. Systematic review and meta-analysis of the clinical effectiveness of shock wave lithotripsy, retrograde intrarenal surgery, and percutaneous nephrolithotomy for lower-pole renal stones. *Eur Urol.* 2015;67(4):612-616.
27. El-Assmy A, El-Nahas AR, Abou-El-Ghar ME, et al. Kidney stone size and hounsfield units predict successful shockwave lithotripsy in children. *Urology.* 2013;81:880.
28. McAdams S, Kim N, Dajusta D, et al. Preoperative stone attenuation value predicts success after shock wave lithotripsy in children. *J Urol.* 2010;184:1804.
29. Yucel S, Akin Y, Danisman A, et al. Complications and associated factors of pediatric extracorporeal shock wave lithotripsy. *J Urol.* 2012;187(5):1812-1816.
30. Krambeck AE, LeRoy AJ, Patterson DE, et al. Long-term outcomes of percutaneous nephrolithotomy compared to shock wave lithotripsy and conservative management. *J Urol.* 2008;179:2233.
31. Seklehner S, Laudano MA, Jamzadeh A, et al. Trends and inequalities in the surgical management of ureteric calculi in the USA. *BJU Int.* 2014;113(3): 476-483.
32. Seklehner S, Laudano MA, Del Pizzo J, Chughtai B, Lee RK. Renal calculi: trends in the utilization of shockwave lithotripsy and ureteroscopy. *Can J Urol.* 2015;22(1):7627-7634.
33. Ishii H, Griffin S, Somani BK. Ureteroscopy for stone disease in the pediatric population: a systematic review. *BJU Int.* 2015;115(6):867-873.
34. Assimos D, Krambeck A, Miller NL, et al. Surgical management of stones: American Urological Association/Endourological Society Guideline. *J Urol.* 2016;196(4):1161-1169.
35. Tasian GE, Copelovitch L. *Management of Pediatric Kidney Stone Disease.* In: Partin AW, Dmochowski RR, Kavoussi LR, Peters CA, Wein AJ, eds. *Campbell-Walsh-Wein Urology.* Elsevier; 12th ed. 2020.
36. Borghi I, Meschi T, Amato F, et al. Urinary volume, water and recurrences in idiopathic calcium nephrolithiasis: a 5-year randomized prospective study. *J Urol.* 1996;155(3):839-843.
37. Borghi I, Meschi T, Maggiore U, et al. Dietary therapy in idiopathic nephrolithiasis. *Nutr Rev.* 2006;64(7 Pt 1):301-312.

38. Taylor EN, Curhan GC. Diet and fluid prescription in stone disease. *Kidney Int.* 2006;70(5):835-839.
39. Curhan GC, Willett WC, Spetzer FE, et al. Comparison of dietary calcium with supplemental calcium and other nutrients as factors affecting the risk for kidney stones in women. *Ann Intern Med.* 1997;126(7):497-504.
40. Taylor EN, Stampfer MJ, Curhan GC. Dietary factors and the risk of incident kidney stones in men: new insights after 14 years of follow-up. *J Am Soc Nephrol.* 2004;15(12):3225-3232.
41. Domrongkitchaiporn S, Stitchantrakul W, Kochakarn W. Causes of hypocitraturia in recurrent calcium stone formers: focusing on urinary potassium excretion. *Am J Kidney Dis.* 2006;48(4):546-554.
42. Barcelo P, Wuhl O, Servitge E, et al. Randomized double blind study of potassium citrate in idiopathic hypocitraturic calcium nephrolithiasis. *J Urol.* 1993;150(6):1761-1764.
43. van Woerden CS, Groothoff JW, Wijtburg FA, et al. Clinical implications of mutation analysis in primary hyperoxaluria type 1. *Kidney Int.* 2004;66(2):746-752.
44. Lao M, Kogan BA, White MD, et al. High recurrence rate at 5-year follow up in children after upper urinary tract stone surgery. *J Urol.* 2014;191(2):440-444.
45. Tasian GE, Kabarriti AE, Kalmus A, et al. Kidney stone recurrence among children and adolescents. *J Urol.* 2017;197(1):246-252.
46. Tekin A, Tekgul S, Atsu N, et al. Oral potassium citrate treatment for idiopathic hypocitruria in children with calcium urolithiasis. *J Urol.* 2002;168(6):2572-2574.
47. Pietrow PK, Pope JC IV, Adams MC, et al. Clinical outcome of pediatric stone disease. *J Urol.* 2002;167(2 Pt 1):670-673.

Pediatric Voiding Function and Dysfunction

Dana A. Weiss, MD, and Stephen Zderic, MD

Basic Embryology

The urinary bladder and rectum arise from the primitive hindgut (the cloaca), which is partitioned by the urorectal septum. As a result of this common embryologic origin, the bladder and rectum share a substantial overlap in sensory innervation within the S2, S3, and S4 sacral segments. This is the reason that clinically, constipation is often seen in patients with voiding dysfunction, and treating the constipation often cures the voiding symptoms.

The ureteral buds develop from the wolffian ducts and penetrate the blastema to start formation of the kidney. In females, the ureteral bud takes off from the wolffian duct and may enter the lower urinary tract in an ectopic position that is distal to the urinary sphincter. Locations for such an ectopic ureter include the urethra, periurethral folds, or vagina along the lines of Gartner ducts. This embryology is important as in young girls with severe and continuous urinary incontinence, an ectopic ureter must be suspected as a possible anatomic cause.

Anatomy and Physiology

The cerebral cortex is involved in the perception of bladder fullness and, in the mature child and adult, exerts volitional control over micturition by regulating the pontine micturition center. In adults, the sensation of a full bladder has been localized to the pons, midcingulate cortex, insular cortex, and the bilateral prefrontal area using positron emission tomography (PET) and functional magnetic resonance imaging (fMRI) scanning studies. Coordination of micturition is centered in the brain stem in a cluster of neurons referred to as Barrington nucleus.

Under conditions of bladder storage, one population of neurons that express the stress neuropeptide corticotrophin-releasing factor (CRF+) descend from Barrington nucleus to inhibit the sacral reflex (located at segments at S2, S3, and S4). Another distinct set of neurons in Barrington nucleus that do not express CRF (CRF−) can trigger a bladder contraction. Yet another distinct subset that express the estrogen receptor activate the striated external sphincter.

With bladder filling, afferent sensory nerves enter the posterolateral region of the sacral segments. These synapse with a short interneuron, which crosses the cord to synapse with the motor nuclei in the anterior horn. The activity of this interneuron is modulated by descending influences from Barrington nucleus in the brain stem. With the loss of the tonic inhibitory influences, the motor neuron is activated and voiding is initiated with the contraction of the detrusor. The contraction of the detrusor is mediated by acetylcholine binding to muscarinic receptors. The M_3 and M_4 subtypes are found in bladder. Concurrent with the rise in detrusor pressure, there must also be a funneling and opening of the bladder neck. This process is under autonomic control and this region of the bladder is rich in alpha-adrenergic receptors. It is also a region of the bladder that is rich in nitric oxide (NO) synthase; multiple studies have shown that NO serves as an important neurotransmitter in this area. It is because of this that relaxation of the bladder neck can be achieved with an alpha antagonist in order to facilitate bladder emptying in patients with proven internal sphincteric dyssynergia.

Concurrent with the rise in detrusor pressure, there must also occur a relaxation of the striated external sphincter located distal to the bladder neck. These striated muscle fibers are under voluntary control. The striated external sphincter contractions are mediated by the neurotransmitter acetylcholine, which binds to nicotinic receptors. This is clinically relevant as botulinum toxin (BOTOX) locally injected to the striated sphincter can produce relaxation because BOTOX is a selective inhibitor of the nicotinic receptor family.

The Normal Voiding Cycle

1. Bladder filling proceeds under conditions of low storage pressures.
2. At a certain volume, the sensation of fullness is noted.
3. Barrington nucleus removes its inhibitory influences.
4. The sacral reflex arc is activated.
5. With detrusor contraction, there is a rise in intravesical pressure.
6. This sustained rise in detrusor pressure is accompanied by a funneling of the bladder neck and a relaxation of the striated external sphincter.

NEONATE AND INFANT

In the traditional view, neonates and infants voided to completion via activation of the sacral reflex arc, and it was assumed that there was no suprasacral control of micturition at this time. It is now accepted that neonates and infants have some degree of suprasacral control over micturition based on the following observations:

1. Evidence for residual urine on voiding cystourethrography (VCUG).
2. Evidence of a contracting striated external sphincter on VCUG.
3. Evidence of postvoid residuals following spontaneous voids.

Voiding in the neonate and infant is related to the sleep cycle. Sillen has shown that 90% of neonates and infants will awaken from sleep in the minute preceding micturition.

TRANSITIONAL PHASE

In time, the toddler begins to gain the sensation of bladder distention with filling. The toddler begins to spend more time in the storage phase. During this time, parents will report an increase in the number of dry diapers. Parents may also note dry diapers in the morning. Bladder capacity begins to increase as evidenced by increased urinary volumes and increased time of storage. Bowel continence then appears. Finally, the toddler expresses an interest in the commode and ultimately a preference is expressed by the child for underwear.

MATURATION

Even in the middle phases of the transition, a child may be dry by day, and yet the voiding cycle is incomplete. The child has learned to fire the external sphincter to prevent an episode of incontinence.

Often the child is also contracting the external sphincter during voiding phase and thus fails to empty completely. In time, there is better "fine-tuning" of the voiding cycle by the child, and continence is achieved with a minimal postvoid residual urine.

The Clinical Manifestations of Voiding Dysfunction

Pediatric patients with voiding dysfunction have a wide spectrum of presentations.

1. Urinary tract infections ([UTIs] including cystitis, pyelonephritis)
2. Infrequent voider
3. Daytime incontinence
4. Diurnal incontinence
5. Nocturnal enuresis

The degree of symptoms spans a spectrum from mild dysfunctional voiding (occasional "accident") to severe dysfunctional voiding (Hinman syndrome).

HINMAN SYNDROME

Hinman syndrome is caused by severe detrusor sphincter dyssynergia in the neurologically intact child—one with a normal clinical examination and MRI of the spinal cord. It manifests with incontinence—often day and night; fecal soiling; recurrent cystitis; pyelonephritis and vesicoureteral reflux. In extreme cases, it may progress to renal failure. There are inherited familial cases of Hinman syndrome that were initially described in Medellin, Colombia, by Dr. Bernardo Ochoa as an autosomal recessive trait. These patients also have a characteristic downturned smile, and hence this is referred to as the Ochoa urofacial syndrome.

Based on their original genetic pedigrees, over two decades, the gene was mapped to chromosome 10q and subsequently identified as the heparanase 2 gene (HPSE2). Deletion of HPSE2 in mice recapitulates a voiding phenotype with poor bladder emptying that leads to death from renal failure.

The Clinical Approach to the Patient

The efficient management of the pediatric patient with voiding dysfunction calls for a clear strategy that begins by gathering information, an assessment of severity, and the formulation of a therapeutic plan. Despite the technologic age we practice in, this process must begin with a careful history. In cases where simple therapies have failed, the history must always be revisited.

HISTORY

Physicians must approach such visits with ample time and patience. Time and again, families and patients will give us a first-rate history if we simply let them speak in their words and at their pace (Dr. Barry Belman has coined the term audio-uro-dynamics for this "procedure"). Simply giving the family and patient free rein and "letting them go" will provide many of the answers we seek. For some families, this may seem daunting, and a prompt, such as, "How does your child's bladder problem affect you on a car trip or a visit to the mall?" will get them to relay the information needed **in their terms**. This may at times be much easier said than done within a busy clinic. However, we all need to be reminded that *an ounce of active listening validates the family's concerns* far more than a pound of hastily given therapy no matter how accurate it may be. All of us need to remember that among our seemingly endless stream of day and night wetters lurks the rare (1%–3%) patient with an ectopic ureter or a posterior urethral valve whose cure and well-being can only be ensured by a surgical procedure.

QUESTIONS A CONSULTING PHYSICIAN MUST CONSIDER

1. Age and sex of the patient.
2. Age at which training was attempted.
3. Was the patient ever dry? Do parents ever remember a dry diaper in infancy?
4. Fluid intake—is your child thirstier than other children their age?
5. How frequently does your child void? What is the child's maximal dry interval?
6. Does your child make a last-minute rush to get to the bathroom (urgency)?
7. Does your child ever squat en route to the bathroom? (Vincent curtsy—on occasion a parent will demonstrate this maneuver in which the child stops an episode of urgency by dropping

down and tucking their heel into their perineum to create a compression.)

8. What does it sound like when your child is urinating? Many parents will relay the classic features of a starting and stopping staccato stream characteristic of detrusor sphincter dyssynergia.
9. Is urination painful?
10. Is your child constipated? What is the frequency of stooling? Are the stools hard or soft? Is defecation painful? Is there fecal soiling of the underwear?
11. Has your child ever had a UTI? If yes, was this associated with a high fever? How the urine specimen was collected (bag, voided, or catheter)?
12. Have any radiology studies been done?
13. Was your child imaged with in utero sonography? Keep in mind that most (although not all) major congenital obstructive uropathies will be detected in utero. For many expectant mothers only one sonogram is performed at the 19- to 22-week time point. Although this screening sonogram will pick up major problems, hydronephrosis may be progressive, and not identified early in gestation. Remember that despite widespread fetal sonography, about 30% of posterior urethral valve patients are diagnosed based on a presentation of abnormal voiding or infection.
14. Is there a history of maternal diabetes? In such cases, the child is at risk for the development of sacral agenesis and may present some time later with a neurogenic bladder.
15. General social developmental questions should include any history of developmental delay, grade in school, scholastic performance, social stressors (death of family member or friend, divorce).
16. What are the restrooms at school like? Does your child have unrestricted bathroom privileges? Are the restrooms safe?
17. Does your child wet the bed? If so, how many nights within a week/month? Is your child difficult to arouse from sleep? Does your child snore? How loud? Does your child ever stop breathing at night and awaken only to fall back into a deep sleep? Is your child falling asleep during the daytime hours?

SELF AND FAMILY ASSESSMENT TOOLS

These are also critical measures at the time of intake. In some practices, a family whose child is being scheduled for a wetting complaint will be mailed or emailed an information packet that includes a voiding diary and a self-assessment tool that translates into a symptom score.

These additional self-reported data that should be reviewed by the physician include:

1. Voiding and elimination diaries.
   a. Times of voids
   b. Volumes
   c. Fluid intake
   d. Bowel habits
2. Voiding questionnaire with scoring system—at least two such questionnaires have been developed for voiding dysfunction and serve as a pediatric version of the American Urological Association (AUA) symptom score. These scales provide a practitioner with a sense of how many resources a patient will require during therapy. In addition, if a patient's score fails to improve, these scores may indicate the need for more advanced, expensive, and invasive testing. We have incorporated our parent/patient self-reported symptom score into our electronic medical record and have access to this information before we start the visit.

THE PHYSICAL EXAMINATION

1. General appearance—evidence of neurologic or developmental issues?
2. Unusual facies (downturn of smile)—Ochoa syndrome—described by Dr. Ochoa as an inherited syndrome of urinary and fecal incontinence. The pontine micturition center is localized near the cranial nerves controlling facial expression, which accounts for this association. Autosomal recessive and localized to chromosome 10q23–24 and has been mapped to an area corresponding to the HPSE2 (Online Mendelian Inheritance in Man [OMIM] entry # 613469).
3. Gait and general neurologic assessment—does the patient favor one limb over another? Do the shoes wear evenly?
4. Spine—a careful examination of the lumbar-sacral region is crucial. Look for lipomas, hair tufts, or dimpling in this

region. These are clues to the possible presence of a tethered cord.

5. Abdomen—distended from constipation?
6. Genitalia.
7. In female patients, check for continuous leakage; if this is present, suspect ectopic ureter.

Observe the Patient Void

Direct observation of a void can be crucial. A patient who is voiding normally should be able to converse with ease. In contrast, a thin and weak yet steady stream with the patient unable to converse while applying a Valsalva maneuver would be indicative of a possible stricture or an underactive bladder. In contrast, a staccato stream with a start and stop pattern would be indicative of striated detrusor sphincter dyssynergia.

LABORATORY TESTING

The following laboratory studies are inexpensive and may be read from a dipstick analysis in the office and provide useful clues:

1. Urinalysis
   a. Urine culture—to be ordered if the urinalysis is positive for leukocytes and nitrates
2. Urine specific gravity—the first morning urine is especially helpful because the specific gravity should be high. A low specific gravity in the morning should trigger suspicion of diabetes insipidus (DI), and prompt careful questioning about water intake.

In severe cases with abnormal imaging, or recurrent pyelonephritis, a blood urea nitrogen (BUN)/creatinine (Cr) should be checked.

IMAGING

In many instances, no imaging is needed. A well-conducted history and physical examination followed by simple recommendations such as a timer watch and a voiding diary and treatment of constipation (if it is present) are all required to produce continence. However, in selected cases, imaging should be obtained beginning with the more simple, less invasive, and less expensive studies and proceeding to the more invasive and advanced studies only if required.

1. **Kidney ureter bladder (KUB) x-ray**—a simple and inexpensive study that demonstrates for physician, family, and patient alike the presence of significant constipation. This is probably the only imaging the majority of these patients will need unless there is an associated history of UTIs.
2. **Ultrasound**—increased expense but noninvasive; offers the benefit of reassurance to physician, patient, and family that the anatomy is set correctly. It is okay to have a lower threshold for ordering an ultrasound given that it is profoundly frustrating for a family and patient to attempt behavioral management methods for a long time, only to discover after months of futility that the underlying problem was anatomic. Critical to order in situations in which one suspects anatomic incontinence in a female on the basis of ectopic ureter. This imaging must include renal *and* bladder views.
   a. Suspect ectopic ureter based on:
      1) Hydronephrosis most often in upper pole system.
      2) Dilated ureter behind the bladder with ureter dropping below the level of the bladder neck.
   b. Although rare, even a well-done ultrasound may miss an ectopic ureter, and if the history is compelling enough, further imaging with an MRI-IVP (intravenous pyelogram) is warranted. (Though an old-fashioned IVP may be ordered, the MRI-IVP is more sensitive in this setting.)
3. **VCUG**—increased expense, invasive, and potentially traumatic to the child. This can be done via a traditional fluoroscopic approach or contrast-enhanced ultrasound modality. Today there is a growing movement to limit the number of VCUGs being done except in those cases in which there simply is no alternative to searching for vesicoureteral reflux or excluding bladder outlet obstruction. The following are indications for a VCUG study in patients with voiding dysfunction:
   a. Febrile UTI—this can evaluate for vesicoureteral reflux as well as evidence of severe detrusor external sphincter dyssynergia, as demonstrated by a classic "spinning top" urethra during voiding (Fig. 29.1).
   b. A male patient with a thick-walled bladder and upper tract changes—to rule out the presence of posterior urethral valves or a urethral stricture.

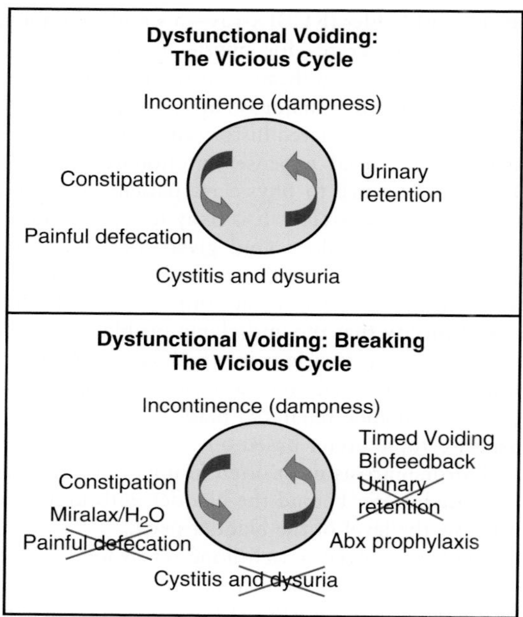

FIGURE 29.1 (A) A fluoroscopic and (B) contrast-enhanced ultrasound voiding cystourethrogram images demonstrating a classic "spinning top" urethra. This reveals detrusor external sphincter dyssynergia in these patients.

Imaging That Is Less Frequently Indicated for Voiding Dysfunction

1. **IVP**—this study **was** the gold standard for detecting the presence of ectopic ureters and duplication anomalies. Certainly in the presence of adequately functioning renal parenchyma, there will be accumulation of contrast within a dilated system that provides a clue of possible ectopia. *Delayed views are essential and this study must be monitored closely by the radiologist, as well as the urologist ordering the study*. Failure to obtain the proper views will render the study worthless, hence the importance of communication between urologist and radiologist.

2. **Computed tomography (CT) scan or MRI-IVP**—in recent years advances in technology have expanded the use of rapid scanning using either the CT scan or the MRI, and these have been applied to the search for ectopic ureters. For small, poorly functioning systems, the use of the CT with contrast or MRI with gadolinium will allow for detection of contrast within nondilated ureters that can escape detection with sonography or a conventional IVP.
3. **Lumbar-sacral MRI**—this study is indicated for any patient with focal neurologic signs (abnormal gait, foot drop) or findings on examination of the lumbar-sacral spine (hair tuft, lipoma, abnormal dimple). In the absence of these findings, and in situations in which the patient fails to improve, this study may also be considered to rule out a tethered cord.

URODYNAMIC MEASUREMENTS

1. **Uroflow and measurement of postvoid residual with handheld ultrasound unit**—this simple and easy-to-use technique is complementary to direct observation of the void. A sawtooth flow pattern suggests the firing and relaxation of the external sphincter seen with classic dysfunctional voiding. A slow, flat, and prolonged curve suggests outflow obstruction on an anatomic basis. For most patients, this is the only urodynamic study needed.
2. **Cystometrogram**—indicated to rule out uninhibited bladder contractions. While the administration of anticholinergic medications may be initiated on an empiric basis, cystometry should be done prior to BOTOX therapy (into either the striated external sphincter or the detrusor), which is an invasive procedure.
3. **Videourodynamics**—indicated to rule out uninhibited contractions and also to assess the bladder neck in complex cases.

In our experience, cystometry and videourodynamics are rarely indicated in the assessment of pediatric voiding dysfunction. These studies will usually be limited to less than 5% of patients presenting to a pediatric voiding dysfunction clinic and should be restricted to those patients who fail the basic treatment protocols or anticholinergic therapy or those in whom internal sphincteric dyssynergia is suspected. This is in marked distinction to those patients in whom a clear-cut neurogenic bladder is present as in spina bifida patients, all of whom must undergo urodynamic testing. When urodynamic or videourodynamic studies are indicated, the best information will be obtained when the urologist ordering the study is present and communicates with the patient so as to best recreate in the laboratory setting the symptoms that the patient experiences.

Treatment of Dysfunctional Voiding/ Elimination by Category

Selection of the optimal treatment calls for an understanding of the cycle of failure (Fig. 29.2). Based on this, one can begin to design a program for the patient that addresses the patient's unique needs.

URINARY TRACT INFECTIONS

For many patients the sole manifestation of voiding dysfunction is recurrent cystitis. A careful voiding history often reveals a patient who is dry by day and night but who voids infrequently (two to three times per day), has poor water intake, and is constipated. Often these patient are treated for 3–5 days with antibiotics, and then the cystitis recurs within weeks, and the cycle is repeated.

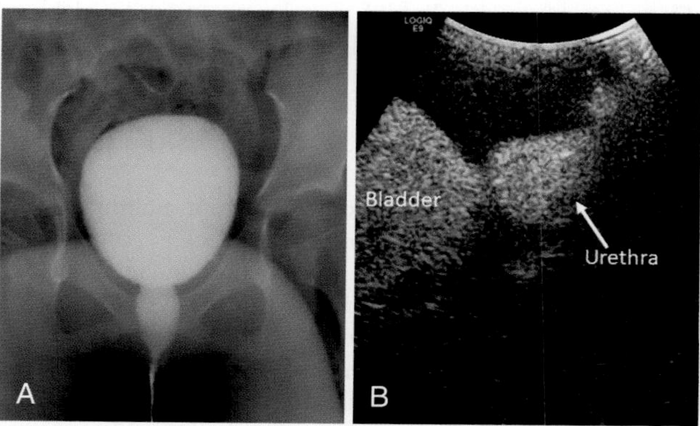

FIGURE 29.2 The cycle of dysfunctional voiding in which constipation leads to cystitis and dysuria, followed by retention and wetting, and the "menu" of choices by which the cycle is broken.

This is a call for the use of antibiotic prophylaxis to help break the cycle. Treatment should consist of:

1. Antibiotic prophylaxis
2. Timed voiding regimen (2-hour intervals) using a timer watch with alarms
3. Increased free water intake
4. Treat associated constipation
5. Voiding diaries

INFREQUENT VOIDER

These patients may void two to three times per day and often present with dampness as the primary complaint. In many instances, these are high-achieving children who just cannot break away from what they are doing to "listen to their bladder." In other instances, these children are reluctant to use the restrooms at school because of fear of sanitation and/or safety. These children should be treated the same as those with UTIs except they do not need the antibiotic prophylaxis. A note should be provided to the school nurse/teacher for unrestricted bathroom privileges.

CONSTIPATION

Constipation is the enemy of continence. Time and again patients present with mild to moderate voiding dysfunction and/or UTIs with significant constipation, and on institution of a bowel regimen all voiding complaints cease. Basic and clinical science back this up as studies show that rectal wall distention with a balloon alters urodynamic patterns most likely by altering the sacral reflex arc. Recall the common shared origin of the bladder and rectum from the cloaca.

Treatment should consist of the simplest approach and progress to the more invasive based on a lack of response:

1. Increase water intake
2. Increase fruits and vegetable intake; increase fiber-based cereals
3. Stool-softening regimens: lactulose, MiraLAX
4. Enemas
   a. Retrograde, administered per rectum
   b. Antegrade administration of enema via surgically created appendiceal access for medically refractory cases (cecostomy tube, antegrade colonic enema [ACE] procedure)

DYSFUNCTIONAL VOIDING WITH DETRUSOR SPHINCTER DYSSYNERGIA

For patients in whom the diagnosis of detrusor sphincter dyssynergia is suspected, confirmation with a uroflow may be helpful to confirm the rising and falling or consistently depressed flow rate. There are two types of detrusor sphincter dyssynergia to consider, and their treatments differ markedly.

Striated External Sphincter Dyssynergia

This is the most common form, and their uroflow shows a characteristic notching as the flow rises and falls according to the firing of the external sphincter. This may be treated with the same standard urotherapy, including the addition of biofeedback therapy to coach the patient into relaxing the pelvic floor. Only if these less invasive means of treatments fail would one proceed to the remaining options (usually following a carefully performed videourodynamic assessment):

1. Clean intermittent catheterization
2. Cystoscopy and direct injection of BOTOX into striated external sphincter

Internal Sphincteric Dyssynergia

This is the less common form. These patients demonstrate a diminished flow rate with a flattened curve. To make this diagnosis accurately, videourodynamics are essential. The low flow rate, silent pelvic floor electromyogram (EMG), and increased voiding pressures correlate with the closed bladder neck on fluoroscopy to clinch this diagnosis.

1. Treat with alpha blocker (terazosin, doxazosin, tamsulosin) to lower the resistance at the level of the bladder neck.

HINMAN SYNDROME

These rare patients represent the extreme end of the dysfunctional voiding spectrum. The syndrome has also been labeled as the nonneurogenic neurogenic bladder. Hinman noted, in their original description of these patients, the presence of urinary incontinence, fecal soiling, UTIs, and upper tract changes often associated with pyelonephritis, and, in some cases, renal failure developed. These patients will require imaging consisting of a renal bladder ultrasound, and videourodynamics should be done to understand if the bladder is capable of low-pressure storage. Renal function must be assessed. A lumbar-sacral MRI and neurosurgical consultation are warranted to completely exclude any spinal cord lesion. Treatment options for this complex group of patients may include:

1. Timed voiding.
2. Antibiotic prophylaxis.
3. Biofeedback.
4. An assessment of renal function.
5. Bowel regimen ranging from MiraLAX to enemas. In the event that these simpler measures fail, more aggressive approaches may be indicated to preserve renal function.
6. Clean intermittent catheterization (CIC)—in many of these cases, the use of CIC will actually teach the child how to relax the external sphincter.

In rare instances, patients with Hinman syndrome may become surgical candidates to preserve their renal function.

1. Vesicostomy—if the patient is noncompliant with CIC or the social situation is poor and the patient might be lost to follow-up.
2. Appendicovesicostomy with or without bladder augmentation.
3. Antegrade continence enema procedure for constipation.

NOCTURNAL ENURESIS

This common problem often presents as a seemingly isolated finding. In fact, in taking a careful history, one can often elicit evidence for daytime voiding dysfunction. This is critical because more often than not, addressing the daytime voiding dysfunction will result in nighttime dryness as the child is actually going to bed with an empty bladder.

Additional Background

1. Twenty percent of all 5-year-olds wet the bed. This drops by 50% each year. By about age 10, 1% are still experiencing some degree of enuresis. In a Swedish study, 90% of all neonates would awaken in the minute prior to urination, but 10% slept right on through their voiding. These investigators will ultimately tell us whether these 10% of neonates are the ones presenting at age 5 and beyond with persisting enuresis.

2. Consider the possibility of upper airway obstruction and sleep apnea; these patients need a sleep study and ear, nose, and throat (ENT) evaluation.
3. Consider the degree of thirst. Most children with enuresis will not get up to drink at night.
   If this is happening frequently, consider the possibility of DI.
      Measure the specific gravity (cheaply done via dipstick) and/or check an osmolality on the first morning urine if you suspect DI.
4. Collect voided volumes and assess the child's bladder capacity. Are they voiding volumes that are about 50% of their expected bladder capacity (EBC; where EBC can be estimated from the formula: EBC [in cubic centimeters] = weight [kilograms] × 7)? Consistent low volumes offer an opportunity to use Ditropan to help grow capacity.

Treatments for Nocturnal Enuresis

1. Double void in the 1 hour before bedtime.
2. Aim to consume two-thirds of water and fluid intake before noon time. This helps to grow bladder capacity, and also assures the child is better hydrated later in the day. This practice has scientific backing as experimental studies in mice and rats show that administration of Lasix in the drinking water leads to increased water consumption, which after a month led to increased voided volumes and urodynamic capacity. Many children come home from school and sports and are dehydrated, consume their required fluids and then immediately go to bed. Children must satiate their thirst especially after sweating in a sporting event. Fluid deprivation after sports is dangerous, and hence the argument for hydration in the morning.
3. Alarm—this simple electrical circuit is placed in the pajamas and makes a buzzing sound if the contact is established by fluid. Alarms work in 80% of cases after 3 months of work. If the child sleeps through the alarm, the parent must awaken and arouse the child to void. Otherwise, the approach will fail. Alarms work best in cases in which the child is a lighter sleeper or the parents are highly motivated to awaken with the alarm and in turn wake up their child. Alarms function as a biofeedback tool—the child learns to associate the sensation

of a full bladder during sleep with the need to arouse and then void. Waking the child up at set hours during the night to void is not the same as using an alarm because the bladder may not be full at the time the child is awakened.

Pharmacologic Options for Enuresis

1. Desmopressin (DDAVP)—nasal spray (rarely used today) or tablet (0.2-mg tablets)
   a. One to three tablets at bedtime
2. Oxybutynin or Ditropan—this anticholinergic can be used for those patients who demonstrate consistent low bladder volumes on their voiding diary such as those children who consistently void less than 50% of their expected capacity.
3. Imipramine—25 up to 75 mg orally at bedtime (PO QHS)
   a. Rarely used today, only for the most refractory cases in older children

ANTICHOLINERGIC THERAPY IN PEDIATRIC VOIDING DYSFUNCTION

The purpose of anticholinergic therapy is to enhance bladder capacity by eliminating the presence of uninhibited bladder contractions. Most children with dysfunctional voiding have excellent bladder capacity, and thus anticholinergic therapy is rarely indicated in this population. On occasion, we will identify children with severe urgency and frequency for whom a trial of oxybutynin (Ditropan) is indicated; however, this is a small percentage of patients. In these instances, empiric therapy is reasonable, although some might advocate urodynamic or videourodynamic studies prior to such therapy. There are pediatric patients with overactive bladder who fail anticholinergic therapy and who on vidoeurodynamic studies demonstrate uninhibited bladder contractions. These highly selected patients may respond to submucosal injections of BOTOX with an increase in bladder capacity and a drop in their urinary frequency and symptom scores.

VOIDING DYSFUNCTION AND VESICOURETERAL REFLUX

Many patients with vesicoureteral reflux will prove to have significant dysfunctional voiding. Treating the dysfunctional voiding is also treating the reflux. Patients with dysfunctional voiding and reflux have a better prognosis for spontaneous resolution than those without voiding dysfunction on a grade for grade basis. Ureteral reimplantation (by open or robotic surgery) in the face of dysfunctional voiding has a higher complication rate and is to be avoided until the voiding dysfunction has been treated.

Diabetes Insipidus

Rarely, patients with DI will present to a urologist with "voiding dysfunction." These patients have the following characteristics: thirsty; crave cold water; they will wake up at night to drink; they will resist vigorously any attempt to deprive them of water; polyuria (accompanied by a low specific gravity on the first morning urine analysis); fabulous flow rates with no residual urine.

In this setting, the following studies are indicated:

1. First morning urine for specific gravity
2. Water deprivation study with serum and urine osmolarities—this is a difficult study to perform correctly, and it is done in a specialized inpatient unit and is supervised by the endocrinology service
3. Treated by endocrinologists with DDAVP

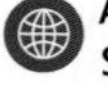

Additional content, including Self-Assessment Questions and Suggested Readings, may be accessed at www.ExpertConsult.com.

Transitional Urology

Zoe S. Gan, MD, Sameer Mittal, MD, MS, FAAP,
and Robert C. Kovell, MD

Introduction

For many adult urologists, the nuances of pediatric urology are unfamiliar territory. Conditions such as spina bifida, exstrophy, hypospadias, and posterior urethral valves often take a back seat to conditions like prostate cancer, benign prostatic hyperplasia (BPH), and erectile dysfunction (ED), both in training and in the adult urologist's clinic. As patients with congenital urologic issues live longer, fuller, more productive lives, more of these individuals transition to the care of adult providers. While the complexity of their conditions can be daunting at first, we as urologic providers can have a tremendous impact on their overall health throughout the course of their lifetime. In this chapter, we provide an overview of the unique challenges and conditions these individuals face and the clinical management related to these issues.

OUR APPROACH TO TRANSITION

The ideal method of transitioning patients from pediatric to adult urologic care has not been defined. At our institution, we pair an adult reconstructive urologist with the patient's pediatric urologist to form the foundation of a urologic care team for each patient. The adult urologist begins to partake in visits during the adolescent years, building a sense of familiarity and trust over time. This also gives the urologists plenty of time to discuss the patient's unique anatomy/history, review images, and discuss goals of care going forward. If surgeries are undertaken during this time, every effort is made to do them together so that the adult provider will be familiar with the patient's particular anatomy.

As patients progress through adolescence, we make individual decisions on timing of moving patients from our pediatric facility to the adult facilities based on both medical and social factors. We try to provide an early "foot in the door" at the adult facilities, addressing patient concerns that no one will understand their condition as they transition part of their care to the adult world. While the role of the pediatric urologist may diminish over the years, they remain a vital part of the team, available for consultation and discussion.

At many other institutions and clinics, the optimal plan may look very different than ours. In any case, every effort should be made to obtain previous records, especially operative notes and previous imaging studies when available. If possible, discussion with the patient's pediatric urology team or treating adult urologists (and other relevant specialists) can be invaluable in terms of understanding the patient and saving time piecing together records. Social work assistance is vital to help with logistical issues such as insurance and transportation, which remain major barriers to care. Finally, trust is key. Patients and families have generally developed a very strong bond with their pediatric providers over many years. This will never be replaced nor should it. We have found that creating a team-based approach allows for a slow, but deliberate incorporation of the adult urologist with the "endorsement" of the pediatric urologist, which often goes a long way with many families. Such continuity is important for the successful transition from pediatric to adult care for various urologic conditions. In this chapter, we address several of these conditions and discuss long-term management. Overview tables are provided regarding general long-term considerations (Table 30.1), as well as those specific to sexual function and fertility (Table 30.2).

Spina Bifida

BACKGROUND

Spina bifida is a congenital neural tube defect that exists on a spectrum. In the most severe form, myelomeningocele, both meninges and neural tissue herniate through the spinal defect, and nearly all patients have neurogenic bladder dysfunction. Myelomeningocele has a prevalence of 30 cases per 100,000 live births in the United States, and due to advances in care, 80%–90% of these individuals will live well into adulthood. Urologic issues tend to have a substantial impact on both the quality and quantity of life of

TABLE 30.1 Adult Considerations for Pediatric Conditions

	Upper Tract	Lower Tract	Infection
Spina bifida	• Assess for signs of decompensation (RUS) • Kidney function: GFR[a]	• Assess for low/safe pressures (UDS) • Manage continence (meds, CIC, etc.)	• Atypical symptoms • High stone rate
Exstrophy/ epispadias	• Assess for signs of decompensation (RUS) • Kidney function	• Assess for low/safe pressures (UDS) • Manage continence (meds, CIC, etc.) • Avoid deflux, slings, sphincters	• May see epididymitis due to high urethral pressures
Hypospadias	• Unaffected in most patients • Assess selectively if severe strictures or concern for bladder decompensation	• Assess for voiding dysfunction (may be secondary to stricture or urethrocutaneous fistula) • Consider uroflow, PVR, RUG, VCUG and/ or cystoscopy	• May occur with stricture, diverticulum, or utricle
Posterior urethral valves	• Assess for signs of decompensation (RUS) • Kidney function	• Assess for low/safe pressures (UDS) • Manage continence (meds, CIC, etc.)	• At high risk due to reflux, incomplete emptying, CIC

Continued

TABLE 30.1 Adult Considerations for Pediatric Conditions—cont'd

	Upper Tract	Lower Tract	Infection
Prune belly syndrome	• Assess for signs of decompensation (RUS) • Kidney function • Ureters typically dilated due to peristaltic abnormalities; avoid reimplantation • Surgical fixation of kidney at transplantation	• Assess for low/safe pressures (UDS) • Manage continence (meds, CIC, etc.) • Caution with CIC • May have stenotic urethra	• At risk due to urinary stasis • Avoidance of instrumentation may decrease risk of infection

[a]Serum creatinine alone may be inaccurate in this population due to muscle wasting.
CIC, Clean intermittent catheterization; *GFR*, glomerular filtration rate; *meds*, medicines; *PVR*, postvoid residual, *RUG*, retrograde urethrogram, *RUS*, renal ultrasound; *UDS*, urodynamic studies; *VCUG*, voiding cystourethrogram.

TABLE 30.2 Adult Sexual Function and Fertility Considerations for Pediatric Conditions

	Sexual Function	Fertility	Other
Spina bifida	• More likely to be intact with lesions below L3 • Consider issues with dexterity & sensation	• Decreased with ED or ejaculatory function • Testes/sperm production generally intact	• Multispecialty management • Higher risk for sexual abuse

TABLE 30.2 Adult Sexual Function and Fertility Considerations for Pediatric Conditions—cont'd

	Sexual Function	Fertility	Other
Exstrophy/ epispadias	• Men: erectile function and sensation typically preserved. May have small penis size, chordee • Women: may have decreased clitoral size and sensation, narrow vaginal introitus	• Decreased • May need ART • Women: pregnancy high risk, cesarean section recommended	• Psychosocial concerns
Hypospadias	• May have difficulty with ejaculation (collapsed neourethra with penile engorgement) • May have recurrent ventral chordee	• Generally unaffected in mild cases • Ejaculation can be affected by stricture or diverticulum • Proximal location of meatus may affect conception • Concomitant bilateral UDT/proximal hypospadias may warrant further work-up	• Psychosocial concern for some men with penile appearance, ongoing ventral curvature

Continued

TABLE 30.2 Adult Sexual Function and Fertility Considerations for Pediatric Conditions—cont'd

	Sexual Function	Fertility	Other
Posterior urethral valves	• Higher rates of ED in patients who develop CKD/ESRD	• Generally preserved	
Prune belly syndrome	• Higher rates of ED in patients who develop CKD/ESRD	• Decreased • May be improved with early orchiopexy • Normal testosterone	

ART, Assisted reproductive technology; *CKD*, chronic kidney disease; *ED*, erectile dysfunction; *ESRD*, end-stage renal disease; *UDT*, undescended testicle.

these individuals, and the transition into adulthood represents an area of increased risk. Renal deterioration, urinary incontinence, difficulty with catheterization, recurrent urinary tract infections (UTIs), kidney and bladder stones, concomitant bowel issues, sexual function, fertility potential, and potential risk of malignancy are just some of the issues urologists may help this patient population manage and optimize over the course of their lifetimes. Priorities of urologic management include:

- Maximize renal function—assure upper tract drainage at low pressures
- Optimize continence based on patient goals
- Minimize UTIs and stone formation
- Discuss sexual health issues and offer treatment/counseling as needed
- Coordinate care with other specialists

UPPER TRACT PROTECTION

For patients with spina bifida, renal dysfunction can be a major source of morbidity and even mortality. As the kidneys are often normal at birth, upper tract deterioration in spina bifida is primarily driven by high pressures in the lower tract. With optimal management throughout lifetime, this risk can often be significantly mitigated.

Assessing the upper tracts for signs of decompensation is paramount. Upper tract imaging, (usually with renal ultrasound) can show signs of dilation (hydroureteronephrosis) or parenchymal changes (cortical thinning, hyperechogenicity) that signal potential damage to the upper tracts. Additionally, assessment of glomerular filtration rate (GFR) should be undertaken periodically to look for changes in renal function. Serum creatinine testing alone may be inaccurate at predicting GFR in this patient population due to decreased muscle mass, and alternative biomarkers (e.g., cystatin C) may need to be considered.

Periodic assessment of the lower tract should be undertaken with videourodynamics (VUDS) to assure a low-pressure system. VUDS can be used to evaluate the volume range of the bladder over which the pressures remain in a low, stable range, otherwise known as the patient's "safe zone." This can be used to guide optimal catheterization or voiding schedules, as well as suggest the need for further medical or surgical interventions. Sample urodynamics tracings that may be found in cases of neurogenic bladder are shown in Fig. 30.1.

LOWER TRACT MANAGEMENT/CONTINENCE

Urinary continence is an important consideration for many individuals with spina bifida. Continence is associated with independence and patient-reported quality of life metrics.

Successfully optimizing continence issues requires a detailed understanding of the patient's bladder, bladder neck, urethra, and goals of care. Medications such as antimuscarinics, beta-3 agonists, or botox instillation may be used to help improve compliance and ultimately may have a positive effect on continence for some. Ultimately, many patients will consider surgical options to help improve capacity/continence (e.g., augmentation cystoplasty), bladder neck incompetence (e.g., bladder neck reconstruction or closure, sling procedures, artificial urinary sphincter). In select situations, alternative procedures such as vesicostomy or urinary diversion may also be utilized. The risks and benefits of each of these options must be carefully weighed in light of the patient's individual situation.

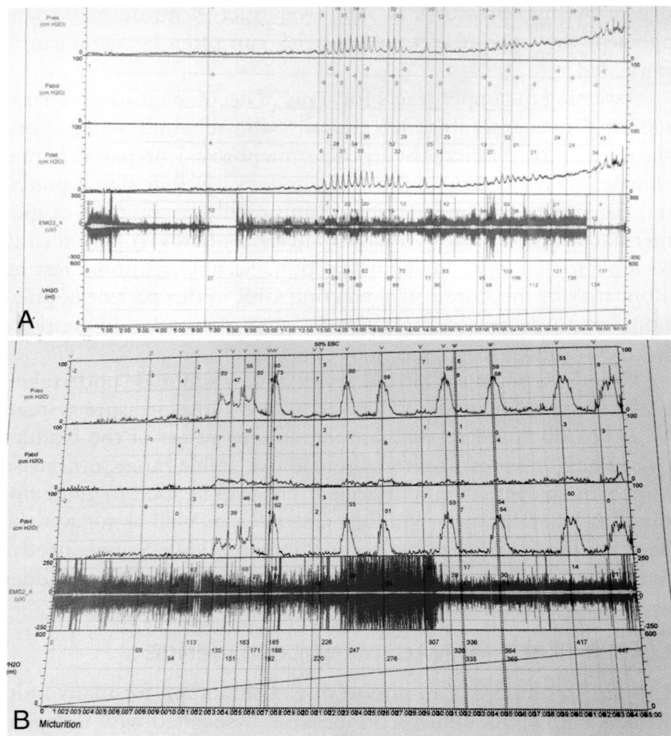

FIGURE 30.1 Sample urodynamic tracings during the filling phase in cases of neurogenic bladder dysfunction, which may show (A) loss of compliance and/or (B) detrusor overactivity.

Additionally, the urologist should help design regimens for these individuals to prevent and manage UTIs and stones as much as possible. Stones tend to occur at higher rates in these individuals due to bone demineralization, stasis of urine, infections, and mucus formation. Differentiating between chronic bacteriuria and true infection can be challenging for patients and providers alike, as symptoms rarely are classic. Antibiotics should be used judiciously to prevent morbidity and resistance associated with treating colonization.

SEXUAL HEALTH/FERTILITY

Like their age-matched peers, sexual health is often a significant concern for patients with spina bifida as they reach adolescence and adulthood.

For male patients with lower spinal cord lesions (below L3), spontaneous erections and sensation are more likely to be intact, whereas higher lesions tend to be associated with a much higher degree of sexual dysfunction. For female patients, appropriate counseling on sexual health issues and referral to gynecology when appropriate is recommended. Phosphodiesterase-5 inhibitors are reasonably effective in this population and should be considered first-line management when possible. Second-line options such as vacuum devices, intraurethral suppositories, intracorporeal injections, and prosthetic surgery can be considered as well, but may be challenging due to issues with dexterity and sensation and should be used with caution. Providers should be aware of the higher risk for abuse in this vulnerable population.

MULTISPECIALTY MANAGEMENT

Effective management of patients with spina bifida generally requires a multispecialty approach. These patients may require care from neurologists, neurosurgeons, orthopedists, gastroenterologists, general or colorectal surgeons, plastic surgeons, and wound specialists to name a few. While multispecialty spina bifida clinics are ideal, these are currently rare in adult facilities. Identifying primary care physicians, pediatricians, or other providers who can coordinate their overall care and help them sort through significant barriers to care (e.g., insurance, transportation, etc.) is essential to optimizing their medical management.

Exstrophy-Epispadias Complex

BACKGROUND

Exstrophy-epispadias is a complex disease that has a spectrum of presentation from epispadias (30%) to bladder exstrophy (60%) to the most complex being cloacal exstrophy (10%). The incidence of bladder exstrophy is 1 in 10 to 50,000 live births. These anomalies are associated with abnormalities of the entire genitourinary tract and the musculoskeletal system.

At presentation in bladder exstrophy, the bladder is open and exposed through the lower abdominal wall and the urethra is open on the dorsum of the penis or in between the right and left halves of the clitoris. Isolated urethral anomalies are consistent with epispadias. In all cases, the pubic bones are separated in the midline (pubic diastasis). The need for correction of this diastasis is controversial and being actively researched. Like most congenital urologic problems, the major focus of reconstruction in the short- and long-term are:

- Preservation of renal function
- Bladder storage
- Urinary continence
- Acceptable functional and cosmetic appearance of the genitals
- Prevention of infection and stones

INITIAL APPROACH AND LONG-TERM MANAGEMENT

In patients with a history of exstrophy-epispadias who are seeking to establish care with a new provider, it is vital to clinical care that previous records are obtained and direct correspondence with previous providers/surgeons is attempted. With little consensus on surgical approach, variations in technique and thought process make this exercise crucial to establishing and continuing care for these patients. If assuming care of these patients, a multidisciplinary approach with consultation with a pediatric urologist experienced in exstrophy-epispadias and/or a reconstructive urologist should be taken prior to major surgical reconstruction.

INFECTION

Infection is commonly seen in patients with exstrophy-epispadias. The incidence of UTI is related to urinary stasis, instrumentation/catheterization, and/or bladder substitution or augmentation. Risk factors for UTI such as vesicoureteral reflux, which is a common finding, and bladder stones can be identified and addressed in instances of recurrent UTI. Epididymitis can also be seen in adult male patients due to high urethral pressures and may require management of the urethra/bladder neck or potentially vasectomy, epididymectomy, or even orchiectomy in refractory cases for treatment and pain relief.

CONTINENCE

Continence rates can vary from 30% to 90% in these patients. This broad range is due to the variability in defining continence (i.e., many studies include patients who underwent a bladder neck closure, bladder augmentation with appendicovesicostomy). Understanding the concept of "social continence" and the patient's desire to improve continence should guide a stepwise surgical approach if pursued. Experience with Hyaluronic Acid/Dextranome (Deflux) to the bladder neck and artificial urinary sphincters to assist with urinary continence have been limited in success and follow-up.

RENAL PRESERVATION

Close upper tract monitoring is essential for long-term care of patients with bladder exstrophy. Periodic renal and bladder ultrasounds and as-needed nuclear medicine scans and urodynamics are important to identify lower tract findings prior to the onset of upper tract renal deterioration.

SEXUAL FUNCTION

Most male patients with exstrophy maintain erectile function and sensation despite limited phallic length and variable degrees of chordee. This can also impact the ability to engage in intercourse, although a majority of postpubertal males report successful intercourse. In cases where penile size is severely limited, surgical options including scar release or neophallus formation may be considered.

Ejaculation rates are also noted to be ~85%, but retrograde ejaculation can commonly occur. Fertility rates may be decreased due to oligospermia, azoospermia, decreased sperm motility, and/or low ejaculate volumes. Patients seeking counseling on fertility may need assistive reproductive technology and co-management with a reproductive endocrinologist.

Women with exstrophy may experience decreased clitoral sensation or clitoral atrophy. Intercourse may be limited due to narrowing of the vaginal introitus, which may require serial dilations or vaginoplasty for correction. Fertility is reduced, with worse fetal/neonatal outcomes. Pregnancy is considered high risk and needs appropriate urologic and maternal-fetal medicine consultation. Due to the aberrant pelvic floor, prolapse can be common requiring further treatment postpartum. Cesarean section is generally recommended over vaginal delivery.

PSYCHOSOCIAL CONCERNS

A notable body of literature continues to emerge on the psychological outcomes in patients with bladder exstrophy. Inquiring about and working with behavior specialists to address anxiety, depression, psychosocial interactions, genitalia, and body appearance are paramount as these patients continue to age.

Long-Term Consideration of Complex Urologic Reconstruction

In pediatric populations with impaired bladder capacity, compliance, or continence (secondary to spina bifida, exstrophy, etc.), major urologic reconstructions including catheterizable channels, bladder augmentations, and/or urinary diversions are common.

Bladder augmentation (augmentation cystoplasty) involves the integration of ileum and/or cecum, sigmoid colon, or stomach into the native bladder. Many adult providers favor augmenting the bladder with a segment of reconfigured ascending colon/cecum as a pouch for urine storage while utilizing the ileocecal valve as a built-in continence mechanism with the segment of tapered distal ileum utilized as a catheterizable channel (hemi-Indiana catheterizable ileocystoplasty). Alternatively, the channel may be created in a more standard fashion from the appendix (appendicovesicostomy) or reconfigured ileum (Monti procedure) and tunneled into the native bladder (Mitrofanoff procedure). Alternatively, in very selected cases, a continent catheterizable channel may be constructed from the native bladder to the abdominal wall, with tunneling of the channel at the bladder end to create a continence mechanism for self-catheterization.

COMPLICATIONS OF UROLOGIC RECONSTRUCTION

Complications associated with augments and diversions can occur years after initial creation, warranting lifelong monitoring in these patients. Complications including metabolic abnormalities, mucus production, urinary stone formation, recurrent UTI, secondary malignancy, bowel obstruction, or bladder perforations are important to consider and manage.

PERFORATION

One of the most feared complications in patients undergoing lower urinary tract reconstruction is bladder perforation. These patients often present with abdominal pain, distention, fever and/or sepsis. As many neurogenic patients (i.e., myelomeningocele) undergo lower urinary tract reconstruction, their abdominal sensation may be impaired. The clinician must therefore maintain a high-degree of suspicion to rule out perforation in equivocal cases.

Early postoperative perforation can occur along the bowel to bladder anastomosis due to ischemia at the edges of these tissues, but delayed perforation generally occurs within the bowel segment secondary to chronic overdistention, ischemia, and ultimately necrosis. Multiple large series have reported varying incidences of perforation, which is likely around 9%. Obtaining a cystogram will identify the area and degree of perforation, although false-negative studies have suggested that computed tomography plays an important role in diagnosis. If identified, the treatment is abdominal exploration with surgical repair. This allows for bladder closure and abdominal washout to treat the peritonitis. Small case series have reported limited experience with conservative management with continuous catheter drainage, antibiotics, and serial examinations. This approach is not well characterized and should be considered judiciously.

Patients with a history of cognitive issues, substance abuse, or mental health issues may be at a higher risk for perforation and should be monitored closely.

METABOLIC COMPLICATIONS

Metabolic complications arise both from the integration of bowel into the urinary tract and the removal of native bowel. Ileal and sigmoid mucosa absorb ammonia from urine, leading to a hypokalemic, hypochloremic metabolic acidosis; bicarbonate treatment may be considered in patients developing chronic acidosis. In addition, removal of distal ileum can contribute to vitamin B_{12} deficiency. Care should be taken with ileocecal valve removal in neurogenic patients as this may increase the risk of diarrhea.

Gastric mucosa in the urinary tract is commonly associated with hematuria-dysuria syndrome in sensate patients, characterized by hematuria, dysuria, and/or suprapubic pain. This is thought to be secondary to acid production and possibly *Helicobacter pylori*. While most patients have intermittent, mild symptoms that do not require treatment, Histamine H2 blockers and proton pump inhibitors are effective treatment options if needed. This makes gastric mucosa a less attractive choice for augmentation.

URINARY TRACT INFECTIONS AND STONES

Incomplete urinary drainage, stasis of urine, and using bowel substitutions contribute to mucus production, which ultimately serves as a nidus for stone formation and infection (Fig. 30.2). Both the bowel segment and the use of clean intermittent catheterization (CIC) lead to increased rates of bacteriuria. Differentiating colonization and a clinical infection will remain a lifetime dilemma requiring a careful examination of all associated symptoms and presentations, as the urinalysis and urine culture may be misleading. In cases of recurrent infections or stones, complete bladder drainage and daily irrigations of the bladder with water, saline, or selective antibiotic solutions are effective at decreasing its incidence and should be recommended and reinforced. The presence of urea-splitting organisms on urine culture may warrant empiric treatment in the setting of recurrent calculi.

MALIGNANCY

The incidence of tumor formation, particularly adenocarcinoma, during long-term follow-up of patients undergoing ureterosigmoidostomy and enterocystoplasty has been reported. Time

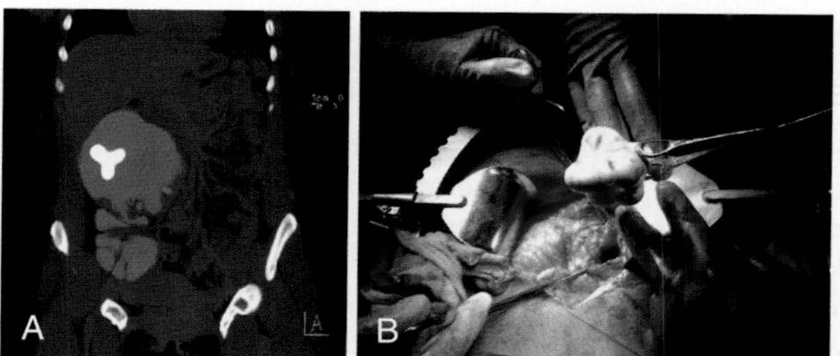

FIGURE 30.2 (A) Computed tomography (CT) scan shows a bladder stone in a previously augmented bladder. (B) Stone removed in an open approach.

latency has been reported to range from 4 to 20+ years after initial diversion. Due to variations in sample size and follow-up in the reported cohorts, the precise incidence that this occurs has not been well established. This has made development of surveillance guidelines difficult. This is an area of particular importance for the transitional and adult reconstructive urologist assuming care for these patients as the life expectancy for these patients is extended.

Hypospadias

Patients who present later in life with a new diagnosis of hypospadias (urethral opening on the ventral side of the penis) or history of previous hypospadias repair present a unique challenge to the reconstructive or pediatric urologist. As discussed in Chapter 26, the spectrum of disease can vary widely. Although limited at this time, there is a growing body of literature characterizing adult outcomes after prepubertal hypospadias repair which will help guide care for these patients. During evaluation as an adolescent or adult, it becomes important to characterize the patient's bother with respect to voiding dysfunction, sexual function/sexual satisfaction and/or cosmesis as these will be the main determinants to help tailor the work-up and treatment. Adult men presenting with other primary concerns who are incidentally noted to have a distal hypospadias without bother emphasizes the importance of patient-specific management in older patients.

URINARY FUNCTION

Voiding dysfunction remains the most common complaint in patients with previous history of hypospadias repair undergoing evaluation likely secondary to the presence of urethral stricture, urethral diverticulum and/or urethrocutaneous fistula (UCF). Additionally, it has been hypothesized that the reconstructed neourethra after hypospadias repair may not be distensible as a normal urethra leading to worsening voiding dysfunction. These etiologies lead to symptoms of dysuria, slow urinary stream, post-void dribbling, spraying, deflected urinary stream and/or urinary retention.

Identification of a UCF may be difficult to locate on physical exam, and utilization of micturition photos and/or videos may be of assistance. Patients suspected to have a stricture or UCF should be evaluated with uroflowmetry and postvoid residual. Interpretation of uroflowmetry may be difficult in this population, as "normal" uroflowmetry in patients with hypospadias have not been fully characterized. Retrograde urethrogram and cystoscopy are helpful tools in the work-up allowing for surgical planning. Sample findings for adult patients with prior hypospadias repair are presented in Fig. 30.3.

Prostatic utricle should also be suspected in patients with a history of more proximal hypospadias who present with urinary incontinence (especially postvoid dribbling) and recurrent UTIs.

SEXUAL FUNCTION AND RECURRENT CHORDEE

Men with a history of hypospadias repair may have difficulty with ejaculation (including milking of semen and poor force), recurrent ventral chordee, and overall decreased sexual satisfaction compared to controls. During ejaculation, without normal corporal spongiosum tissue around the neourethra, the urethra tends to be collapsed with penile engorgement leading to decreased force of emission. Recurrent ventral chordee tends to occur after puberty as the ventral tissue deficiency becomes more disproportionate during penile elongation. The rate at which this phenomena occurs and its association with initial hypospadias

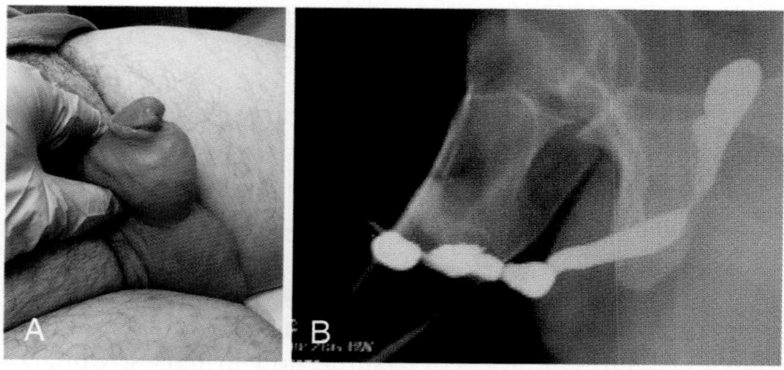

FIGURE 30.3 (A) Prior hypospadias repair with development of large ventral swelling concerning for diverticulum formation or large inclusion cyst. (B) Another patient with a history of prior hypospadias repair. Retrograde urethrogram showing multiple urethral strictures in the area of previous repair and back filling of a prostatic utricle.

severity and repair type are unknown. If recurrent chordee is noted, patient bother should guide pursuit of treatment and expectations moderated.

SURGICAL CONSIDERATIONS

There are few topics in pediatric urology more satisfying and humbling than hypospadias surgery. Hypospadias reoperations are covered in Chapter 26 of this text. In adults with recurrent strictures, repair can be challenging but can often be undertaken with reasonable success rates. Tissue quality may be compromised due to decreased blood supply and increased scar tissue which may compromise graft take and vascularized layers for coverage. For some patients, staged approaches may be necessary. Outcomes data in this population is building and should get better with more studies and follow-up. In older patients or more severe cases, perineal urethrostomy can also be considered.

Posterior Urethral Valves

ETIOLOGY

Posterior urethral valves (PUVs) are membranous folds within the posterior urethra that obstruct the lumen and are the most common congenital cause of lower tract obstruction in young males (see subsection "Posterior Urethral Valves" in Chapter 26). Initial surgical management is usually endoscopic transurethral incision or ablation of the valves, although temporary vesicostomy may be performed in select cases until valve incision can be undertaken safely.

BLADDER MANAGEMENT

Chronic obstruction from PUVs and subsequent bladder overdistension may lead to poor bladder compliance and contractility. These maladaptive changes commonly manifest as lower urinary tract symptoms when patients reach adulthood. Bladder function may be assessed with urodynamic studies. Strategies such as timed voiding, double voiding, overnight catheter drainage, and/or intermittent catheterization may be employed as appropriate. Primary goals are to (1) minimize patient symptoms (e.g., incontinence, incomplete emptying) and (2) keep bladder volumes and pressures low to reduce the risks of vesicoureteral reflux and upper tract damage.

RENAL FUNCTION

About one-third of these patients develop chronic kidney disease by adulthood. This pathway is often set in motion early in development with obstruction from the PUVs leading to renal dysplasia. Additionally, as some patients mature, a loss of the renal concentrating mechanism coupled with a degree of myogenic dysfunction of the bladder and decreased compliance can lead to worsening upper tract dilation and dysfunction (i.e., the valve bladder syndrome). Aggressive monitoring and intervention may help delay this progression. Despite appropriate therapy, some develop end-stage renal disease requiring dialysis and may ultimately undergo transplantation. Thus monitoring kidney function (serum creatinine) and upper tract morphology (imaging) may identify changes warranting urologic intervention and nephrology referral.

Prune Belly Syndrome

Prune belly syndrome is characterized by a triad of bilateral undescended testes, underdeveloped or absent abdominal wall musculature, and urinary tract abnormalities, all of which can exist over a wide spectrum of severity.

Urinary tract anomalies can include:

- Bladder—normal or enlarged in capacity often coupled with poor emptying
- Ureters—tend to be dilated due to peristaltic abnormalities without anatomic obstruction
- Urethra—may be narrowed/stenotic in some patients, bladder neck elevation

Management of the upper tracts is vital as these patients are at high risk for renal failure over the course of their lifetimes. This may be secondary to poor drainage leading to dilation, reflux, and/or infection. As upper tract dilation is often secondary to lower tract issues and poor ureteral peristalsis, ureteral reimplantation should be avoided or undertaken with the greatest of care due to risk of creating obstruction, reflux, or poor drainage as surgery can worsen an already tenuous system if performed imprudently.

In patients with progressive renal failure, lower tract issues should be addressed and managed before renal transplantation is undertaken. Due to lack of abdominal musculature support, surgical fixation of the transplanted kidney is required at the time of transplantation to decrease the risk of renal pedicle torsion.

Stenotic urethras are often managed initially with a progressive augmentation by dilating the urethra anterior (PADUA) procedure. Should stenosis recur, urethroplasty or catheterizable channel creation can be considered. Care should be taken with CIC in this patient population due to the high susceptibility for infection and urethra/bladder neck abnormalities.

Fertility potential is limited in these patients but has been reported in select individuals. Sperm production tends to be of poor quality in the testes of these patients, but with early orchiopexy, fertility may still be possible. Ejaculation can be affected by urethral or bladder neck issues. Testosterone production tends to be reasonably normal leading to normal libido and orgasmic function.

Urologic Issues in Childhood Cancer Survivors

Pediatric cancer mortality has declined substantially with advancements in cancer treatments, with 5-year survival rates over 80% for patients under age 20 and over 400,000 childhood cancer survivors in the United States alone. With this increased lifespan comes additional urologic quality of life considerations, most notably infertility and sexual health, as chemotherapy and radiation treatments are highly destructive to gonadal tissue.

INFERTILITY

Pediatric cancer survivors have two to three times the chance of having infertility compared to their siblings without cancer. However, out of survivors with infertility, about one-third reported at least one previous pregnancy resulting in a live birth, suggesting that infertility may be episodic. Risk factors include exposure to higher doses of alkylating agents or testicular radiation, exposure to bleomycin, surgical removal of any genital tract organ, or compromised ejaculation. On semen analysis, up to a quarter of male survivors may have severe oligospermia or persistent azoospermia.

Cryopreservation of sperm prior to cancer treatment, when possible, has been shown to be effective in fertility preservation. Up to 86% of pediatric cancer survivors referred for sperm banking can produce viable semen samples for cryopreservation, even those as young as 12 years old. Using in vitro fertilization (IVF) or intracytoplasmic sperm injection (ICSI), clinical pregnancy rates using pretreatment cryopreserved sperm can be up to 57%. Therefore the American Society of Clinical Oncology recommends that sperm cryopreservation be offered in all eligible cases.

SEXUAL HEALTH

The prevalence of ED in pediatric cancer survivors (many in their mid-30s) has been reported at anywhere from 10% to 30%. Risk factors for ED in this population include higher doses of testicular radiation, testosterone < 250 ng/dL, prior surgery on the spinal cord or nerves, prostate surgery (rhabdomyosarcoma), pelvic surgery, and greater body image dissatisfaction. A comprehensive evaluation is warranted to identify appropriate multimodal treatments of ED for these individuals.

Additional content, including Suggested Readings, may be accessed at www.ExpertConsult.com.

Geriatric Urology

George W. Drach, MD

Urology and Aging Patients

Our growing geriatric population will impact urology in major ways over the next 2 to 3 decades. General urologists will have nearly 50% of their patients in the over-65 age group (Table 31.1). Urologists will also face difficult management decisions opting for or against major surgery in these patients. This is especially true for patients with bladder and prostatic cancer because they often do not reach the stage of invasive cancer until over age 60 (Fig. 31.1). Some of these surgical candidates remain relatively healthy. Others demonstrate poor surgical risk because of their general condition and comorbidities.

Should we in urology approach these elderly patients differently from our younger, healthier patients? Yes, but the response to this question comes in modification of three elements of our usual "evaluation and management" algorithm: steps in initial evaluation of the elderly patient differ; decision processes regarding further evaluation and recommendation for treatment require alteration; and decisions on management of definitive therapy require additional thought integrated into the milieu of aging.

There are several excellent resources for geriatric urology. Throughout this chapter I refer to a small text, *Geriatrics at Your Fingertips* (GAYF), which is of great assistance in management of all geriatric patients. Another source is the text *Geriatrics Syllabus for Specialists*. Both are available from the American Geriatrics Society, and both should be on the office bookshelf of every urologist who treats adults. In addition, the text *Primer of Geriatric Urology* has recently been published.

To summarize, for our geriatric urology patients, initial evaluation must be altered to include careful drug history, obtain necessary old records, and evaluate functional abilities. Therapeutic decisions must be based upon presence or absence of comorbidities

TABLE 31.1 Outpatient Visits by Medicare Patients (2006)

Specialty	Percentage (%)
Cardiology	58.4
Ophthalmology	48.5
Urology	47.9
General internal medicine	42.7
General surgery	35.8
Neurology	28.6
Dermatology	28.1
Otolaryngology	22.5
Orthopedic surgery	25.0
Family practice	25.9
Psychiatry	9.9
Gynecology	7.1

(Adapted from Drach GW, Forciea MA. Geriatric patient care: basics for urologists. *AUA Update Series*. 2005;24:286-296.)

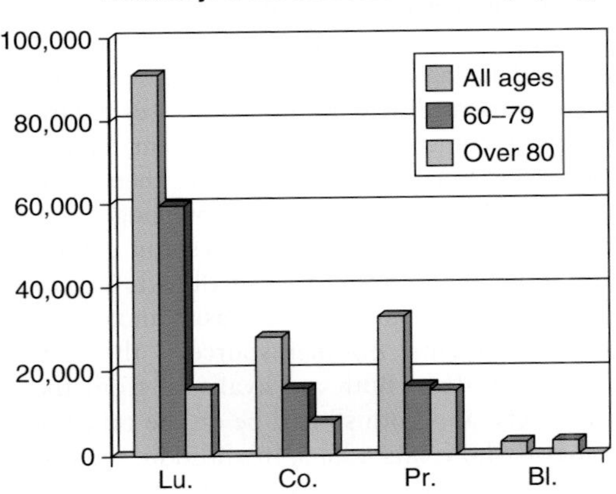

FIGURE 31.1 Most prostate cancer deaths occur after age 60. Bladder cancer deaths do not become noticeable until after age 80. *Bl*, Bladder; *Co*, colon; *Lu*, lung; *Pr*, prostate. (Adapted from Hollenbeck BK, Miller DC, Taub D, et al. Aggressive treatment for bladder cancer is associated with improved overall survival among patients 80 years old or older. *Urology*. 2004;64:292-297.)

along with total functional capacity, rather than chronological age. Finally, the perioperative period must include concern for optimization of comorbidities, attention to pain control, fall prevention, and early discharge planning. All possible steps to prevent or ameliorate mental status change are necessary. With these details accomplished, care of our aged patients will be more beneficial.

CLINICAL PEARLS

1. At the beginning of your evaluation of the geriatric urology patient, you must assess and integrate the patient's cognitive ability.
2. High functional ability of the older patient predicts a likely successful outcome of your treatment program.
3. Decisions on advising therapeutic intervention must be based on physiologic age, not chronologic age.
4. Discharge planning should begin before any hospital admission and must include the social conditions of the patient.

Additional content, including Self-Assessment Questions and Suggested Readings, may be accessed at www.ExpertConsult.com.

Quality and Safety Considerations in Urology

Ankur A. Shah, MD, MBA, and Justin B. Ziemba, MD, MSEd

Introduction: What Is Patient Safety and Quality Improvement?

1. The Committee on the Quality of Healthcare in America was formed in June 1998. This was an independent committee of experts supported by the Institute of Medicine. They created the landmark document, *To Err Is Human* (published in 200), that renewed America's focus on quality improvement and patient safety. *To Err Is Human* has since shaped the landscape for efforts to improve the quality of health care in America.
2. The purpose of *To Err Is Human* was to provide a comprehensive set of recommendations that help create external pressure on key stakeholders in order to restructure the fragmented American health care system. The document demonstrates the harm caused by medical errors with regard to patients and lost revenue. It also showed that blame for errors in the health care system goes beyond individuals and is, in fact, dependent on the structure and processes in place within our health care system. By changing organizational culture to make error prevention a priority and providing incentives that align all involved stakeholders, we can strive to improve the quality of care we provide, reduce waste, decrease unnecessary costs, and keep patients safe.
3. In order to understand the principles of patient safety and quality improvement, we must first understand the key terms.
   a. **Error** is defined as "the failure of a planned action to be completed as intended or the use of a wrong plan to achieve an aim." Errors can be active or latent. **Active errors** are a

result of a direct action; however, they do not speak to the intent of a person. Whereas **latent errors** occur due to underlying structural or process-based issues.

b. The term **adverse event (AE)** is often used interchangeably with medical error; however, they are not synonyms. AEs include miscommunications affecting patient care, missed diagnoses as well as the provision of inadequate or negligent care to patients in a variety of settings (i.e., emergency room triage, postoperative care, etc.). While AEs do result from medical intervention, not all are due to medical error, which is an important distinction to realize.
   1) For example, the development of a pulmonary embolism (PE) after radical cystectomy and urinary diversion is an AE, but it may or may not be due to medical error. If investigation of the AE found that the patient was not ordered for subcutaneous heparin prophylaxis postoperatively and subsequently developed a PE, the AE was preventable and clearly due to medical error. However, if the patient developed a PE postoperatively without any identifiable causes, this would be called an AE attributed to a highly morbid surgery for which PE is a known complication and therefore not due to medical error.

c. While **patient safety** is based on an amalgamation of several concepts, it has been defined more generally as "freedom from accidental injury." One of the fundamental concepts in patient safety is reliability. Reliability references the fact that patients should be guaranteed the necessary services (i.e., surgery) in a time-sensitive manner appropriate for their underlying diagnosis.

d. **Quality improvement** is based on a number of terminologies and concepts adapted from nonmedical industries such as aviation and manufacturing. It consists of data-driven actions that lead to the tangible improvement of both individual patient care and health services delivery within an organization.

e. A **near miss** is a potential medical error that ultimately does not result in harm to the patient due to either intervention or by chance.

f. A **never event** quite literally refers to an event that should never happen. A never event in urology, for example, would be wrong-site nephrectomy, where the kidney with the mass was *not* removed and the healthy kidney was removed instead.

g. A **sentinel event** is defined by the Joint Commission as "any unexpected occurrence involving death or serious physical or psychological injury, or risk thereof."

Medical Error: Consequences and Contributing Factors

CONSEQUENCES OF MEDICAL ERROR

1. As first established by *To Err Is Human* and commonly cited in the literature, it is estimated that 44,000 to 98,000 Americans die each year as a result of medical error. In addition, about 400,000 hospital inpatients are impacted by preventable medical error.
2. The costs to our health care system associated with these staggering numbers are estimated to be in the range of $8.5 to $14.5 billion. Moreover, this does not account for the total costs to society with regard to lost income, lost productivity, and disability.
3. There are also opportunity costs from medical error. There are errors that require additional testing, medications, and procedures to reverse their outcomes. The costs of these errors are passed onto the consumer in the form of higher medical bills, copayments, and insurance premiums.
4. And finally, there are intangible costs manifested through the faith lost in providers and the health care system overall by patients as a result of preventable medical errors. This, in turn, can lead to decreased job satisfaction from health care workers, which can subsequently decrease productivity and result in further costs to the system.

FACTORS CONTRIBUTING TO MEDICAL ERROR

1. A significant contributing factor to medical error in American health care is the fragmented nature of the system in the setting of a rapidly changing technological landscape and an increasing demand for services. While the *Patient Protection and Affordable Care Act* has caused a shift in the landscape of

American health care from solo practitioners to large hospital systems and group practices, the fundamental methods by which health care is delivered have not changed.

2. Prior to the publication of *To Err Is Human*, the focus of health care organizations was on an individual level. It sought to catch isolated errors and reprimand practitioners for their actions. Thus quality assurance was not evidence based, and it was more punitive than innovative.
3. The Committee on Healthcare Quality in America changed the American health care system by placing a focus on quality improvement (as opposed to assurance), thereby promoting the use of data to measure the effectiveness of processes in attaining desired outcomes. It also recognized that the majority of medical errors are not due to individual providers but instead due to systems-based issues.
4. In fact, it has been estimated that 80% of medical errors are due to a system failure. Improvements in our health care system will come with evidence-based, systems-focused changes where we recognize that humans are fallible; thus while medical errors are inevitable, the goal is to design processes that maximally prevent serious harm from befalling patients.
5. A model that aptly demonstrates organizational error is British psychologist James Reason's **Swiss cheese model**, which describes the supposition that individual error is typically not the basis for harm (Fig. 32.1). Instead, multiple errors must align through a number of layers ("of cheese") in order to cause a poor outcome. This model thereby reinforces systems-based thinking and promotes the goal of "shrinking the holes" within organizations so that the chance of the holes aligning and causing harm is minimal. By restructuring systems, institutions can focus on the processes that led to the ultimate AE instead of focusing on the end result alone.

Creating Safety Culture in the Workplace

ESTABLISHING A CULTURE THAT SUPPORTS PATIENT SAFETY

1. We have thus far discussed what medical errors are and the factors that contribute to them. We have established that

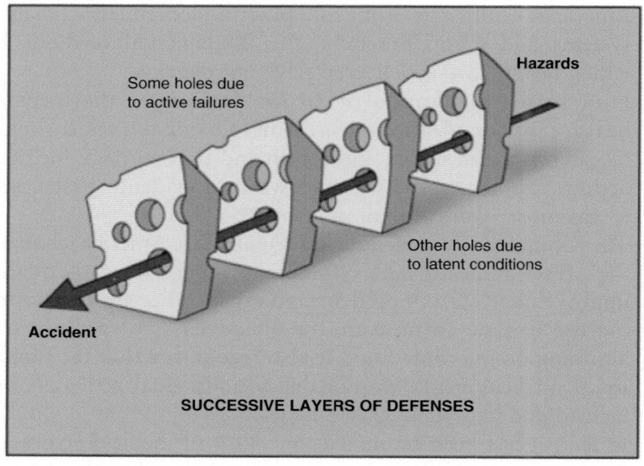

FIGURE 32.1 Swiss cheese model. (From Jhugursing M, Dimmock V, Mulchandani H. Error and root cause analysis. *BJA Educ*. 2017; 17[10]:323-333.)

medical errors and AEs occur daily in the American health care system as a result of a variety of failures on a systems-based or individual level. Health care organizations differentiate themselves not by the presence of medical errors but in how they respond to them. The response of a hospital or health care organization to a serious clinical AE is largely dependent on their culture of safety, which is a significant contributor to safety and quality outcomes.

2. We define the **culture of safety** as fostering an environment where involved stakeholders are willing to speak up on matters involving patient safety without fear of repercussion and with the knowledge that they will receive feedback on the actions taken regarding their opinions. As we will discuss next, a culture of safety is created from the top down and bottom up.
3. It goes without saying for the vast majority of physicians, nurses and other clinical staff within health care organizations, the safety and care of patients always comes first. Similarly, organizational leadership must emphasize patient safety as a priority in order to help create a culture of safety.

4. An organization's strategic agenda must reflect a strong focus on patient safety in order to maintain patient safety as an organizational priority.
5. While safety culture fundamentally involves placing patients at the top of the priority list, it also must focus on fostering trust among staff, which is more formally known as establishing **psychological safety** within an organization. British psychologist James Reason, the intellectual father of patient safety and creator of the Swiss cheese model for medical error that was discussed previously, created the concept of psychological safety. It is informally thought of as the ability of employees to speak up regarding their concerns. Formally, psychological safety has four important attributes, which are described as follows:
   a. Anyone can ask questions without looking stupid.
   b. Anyone can ask for feedback without looking incompetent.
   c. Anyone can be respectfully critical without appearing negative.
   d. Anyone can suggest innovative ideas without being perceived as disruptive.

ADDRESSING ORGANIZATIONAL INFRASTRUCTURE

1. The purpose of most health care organizations is to deliver safe, reliable, and effective care to patients. The performance of health care organizations is dependent upon leaders throughout various levels of management who all contribute to the overall success of an organization. Upper-level management creates policy and directs the organization, middle-level managers oversee nonclinical staff who are essential to the success of the organization, and clinical leaders use their knowledge to help their teams deliver optimal care.
2. Creating an environment that promotes psychological safety is the responsibility of hospital leaders. Another role is that of the **patient safety officer**. The patient safety officer is an essential part of health care organizations' fundamental goal of providing safe and reliable care through the implementation of best practices throughout the hospital. By designating an individual who is responsible for overseeing the implementation of new programs and educating staff on safety efforts

such as reporting mechanisms, an organization can demonstrate their priorities and reinforce safety culture.

3. Communication and accountability are key facets of successful health care organizations. Managers should regularly meet with their staff—both clinical and nonclinical—to assess their opinions on how operations are functioning, to help identify areas for improvement and to receive feedback on their own actions. In certain situations, such as in the morning outside of the operating room, appropriate clinical leaders can hold **huddles,** which are brief meetings that allow information to be quickly shared among key stakeholders. The purpose of these huddles is to ensure that representatives from the operating room staff, nurses, and surgeons are on the same page and to allow a brief forum for discussion. By demonstrating through their actions that feedback and continuous improvement is an expectation, leaders can create a psychologically safe environment and promote teamwork and communication, which are essential to the success of any organization.
4. An effective way to develop trust and enhance psychological safety within organizations is to reward individuals for filing incident reports, sharing the analysis of these reports with staff, and regularly meeting with middle managers and individuals to address their concerns and/or the feedback from their reporting. This promotes teamwork and communication, and demonstrates that the leadership's values align with those of the organization.

Standardizing Health Care Systems and Improving Reliability

1. As mentioned several times previously, *To Err Is Human* helped the field of medicine improve the quality of care significantly since the year 2000. Deaths from preventable medical error have gone from 98,000 Americans a year to 35,000. While these are only estimates, the data show there have been significant improvements in the care we deliver.
2. The improvement we have seen in surgery can be classified into three distinct waves: technical advancements, standardization of procedures, and high-reliability organizing. These

classifications represent the change in ideology within the field of quality improvement over the years.

a. **Technical advancements** refer to the improvement in surgical technique and technology that has made surgery more effective and less morbid. For example, laparoscopic and, more recently, robotic surgery have dramatically changed the surgical specialty. It was previously not unusual for patients to have blood loss estimated at 1 L or more in a radical retropubic prostatectomy. Due to widespread adoption of robotic surgery in urology, patients undergoing robotic-assisted radical prostatectomy typically have blood loss less than 200 mL; this is mostly due to the visualization and dexterity provided deep in the pelvis by the da Vinci robot.
b. The **standardization of procedures** was largely inspired by *To Err Is Human*. It involves identifying best practices in specific clinical scenarios that when performed consistently improve patient care. These practices, established through multidisciplinary collaboration and rooted in strong evidence, are then implemented through a variety of methods such as checklists and care bundles. Compliance to the standardized process is then measured (goal of greater than 95%) and the resultant impact on patient care is determined.
    1) A prime example of standardization is the Ventilator Bundle Checklist created by the Institute for Healthcare Improvement (IHI). It includes basic measures to help prevent the most common complications of mechanical ventilation, such as elevation of the head of the bed to between 30 and 45 degrees, daily sedation vacations to assess extubation potential, peptic ulcer disease prophylaxis, deep venous thrombosis prophylaxis, and daily oral care with chlorhexidine. There is an abundance of evidence demonstrating that the use of bundles as the foundational blocks to improve patient care results in high levels of reliability across teams and organizations.
c. The third wave of innovation is coined **high-reliability organizing,** which is based on the **Safety II** movement. While the movement to promote standardization was largely the result of *To Err Is Human*, Safety II is a contemporary movement within high-performing health care organizations. Safety II,

which is often referred to as high-reliability organizing, came about because standardization in health care has seemed to reach a point of diminishing returns with regard to improving outcomes, likely due to the inherent complexity in caring for patients as individuals. It focuses on making sure "as many things as possible go right" as opposed to Safety I, which ensured "as few things as possible go wrong."

1) The Safety II concept recognizes that there is variability in performance on a day-to-day basis given that we are all human. The important thing to realize is how individuals and organizations adapt to those changes in order to succeed. In fact, there is evidence that demonstrates hospitals with low mortality rates have comparable rates of surgical complications to hospitals with high mortality rates, but it is their response to these complications that differentiates them.

Methods of Patient Safety Investigation

INTRODUCTION

As discussed extensively in this chapter, preventable medical error is prevalent within the American health care system with significant economic, emotional, and indirect consequences on patients, families, providers, and the system overall. Quality improvement and patient safety efforts have been adopted across the system, thanks to the efforts of the IHI and numerous other organizations. In the previous section we discussed the principles of quality improvement efforts, which aim to optimize health care delivery in a safe manner. However, medical errors still occur. In this section, we will discuss the primary methods of patient safety investigation that have been implemented across the American health care system.

ROOT CAUSE ANALYSIS

1. **Root cause analysis (RCA)** is a technique originally developed in psychology and systems engineering before being adopted by the health care industry. The Veterans Affairs system and Joint Commission are responsible for introducing the concept of RCA to the health care industry. The purpose of an RCA is to retrospectively analyze errors in order to prevent similar

additional errors from occurring. The RCA process addresses three questions:

a. What happened?
b. Why did it happen?
c. How can we prevent this from happening again?

2. In the modern era, the vast majority of hospitals require RCAs to be performed with any sentinel event, and in some states, these events must be reported to state health departments. However, many thought leaders within the quality improvement and patient safety sphere criticize the efficacy of RCAs, particularly in smaller hospitals, as there is little evidence to suggest RCAs improve patient safety. Moreover, data suggest that the quality of RCAs varies notably among organizations. In many RCAs, the follow-up on outcomes is rare, which leads to repeat events in hospitals and health care organizations. Experts suggest that there needs to be renewed emphasis on the follow-up of outcomes, and that RCAs should be recalibrated to focus on larger scale collaborative efforts to analyze "big data" as opposed to focusing on individual events. In this way, trends across hospitals can be identified and preventive measures can be implemented on a larger scale with appropriate follow-up.

MORBIDITY AND MORTALITY CONFERENCE

1. **Morbidity and mortality conference**, colloquially referred to as **M&M** by residents and surgeons alike, has difficult roots to trace. Nonetheless, one of the early precursors to M&M was actually founded in Philadelphia by the Philadelphia County Medical Society. The group was called the Anesthesia Mortality Committee that met to discuss fatalities surrounding anesthesia and interesting cases to improve their standards of care. This committee eventually morphed into the Anesthesia Study Commission and included anesthesiologists, surgeons, and internists and was not limited only to fatalities. This commission also began publicly reporting some of their data. The fundamentals of the Anesthesia Study Commission have been adopted by institutions all over the country as the guiding principles of M&Ms.
2. M&M conferences serve as a forum for departments to identify and learn from internal errors. While M&Ms throughout history have often been contentious given the sensitive nature of publicly acknowledging individuals' mistakes,

many high-reliability organizations have shifted the mindset from "blame" to constructive self-reflection.

a. The keys to an effective M&M involve appropriate case selection and high attendance. Attendees should include individuals from within the department as well as relevant stakeholders from the hospital administration and/or those who were involved in the AEs being discussed. The case selection and moderation should be performed by a senior physician who can take control of the meeting and ensure all participants feel supported.
b. According to Orlander, Barber, and Fincke (2002), a successful M&M should
   1) Identify the events that led to undesirable patient outcomes
   2) Promote discussion of the errors made
   3) Identify insights regarding patient care as a result of the experience being discussed
   4) Reinforce accountability for providing high-quality care
   5) Create an environment where surgeons are comfortable taking responsibility and discussing potential causative factors for their mistake(s)

SAFETY EVENT ANALYSIS

1. In early 2019, the Accreditation Council for Graduate Medical Education (ACGME) began the process of identifying new ways for integrating patient safety into the clinical learning environment (CLE) for residents and fellows. One of the tools developed to engage residents and fellows in patient safety activities was the **safety event analyses (SEAs)**. SEAs were created to move the focus from reporting sentinel events (i.e., in M&M, RCA, etc.) to analyzing all events, including near misses in order to create organizational change and ultimately improve patient care (Fig. 32.2).
2. SEAs are small group sessions conducted within the CLE either in the ambulatory clinics, inpatient units, or in the operating room. These sessions last approximately 15 to 30 minutes and can occur separately or as part of a regularly scheduled safety meeting. They are meant to be interdisciplinary sessions involving all relevant and available stakeholders. Again, these SEAs usually focus on near misses or events with minimal harm. In this way, future events of the same nature

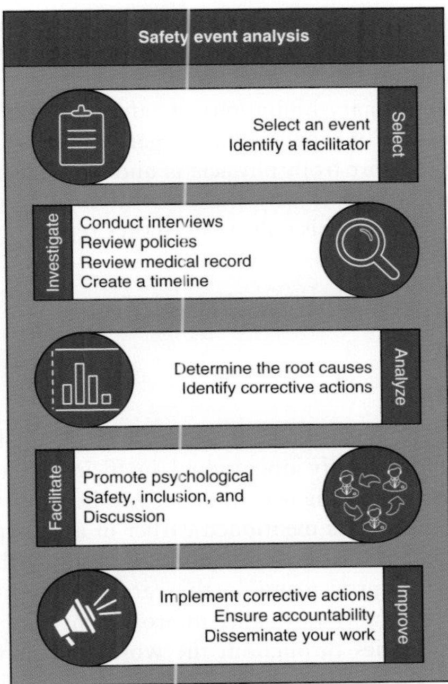

FIGURE 32.2 Safety event analysis.

can be prevented from progressing into sentinel events and can serve as a learning tool to guide immediate process change.

SAFETY REPORTING SYSTEMS

1. The Institute of Medicine initially recommended the utilization of patient safety reporting systems within hospitals and organizations in order to evaluate reasons for patient harm from medical care. The Joint Commission now requires hospitals to report mistakes.
2. Many hospitals have developed web-based patient safety reporting systems.
3. Within these systems, harm is graded low to high by scoring mechanisms, which are typically based on the level of intervention required to correct any harm that has come to

the patient. Each submitted event is also localized to a floor or department within the hospital. Submissions can be anonymous.

4. One of the primary limitations of safety reporting systems is the submission of events. Many organizations find it difficult to gather support from physicians and employees in submitting events, which is why the cultivation of a robust safety culture is critical. This culture promotes reporting.

Quality Improvement: Principles and Methods

INTRODUCTION

1. As the cost of medical care increases in the United States, it is important to identify operational inefficiencies to eliminate waste so that spending is used directly to benefit patients in an effective manner. As mentioned earlier in the chapter, **quality improvement** is a series of continuous actions that leads to quantifiable improvements in the care provided to patients. There are a number of quality improvement methods used in various industries throughout the world that have been applied to medicine. To maximize efficiency, organizations can address one or more of three key factors: inputs, processes, and/or outcomes. In this section, we will review a few of the fundamental methods for quality improvement that review the three key factors described previously.

THE MODEL FOR IMPROVEMENT

1. The **Model for Improvement** is a quality improvement methodology widely employed by health care organizations to achieve optimal outcomes. It focuses on continuous quality improvement as testing change is an iterative process.
2. There are three fundamental questions that are asked as part of the Model for Improvement:
   a. What are we trying to accomplish?
   b. How will we know that a change is an improvement?
   c. What changes can we make that will result in improvement?
3. Based on the answers to the aforementioned questions, teams can employ the **Plan-Do-Study-Act (PDSA) cycle** to test their

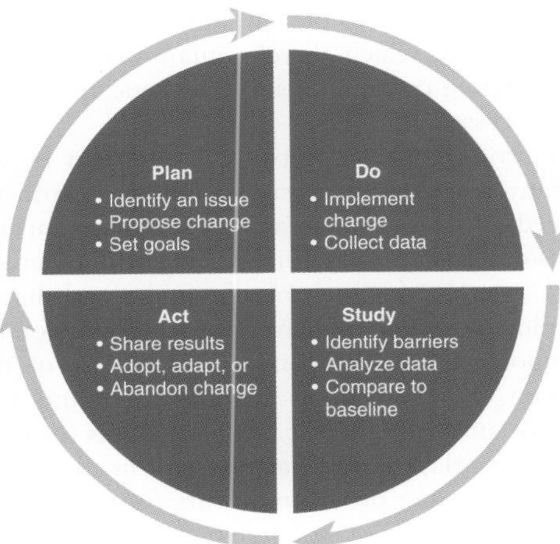

FIGURE 32.3 Plan-Do-Study-Act cycle. (From Berman L, Raval MV, Goldin A. Process improvement strategies: designing and implementing quality improvement research. *Semin Pediat Surg*. 2018;27[6]:379-385 [figure 1].)

desired changes in order to determine whether their interventions are creating improvements (Fig. 32.3).

a. As part of the PDSA cycle for continuous improvement, teams must *p*lan an intervention, *d*o or actually try the intervention, *s*tudy the effects of the intervention, and *a*ct on the lessons learned. This is an iterative process.

LEAN AND SIX SIGMA

1. **Lean** is a concept that began in the early 1900s and was popularized by Toyota Production Systems in the 1940s. As stated by Koning et al., "Lean is an integrated system of principles, practices, tools and techniques focused on reducing waste, synchronizing workflows and managing variability in production flows." The strengths of Lean are its focus on value-added activities that benefit the customer and its set of standard solutions to common problems. The core principles of Lean are responsible for its success. Three of the fundamental concepts of Lean Thinking are defined as follows:
   a. **Jidoka** is translated as "automation with a human touch" and refers to halting the assembly line as soon as a problem

occurs. The goal is to prevent any defective products from being created, which thereby guarantees quality through incorporating continuous improvement into daily production processes.

1) In urology, the concept of Jidoka can be applied to many scenarios. One such example is with the use of needle guides during magnetic resonance imaging (MRI) fusion prostate biopsies. If a high-volume practice relies on a vendor for their needle guides and that vendor is suddenly unable to deliver due to production issues, it is important for the managers in charge of the supply chain to have backup manufacturers and a safety reserve. In this manner, cancer diagnoses for patients will not be delayed, and patients will not lose trust in the ability of their providers to care for them.

b. **Kaizen** translates as "good change" and incorporates the philosophy of continuous improvement. It refers to the PDSA cycles performed as part of the troubleshooting process during Lean Thinking. In keeping with the example of supply chain issues regarding needle guides, the entire issue could have been prevented if there was a mechanism in place to communicate with the manufacturer to anticipate production issues. For example, the shortage of needle guides could have been prevented from reaching patients (i.e., delaying prostate biopsies) by having contracts with multiple companies as an anticipatory step. Kaizen is an integral aspect of the Lean philosophy and can prevent issues from reaching the customer (i.e., patients) through continuous improvement.

c. **Just-in-time** (**JIT**) describes an ideal production system with no waste. It refers to a system where each step of the production process produces only what is essential for the next step to continue thereby maximizing value and eliminating waste.

1) In health care, JIT has been used for quite some time with regard to the supply chain. As demonstrated in the situation with prostate biopsy needle guides, JIT is cost efficient when there are no production issues as hospitals are not required to maintain an inventory. Another example that is relevant to the Coronavirus 2019 (COVID-19)

pandemic is that of personal protective equipment such as N95 masks. Most hospitals prior to the pandemic used JIT to ensure N95s were available as necessary in specific situations. This was again financially advantageous as hospitals were not responsible for the cost of inventory and there were no supply chain issues.

b. However, JIT has intrinsic risks when supply is limited, as demonstrated in the situation of the needle guide shortage. In addition, during the COVID-19 pandemic, very few hospitals had strategic stockpiles of N95 masks that were available when the pandemic required the majority of frontline providers to don these masks, which created a critical shortage of N95 masks across the country. The COVID-19 pandemic may forever change the health care industry's reliance on the concept of JIT.

2. **Six Sigma** provides a conceptual framework for the implementation of quality improvement projects. It was originally created by Motorola in 1987, furthered by General Electric and eventually adopted by the health care industry due to its success. The term Six Sigma refers to the fact that Motorola committed to reduce their defect rate to within six standard deviations (sigma). While the exact math remains up for debate, the philosophy Motorola created continues to be referred to as Six Sigma in the literature to this day.
   a. Six Sigma provides a detailed structure on how to carry out quality improvement projects. Briefly, it utilizes project leaders and project owners. Project leaders are referred to as Black Belts and Green Belts, and project owners are called Champions. Six Sigma therefore requires buy-in from both upper management and workers in order to be successful. Its goal is to reduce costs while creating a reliable product that satisfies customers. When applied to health care, its goals are in line with the principles of evidence-based medicine: diagnoses are made cautiously based on all available data, and treatment plans are implemented with continuous checks to ensure they are truly effective.
   b. The problem-solving approach of Six Sigma employs the **DMAIC** framework, which refers to the steps involved in

the process: *d*efine, *m*easure, *a*nalyze, *i*mprove, and *c*ontrol.

1) **Define**—this is the initial step in the problem-solving process. In the "define" stage, the problem at hand and relevant stakeholders are identified in order to establish the purpose of the quality improvement project.
2) **Measure**—in this phase of the problem-solving cycle, the baseline data are gathered and examined to determine the necessary future steps of the project. Then a data collection plan must be created and the specific process metrics that will be utilized in the project should be ascertained. One way to depict key process metrics is the Ishikawa (fishbone) diagram in which the bones of the fish are the drivers of the process under investigation (Fig. 32.4).
3) **Analyze**—in this step, the key metrics identified in the "measure" phase are analyzed using the appropriate statistical tools. The primary drivers of error are delineated so that interventions can be designed to target them.
4) **Improve**—this phase of the process consists of three steps. First, brainstorming sessions involving all key members of the project generate creative solutions. Next, the ideas are used to collect stakeholder buy-in throughout the department or organization. And lastly, the change(s) are actually implemented.

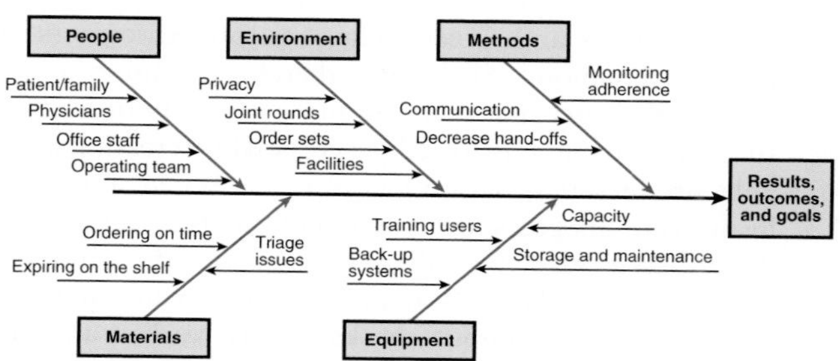

FIGURE 32.4 Fishbone diagram. (From Berman L, Raval MV, Goldin A. Process improvement strategies: designing and implementing quality improvement research. *Semin Pediat Surg*. 2018;27[6]:379-385 [figure 2].)

5) **Control**—once a change has been implemented in the "improve" phase of the DMAIC cycle, the control phase is used to ensure the intervention is successful in the long term by continuous monitoring of key metrics. Therefore positive changes from the implementation will be perpetuated through continuous quality improvement.

3. **Lean Six Sigma**
   a. Sometime after the adoption of both Lean Thinking and Six Sigma in the health care sphere, many experts and organizations began synthesizing the two into their efforts for quality improvement, thereby coining the term Lean Six Sigma. The two approaches are complementary as Lean provides a conceptual framework and set of best practices to maximize value while Six Sigma provides an analytic framework for problem-solving. The combination of the two concepts into Lean Six Sigma combines the best aspects of both in order to maximize efficiency, innovation and quality within health care. As George (2002) states, Lean Six Sigma allows organizations to "[do] quality quickly."

Conclusion

Quality improvement is a fundamental concept in medicine and critical to maintaining the highest standards of patient safety within our health care system. Over the last two decades, the fields of quality improvement and patient safety have developed significantly. The medical field has adopted principles from a variety of industries (i.e., aviation and automobile) in order to remain dynamic and best serve our patients. Throughout this chapter we have explored these theories and methods. Ultimately, the responsibility to promote safety is shared by all members of the health care team—ranging from the chief executive officer to patient care associates. By promoting a culture of safety, striving for continuous improvement, being aware of the financial implications of clinical decisions, and most importantly, maintaining focus on the patient as the center of all care, we can provide the best medical care possible and strive to maintain the oaths we took as physicians to keep patients from harm.

Additional content, including Suggested Readings, may be accessed at www.ExpertConsult.com

Clinical Research Design and Statistics

Gregory E. Tasian, MD, MSc, MSCE, and
John K. Weaver, MD

Research Question

All clinical research starts with a research question. The research question is the objective of the study, the specific uncertainty the investigator wants to resolve. Research questions often begin with a general concern that must be narrowed down to a concrete, researchable issue. The question must be focused before study planning efforts can begin. Often, this involves breaking the question into specific components and singling out one or two of those to build the protocol around.

A good research question should pass the "so what?" test. Getting the answer to the research question should contribute usefully to the current state of knowledge. The acronym FINER denotes fives essential characteristics of a good research question: it should be **F**easible, **I**nteresting, **N**ovel, **E**thical, and **R**elevant.[1] The challenge in finding a research question is defining an important one that can be transformed into a feasible and valid study that tests the associated hypothesis.

Errors in Research

The goal of any study is to maximize the validity of inference from what was observed in the study sample to what is happening in the population. However, no study is entirely free of errors. There are two main errors that interfere with research inferences: random error and systematic error.

Random error is a wrong result due to chance. Several techniques exist for reducing random error, but the simplest is to increase the sample size of a study. The use of a large sample diminishes the likelihood of a substantially wrong result by increasing the precision of the estimate. Systematic error is a wrong result due to bias. These are sources of variation that distort the study findings in one direction. The best way to improve the degree to which a result approximates the true values is to design the study in a way that reduces the size of the various biases.

With respect to measurement, random error would be variations in responses to a questionnaire by the same respondent on several occasions. A systematic error would result from a questionnaire that is unclear and leads to respondents providing inaccurate answers, particularly by certain groups of respondents. It is critical for investigators to constantly be cognizant of how they can minimize error throughout a study.

Study Design

The design of a study is the most important component of clinical research. Broadly, study designs can be broken into two classes: observational studies and clinical trials, which differ in their capacity to establish causality and the degree to which confounding and bias could decrease the validity of results. Causal inference is highest for clinical trials and generally lower for observational studies. Similarly, the risk of bias and confounding is generally lower in clinical trials. In clinical trials, researchers apply an intervention to one group and examine its effects by comparing outcomes to those of a group that did not receive the intervention (i.e., the control group). On the other hand, observational studies are those studies in which researchers observe how a risk factor, diagnostic test, treatment, or other intervention is associated with an outcome without changing who is exposed to it. While there a many types of observational studies, the three most common are cross-sectional studies, cohort studies, and case-control studies.[2]

COHORT STUDIES

In cohort studies, participants are selected based on presence of a specific factor, called the exposure, and then followed for the occurrence of an outcome.[1]

[1]The term "cohort" is derived from the Latin word *cohors*. Roman legions were composed of 10 cohorts. During battle each cohort, or military unit, consisting of a specific number of warriors and commanding centurions was traceable. The word "cohort" has been adopted into epidemiology to define a set of people followed over a period of time.[3]

In a cohort study, an outcome- or disease-free study population is first identified by the exposure or event of interest and followed in time until the disease or outcome of interest occurs. Because exposure is identified before the outcome, cohort studies provide a temporal framework and thus have higher causal inference. Cohort studies are particularly advantageous for examining rare exposures because subjects are selected by their exposure status. Additionally, the investigator can examine multiple outcomes simultaneously. A disadvantage includes a potentially long follow-up duration, which can make a cohort study a costly endeavor.[2] Cohort studies can be further divided into prospective studies that begin in the present and follow subjects into the future and retrospective studies that examine information collected over a period of time in the past.

CASE-CONTROL STUDIES

Case-control studies compare a group of people who have a disease or other outcomes with another group who do not. Case-control studies identify subjects by outcome status at the outset of the investigation. Once outcome status is identified and subjects are categorized as cases, controls (subjects without the outcome but from the same source population) are selected. Data about exposure to a risk factor or several risk factors are then collected. This collection is often retrospective but can be ascertained at the time of the study. Case-control studies are well suited to investigate rare outcomes or outcomes with a long latency period because subjects are selected from the outset by their outcome status. Thus, in comparison to cohort studies, case-control studies are generally faster, relatively inexpensive to implement, require comparatively fewer subjects, and allow for multiple exposures or risk factors to be assessed for one outcome.[4]

CROSS-SECTIONAL STUDIES

In cross-sectional studies, observations are made on a single occasion. Cross-sectional studies, also known as prevalence studies, examine the data on disease and exposure at one time point. Causal inference is reduced because the temporal relationship between disease occurrence and exposure cannot be established. Cross-sectional designs are well suited for describing variables and their distribution patterns. Like all other observational studies, cross-sectional studies can establish associations, but the choice of which variables to label as exposures and which as outcomes depends on the presumed causal pathway that needs to be determined a priori by the investigator rather than on the study design. They provide information about prevalence, the proportion who have a disease, or condition at one point in time, but generally cannot be used to estimate incidence or the proportion who develop a disease or condition over time.

CLINICAL TRIALS

The randomized, controlled blinded trial is the best design for establishing causality and efficacy of interventions. However, clinical trials are generally expensive, time consuming, and often only address a narrow question. For these reasons, trials are generally reserved for mature research questions when observational studies have already suggested that an intervention might be effective, but stronger evidence is required before it can be approved or recommended. Not every research question is amenable to the clinical trial design. Additionally, nonrandomized or unblinded trials may be all that is feasible for some research questions.[1]

The classic randomized controlled trial is a parallel, between-group design that includes a group that receives an intervention to be tested, and a control group that receives either no active treatment (preferably a placebo) or a comparison treatment. The investigator applies the intervention and control, follows both groups over time, and compares the outcome between the intervention and control groups. This design allows an investigator to observe the effects of their intervention on the outcome variable while using randomization to minimize the influence of confounding variables.

Study Population

Inclusion and exclusion criteria are initially specified that define the target population. These criteria identify the kinds of people best suited to answer the research question. A population is a complete set of people with specified characteristics, and a sample is a subset of the population. The group of individuals identified for a study can only be a sample of the population of interest because there are practical barriers to studying the entire population. Decisions need to be made on how to recruit an appropriate number of people from an accessible subset of this population to be the participants in the study. Recruitment often involves certain trade-offs. For example, recruiting patients from many clinics across the country would result in greater generalizability than recruiting from a single clinic, but enhancing generalizability must be weighed against increased cost and complexity.

Variables

Another major set of decisions in designing any study concerns the choice of which variables to measure. In considering the association between two variables, the one that occurs first or is more likely on biologic grounds to be causal is called the exposure and the other is called the outcome variable or endpoint.

EXPOSURE

Most observational studies may have many variables that could be considered exposures (age, race, sex, smoking history). However, it is important to specify the variable of interest (primary exposure) and those variables that are confounders.

OUTCOME

Observational studies and clinical trials may include many outcome variables. However, it is critical to specify the primary outcome in any type of study as that will determine the power or sample size required. The ultimate goal of any study is to flesh out the relationships of each individual exposure with each of the outcomes of interest.

CONFOUNDERS

Confounders are "nuisance" variables that are associated with the primary exposure and the outcome but not on the causal pathway. Confounders complicate the interpretation of the findings of a study. For example, in a study designed to determine the effect of poor hydration on kidney stone development, if the group of patients with poor hydration also have a high sodium intake it will be difficult to determine if poor hydration or a high sodium-diet is driving kidney stone development. Thus high-sodium diet is one of many potential confounders that would need to be accounted for. In a randomized trial, the process of randomization balances sodium intake between the groups; however, sodium intake would have to be measured and adjusted for in an observational study.

TYPES OF VARIABLE

The measurement scales of variables are critical to consider when designing a study. Variables can be classified as continuous or categorical. There are two major types of categorical variables: dichotomous and ordinal. Dichotomous reflects two mutually exclusive groups (e.g., male/female, present/absent). Ordinal implies an order to the categories (e.g., pathologic grading scale). When given the choice, generally choose continuous variables over categorical variables because the additional information they contain improves statistical efficiency.

Statistical Analysis

SAMPLE SIZE CALCULATIONS

The investigator must develop plans for estimating sample size. As with the study design, the statistical analysis plan arises from the specified hypothesis. For prospective studies, it is critical to determine the number of subjects needed to observe the expected difference in the outcome between study groups with reasonable probability (an attribute known as power).[5] Any discussion of power must start with a brief overview of estimated effect size, type 1 error, and type 2 error.

TYPE 1 AND TYPE 2 ERRORS

Hypothesis testing requires constructing a statistical model of what the data would look like if chance or random processes alone were responsible for the results. A hypothesis that chance alone is responsible for the results is called the null hypothesis. Thus if a proposed study does not identify a statistically significant association between the variables being studied, then the null hypothesis is accepted.[6] On the other hand, if the result is found to be statistically significant, then the null hypothesis is rejected and the alternative hypothesis is accepted. For example, if the hypothesis of a study states "We hypothesize that smoking is associated with bladder cancer" then the null hypothesis would be that there is no association between smoking and bladder cancer and the alternative hypothesis would be that there is an association.

If the study shows an association between smoking and bladder cancer, then the null hypothesis would be rejected.

Type 1 error (alpha) occurs when the null hypothesis is rejected incorrectly. In other words, the researcher states a statistically significant finding was present when it actually was not. In clinical research a predefined convention is to set the limit of type 1 error in a study at 5%. This error rate is illustrated using a *P* value. A *P* value under .05 indicates that the risk of making a type 1 error is less than 5%.

Type 2 error (beta) occurs when the null hypothesis is accepted incorrectly. In other words, the researcher states that a statistically significant finding was not present when it actually was. Type 2 error occurs when the researchers fail to see a statistically significant difference when one does in fact exist. This is often a result of an underpowered study in which a small sample size prevented the researcher from seeing the true relationship between the variables in question.

POWER

The power of a study is 1−beta (beta = type 2 error). When clinicians approach statisticians with concerns about the power of their study they often ask the question: how many patients do I need in my study in order to have enough power to find a statistically significant difference? They do not ask how much power their study needs, as the amount of power needed is another predefined convention, but instead they ask how large of a sample size or (n) they need.

The relationship between power and sample size can be demonstrated using the sample size equation for two arm studies: $n_1 = n_2 = ([f(alpha) + f(beta)]^2/delta^2)$, where n_1 is the number of patients in one arm of the study and n_2 is the number of patients in the other arm of the study. Delta is the effect size that the researcher would like to capture. Because delta is in the denominator of this equation an increase in effect size results in a decrease in the number of patients required to reach sufficient power. For example, if a new cancer drug decreases the risk of death by 80% you would need fewer patients to power a study to show a change in survival of 80%. But if a cancer drug only decreases the risk of death by 1% you would need a much larger sample size to accurately show that result.

The variable f(alpha) corresponds to the preselected acceptable type 1 error (alpha), which is set to 5% or .05. The variable f(beta) corresponds to the preselected acceptable type 2 error (beta), which is often set to .2. Setting beta to .2 results in a power of .8 or 80% as power is equal to 1−beta. A power cutoff of 80% is another predefined convention. Thus if the effect size is provided, the calculation of sample size is straightforward.

Although a useful guide, sample size calculations give a deceptive impression of statistical objectivity. They are only as accurate as the data and estimates on which they are based, which are often just informed guesses. Sample size planning is best thought of as a mathematical way of making a ballpark estimate. It may reveal that the research design is not feasible or that different predictors or outcome variables are needed. Thus the sample size should be estimated early in the design phase of a study, when major changes are still possible.

SENSITIVITY AND SPECIFICITY

Sensitivity and specificity are statistical measures that are widely used in clinical research. They are used to describe the performance of a binary classification test.

Sensitivity

Sensitivity is the ability of a test to correctly identify individuals with a disease. In other words, if a test is highly sensitive, the test will accurately identify all patients who have the disease (true positives) and will not misclassify any patients who have the disease as not having the disease (false negative). Sensitivity testing only looks at patients who have the disease (true positives, false negatives) and determines how well the test did in classifying these patients. The formula is true positive/(true positive + false negative). If the false-negative rate of a test is low (the number of people who have the disease and were incorrectly classified by the test as not having the disease), then the denominator will be smaller and the ratio will approach 1 indicating a very sensitive test.

Specificity

Specificity is the ability of a test to correctly identify individuals without a disease. Specificity testing only looks at patients who do not have the disease (true negatives, false positives) and determines how well the test did in classifying these patients. The formula is true negative/(true negative + false positive). If the false-positive rate of a test is low (the number of people who do not have the disease and were incorrectly classified by the test as having the disease), then the denominator will be smaller and the ratio will approach 1, indicating a very specific test.

Implementing The Study

An investigator designs a study plan in which the choice of research question, subjects, and measurements enhances external validity of the study and is conducive to implementation with a high degree of internal validity. Internal validity assesses the degree to which the investigator draws the correct conclusions about what actually happened in the study. External validity (also called generalizability) assesses the degree to which these conclusions can be appropriately applied to people and events outside the study.

Implementation is the degree to which the actual study matches the study plan. If a study is not implemented properly, there is risk that the conclusions of the study could be inaccurate. Countless errors can occur in patient enrollment and measurement acquisition that can negatively affect a study. For example, significant bias can be introduced to a study if a study seeks to include all eligible clinic patients, but only patients with functional e-mail addresses respond and consent to the study. Additionally, if a questionnaire is unclear, it may result in confusion and incorrect responses.

A special kind of validity problem arises in studies that examine the association between a predictor and an outcome variable in order to draw causal inference. This is common in observational studies. For example, if a cohort study identifies an association between exercise and kidney stones, does this represent cause and effect, or is exercise just an innocent bystander in a web of causation that involves other variables? As previously discussed, reducing the likelihood of confounding is one of the major challenges in designing an observational study. Randomization that occurs in clinical trials has the highest causal inference because it balances measured and unmeasured confounders between the groups.

There are many sophisticated statistical methods that can address confounders in observational studies. These include effect modification, statistical adjustments such as multivariable regression, and propensity scoring.[7][2] Effect modification ensures that only cases and controls with similar levels of a potential confounding variables are compared. It involves segregating the subjects into subgroups according to the level of a potential confounder and then examining the relation between the predictor and outcome separately in each subgroup.

Statistical methods are often used to adjust for confounders. These techniques model the association between the primary exposure and the outcome by accounting for how other variables may influence these results. For example, if an investigator wants to understand the association between diet and kidney stones, they must adjust simultaneously for several potential confounders such as age, sex, race, and education. This adjustment is most often accomplished using multivariable regression models. The particular type of regression model is determined by the type of outcome (e.g., continuous versus dichotomous), structure of data, and the consideration of time. Building the model requires identification of the potential confounders and assessment of the variables to ultimately have a parsimonious but comprehensive model that accounts for all the factors that are associated with the exposure and the outcome.

Propensity scores are another method available to adjust for confounders. Propensity scores can be particularly useful for observational studies analyzing treatment efficacy. The problem that patients for whom a treatment is indicated are often at higher risk, or otherwise different from those who do not get the treatment. Instead of adjusting for all factors that predict outcome, use of propensity scores involves creating a multivariable model to estimate the probability of receipt of the intervention. Each subject can then be assigned a predicted probability of treatment or a propensity score. This single score can be used as the only confounding variable in a stratified or multivariable analysis. Alternatively, subjects who did and did not receive the treatment can be matched by propensity score, and outcomes compared between matched pairs.

Additional content, including Suggested Readings, may be accessed at www.ExpertConsult.com

[2]This chapter is not comprehensive as a full discussion of statistical methods is beyond the scope of the chapter.

Note: Page numbers followed by *b* indicate boxes, *f* indicate figures, and *t* indicate tables.

A

C

D

E

F

G

H

I

J

K

L

M

O

P

Q

R

S

T

U

V

W

X

Y

Z

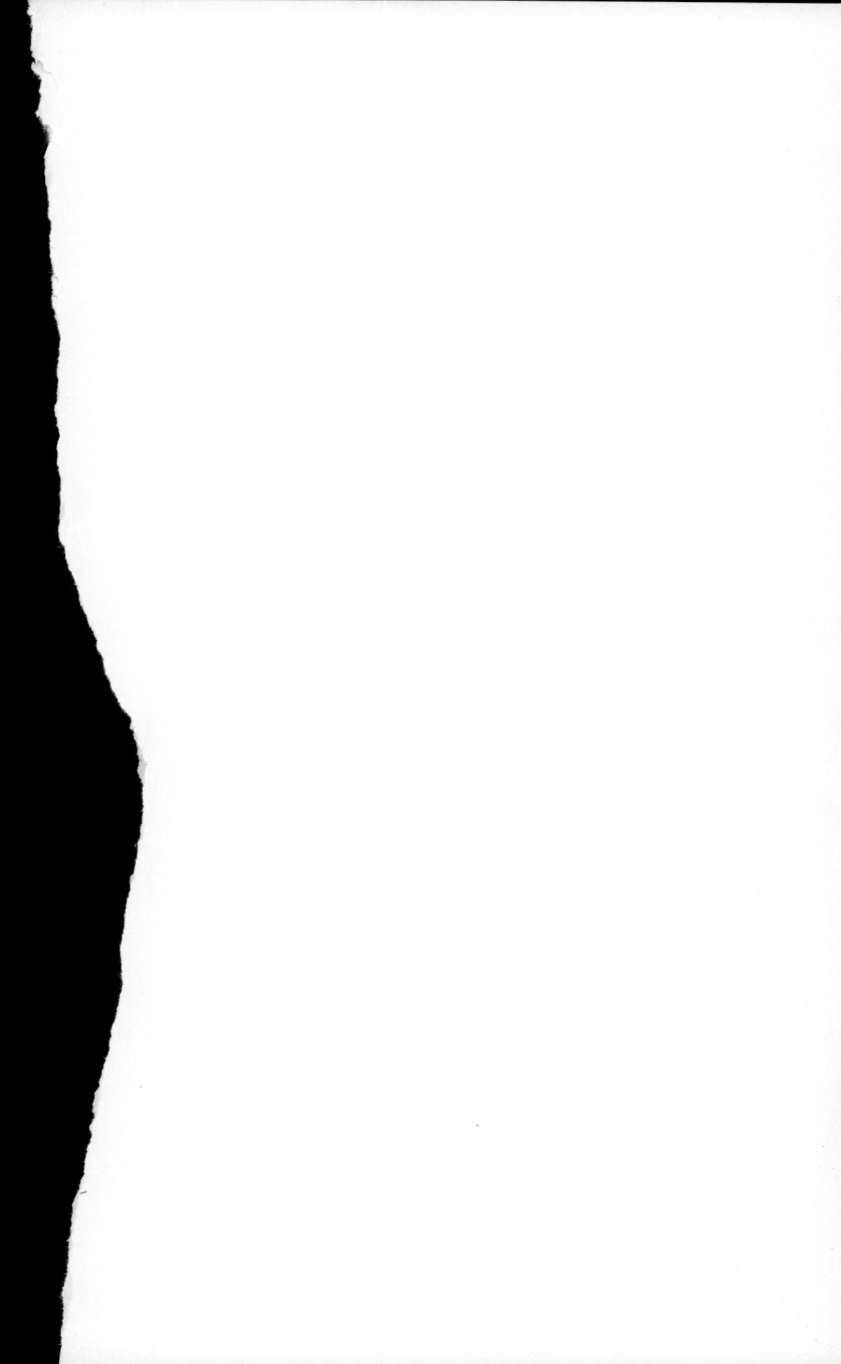